Christensen's
Physics of
Diagnostic Radiology

Christensen's
Physics of
Diagnostic Radiology

THOMAS S. CURRY III, M.D.

Professor of Radiology, University of Texas
Southwestern Medical Center at Dallas
and Parkland Memorial Hospital

JAMES E. DOWDEY, Ph.D.

Associate Professor of Radiology (Physics),
Southwestern Medical Center at Dallas
and Parkland Memorial Hospital

ROBERT C. MURRY, Jr., Ph.D.

Associate Professor of Radiology (Physics)
Southwestern Medical Center at Dallas
and Parkland Memorial Hospital

4th Edition

Lea & Febiger • Philadelphia • London

Lea & Febiger
200 Chester Field Parkway
Malvern, Pennsylvania   19355-9725
U.S.A.
(215) 251-2230
1-800-444-1785

Library of Congress Cataloging-in-Publication Data

Curry, Thomas S., 1935–
    Christensen's physics of diagnostic radiology.—4th ed. /
Thomas S. Curry III, James E. Dowdey, Robert C. Murry, Jr.
        p.   cm.
    Rev. ed. of: Christensen's introduction to the physics of
diagnostic radiology. 3rd ed. / Thomas S. Curry III, James E.
Dowdey, Robert C. Murry, Jr. 1984.
    Includes bibliographical references.
    ISBN 0-8121-1310-1
    1. Diagnosis, Radioscopic. 2. Medical physics. I. Dowdey, James E.
II. Murry, Robert C.   III. Christensen, Edward E., 1929–
Introduction to the physics of diagnostic radiology. IV. Title.
V. Title: Physics of diagnostic radiology.
    [DNLM: 1. Physics. 2. Radiography. 3. Radiology. 4. Technology,
Radiologic. WN 110 C976c]
RC78.C87   1990
616.07′57—dc20
DNLM/DLC
for Library of Congress   90-5586
                                                             CIP

        1st Edition, 1972
            Reprinted 1973, 1975, 1976, 1977
        2nd Edition, 1978
            Reprinted 1979, 1981, 1982, 1983
        3rd Edition, 1984
            Reprinted 1985, 1987
        4th Edition, 1990

Reprints of chapters may be purchased from Lea & Febiger in quantities of 100 or more.

PRINTED IN THE UNITED STATES OF AMERICA
Print Number: 6   5   4   3   2

Dedicated to: ————————————————————

      MISS WINN

      VAUDA

      BARBARA

PREFACE

Why a new edition of a physics book? Physics does not change. But our understanding and use of physics continues to develop.

The competent radiologist must know something about the physics of diagnostic imaging. The tough question is exactly what physics should the radiologist know to function competently in the environment in which he finds himself. As we sit in our little room in Dallas and ponder this question we realize that we will fail to include information that should be known, and undoubtedly we will include some things that need not be known. It is obvious that one individual is unlikely to become and remain an expert in physics and technology, plus diagnostic imaging. There is just too much to learn in each field, and learned information becomes obsolete too fast. We applaud the developing trend that pairs a radiologist and a radiologic physicist as a team that provides the maximum patient benefit from diagnostic imaging studies. Thus, our goal is not to turn radiologists into physicists, but rather to allow radiologists to understand and appreciate

the amazing technology available, and let the physicist worry about the technical details.

In our quest to include information that should be known, and reduce the amount that need not be known, we have in this edition eliminated the material on copying radiographs and subtraction techniques. We have reduced the amount of information on cinefluorography and non-image-intensified fluoroscopy, and consolidated fluoroscopic imaging and recording into a single chapter. Several areas, such as attenuation and grids and beam restrictors, remain essentially unchanged. In other areas we have tried to update the material to indicate new technology. These areas include x-ray generators (solid-state devices), xerography (liquid toner), CT scanners (fast-imaging technology) and ultrasound (color Doppler). Obviously, the needed addition was in MRI, and a new chapter was added to expand this topic.

We certainly appreciate the positive response to this text, and hope the current edition will continue to fill the needs of radiology residents and student technologists.

Dallas, Texas

Thomas S. Curry, III
James E. Dowdey
Robert C. Murry

ACKNOWLEDGMENTS _____

Another edition is about wrapped up, causing us once again to reflect on those who contributed so much time and talent.

Our friends at E.I. du Pont de Nemours and Company, Eastman Kodak Company, and Philips Medical Systems continued to offer support.

Marty Burgin once again prepared all the new illustrations, and introduced us to the wonders of computer graphics. Marty did much more than draw the pictures. She spent time helping us improve and refine many of the illustrations, especially those dealing with electronics and MRI. We recognize and appreciate her considerable talent and kindness.

An amazing stroke of good fortune guided a remarkable individual to our photography department. Only a few weeks after she joined our department, Claudia Wylie had assumed responsibility for almost all our photographic support. Claudia took great pictures, but her effort did not stop there. She organized the entire book, chapter by chapter, and served as liaison between the authors and artist as additions, alterations, and corrections required attention. The enormous amount of time and dedication Claudia provided was one of the delightful surprises one hopes for but seldom finds. Thank you, Claudia.

This textbook is made possible by the entire Department of Radiology, University of Texas Southwestern Medical Center at Dallas. Everything in this edition has been prepared by a physicist and a radiologist sitting at a long table to compose and revise the manuscript together. It was necessary for the authors to distance themselves from the demands and invasions of other academic and clinical responsibilities for several months. The understanding and support of our friends and colleagues was absolutely spectacular, and this attempt to say thinks will fall far short of the genuine affection we hold for each of these splendid individuals. We can name only a few, and chose to single out those who were most directly inconvenienced because of our absence. In the physics department, graduate students Tom Lane, Tim Blackburn, and Jerome Gonzales provided research effort and critical review of manuscripts. Our friend, John Moore, continued to come up with ideas and suggestions. Our senior residents in diagnostic radiology must be the most understanding residents in the cosmos. The seven who functioned in an exemplary manner during the seven months they were being given little attention from their assigned staff radiologist were Drs. Lori Watumull, Jim Fleckenstein, Tom Fletcher, Christine Page, Diane Twickler, Mark Girson, and Brian Bruening. All our residents are wonderful people. Our colleagues on the teaching staff continued with their enthusiastic support and encouragement. Drs. Helen Redman and George Miller absorbed most of the increased clinical work caused by the frequent unavailability of T.S.C. Drs. Georgiana Gibson and Bill Erdman helped with clinical MRI information and illustrations, as did Drs. Hortono Setiawan and Rebecca Harrell in CT and Ultrasound. We must mention those faculty members who really helped with encouragement when things didn't go smoothly. These include Drs.

Robert Parkey, George Curry, Peter Antich, Geral Dietz, Robert Epstein, Mary Gaulden, William Kilman, Michael Landay, and Jack Reynolds, who has suffered through four editions with us. A special thanks goes to Geoffrey Clarke, Ph.D., who spent many hours guiding us through the complexities of MRI.

Our search for help with word processing provided a second delightful surprise. Eula Stephens had been with us only a few days when we approached her about typing the manuscript. She accepted this challenge, and has shown great skill and dedication as work has progressed. Equally important, she has been friendly and patient as we return page after page marked up with changes after we had promised that the final version was done. Eula has been a genuine pleasure to work with.

As always, the final thanks must go to our wives and families for continuing to support us and take care of us.

TSC
JED
RCM

CONTENTS _____

CHAPTER

1 *Radiation*

Wilhelm Conrad Roentgen, a German physicist, discovered x rays on November 8, 1895. Several fortunate coincidences set the stage for the discovery. Roentgen was investigating the behavior of cathode rays (electrons) in high energy cathode ray tubes, which consisted of a glass envelope from which as much air as possible had been evacuated. A short platinum electrode was fitted into each end and when a high-voltage discharge was passed through this tube, ionization of the remaining gas produced a faint light. Roentgen had enclosed his cathode ray tube in black cardboard to prevent this light from escaping to block any effect the light might have on experiments he was conducting. He then darkened his laboratory room to be sure there were no light leaks in the cardboard cover. On passing a high-voltage discharge through the tube, he noticed a faint light glowing on a work bench about 3 ft away. He discovered that the source of the light was the fluorescence of a small piece of paper coated with barium platinocyanide. Because electrons could not escape the glass envelope of the tube to produce fluorescence, and because the cardboard permitted no light to escape from the tube, he concluded that some unknown type of ray was produced when the tube was energized. We can imagine his excitement as he investigated the mysterious new ray. He began placing objects between the tube and the fluorescent screen: a book, a block of wood, and a sheet of aluminum. The brightness of the fluorescence differed with each, indicating that the ray penetrated some objects more easily than others. Then he held his hand between the tube and the screen and, to his surprise, the outline of his skeleton appeared on the screen. By December 28, 1895, he had thoroughly investigated the properties of the rays and had prepared a manuscript describing his experiments. In recognition of his outstanding contribution to science, Wilhelm Conrad Roentgen was awarded the first Nobel Prize for Physics in 1901.

ELECTROMAGNETIC SPECTRUM

X rays belong to a group of radiations called electromagnetic radiation. **Electromagnetic radiation is the transport of energy through space as a combination of electric and magnetic fields** (hence the name electromagnetic). Familiar members of the family of electromagnetic radiation include radio waves, radiant heat, visible light, and gamma radiation.

Electromagnetic (EM) radiation is produced by a charge (usually a charged particle) being accelerated. The converse is also true; that is, a charge being accelerated will emit EM radiation. Right here at the beginning we run into our first problem. Physics, our beloved exact science, presents a contradiction. The problem is just this: in our discussion of atomic structure (see Chap. 2) we will discuss electrons (charged particles) revolving around the nucleus in circular orbits while maintaining a precise energy. (This is a result of the Bohr theory of the hydrogen atom.) This picture of atomic structure violates the converse statement above. First, if an electron moves in a circular orbit, it must have centripetal acceleration (an acceleration toward the cen-

1

ter of the circular path); therefore, it should emit EM radiation. The loss of energy would require the electron to change its orbit and energy. As a matter of fact, there was some heated discussion when Bohr first introduced his theory that electrons could not possibly be in circular orbits because, being accelerated, they would emit energy and spiral into the nucleus. Shifty-eyed physicists easily get around this argument by saying that electrons, after all, are standing waves about the nucleus and therefore do not represent accelerating charges. It is fair to say, however, that outside the atom a charge being accelerated will emit EM radiation. The energy that charged particles obtain in circular particle accelerators is limited by the energy loss to EM radiation as the particles move about the accelerator. A cyclotron is a good example of an accelerator type that is EM-radiation-limited.

But we haven't finished. In the same atomic structure discussion, we allow electronic transitions from one energy state to another with emission of EM radiation energy, but with no mention of acceleration. In fact, we really think of instantaneous transitions across regions in which electrons cannot possibly exist. This concept of energy level transitions seems to contradict the first statement that EM radiation is produced by an accelerated charge.

There are a couple of observations that must be made. First, the world of quantum physics (represented here by Bohr's theory) does not always behave as we, living in a somewhat larger world, might expect. Because x rays are produced in the quantum physics world, we must understand some of the laws governing that world. Second, in this book we have endeavored to be as physically accurate as possible while emphasizing those points that we feel clinicians should understand.

Perhaps we should then rephrase the statement: EM radiation, except for that produced in energy level transitions (including nuclear transitions), is produced by an

accelerating charge. Any accelerating charge not bound to an atom (including the nucleus) will emit EM radiation.

Some time should be spent here discussing the production and structure of EM radiation. To do that, we will start with a single small charged ball. (Because we recognize the electron as a charged particle, we can put a charge on a ball by adding or taking away electrons. If we add electrons, we will charge the ball negatively. Subtraction of electrons results in a positively charged ball.) We can only determine if we are successful in placing a charge on the ball by observing its interactions with the world around it. Coulomb studied the forces that exist between two charged balls, and today we call the forces between charged objects "Coulomb forces." The force between two small balls having charges q_1 and q_2 is

$$F = \frac{kq_1q_2}{r^2}$$

F = force (a vector)
k = a constant whose value depends on the system of units
q_1 and q_2 = charge on balls
r = distance between balls.

This force is always along the line joining the two balls. (More accurately, it is the line joining the centers of the two charge distributions. If we use "point" charges we don't have to worry about the charge distribution.) If q_1 and q_2 are like charges (same sign; positive and positive or negative and negative), the force is a repelling force. If q_1 and q_2 are unlike charges, the force is attractive. Gravitational force also has this mathematical form, but it is always attractive.

We nearly always introduce the electric field (E) to describe the possible interactive forces. We define the electric field for a charge distribution (q_1) as the force that q_1 would exert on a positive unit charge (q_2 equals 1). Note that E has a unique value and direction at each point surrounding a charge. Figure 1–1 shows the E field sur-

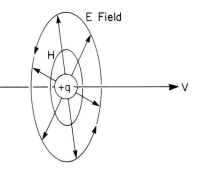

Figure 1–2 Electric and magnetic fields surrounding a positive charge moving with constant velocity

Figure 1–1 Electric field surrounding a positive charge at rest

rounding a point positive charge. Note that E is radially directed and falls off (decreases in size) as $1/r^2$. The electric field for more complicated charge distributions could be more or even less complicated. (The electric field for an infinite plane uniformly charged is constant everywhere.) This electric field is sometimes called the static (electric is implied) field because the charge is at rest.

If the charge moves with a constant velocity, we not only see an electric field (E) moving with the charge, but also a magnetic field (H) surrounding the line (path) along which the charge is moving. (A more detailed discussion of magnetic fields will be found in Chapter 23.) Figure 1–2 shows the electric field radially directed and the circular magnetic field (H). Here E and H (both vectors) are perpendicular at any one point.

The next thing to do is to let the charge accelerate. Here we have conceptual problems. At constant velocity, the electric field moves along with the charge. But, with acceleration, the charge moves to a new location before the outer regions of the electric field realize that the charge is at a different place than it should be. The electric field lags behind the charge, as does the magnetic field. The lagging behind produces a "kink" in the electric field lines that moves outward from the charge with a finite (but large) velocity. We can think of this kink as being the EM radiation. We don't know any better way to describe this rather complex concept.

EM radiation is made up of an electric field and a magnetic field that mutually support each other. Figure 1–3 shows the E and H fields and the direction of propagation of the EM radiation. Note that E and H are perpendicular, that they reverse together, and that both E and H are perpendicular to the direction of propagation. The concept to be visualized is that E and H interact to build each other up to some value, then collapse together and build each other up in the opposite direction. Energy is transmitted through space by the EM radiation.

The radiation depicted in Figure 1–3 was produced by a charge oscillating back and forth. Suppose we consider a radio

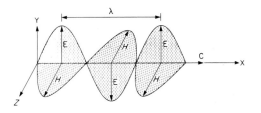

Figure 1–3 Representation of electromagnetic radiation

transmission tower. The purpose of the tower is to transmit radio signals that, as you might have guessed, are EM radiation. The transmission is accomplished by accelerating charge up and down a conductor in the tower. As the charge is accelerated up the tower, we might get one section of the EM radiation shown in Figure 1–3. As the charge moves down the tower, the following section of the EM radiation is produced. When the charge changes direction, so do the E and H fields. Thus, a radio wave can be produced by forcing charge to move up and down the tower by applying an alternating voltage to the tower. The frequency of the radio wave is just how many times per second the charge changes direction. Of course, we tune our radios at home to a given frequency to find a particular station. The information we obtain from the radio, perhaps music, is superimposed on the EM radiation generated by the tower. How that is done is another story.

We would be in excellent shape if EM radiation didn't interact with the particles of our old world. Obviously, without such interaction we wouldn't be here to wonder about EM radiation anyway. Life-giving energy from the sun gets here by EM radiation.

Maybe it would be instructive to see how radio waves interact with your radio. Just a little while ago we talked about EM radiation in the form of radio waves being emitted from a radio tower. (We didn't say there that the energy emitted was emitted outward from the tower in something of a doughnut-shaped pattern. The maximum intensity is emitted perpendicularly to the tower, while there is no intensity directly above the tower. That pattern is best for us, because most of us don't listen to a radio while directly above the tower.) What we need to detect the radio wave is some antenna (an electrical conductor) in the radio radiation pattern. When the radio wave (the E and H fields) passes the antenna, the E-field part of the EM radio wave exerts a force on the electrons in the antenna,

which makes the electrons oscillate back and forth in the antenna at the frequency of the radio wave. Consequently, the antenna detects the EM radiation by the electrons moving under the influence of the E field in the EM radiation. In this type of detection, the EM radiation looks and behaves as a wave. As the frequency of the EM radiation increases, however, a point is reached in the frequency range (not a single precise frequency) at which the electron can no longer follow the electric field. At frequencies in this range and higher, the electrons interact with the EM radiation as if the EM radiation were an energy bundle, rather than made up of waves. Later, we will see that coherent scattering of x rays is by an interaction of the wave type, while photoelectric absorption is an interaction of the energy bundle (called a photon) type. To stay away from exotic physics, it is necessary to discuss EM radiation as if it were comprised of both particles (photons) and waves. Let us hasten to add that EM radiation will behave as only one of the two, and that this behavior is always the same for a given interaction (or experimental measurement).

To finish the radio detection, we note one problem: there are a number of radio stations broadcasting at the same time. We must pick one frequency (the station we want to listen to) and discard the rest. This selection is done by a "tank" circuit on the end of the antenna. We tune the tank circuit (by the station selection knob) to keep only one frequency. What we hear on the radio is the second part of the other story introduced in the paragraph on radio transmission.

In the first chapters in this text, we will be interested in how the E part of the EM radiation reacts with electrons. Later, when discussing nuclear magnetic resonance, we will consider reactions with the H (magnetic) part of the field that are produced by oscillating electrons.

The interactions of different kinds of EM radiation are difficult to understand.

Some are explained only if they are assumed to be particles, while others are explained only by theories of wave propagation. **It is necessary to discuss electromagnetic radiation as if it were composed of both particles and waves.**

Wave Concept of Electromagnetic Radiation

Electromagnetic radiation is propagated through space in the form of waves. They may be compared to waves traveling down a stretched rope when one end is moved up and down in a rhythmic motion. While the waves with which we are familiar must be propagated in a medium (such as the example of the rope, waves traveling in water, or sound waves traveling in air), electromagnetic waves need no such medium; that is, they can be propagated through a vacuum. Waves of all types have an associated wavelength and frequency. The distance between two successive crests, or troughs, is the wavelength of the wave, and is given the symbol λ (the Greek letter *lambda,* the initial for length). The number of waves passing a particular point in a unit of time is called the frequency, and is given the symbol ν (the Greek letter *nu,* the initial for number). If each wave has a length λ, and ν waves pass a given point in unit time, the velocity of the wave is given by

$$V = \lambda \times \nu$$

For example, if the wavelength is 4 ft and the frequency is 60 waves/min, then

$$V = 4 \text{ ft} \times 60/\text{min}$$
$$V = 240 \text{ ft/min}$$

EM radiation always travels at the same velocity in a vacuum. This velocity is 186,000 miles per second (3×10^8 meters per second), which is usually referred to as the velocity of light and given the symbol c. Therefore, we may express the relationship between velocity, wavelength, and frequency as

$$c = \lambda \nu$$

c = velocity of light (m/sec)
λ = wavelength (m)
ν = frequency (per sec).

Because all types of electromagnetic radiation have the same velocity, the frequency of the radiation must be inversely proportional to its wavelength. All types of radiation in the electromagnetic spectrum differ basically only in wavelength. The wavelength of a radio wave may be 5 miles long, while a typical x ray is only 1 billionth of an inch. The wavelength of diagnostic x rays is extremely short, and it is usually expressed in angstrom units (Å) or nanometers (nm). An angstrom is 10^{-10} m, while a nanometer is 10^{-9} m. Therefore, one nm is equal to 10 Å. Or, if you prefer, one Å is equal to 0.1 nm. You may wish to refresh your memory of various prefixes by referring to Table 1–1. The wavelength of most diagnostic x rays is between 1 and 0.1 Å. The wavelength of an electromagnetic wave determines how it interacts with matter. For example, an electromagnetic wave 7000 Å (700 nm) long can be seen by the human eye as red light, and a wavelength of 4000 Å is seen as blue light. The frequency of blue light may be calculated by knowing its wavelength (4000 Å = 4×10^{-7} m):

$$c = \lambda \nu \text{ or } \nu = \frac{c}{\lambda}$$
$$\nu = \frac{3 \times 10^8 \text{ m/sec}}{4 \times 10^{-7} \text{ m}}$$
$$\nu = 7.5 \times 10^{14}/\text{sec}$$

Blue light, with a wavelength of 4000 Å, has a frequency of 7.5×10^{14} vibrations per second. Similarly calculated, the frequency of an x ray of wavelength 0.1 Å is 3×10^{19} vibrations per second.

The complete spectrum of electromag-

Table 1–1. Prefixes

FACTOR	PREFIX	SYMBOL
10^9	giga	G
10^6	mega	M
10^3	kilo	K
10^{-1}	deci	d
10^{-3}	milli	m
10^{-6}	micro	μ
10^{-9}	nano	n
10^{-12}	pico	p

netic radiation covers a wide range of wavelengths and frequencies. The various parts of the spectrum are named according to the manner in which the type of radiation is generated or detected. Some members of the group, listed in order of decreasing wavelength, are

Radio, television,	
radar:	3×10^5 to 1 cm
Infrared radiation:	0.01 to 0.00008 cm
	(8000 Å)
Visible light:	7500 (0.000075 cm) to
	3900 Å
Ultraviolet radiation:	3900 to 20 Å
Soft x rays:	100 to 1 Å
Diagnostic x rays:	1 to 0.1 Å
Therapeutic x ray and	
gamma rays:	0.1 to 10^{-4} Å

There is considerable overlap in the wavelengths of the various members of the electromagnetic spectrum; the numbers listed are rough guides. It is again stressed that the great differences in properties of these different types of radiation are attributable to their differences in wavelength (or frequency).

The wave concept of electromagnetic radiation explains why it may be reflected, refracted, diffracted, and polarized. There are some phenomena, however, that cannot be explained by the wave concept.

Particle Concept of Electromagnetic Radiation

Short electromagnetic waves, such as x rays, may react with matter as if they were particles rather than waves. These particles are actually discrete bundles of energy, and each of these bundles of energy is called a **quantum,** or **photon.** Photons travel at the speed of light. The amount of energy carried by each quantum, or photon, depends on the frequency (v) of the radiation. If the frequency (number of vibrations per second) is doubled, the energy of the photon is doubled. The actual amount of energy of the photon may be calculated by multiplying its frequency by a constant. The constant has been determined experimentally to be 4.13×10^{-18} keV·sec, and is

called Planck's constant. (Planck's constant in SI units is 6.62×10^{-34} joules seconds [J·s]). Planck's constant is normally given in the SI units. We made the conversion to keV·sec to make the calculation of the energy of x-ray photons have the units of kiloelectron volts.) The mathematical expression is written as follows:

$$E = hv$$

E = photon energy
h = Planck's constant
v = frequency.

The ability to visualize the dual characteristics of electromagnetic radiation presents a true challenge. But we must unavoidably reach the conclusion that EM radiation sometimes behaves as a wave and other times as a particle. The particle concept is used to describe the interactions between radiation and matter. Because we will be concerned principally with interactions, such as the photoelectric effect and Compton scatter, we will use the photon (or quantum) concept in this text.

The unit used to measure the energy of photons is the electron volt (eV). An electron volt is the amount of energy that an electron gains as it is accelerated by a potential difference of 1 V. Because the electron volt is a small unit, x-ray energies are usually measured in terms of the kiloelectron volt (keV), which is 1000 electron volts. We will usually discuss x rays in terms of their energy rather than their wavelengths, but the two are related as follows:

$$c = \lambda v \text{ or } v = \frac{c}{\lambda}$$

and

$$E = hv$$

Substituting $\frac{c}{\lambda}$ for v,

$$E = \frac{hc}{\lambda}$$

The product of the velocity of light (c) and Planck's constant (h) is 12.4 when the unit of energy is keV and the wavelength is in angstroms. The final equation showing the relationship between energy and wavelength is

$$E = \frac{12.4}{\lambda}$$

E = energy (in keV)
λ = wavelength (in Å).

Table 1–2 shows the relationship between energy and wavelength for various photons.

If a photon has 15 eV or more of energy it is capable of ionizing atoms and molecules, and it is called "ionizing radiation." An atom is ionized when it loses an electron. Gamma rays, x rays, and some ultraviolet rays are all types of ionizing radiation.

UNITS

While writing this text we encountered a problem regarding the units used to measure various quantities. Whenever possible we have tried to use SI units. Sometimes this resulted in very large or very small numbers, and often in such cases we used cgs system units. A brief description of units will help you to follow the various units used in this text.

The SI system (Systéme Internationale d'Unités) is a modernized metric system based on the MKS (meter-kilogram-second) system. The SI system was originally defined and given official status by the Eleventh General Conference on Weights and Measures in 1960. (A complete listing of SI units can be found in the National Bureau of Standards Special Publication 330, 1977 edition.) There are only seven base units and two supplementary units.

All others are derived from these nine units, although some are given special names. Table 1–3 gives the seven fundamental quantities to which the seven base SI units refer. The MKS units for these seven quantities are identical to the SI units. For comparison, Table 1–3 also lists those common cgs (centimeter-gram-second) units that have been used elsewhere in this book. A blank entry does not mean that there is no cgs equivalent, but that we have not used those units elsewhere and do not wish to add complications. Note that the two supplementary units at the bottom of Table 1–3 (radians and steradians) merely formalize the use of radians for angular measurements. There are 2π radians in 360° (i.e., in a complete circle), so one radian is about 57.3°; there are 4π steradians in a sphere.

Units for any physically known quantity can be derived from these nine SI units. Table 1–4 lists some quantities mentioned in this book, and all but one also have a name in SI units. Again, those common units used elsewhere are also listed. Of course, each unit in the table can be expressed in SI base units only, and a column is included to show this. Sometimes expressing one derived SI unit in terms of other derived SI units reveals some underlying principles of physics. For instance, we note that the SI unit of power is the watt, which in base SI units equals 1 $\frac{m^2kg}{s^3}$. The meaning of the base SI units might be immediately apparent to a physicist, but J/s (joules per second) is a little easier to comprehend. This is just energy per unit time, or power. Electrical power would be even harder to understand in base SI units, but V · A (volts times amps) is our comfortable definition.

The SI unit of radionuclide activity is the becquerel (Becquerel has finally made the big time, after discovering radioactivity in 1896, the same year that Roentgen discovered x rays). The fact that one Bq is the

Table 1–2. Correlation Between Wavelength and Energy

WAVELENGTH (Å)	ENERGY (keV)
0.0005	24,800
0.08	155
0.1	124
1.24	10

Table 1–3. SI Base and Supplementary Units

QUANTITY	SI UNIT NAME	SI SYMBOL	FAMILIAR cgs UNIT	cgs SYMBOL
SI base units:				
Length	meter	m	centimeter	cm
Mass	kilogram	kg	gram	g
Time	second	s	second	s
Electric current	ampere	A		
Temperature	kelvin	K		
Amount of substance	mole	mol		
Luminous intensity	candela	cd		
SI supplementary units:				
Plane angle	radian	rad		
Solid angle	steradian	sr		

Table 1–4. SI Derived Units with Special Names

QUANTITY	SI UNIT NAME	SI SYMBOL	EXPRESSED IN SI BASE UNITS	EXPRESSED IN OTHER SI UNITS	MORE FAMILIAR UNIT
Frequency	hertz	Hz	$\dfrac{1}{s}$		
Force	newton	N	$\dfrac{m \cdot kg}{s^2}$		
Energy	joule	J	$\dfrac{m^2 kg}{s^2}$	$N \cdot m$	erg (cgs)
Power	watt	W	$\dfrac{m^2 kg}{s^3}$	$\dfrac{J}{s}$ or $V \cdot A$	
Charge	coulomb	C	$A \cdot s$		
Radioactivity	becquerel	Bq	$\dfrac{1}{s}$		curie
Absorbed dose	gray	Gy	$\dfrac{m^2}{s^2}$	$\dfrac{J}{kg}$	rad
			$\dfrac{A \cdot s}{kg}$	$\dfrac{C}{kg}$	roentgen
Electric potential	volt	V	$\dfrac{m^2 \cdot kg}{s^3 \cdot A}$	$\dfrac{W}{A}$	
Capacitance	farad	F	$\dfrac{A^2 s^4}{m^2 kg}$	$\dfrac{C}{V}$	
Magnetic flux	weber	Wb	$\dfrac{m^2 kg}{s^2 \cdot A}$	$V \cdot s$	
Magnetic flux density (magnetic induction)	tesla	T	$\dfrac{kg}{s^2 \cdot A}$	$\dfrac{Wb}{m^2}$	gauss

decay of one nucleus per second may be a little inconvenient, but even simplicity has its price. The SI unit of radiation absorbed dose is the gray, which again refers to the quantity of ionizing radiation energy absorbed per unit of mass. There is no special SI unit corresponding to the familiar radiation exposure unit of the roentgen. The roentgen was originally defined as the charge produced in a given mass of air, and comparable SI units are C/kg (C = coulomb).

A good table is needed to convert the older units and United States units (based on the British engineering system) to SI units. A foot is about 0.305 m, a joule is 10 million ergs, and so forth. We will undoubtedly continue to use a combination of units from different systems for some time. For instance, we purchase electric power in kilowatts (SI units), potatoes in pounds (British engineering unit), and heat energy in BTUs (British thermal units), all different systems. An increasingly complex world should uniformly use something like SI units. A sixteenth-century English peasant may not have needed to convert a speed of furlongs per fortnight into inches per second, and we should not have to either.

SUMMARY

Wilhelm Conrad Roentgen discovered x rays on November 8, 1895. X rays are members of a group of radiations known as electromagnetic radiations, of which light is the best-known member. They have a dual nature, behaving in some circumstances as waves and under different conditions as particles. Therefore, two concepts have been postulated to explain their characteristics. A single particle of radiation is called a photon, and we will discuss x rays in terms of photons.

REFERENCE

1. Glasser, O.: Wilhelm Conrad Roentgen and the Early History of the Roentgen Rays. Springfield, IL, Charles C Thomas, 1934.

CHAPTER

2 *Production of X Rays*

DIAGNOSTIC X-RAY TUBES

X rays are produced by **energy conversion** when a fast-moving stream of electrons is suddenly decelerated in the "target" anode of an x-ray tube. The x-ray tube is made of Pyrex glass that encloses a vacuum containing two electrodes (this is a diode tube). The electrodes are designed so that electrons produced at the cathode (negative electrode or filament) can be accelerated by a high potential difference toward the anode (positive or target electrode). The basic elements of an x-ray tube are shown in Figure 2–1, a diagram of a stationary anode x-ray tube. Electrons are produced by the heated tungsten filament and accelerated across the tube to hit the tungsten target, where x rays are produced. This section will describe the design of the x-ray tube and will review the way in which x rays are produced.

Glass Enclosure

It is necessary to seal the two electrodes of the x-ray tube in a vacuum. If gas were present inside the tube, the electrons that were being accelerated toward the anode (target) would collide with the gas molecules, lose energy, and cause secondary electrons to be ejected from the gas molecules. By this process (ionization), additional electrons would be available for acceleration toward the anode. Obviously, this production of secondary electrons could not be satisfactorily controlled. Their presence would result in variation in the number and, more strikingly, in the reduced speed of the electrons impinging on the target. This would cause a wide variation in tube current and in the energy of the x rays produced. Actually, this principle was used in the design of the early so-called "gas" x-ray tubes, which contained small amounts of gas to serve as a source of secondary electrons. The purpose of the vacuum in the modern x-ray tube is to allow the number and speed of the accelerated electrons to be controlled independently. The shape and size of these x-ray

Figure 2–1   The major components of a stationary anode x-ray tube

tubes are specifically designed to prevent electric discharge between the electrodes.

The connecting wires must be sealed into the glass wall of the x-ray tube. During operation of the x-ray tube, both the glass and the connecting wires are heated to high temperatures. Because of differences in their coefficients of expansion, most metals expand more than glass when heated. This difference in expansion would cause the glass-metal seal to break and would destroy the vacuum in the tube if special precautions were not taken. Because of this problem, special alloys, having approximately the same coefficients of linear expansion as Pyrex glass, are generally used in x-ray tubes.

Cathode

The negative terminal of the x-ray tube is called the cathode. In referring to an x-ray tube, the terms **cathode** and **filament** may be used interchangeably, a statement that is not true for other types of diode tubes. In addition to the **filament,** which **is the source of electrons** for the x-ray tube, the cathode has two other elements. These are the connecting wires, which supply both the voltage (average about 10 V) and the amperage (average about 3 to 5 A) that heat the filament, and a metallic focusing cup. The number (quantity) of x rays produced depends entirely on the number of electrons that flow from the filament to the target (anode) of the tube. **The x-ray tube current, measured in milliamperes (1 mA = 0.001 A), refers to the number of electrons flowing per second from the filament to the target.** It is important to understand where these electrons come from, and to remember that the number of electrons determines x-ray tube current. For example, in a given unit of time, a tube current of 200 mA is produced by twice as many electrons as a current of 100 mA, and 200 mA produces twice as many x rays as 100 mA.

The filament is made of tungsten wire, about 0.2 mm in diameter, that is coiled to form a vertical spiral about 0.2 cm in diameter and 1 cm or less in length. When current flows through this fine tungsten wire, it becomes heated. When a metal is heated its atoms absorb thermal energy, and some of the electrons in the metal acquire enough energy to allow them to move a small distance from the surface of the metal (normally, electrons can move within a metal, but cannot escape from it). Their escape is referred to as the process of **thermionic emission,** which may be defined as the emission of electrons resulting from the absorption of thermal energy. The electron cloud surrounding the filament, produced by thermionic emission, has been termed the "Edison effect." A pure tungsten filament must be heated to a temperature of at least 2200° C to emit a useful number of electrons (thermions). Tungsten is not as efficient an emitting material as other materials (such as alloys of tungsten) used in some electron tubes. It is chosen for use in x-ray tubes, however, because it can be drawn into a thin wire that is quite strong, has a high melting point (3370° C), and has little tendency to vaporize; thus, such a filament has a reasonably long life expectancy.

Electrons emitted from the tungsten filament form a small cloud in the immediate vicinity of the filament. This collection of negatively charged electrons forms what is called the **space charge.** This cloud of negative charges tends to prevent other electrons from being emitted from the filament until they have acquired sufficient thermal energy to overcome the force caused by the space charge. The tendency of the space charge to limit the emission of more electrons from the filament is called the **space charge effect.** When electrons leave the filament the loss of negative charges causes the filament to acquire a positive charge. The filament then attracts some emitted electrons back to itself. When a filament is heated to its emission temperature, a state of equilibrium is quickly reached. In equilibrium the number of electrons returning to the filament is equal to the number of electrons being emitted. As a result, the number of electrons in the space charge remains constant, with the actual number depending on filament temperature.

The high currents that can be produced by the use of thermionic emission are possible because large numbers of electrons can be accelerated from the cathode (negative electrode) to the anode (positive electrode) of the x-ray tube. The number of electrons involved is enormous. The unit of electric current is the ampere, which may be defined as the rate of "flow" when 1 coulomb of electricity flows through a conductor in 1 sec. The coulomb is the equivalent of the amount of electric charge carried by 6.25×10^{18} electrons. Therefore, an x-ray tube current of 100 mA (0.1 A) may be considered as the "flow" of 6.25×10^{17} electrons from the cathode to the anode in 1 sec. **Electron current across an x-ray tube is in one direction only** (always cathode to anode). Because of the forces of mutual repulsion and the large number of electrons, this electron stream would tend to spread itself out and result in bombardment of an unacceptably large area on the anode of the x-ray tube. This is prevented by a structure called the cathode **focusing cup,** which surrounds the filament (Figs. 2–2 and 2–4). When the x-ray tube is conducting, the focusing cup is maintained at the same negative potential as the filament. The focusing cup is designed so that its electrical forces cause the electron stream to converge onto the target anode in the required size and shape. The focusing cup is usually made of nickel. Modern x-ray tubes may be supplied with a single or, more commonly, a double filament. Each filament consists of a spiral of wire, and they are mounted side by side or one above the other, with one being longer than the other (Fig. 2–2). It is important to understand that only one filament is used for any given x-ray exposure; the larger filament is generally used for larger exposures. The heated filament glows and can be easily ob-

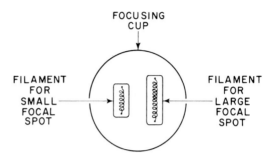

Figure 2–2 A double filament contained in a focusing cup

served by looking into the beam exit port of an x-ray tube housing (do not forget to remove the filter).

Two additional filament arrangements may be seen in highly specialized x-ray tubes. A tube with three filaments (triple-focus) is available. Another special application is a stereoscopic angiographic tube. In this tube the two focal spots are widely separated (about a 4-cm separation). When two films are exposed, using a different focal spot for each film, a stereoscopic film pair is produced. This tube is useful in angiography when rapid exposure of multiple stereoscopic film pairs is desired. Intervals as short as 0.1 sec between exposures can be obtained with stereoscopic tubes.

Vaporization of the filament when it is heated acts to shorten the life of an x-ray tube, because the filament will break if it becomes too thin. The filament should never be heated for longer periods than necessary. Many modern x-ray circuits contain an automatic filament-boosting circuit. When the x-ray circuit is turned on, but no exposure is being made, a "standby" current heats the filament to a value corresponding to low current, commonly about 5 mA. This amount of filament heating is all that is required for fluoroscopy. When exposures requiring larger tube currents are desired, an automatic filament-boosting circuit will raise the filament current from the standby value to the required value before the exposure is made, and lower it to the standby value immediately after the exposure.

Tungsten that is vaporized from the filament (and occasionally from the anode) is deposited as an extremely thin coating on the inner surface of the glass wall of the x-ray tube. It produces a color that becomes deeper as the tube ages. Aging tubes acquire a bronze-colored "sunburn." This tungsten coat has two effects: it tends to filter the x-ray beam, gradually changing the quality of the beam, and the presence of the metal on the glass increases the possibility of arcing between the glass and the electrodes at higher peak kilovoltage (kVp) values, which may result in puncture of the tube. One of the reasons metal, as opposed to glass, x-ray tube enclosures have been developed is to minimize the effect of deposition of tungsten on the tube wall. We will discuss metal tubes later in this chapter.

Line Focus Principle

The focal spot is the area of the tungsten target (anode) that is bombarded by electrons from the cathode. **Most of the energy of the electrons is converted into heat,** with less than 1% being converted into x rays. Because the heat is uniformly distributed over the focal spot, a large focal spot allows the accumulation of larger amounts of heat before damage to the tungsten target occurs. The melting point of tungsten is about 3370° C, but it is best to keep the temperature below 3000° C. The problems posed by the need for a large focal spot to allow greater heat loading, and the conflicting need for a small focal area to produce good radiographic detail, were resolved in 1918 with the development of the **line focus principle.** The theory of line focus is illustrated in Figure 2–3. The size and shape of the focal spot are determined by the size and shape of the electron stream when it hits the anode. The size and shape of the electron stream are determined by the dimensions of the filament tungsten wire coil, the construction of the focusing cup, and the position of the filament in the

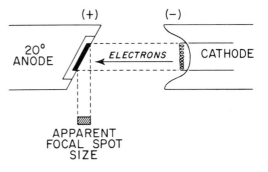

Figure 2–3   The line focus principle

focusing cup. The electron stream bombards the target, the surface of which is inclined so that it forms an angle with the plane perpendicular to the incident beam. The anode angle differs according to individual tube design and may vary from 6 to 20°. Because of this angulation, when the slanted surface of the focal spot is viewed from the direction in which x-rays emerge from the x-ray tube, the surface is foreshortened and appears small. It is evident, therefore, that the side of the effective, or apparent, focal spot is considerably smaller than that of the actual focal spot. If the decrease in projected focal spot size is calculated, it is found that the size of the projected focal spot is directly related to the sine of the angle of the anode. Because sine 20° = 0.342 and sine 16.5° = 0.284, an anode angle of 16.5° will produce a smaller focal spot size than an angle of 20°. Thus, as the angle of the anode is made smaller, the apparent focal spot also becomes smaller.

Some newer 0.3-mm focal spot tubes may use an anode angle of only 6°. Such small angles permit the use of larger areas of the target for electron bombardment (and heat dissipation), yet achieve a small apparent focal spot size. For practical purposes, however, there is a limit to which the anode angle can be decreased as dictated by the heel effect (the point of anode cutoff). For general diagnostic radiography done at a 40-in. focus-film distance, the anode angle is usually no smaller than 15°.

Focal spot size is expressed in terms of the apparent or projected focal spot; sizes of 0.3, 0.6, 1.0, and 1.2 mm are commonly employed.

Anode

Anodes (positive electrodes) of x-ray tubes are of two types, **stationary** or **rotating.** The stationary anode will be discussed first because many of its basic principles also apply to the rotating anode.

Stationary Anode. The anode of a stationary anode x-ray tube consists of a small plate of tungsten, 2- or 3-mm thick, that is embedded in a large mass of copper. The tungsten plate is square or rectangular in shape, with each dimension usually being greater than 1 cm. The anode angle is usually 15 to 20°, as discussed above.

Tungsten is chosen as the target material for several reasons. It has a **high atomic number** (74), which makes it more efficient for the production of x rays. In addition, because of its **high melting point,** it is able to withstand the high temperature produced. Most metals melt between 300 and 1500° C, whereas tungsten melts at 3370° C. Tungsten is a reasonably good material for the absorption of heat and for the rapid dissipation of the heat away from the target area.

The rather small tungsten target must be bonded to the much larger copper portion of the anode to facilitate heat dissipation. In spite of its good thermal characteristics, tungsten cannot withstand the heat of repeated exposures. Copper is a better conductor of heat than tungsten, so the massive copper anode acts to increase the total thermal capacity of the anode and to speed its rate of cooling.

The actual size of the tungsten target is considerably larger than the area bombarded by the electron stream (Fig. 2–4). This is necessary because of the relatively low melting point of copper (1070° C). A single x-ray exposure may raise the temperature of the bombarded area of the tungsten target by 1000° C or more. This

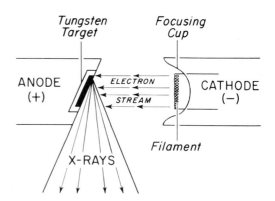

Figure 2–4 Lateral view of the cathode and anode of a stationary anode x-ray tube

high temperature is reached by any metal in the immediate vicinity of the focal spot. If the tungsten target were not sufficiently large to allow for some cooling around the edges of the focal spot, the heat produced would melt the copper in the immediate vicinity of the target.

All the metals expand when heated, but they expand at different rates. The bonding between the tungsten target and the copper anode provides technical problems because tungsten and copper have different coefficients of expansion. If the bond between the tungsten and the copper were not satisfactorily produced, the tungsten target would tend to peel away from the copper anode.

Rotating Anode. With the development of x-ray generators capable of delivering large amounts of power, the limiting factor in the output of an x-ray circuit became the x-ray tube itself. The ability of the x-ray tube to achieve high x-ray outputs is limited by the heat generated at the anode. The rotating anode principle is used to produce x-ray tubes capable of withstanding the heat generated by large exposures.

The anode of a rotating anode tube consists of a large disc of tungsten, or an alloy of tungsten, which theoretically rotates at a speed of about 3600 revolutions per minute (rpm) when an exposure is being made. In practice, the anode never reaches a speed of 3600 rpm because of mechanical factors such as slipping between the rotor and bearings; therefore, to calculate the ability of a tube to withstand high loads, a speed of 3000 rpm is usually assumed. Although the actual speed of anode rotation varies even between new tubes of identical design, it is safe to assume that anode rotation of any functioning rotating anode will never drop below 3000 rpm, and will usually be greater than 3000 rpm, if 60 hertz (Hz) current is used.

The tungsten disc has a beveled edge. The angle of the bevel may vary from 6 to 20°. The bevel is used to take advantage of the line focus principle previously described. **The purpose of the rotating anode is to spread the heat produced during an exposure over a large area of the anode.** Figure 2–5 illustrates this principle. (The dimensions are not drawn to scale.) If we assume that the filament and focusing cup of the x-ray tube produce an electron beam that covers an area of the anode 7-mm high and 2-mm wide, the area of the anode bombarded by electrons is represented by a 14-mm² rectangle. We recognize that a 2-mm focal spot is rarely encountered in modern x-ray tubes, but is a useful way to illustrate a point. If the bevel of the target is 16.5°, the effective or apparent focal spot size in our illustration will be about 2 × 2 mm. If the anode were stationary, the entire heat load would be delivered to this one small 14-mm² area of the target. If the target is made to rotate at a speed of 3600 rpm,

however, the electrons will bombard a constantly changing area of the target. The total bombarded area of tungsten is represented by a track 7-mm wide that extends around the periphery of the beveled rotating tungsten disc. The effective focal spot will, of course, appear to remain stationary. At a speed of 3600 rpm, any given area on the tungsten disc is found opposite the electron stream only once every 1/60 sec, and the remainder of the time heat generated during the exposure can be dissipated. During a 1/60-sec exposure, the entire circumference of the tungsten disc will be exposed to the electron beam.

A comparison between the total and instantaneous target areas will illustrate the tremendous advantage offered by the rotating anode tube (Fig. 2–5). At any instant an area of 14 mm² is bombarded by the electron beam in our example. If we assume the average radius of the bombarded area of the tungsten disc to be 40 mm, which is a typical value, the circumference of the disc at a radius equal to 40 mm will be 251 mm. The total target area will then be represented by the height of the electron stream (7 mm) times the average circumference of the disc (251 mm), or a total of 1757 mm². Even though the total loading area has been increased by a factor of about 125 (14 versus 1757 mm²), the apparent or effective focal spot size has remained the same.

The diameter of the tungsten disc determines the total length of the target track, and obviously affects the maximum permissible loading of the anode. Typical disc diameters measure 75, 100, or 125 mm.

To make the anode rotate, some mechanical problems must be overcome, because the anode is contained within the vacuum of the tube. The power to effect rotation is provided by a magnetic field produced by stator coils that surround the neck of the x-ray tube outside the envelope (Fig. 2–6). The magnetic field produced by the stator coils induces a current in the copper rotor of the induction motor, and

C = 2 π r
C = 2 π 40 mm.
C = 251 mm.

7 × 251 = 1757 mm.

Figure 2–5 A rotating anode increases the total target area

Figure 2–6 The major components of a rotating anode x-ray tube

this induced current provides the power to rotate the anode assembly. The clearance between the rotor and the neck of the tube is made as small as possible to ensure maximum efficiency in utilization of the magnetic force supplied by the stator core and windings. Early in the development of rotating anode x-ray tubes, the life of the tube was quite short because of the lack of durable bearings on which the anode assembly could rotate. Because of the friction produced it was necessary to lubricate the bearings, but commonly available lubricants could not be used. Lubricants such as oil would vaporize when heated and destroy the vacuum in the tube; dry lubricants such as graphite would wear off as a powder and destroy the vacuum. This problem was solved by the use of metallic lubricants (especially silver), which are suitable for use in a high vacuum. In modern rotating anode tubes, bearing wear has become a negligible factor in overall tube life.

Heat dissipation in a rotating anode tube presents an additional problem. Heat generated in a solid tungsten disc is dissipated by radiating through the vacuum to the wall of the tube, and then into the surrounding oil and tube housing. Recall that heat is dissipated in a stationary anode by absorption and conductivity is provided by the massive copper anode. In the rotating anode tube, absorption of heat by the anode assembly is undesirable because heat

absorbed by the bearings of the anode assembly would cause them to expand and bind. Because of this problem the stem (Fig. 2–6), which connects the tungsten target to the remainder of the anode assembly, is made of molybdenum. Molybdenum has a high melting point (2600° C) and is a poor heat conductor. Thus, the molybdenum stem provides a partial heat barrier between the tungsten disc and the bearings of the anode assembly.

The length of the molybdenum stem is another important consideration. As a length of the stem is increased, the inertia (this is really a gyroscopic, rather than inertial, problem) of the tungsten disc increases; this increases the load on the bearings of the anode assembly. It is desirable to keep the stem as short as possible. This problem is reduced in metal tubes by the use of bearings at each end of the anode axle (see Fig. 2–12).

Even if all the factors that affect rotation of the relatively heavy anode assembly are optimally controlled, inertia is still a problem. Because of this inertia there is a short delay between application of force to the anode assembly and the time at which the rotor reaches its full angular velocity. This period usually varies from 0.5 to 1 sec. A safety circuit is incorporated into the x-ray circuit that prevents an x-ray exposure from being made until the rotor has reached its full speed.

The life of a rotating anode x-ray tube may be limited by roughening and pitting of the surface of the anode exposed to the electron beam. These physical changes are the result of thermal stress, and they act to diminish the x-ray output of the tube. The decreased output of the x radiation results from excessive scattering of the x rays (more radiation is directed away from the exit window of the tube) and increased absorption of x rays by the target itself. The combination of short exposure time and fast anode rotation causes very rapid heating and cooling of the surface of the anode disc. The loss of heat by radiation from the disc surface occurs before there is time for any significant amount of heat to be conducted into the main mass of the tungsten disc. Therefore, thermal expansion of metal on the surface is much greater than expansion of metal immediately beneath the surface. This condition causes stresses to develop that distort the target surface of the anode disc. It has been found that an alloy of about **90% tungsten and 10% rhenium** (a heavy metal with good thermal capacity) produces an anode that is more resistant to surface roughening and has a higher thermal capacity than an anode of pure tungsten. With these improved anode discs, roughening of the focal track has ceased to be a major problem.

The usual speed of anode rotation using 60-cycle current varies between 3000 and 3600 rpm. If the speed of rotation is increased, the ability of the anode to withstand heat will become greater because any given area of the target is exposed to the electron beam for a shorter period of time during each revolution of the anode. By use of proper circuits, the speed of anode rotation can be increased to about 10,000 rpm. Three modifications of the tube help to overcome the problem associated with this increased velocity; the length of the anode stem is made as short as possible to decrease the inertia of the anode; the anode assembly rotates on two sets of bearings, which are placed as far apart as possible; and finally, the inertia of the anode is reduced by decreasing the weight of the anode itself. This is achieved by employing a compound anode disc in which the largest part of the disc is made of molybdenum (specific gravity 10.2), which is considerably lighter than tungsten (specific gravity 19.3). A relatively thin layer of tungsten-rhenium alloy attached to the disc serves as the actual target for the electron beam. Some laminated discs use carbon (graphite) instead of molybdenum to further decrease disc inertia. Graphite does not conduct heat as well as molybdenum, so a graphite anode disc will become hotter

than a molybdenum disc. There are also some technical problems associated with bonding the tungsten-rhenium layer to the graphite. A laminated disc with a molybdenum substrate has a moment of inertia about 35% less than a solid tungsten disc of equal diameter and heat capacity. A further reduction in moment of inertia of at least 50% can be achieved when the molybdenum is replaced by graphite.

Some anode discs are manufactured with slits or grooves in the target surface of the disc. This allows the material in the focal track to expand without producing the mechanical tension that arises in a solid disc. The back of the anode disc may be coated with a black substance, such as carbon, to aid in heat dissipation from the anode.

Grid-Controlled X-Ray Tubes

Conventional x-ray tubes contain two electrodes (cathode and anode). The switches used to initiate and to stop an exposure with these tubes must be able to withstand the large changes in voltage applied between the cathode and anode. The rather involved topic of dealing with the timers and switches used in the x-ray circuit will be considered in Chapter 3. A grid-controlled x-ray tube contains its own "switch," which allows the x-ray tube to be turned on and off rapidly, as is required with cinefluorography.

A third electrode is used in the grid-controlled tube to control the flow of electrons from the filament to the target. **The third electrode is the focusing cup that surrounds the filament.** In conventional x-ray tubes a focusing cup is electrically connected to the filament. This focusing cup helps to focus the electrons on the target. Because each electron is negatively charged, the electrons repel one another as they travel to the target. As a result, the electron beam (tube current) spreads out. The focusing cup is designed to counteract the spread of the electron beam, which can be accomplished even with the cup and filament electrically connected.

In the grid-controlled tube, the focusing cup can be electrically negative relative to the filament. The voltage across the filament-grid produces an electric field along the path of the electron beam that pushes the electrons even closer together. If the voltage is made large enough, the tube current may be completely pinched off, a condition in which no electrons go from the filament to the target. The voltage applied between the focusing cup and filament may therefore act like a switch to turn the tube current on and off. Because the cup and filament are close together, the voltage necessary to cut off the tube current is not extremely large. For example, to pulse (turn the tube current on and off with the focusing cup), a 0.3-mm focal spot tube operating at 105 kVp requires about −1500 V between the filament and the cup.

Saturation Voltage

When the filament of an x-ray tube is heated, a space charge is produced, as previously discussed. When a potential difference is applied between the cathode and anode, electrons flow from the filament to the anode to produce the tube current. If the potential applied across the tube is insufficient to cause almost all electrons to be pulled away from the filament the instant they are emitted, a **residual space charge** will exist about the filament. As we described earlier in this chapter, this residual space charge acts to limit the number of electrons available, and thus it limits the current flowing in the x-ray tube. From the chart shown in Figure 2–7 it can be seen that, up to about 40 kVp, an increase in kilovoltage produces a significant increase in x-ray tube current even though filament heating remains the same. Above 40 kVp, however, further increases in kilovoltage produce very little change in tube current. In our example, 40 kVp defines the location of the saturation point of this x-ray tube. Below 40 kVp, the current flowing in the tube is limited by the space charge effect (space-charge-limited). Above 40 kVp

(the saturation voltage) the space charge effect, theoretically, has no influence on current flowing in the x-ray tube. In this region the current is determined by the number of electrons made available by the heated filament and is said to be emission-limited or temperature-limited. Reference to Figure 2–7 will show that, in actual practice, a continued increase of kilovoltage above 40 kVp will produce a slight increase in tube current because of a small residual space charge effect. In modern x-ray circuits this slight increase in milliamperes accompanying increased kilovoltage would be undesirable, because the tube current could not be precisely controlled. By the use of resistors the circuit automatically compensates for this change by producing a slight decrease in filament heating as kilovoltage is increased. Note that different x-ray tubes have different saturation voltages and require different amounts of space charge compensation.

Heel Effect. The intensity of the x-ray beam that leaves the x-ray tube is not uniform throughout all portions of the beam. The intensity of the beam depends on the angle at which the x rays are emitted from the focal spot. This variation is termed the "heel effect."

Figure 2–8 shows that the intensity of the beam toward the anode side of the tube is less than that which angles toward the cathode. The decreased intensity of the x-ray beam that is emitted more nearly parallel to the surface of the angled target is

Figure 2–7   Saturation voltage

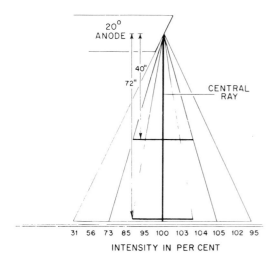

INTENSITY IN PER CENT

Figure 2–8 The heel effect

caused by the absorption of some of the x-ray photons by the target itself. Beam intensity, as related to the angle of emission, varies depending on the physical characteristics of individual x-ray tubes. Figure 2–8 contains average values taken from charts published in several textbooks and is used for purposes of illustration only. If, for example, a 14- × 17-in. film is oriented so that its long axis corresponds with that of the tube, the heel effect can be studied. At a 40-in. target-film distance, the anode end of the film will receive a relative exposure of 73% and the cathode end will receive a relative exposure of 105%. Thus, there is about a 30% difference in the intensity of exposure between the two ends of the film. If the target-film distance is increased to 72 in., it can be determined from the chart that the difference in exposure intensities will be considerably less, roughly 87 to 104%.

Three clinically important aspects of the heel effect are illustrated with this example. First, **the intensity of film exposure on the anode side of the x-ray tube is significantly less than that on the cathode side of the tube.** This factor can be used in obtaining balanced densities in radiographs of body parts of different thicknesses. The thicker parts should be placed

toward the cathode (filament) side of the x-ray tube. This is usually illustrated by pointing out that an anteroposterior (AP) film of the thoracic spine should be made with the tube oriented so that its anode end is over the upper thoracic spine where the body is less thick; the cathode end of the tube is over the lower thoracic spine where thicker body structures will receive the increased exposure, which they require. Second, it can be seen that **the heel effect is less noticeable when larger focus-film distances are used.** Third, for equal target-film distances, **the heel effect will be less for smaller films.** This is because the intensity of the x-ray beam nearest the central ray is more uniform than that toward the periphery of the beam.

Tube Shielding and High-Voltage Cables. Although we usually think of x rays as being confined to the beam emerging from the tube, they are, in fact, emitted with more or less equal intensity in every direction from the target. In addition, the x rays are scattered in all directions following collisions with various structures in and around the tube. The tube housing is lined with lead and serves to absorb primary and secondary x rays that would otherwise produce a high intensity of radiation around the tube, resulting in needless exposure of patients and personnel, as well as excessive film fogging. The effectiveness of the tube housing in limiting leakage radiation must meet the specifications listed in the National Council on Radiation Protection and Measurements Report No. 49, which states that: "The leakage radiation measured at a distance of 1 meter from the source shall not exceed 100 mR (milliroentgens) in an hour when the tube is operated at its maximum continuous rated current for the maximum rated tube potential."

Another function of the tube housing is to provide shielding for the high voltages required to produce x rays. The high-voltage cables, which are connected to the tube through appropriate receptacles in the tube housing, contain a grounding sheath of wires to provide proper grounding of the tube to the earth. To prevent short-circuiting between the grounding wires and the tube, the space between them is filled with extremely thick mineral oil. Thus, the x-ray tube is contained within the tube housing, and oil inside the housing surrounds the tube. The housing is then carefully sealed to exclude all air, because air would expand excessively when heated and rupture the housing. The oil has good electrical insulating and thermal cooling properties. Because of its insulating properties, the oil allows more compact tubes and housings to be used, because it permits points of high potential difference to be placed closer to each other. In addition, convection currents set up in the oil help to carry heat away from the tube. Heat from the oil is absorbed through the metal of the tube shield to be dissipated into the atmosphere.

As the oil in the tube housing is heated it will, of course, expand. A metal bellows within the tube shield allows the oil to expand without increasing pressures on the tube and shield, thus averting possible damage. In addition, the expanded bellows can be made to operate a microswitch, which will automatically prevent further exposures if maximum heating of the oil has occurred.

TUBE RATING CHARTS

It is customary to speak of the total load that can be applied to an x-ray tube in terms of kilovoltage, milliamperes, and exposure time. The limit on the load that can be safely accepted by an x-ray tube is a function of the heat energy produced during the exposure. The maximum temperature to which tungsten can be safely raised is generally considered to be 3000° C. Above this level considerable vaporization of the tungsten target occurs. The rate at which heat is generated by an electric current is proportional to the product of the voltage (kV) and the current (mA). Thus, the total heat produced is a product of volt-age and current and exposure time. This energy is currently expressed in two different systems:

> Heat units (an artificial system)
> SI units (the watt-second or joule)

It is our task to present both systems and relate their values. Heat units will be eliminated in the near future but are still encountered in manufacturer's charts and the literature.

The heat unit (HU) is defined as the product of current (mA) and kVp and time (sec) for single-phase power supplies—a very artificial and unfortunate definition. Recall that in a single-phase generator the peak voltage (kVp) is not the average voltage; kVp is actually 1.4 (or 1.35) times the average voltage (this is more precisely called the "root mean square," or "r.m.s.," voltage; we will call it "average" and use the conversion factor of 1.4). Modern generators contain a three-phase power supply with an almost constant potential voltage (we will assume constant potential) in which kVp and average voltage are the same. What a mess! The HU is defined using kVp of a single-phase unit, which is 1.4 times the average voltage. To find HU for a constant potential generator, we are required (since kVp and average voltage are the same) to multiply kVp by 1.4 because HU are defined in a system in which kVp = 1.4 times average voltage. An example will help. Using a technique of 70 kVp, 100 mA, and 0.1 sec, calculate HU applied to the x-ray tube for a single-phase and a constant-potential generator:

Single phase
70 kVp × 100 mA × 0.1 sec = 700 HU

Constant potential
70 kVp × 1.4 × 100 mA × 0.1 sec = 980 HU

For identical factors, HU of a constant potential generator are higher, but the x-ray tube produces many more x-rays because of the constant voltage.

A watt (W) is a unit of power, and is defined as the product of 1 V times 1 A:

$$1 \text{ W} = 1 \text{ V} \times 1 \text{ A}$$

Note that 1 KV (1000 V) times 1 A (1/1000 A) is also 1 W:

$$1 \text{ W} = 1000 \text{ V} \times 1/1000 \text{ A}$$

The volt in this definition is the average volt. We realize that power is the instantaneous voltage times current, but using the average voltage will keep us from using integral calculus. Power must do something to produce energy (you have power if you are strong enough to lift a weight; you give the weight energy when you pick it up). The unit of energy in the SI system is the joule (J), and is equal to a watt-second.

$$\text{watt} \times \text{second} = \text{watt-second} = \text{joule}$$

A HU is a unit of energy, and a watt-second or joule is a unit of energy, so we may compare the HU with the joule. Difficulty arises because the HU is defined by kVp of a generator (where kVp and average voltage are not the same), while the watt and joule are defined using average voltage. With a constant potential generator it is easy to calculate energy in the SI system, because joules are simply kVp × mA × time (sec). In a single-phase system a conversion is required because kVp and average voltage are not the same. One converts kVp to average voltage by dividing by 1.4 (or multiplying by 0.7). In an x-ray tube the current (mA) is fairly constant so that we do not need to calculate an average value for mA. Another example: calculate the joules of energy generated by a technique of 70 kVp, 100 mA, and 0.1 sec for a single phase and a constant potential generator:

Single phase:
$$\frac{70}{1.4} \text{ kVp} \times 100 \text{ mA} \times 0.1 \text{ sec} = 500 \text{ J}$$

Constant potential:
$$70 \text{ kVp} \times 100 \text{ mA} \times 0.1 \text{ sec} = 700 \text{ J}$$

Now, let's combine our examples of HU and joule calculations for an exposure of 70 kVp, 100 mA, and 0.1 sec:

	Heat Units	Joules
Single phase	700	500
Constant potential	980	700

See what a mess the artificial term "heat unit" causes? Do not memorize conversion factors. Remember the definition of a HU, a joule, and the relationship of average and peak kilovoltage. Then figure out the answer in the system of units required.

The term **kilowatt rating** (of an x-ray tube) is commonly used to express **the ability of the tube to make a single exposure of a reasonable duration.** The reasonable exposure time is defined as **0.1 sec.** Kilowatt ratings are always calculated for an x-ray tube used with a **constant potential generator and high-speed rotation.** For example, what is the maximum milliamperage that can be used at 70 kVp for a single exposure with a 30-kW (30,000-W) x-ray tube?

$$70 \text{ kVp} \times ? \text{ mA} = 30,000 \text{ W}$$
$$? \text{ mA} = \frac{30,000}{70} = 429 \text{ mA}$$

Similarly, a 150-kW tube could accept a tube current of 2140 mA. Remember, these are defined for 0.1-sec exposures. One can use an x-ray tube rating chart to calculate the approximate kW rating. Look at the theoretical tube rating chart in Figure 2–9. Find the 0.1 sec line and notice where it cuts the 70 kVp curve. These two lines cross at the 500 mA line, indicating that this tube could accept an exposure of 70 kVp and 500 mA at 0.1 sec. The approximate kW rating is:

$$70 \text{ kVp} \times 500 \text{ mA} = 35,000 \text{ W} = 35 \text{ kW}$$

A similar calculation at 100 kVp yields:

$$100 \text{ kVp} \times 350 \text{ mA} = 35 \text{ kW}$$

So this is a 35-kW tube.

To summarize, this section has thus far introduced the heat unit, watt-second (joule), and kilowatt rating as parameters that measure x-ray tube loading.

The amount of heat that can be accepted by an x-ray tube without excessive damage is in part determined by: the type of rectification and type of power supply (see Chap. 3); the surface area of tungsten bombarded by electrons (focal spot size, anode diameter, anode mass, target angle, and speed of rotation); and the length of the exposure.

In considering tube rating, three characteristics are encountered: the ability of the tube to withstand a single exposure; the ability of the tube to function despite multiple rapid exposures (as in angiography); and the ability of the tube to withstand multiple exposures during several hours of heavy use.

The safe limit within which an x-ray tube can be operated for a single exposure can be easily determined by the tube rating chart supplied with all x-ray tubes. An example of such a chart is given in Figure 2–9. For example, if it is determined that an exposure will require 50 mAs (500 mA at 0.1 sec), reference to the rating chart will show that the lines signifying 500 mA and 0.1 sec cross at a point that limits maximum

kilovoltage to about 70 kVp. In similar fashion, the safe loading for any combination of exposure factors can be determined from the tube rating chart. This chart is used as an example only. The manufacturer of the x-ray tube used in any diagnostic installation always supplies tube rating charts for the specific circumstances under which the tube will be used. For instance, tube rating charts for a single-phase power supply are not valid for a three-phase power supply. Tube rating charts contain information for many different kilovoltages.

Angiographic techniques requiring multiple exposures during a short period of time produce large amounts of heat. For any tube used for angiography, appropriate ratings will be made available in the form of graphs or charts. Several special considerations must be kept in mind when a tube is subjected to the stresses of rapid sequence radiography:

1. The surface of the target can be overheated by repeating exposures before

Figure 2–9   An x-ray tube rating chart

the surface heat has had time to dissipate into the body of the anode.

2. The entire anode can be overheated by repeating exposures before the heat in the anode has had time to radiate into the surrounding oil and tube housing.

3. The tube housing can be overheated by making too many exposures before the housing has had time to lose its heat to the surrounding air.

4. The total HU of a series of exposures made in rapid sequence must not exceed the HU permissible for a single exposure of a duration equal to the total elapsed time required to complete the series of exposures.

The chart used to calculate the maximum loading of the x-ray tube for a single exposure can also be used to determine the ability of the tube to withstand multiple rapid exposures (Fig. 2–9). For example, assume exposure factors of 500 mA, 0.1 sec, and 70 kVp, with 10 exposures to be made in 10 sec. First, reference to the chart will show that the single exposure is within the capability of the tube. Each exposure will produce 5000 HU (500 × 70 × 0.1 × 1.4 = 5000). Ten exposures will produce 50,000 HU in the 10-sec interval. The maximum number of heat units the x-ray tube can accept during a 10-sec period can be calculated from the chart. Actually, for an exposure time as long as 10 sec, the number of heat units produced is relatively independent of the kilovoltage used, and the permissible loading of the tube during the 10-sec period can be calculated for any convenient kilovoltage curve. On our chart, this calculation could be made using 70 kVp or 100 kVp. For example, 70 kVp applied for 10 sec could be used with a maximum milliamperage of 160 mA, and 70 × 160 × 10 × 1.4 would allow 156,000 HU input in 10 sec. The same calculation for 100 kVp for 10 sec at approximately 110 mA would allow 154,000 HU input. In our example, the input of 50,000 HU in 10 sec is well within the capability of the tube.

Angiographic rating charts are now frequently available. Such a chart is illustrated in Table 2–1 (this is the angiographic rating chart of a Machlett Dynamax 69 tube used with three-phase rectification, high speed anode rotation, and a 1.2-mm focal spot). Notice the asterisk, which reminds you to correlate this chart with the graph for single-exposure ratings. Let us assume we wish to make 20 exposures at a rate of 2 exposures per second; the chart indicates we can use 8800 J per exposure. This results in heat input of 176,000 J in 10 sec. Reference to the single-exposure graph for this tube (not illustrated) would show that the tube could accept a 10-sec continuous exposure at 70 kVp and 250 mA, or an input of 175,000 J (10 × 70 × 250) in 10 sec. The single-exposure graph would also be checked to ensure that the tube could accept each individual exposure in the series. Both the angiographic rating chart and the single-exposure rating graph must be used to ensure that planned exposure factors will not damage the tube.

The ability of an x-ray tube to withstand heat loading over a period of several hours depends on the anode heat-storage characteristics. Figure 2–10 illustrates an anode capable of storing 110,000 J. Note that anode cooling is much more rapid when the anode has accumulated large amounts of heat. This is a practical application of the physical law stating that **heat loss by radiation is proportional to the fourth power of the temperature.** The rate at which an anode heats during a period of constant exposure is important in fluoroscopy. For example, Figure 2–10 shows that a continuous heat input of 500 J per second will produce an accumulation of the maximum number of J in the anode in about 7 min. Therefore, if the tube is used during fluoroscopy at 100 kVp and 5 mA (100 × 5 × 1 = 500 J each second), continuous fluoroscopy beginning with a cold tube will be limited to 7 min. On the other hand, if fluoroscopy is carried out at 90 kVp and 3.8 mA (about 340 J each second), fluo-

Table 2–1. Dynamix 69 Angiographic Rating Chart

TOTAL NUMBER OF EXPOSURES	MAXIMUM LOAD (IN kVp × mA × SEC PER EXPOSURE)*							
	2	5	10	20	30	40	50	60
EXPOSURES PER SECOND								
1	45,000	27,000	17,500	10,800	7,400	5,500	4,400	3,700
2	30,000	20,000	13,600	8,800	6,600	5,400	4,400	3,700
3	24,000	16,500	11,600	7,600	5,800	4,700	4,100	3,600
4	19,500	14,000	10,000	6,800	5,200	4,300	3,700	3,300
5	17,000	12,200	9,000	6,200	4,800	4,000	3,400	3,000
6	14,800	11,000	8,200	5,700	4,500	3,700	3,200	2,900
8	11,800	9,200	7,000	5,000	4,000	3,400	2,950	2,650
10	10,000	7,800	6,200	4,500	3,600	3,100	2,750	2,400
12	8,600	7,000	5,500	4,000	3,300	2,900	2,550	2,250

*Effective focal-spot size 1.20 mm; stator frequency 180 Hz
Used with permission of Machlett Laboratories, Inc., Stamford, CT, 06907

roscopy can be continued indefinitely without causing excessive anode heating.

One of the most important uses of the anode heat-storage chart is to determine the length of time the tube must be allowed to cool before additional exposures can be made. For example, assume that an angiographic procedure produces 5000 J/exposure. If a rapid filming procedure required 20 exposures, the total anode heating would be 100,000 J. If Figure 2–10 represented the anode heat storage chart for the tube in question, it could be determined from the chart that it would require approximately 6 min for the tube to cool from 100,000 to 10,000 J. Thus, if repeat rapid filming were necessary, a delay of 6 min would be needed because of the limitation imposed by the ability of the anode to store heat.

Additional consideration must be given to the ability of the entire tube housing to

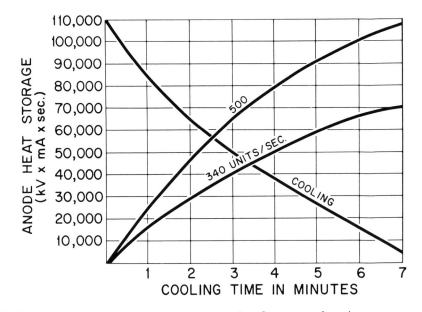

Figure 2–10   A chart of the anode heat storage capacity of an x-ray tube using a constant potential generator

withstand heat. The tube housing can absorb an enormous amount of heat (a figure of 1,500,000 J is not unreasonable). Although the tube housing can absorb large amounts of heat, it also requires considerable time for cooling. Reference to some typical charts will show that it takes, in general, about 30 min for a tube housing to dissipate 600,000 J. If more rapid cooling of a tube housing is required, the use of air circulators will usually double the cooling rate. Cooling rates exceeding 96,000 J per minute are possible.

Metal/Ceramic X-Ray Tubes

A high-performance x-ray tube introduced by Philips Medical Systems* bears the trade name of a ceramic Super Rolatix tube. This tube has a metal casing instead of the usual glass envelope, and has three ceramic insulators. Two insulators provide insulation for the two (positive and negative) high-voltage cables, and one supports the anode stem. We shall explore the advantages of such construction. A picture of this tube is shown in Figure 2–11, and a schematic diagram in Figure 2–12.

Notice in Figure 2–12 that the anode rotates on an axle which has bearings at each end to provide greater stability and reduce stress on the shaft. This additional support allows use of a more massive anode, with anode weights of 2000 g possible. Anodes in conventional x-ray tubes are generally limited to no more than 700 g.

Ceramic insulators are used to insulate the high voltage parts of the x-ray tube from the metal tube envelope. Aluminum oxide is a commonly used ceramic insulator. Ceramic insulators have long been used to attach high-voltage transmission lines to overhead supporting towers. The three ceramic insulators are labeled 4 (high-voltage connectors) and 8 (anode shaft) in Figure 2–12. The use of ceramic insulators allows a more compact tube design.

Using metal as the x-ray tube enclosure

_____
*Philips Medical Systems, Inc., Shelton, CT.

(instead of glass) offers several advantages, the three most important being:

1. Less off-focus radiation
2. Longer tube life with high tube currents
3. Higher tube loading

The metal envelope is grounded; this grounding plus use of ceramic insulation allows adequate electrical safety despite the tube's small size.

Off-Focus Radiation. Off-focus radiation is produced by an x-ray tube when high-speed electrons interact with metal surfaces other than the focal track of the anode (usually other parts of the anode). The main source of off-focus electrons is electron backscatter from the anode. These scattered electrons may then strike the anode a second time and produce x-rays from areas other than the anode focal track.

Off-focus radiation may be partly controlled by placing the collimator, or a lead diaphragm, as close to the x-ray tube as possible. A small port close to the anode will stop more of the widely spread off-focus beam than will a similar sized port placed farther from the anode.

The metal enclosure decreases off-focus radiation by attracting off-focus electrons to the grounded metal wall of the x-ray tube. Since the metal enclosure is at zero potential (i.e., it is grounded), the enclosure is relatively positive as compared to the electrons, which are at a negative potential. Off-focus electrons may be attracted to the anode or to the grounded x-ray tube enclosure. Where the electron goes is in part a function of its distance from the anode or metal wall. Electrons striking the metal wall may produce x-rays, but the low atomic number metal will produce few and low-energy x-rays. The metal enclosure thus decreases off-focus radiation by removing many off-focus electrons.

Longer Tube Life. We have already mentioned the problem of deposition of tungsten (from the anode) on the glass wall of x-ray tubes. This tungsten eventually

Figure 2–11 Photograph of a Super Rolatix ceramic x-ray tube. (Courtesy of Philips Medical Systems, Inc., Shelton, CT)

builds up enough to act as an electrode and cause arcing between the glass and filament. Tungsten deposition is of greatest concern when high tube currents (high mA) are used. A metal enclosed x-ray tube has its metal enclosure connected to ground, and deposition of tungsten will not alter this grounding. For this reason, the useful life of a metal-enclosed x-ray tube will be greater than that of a glass tube, especially when used for high tube currents, such as in angiography.

High Tube Loading. The more massive metal anode of this tube allows significantly higher tube currents (more mAs) to be used because of the larger heat storage capacity of the anode. This allows a higher mAs setting for single exposures. In addition, there is increased capacity for serial exposures because of better cooling that results from more efficient transfer of heat to the oil through the metal enclosure, as compared to a glass enclosure (metal is a much better heat conductor than glass).

INTERACTION OF ELECTRON BEAM WITH X-RAY TUBE TARGET

Atomic Structure

Before attempting to describe the phenomena that occur when fast-moving electrons encounter the tungsten target in an x-ray tube, we must briefly examine the structure of an atom. In 1897, J.J. Thomson discovered a negatively charged particle much smaller than any atom, which came to be called the electron. Based on the work of Rutherford and Bohr, a simple model of an atom may be visualized as a massive positively charged nucleus surrounded by electrons in orbits of specific diameters. The solar system is organized in similar fashion.

Nucleus. The nucleus of an atom is made up of several types of elementary particles, termed **nucleons.** Of the nucleons, only **protons** and **neutrons** will be considered in this discussion, because they are the only ones of importance outside the

1   WHOLE-METAL CASING
2   ANODE DISK
3/6 BALL-BEARINGS
4/8 CERAMIC INSULATORS
5   CATHODE WITH FILAMENT
7   STATOR WINDINGS
9   ANODE SHAFT
10   BERYLLIUM WINDOW

Figure 2–12   Schematic diagram of a Super Rolatix ceramic x-ray tube. (Courtesy of Philips Medical Systems, Inc., Shelton, CT)

field of nuclear physics. The proton has a positive electric charge numerically equal to the charge of the electron, while the neutron has zero electrical charge. The neutron and proton have about the same mass (1.66×10^{-24} g), which is approximately 1836 times greater than the mass of an electron. The number of protons in the nucleus is called the **atomic number** of the atoms, and is given the symbol **Z.** The total number of protons and neutrons in the nucleus of an atom is called the **mass number** and is symbolized by the letter **A.** For example, stable gold (Au) has a nucleus with 79 protons (Z = 79) and 118 neutrons (A = 197). All atoms of an element have the same atomic number (Z), but an element may have several isotopes. All the isotopes of an element have the same number of protons in the nucleus; that is, they have the same atomic number but have different numbers of neutrons and therefore different atomic masses.

In summary, the nucleus of an atom contains protons and neutrons, has a positive electrical charge, and contains almost all the mass of an atom.

Electron Orbits and Energy Levels. The electrons are negative charges revolving around the nucleus. Because an atom is always electrically neutral in its normal state, it must contain an equal number of protons and electrons. The simplest way to describe an atom is to visualize a central positive nucleus with electrons in circular orbits about the nucleus. In this description, the atom resembles a tiny planetary system, with the nucleus as the sun and the electrons as the orbiting planets. Unlike the solar system, with one planet in each orbit, the atomic system allows 2 electrons in the first orbit, up to 8 in the second, up to 18 in the third, up to 32 in the fourth, and up to 50 in the fifth. The electron orbits are designated by letters: K, L, M, N, O, and so on.

The planets of the solar system are all nearly in the same plane, whereas in the description we have given the electrons move about the nucleus in spherical shells. An electron in the shell closest to the nucleus is in the K shell and the electron is called a K electron. L electrons are in the L shell, the second nearest shell to the nucleus. The diameters of the electronic shells are determined by the nuclear force on the electron, and by the angular momentum and energy of the electron. Angular momentum simply indicates that the electron is moving in a curved path. The attractive force between the positively charged nucleus and the negatively charged electron is the force that keeps the electrons in the atom. This force is called the "binding force" of the electron, and is inversely proportional to the square of the distance between the nucleus and electron. Therefore, a K electron has a larger binding force than an L electron. Of course, the binding force of the electron is directed toward the nucleus, and the electron would move toward the nucleus if it were not moving in a curved path. The attractive force caused by the nucleus keeps the electrons moving in a circular path. The earth has a gravitational force toward the sun, but it continues to move around the sun in a stable orbit. Similarly, electrons are in stable orbital shells.

The earth has energy that is the sum of its potential and kinetic energies. The earth's potential energy is a result of the gravitational effect of the sun; its kinetic energy is a result of its motion. By definition, kinetic energy must be positive, but potential energy can be either positive or negative. **Bound particles always have negative energy.** The earth is in a negative energy state, and electrons in an atom are also in negative energy states. To free an electron from an atom, the energy must be raised to zero or to a positive value. The energy that an electron in a shell must be given to raise the energy value to zero is called the **binding energy** of the electron. This is also the energy value designated for the atomic shell that houses the electron. The atomic shells are also called **energy shells.** Tungsten has a K-shell energy of 70 keV and an L-shell energy of 11 keV. Remember, these are negative energy values. To free a K electron from tungsten, the electron must be given 70 keV of energy, while only 11 keV are required to free an L electron. The L electron has 59 keV more energy than the K electron. The binding energy of the electron shells varies from one element to another. For example, tungsten, with an atomic number of 74, has a K-shell binding energy of 70 keV, while copper, with an atomic number of 29, has a K-shell binding energy of only 9 keV.

If a small amount of energy were taken from the earth, it would move a bit closer to the sun. Atomic structural laws, however, prohibit small additions or subtractions of energy from the bound electrons. An electron cannot have any more, or less, energy than that associated with its energy shell, but an electron may jump from one energy shell to another if the shell to which it jumps is not already filled. An electron can move to either a higher or lower energy shell. Electron movement to a lower energy shell (for example, from an L to a K shell) results in the emission of energy. The amount of energy is equal to the difference in the binding energy between the two shells. The energy may take the form of a photon. If the quantity of energy is sufficient, the photon may be called an x ray. Electron movement to a higher energy (for example, from a K to an L shell, or from the K shell to a free electron) requires the addition of energy to the electron. One source of this addition may be the absorption of an x-ray photon.

Each of the atomic energy shells, except the K shell, has subshells of slightly different energies. For example, the L shell has three subshells and an electron in the L shell may have one of three energy values. Of course, a single electron will have only one energy value, but the eight electrons needed to fill the L shell will be divided with two electrons in the lowest, four in the middle, and two in the highest subshells. In a transition from the L shell to the K shell, an electron will emit energy precisely equal to the difference in the energy of the shells. If an L electron leaves the highest subshell and goes to the K shell, it will emit some value of energy. If it leaves the middle shell and goes to the K shell, however, it will emit a slightly different value. An L electron in the lowest subshell may not go to the K shell. This is called a **forbidden transition.**

There are more elaborate models of atomic structure that suggest that the orbits are elliptic (so are the orbits of the solar system) or that the electron is just a standing wave about the nucleus. For diagnostic radiology the circular orbit model is sufficiently accurate.

The diameter of the nucleus of an atom is about 5×10^{-15} m and the diameter of the entire atom is about 5×10^{-10} m. This means that the diameter of the atom is about 100,000 times larger than the diameter of its nucleus. Most of an atom is an empty space, and this explains why a high-speed electron may go through many atoms before colliding with any of the components of an atom. It is interesting to visualize the hydrogen atom in terms of balls. Suppose the hydrogen nucleus (a proton) were a ball 3 in. in diameter. The electron (assuming electron density to be equal to proton density) would be a ball ¼ in. in diameter. The K shell would have a diameter of 1.5 miles. A normal hydrogen atom would be visualized as a 3-inch ball with a ¼-in. ball moving on a spherical shell ¾ of a mile away. More fun, if all the electrons in the atoms of the world could be removed and the nuclei packed together (a condition that exists in the white dwarf stars), the diameter of the earth would be reduced to about 0.1 mile.

The production of x rays makes use of three properties of the tungsten atoms in the target of the x-ray tube: the electric field of the nucleus; the binding energy of orbital electrons; and the need of the atom to exist in its lowest energy state.

Processes of X-Ray Generation

X rays are produced by **energy conversion** when fast-moving electrons from the filament of the x-ray tube interact with the tungsten anode (target). The kinetic energy (E) of the electron in passing across the voltage (V) is increased by

$$E = eV$$

where e is the electronic charge. Because the electric charge (e) of the electron does not change (e = 1.60×10^{-19} C), it is apparent that increasing the voltage across the x-ray tube will increase the kinetic energy of the electron. We define the electron volt as the energy a single electron obtains when crossing one volt. We can write:

$$E = 1.6 \times 10^{-19} \text{ C} \times 1 \text{ V}$$
$$= 1.6 \times 10^{-19} \text{ J}$$

Therefore, one electron volt equals 1.6×10^{-19} J. A joule may be expressed in different units. We previously encountered a joule as a watt-second. We leave it as an exercise in unit management to determine that a watt-second is equal to a coulomb-volt (hint: W = V ·A, A = C/sec). Voltage is expressed as the peak kilovoltage (kVp) applied across the x-ray tube (100 kVp = 100,000 peak volts). **We must clearly distinguish between kVp and keV** (kiloelectron volts). The expression 100 kVp means that the maximum voltage across the tube causing acceleration of the electrons is 100,000 V. The expression keV denotes the energy of any individual electron in the beam (100 keV = 100,000 electron volts). When the x-ray tube is operated at 100 kVp, few electrons acquire a kinetic energy of 100 keV because the applied voltage pulsates between some lower value and the maximum value (kVp) selected. It takes the electrons something like 10^{-10} sec to go from the cathode to the anode, separated by 1 in., when the applied voltage is 100 kilovolts (kV). Each electron will acquire a kinetic energy (eV), where V is the instantaneous voltage across the tube. In a single-phase, full-wave rectified circuit, the voltage varies from 0 to the maximum (kVp) value selected, at a rate of 120 times per second. This will be discussed in more detail in Chapter 3. For the present discussion, it is adequate to state that the voltage (V) providing the potential to accelerate the electrons is pulsating, so that the energy (eV) of electrons that encounter the target (anode of the x-ray tube) covers a broad range. In other words, the **high-speed electrons striking the target do not have the same energy.**

X rays are generated by two different processes when the high-speed electrons lose energy in the target of the x-ray tube. One involves reaction of the electrons with the nucleus of the tungsten atoms, producing x rays that are termed **general radiation,** or **bremsstrahlung.** The second involves collision between the high-speed electrons and the electrons in the shell of the target tungsten atoms, producing x rays that are called **characteristic radiation.** To repeat, when high-speed electrons lose energy in the target of an x-ray tube, x rays are produced by two different processes: (1) general radiation (bremsstrahlung), and (2) characteristic radiation.

General Radiation (Bremsstrahlung). When an electron passes near the nucleus of a tungsten atom, the positive charge of the nucleus acts on the negative charge of the electron. The electron is attracted toward the nucleus and is thus deflected from its original direction. The electron may lose energy and be slowed down when its direction changes. The kinetic energy lost by the electron is emitted directly in the form of a photon of radiation. The radiation produced by this process is called general radiation or bremsstrahlung (from the German for "braking radiation"). Figure 2–13 is a schematic representation of this production of bremsstrahlung.

Most electrons that strike the target give up their energy by interactions with a number of atoms. The electron gives up only part of its energy in the form of radiation each time it is "braked." Electrons penetrate through many atomic layers before giving up all their energy; therefore, not all x-rays are produced on the surface of the target. Occasionally, the electron will collide head-on with a nucleus. In this type of collision all the energy of the electron appears as a single x-ray photon.

Usually an electron will undergo many reactions before coming to rest, and the energy it loses with each reaction is small. In addition, the electrons in the beam striking the target have widely different energies. These two factors cause a wide distribution in the energy of the radiation produced by this braking phenomenon. Most of the radiation will have little energy, and will appear as heat. Few x rays will appear because over 99% of all reactions produce heat. The energy of the radiation is the amount of energy lost by the electrons. As discussed in Chapter 1, the energy of a photon of radiation is inversely related to its wavelength. The wavelength of x-ray photons produced when the electron is braked by the tungsten nuclei in the target is related to the energy (keV) of the electron. The energy of the electron is related to the potential difference (kVp) across the x-ray tube. Consider the case of a head-on collision between the electron and nucleus. All the energy of the electron is given to the resulting x-ray photon. The minimum wavelength (in angstroms) of this x-ray photon can be calculated:

$$\lambda_{min} = \frac{12.4}{kVp}$$

For example, using 100-kVp x-ray potential, the maximum energy (eV) that an electron can acquire is 100 keV. An electron with this energy can produce an x-ray photon with a minimum wavelength of 0.124 Å:

$$\lambda_{min} = \frac{12.4}{100} = 0.124 \text{ Å}$$

Remember, 0.124 Å is the shortest wavelength (highest energy) x-ray photon that can be produced with an x-ray tube potential of 100 kVp. Another way to say this is that 100-keV electrons that strike a target can produce x-ray photons with 100 keV of energy (at most), but this a rather rare event. Most of the x rays produced will

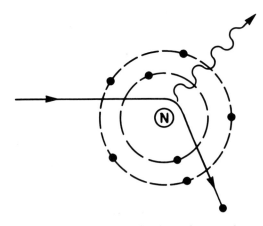

Figure 2–13 The production of general radiation (bremsstrahlung)

have wavelengths longer than 0.124 Å. In fact, the wavelength of over 99% of the radiations will be so long that the radiation will produce only heat.

The energy of the emitted x-ray photon resulting from deceleration of electrons in the electric field of a nucleus depends on how close the electron passes to the nucleus, the energy of the electron, and the charge of the nucleus. Figure 2–14 is a graph of the distribution, or "continuous spectrum," of the wavelengths of x rays resulting from bombardment of the x-ray tube target by electrons. Notice that there will be well defined minimum wavelength (λ_{min}) of x rays produced; this λ_{min} will, of course, depend on the kVp used. The x-ray beam will also contain all wavelengths of x rays longer than the minimum wavelength. Filters (see Chap. 6) are used to remove the long wavelength low energy x rays from the beam. Therefore, the highest energy x-ray photon leaving the x-ray tube depends on the kVp used; the lowest energy x-ray photon leaving the x-ray tube does not depend on kVp, but is determined by the filter used (or by the absorption of low energy x rays by the envelope of the tube if no filter is used).

To review, **the wavelength of x rays in the continuous spectrum varies. The variation is produced by the different energies with which the electrons reach the target, and by the fact that most electrons give up their energy in stages.** The mini-

mum wavelength x-ray photon is dictated by the x-ray tube voltage (kVp). The maximum wavelength (lowest energy) x rays escaping the tube will depend on the filtering action of the enclosure of the x-ray tube and on any added filtration.

Characteristic Radiation. Characteristic radiation results when the electrons bombarding the target eject electrons from the inner orbits of the target atoms. Removal of an electron from a tungsten atom causes the atom to have an excess positive charge, and the atom thus becomes a positive ion. In the process of returning to its normal state, the ionized atom of tungsten may get rid of excess energy in one of two ways. An additional electron (called an Auger electron) may be expelled by the atom and carry off the excess energy. The ejection of Auger electrons does not produce x rays, and so is not of much interest for this discussion. An alternative way to get rid of excess energy is for the atom to emit radiation that has wavelengths within the x-ray range. A tungsten atom with an inner shell vacancy is much more likely to produce an x ray than to expel an electron. X rays produced in this manner are called characteristic x rays because the wavelengths of the x rays produced are characteristic of the atom that has been ionized. For the purposes of illustration we will discuss ejection of an electron from the K shell of tungsten and then apply the principles to electrons in other shells of the tungsten atom.

The binding energy of an electron in the K shell of tungsten is about 70 keV. Therefore, a cathode electron must have energy of more than 70 keV to eject the K-shell electron from its orbit. A 60-kVp electron beam will not contain any electrons with enough energy to eject a K shell electron from tungsten. After an impinging electron uses a 70 keV of its energy to eject the K-shell electron, the remaining energy is shared between the initial electron and the ejected electron. Both these electrons leave the atom (Fig. 2–15). The ionized tungsten

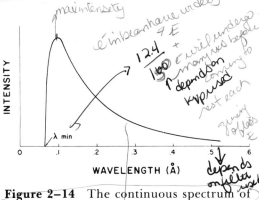

Figure 2–14 The continuous spectrum of x-rays produced by bremsstrahlung

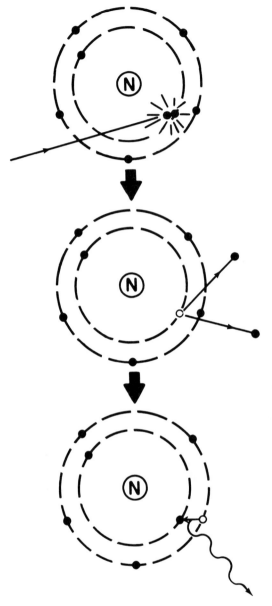

Figure 2–15   The production of characteristic radiation

its excess energy. The energy lost by the L-shell electron is radiated as a single x-ray photon. In tungsten, the energy of this x-ray photon is approximately 59 keV, which is the difference between the binding energy in the K shell (about 70 keV) and that in the L shell (about 11 keV). For tungsten, the energy of this x-ray photon will always be the same, regardless of the energy of the electron that ejected the K-shell electron. Thus, the x-ray photon energy is a "characteristic" of the K shell of a tungsten atom. This process is illustrated in Figure 2–15.

When the L-shell electron moves into the K shell, a vacancy is created. The vacancy may be filled from the M shell, and another x-ray photon will be produced. The energy of the L-characteristic radiation, however, will be much less than that of the K-characteristic radiation. In tungsten, L-characteristic x-ray photons have an energy of about 9 keV (L-shell binding energy is about 11 keV, and that of the M shell about 2 keV). Characteristic radiations will also be generated from transitions involving the outer electron shells of tungsten. The energy of this radiation is small, and ionization in these outer shells produces mostly heat, or x rays that are absorbed by the walls of the x-ray tube.

Figure 2–16 diagrams the energy of the K-characteristic x rays of tungsten, superimposed on the continuous spectrum (bremsstrahlung). There is actually more than one binding energy for each inner shell in the tungsten atom except the K shell, and this causes the appearance of several different energies of characteristic radiation. In Figure 2–16 the α_1 (59.3 keV) and α_2 (57.9 keV) characteristic x rays arise from transition of L-shell electrons to the K shell. The β_1 (67.2 keV) results from an M-shell to K-shell transition, and the β_2 (69 keV) from an N-shell to K-shell transition. The dashed line in Figure 2–16 represents the low energy x rays produced by bremsstrahlung that are removed from the x ray

atom is unstable, and the K-shell electron is rapidly replaced, usually with an electron from the L shell. The replacement electron may, however, come from other shells in the atom. The electron in the L shell has more energy than the K-shell electron, as discussed earlier. In its transition from the L to the K shell, the electron must give up

Figure 2–16   The spectrum of bremsstrahlung and K-characteristic radiation

beam by the enclosure of the x-ray tube and the added filtration.

What contribution does the characteristic radiation make to the total production of x rays by a standard x-ray tube? Below 70 kVp there is no K-shell characteristic radiation. Between 80 and 150 kVp, characteristic radiation (K-shell characteristic) contributes about 10% (80 kVp) to 28% (150 kVp) of the useful x-ray beam. Above 150 kVp the contribution of characteristic radiation decreases, and it becomes negligible above 300 kVp.

Intensity of X-Ray Beams

The intensity of an x-ray beam is defined as the number of photons in the beam multiplied by the energy of each photon. The intensity is commonly measured in roentgens per minute (R/min, or C/kg in the SI system). The intensity of the x-ray beam varies with the kilovoltage, x-ray tube current, target material, and filtration.

Target Material. The target material

used determines how much radiation (the quantity) will be produced by a given applied voltage. (The next section will define the effect of this voltage on the radiation.) **The higher the atomic number of the target atoms, the greater will be the efficiency of the production of x rays.** For example, tungsten (Z = 74) would produce much more bremsstrahlung than tin (Z = 50) if both were used as the target of an x-ray tube and compared at identical tube potential (kVp) and current (mA). Earlier in this chapter we pointed out that tungsten is used as the target material because of its relatively high atomic number (74) and its high melting point (3370° C). Platinum, with a more favorable atomic number of 78, has a melting point of 1770° C, and stable gold (Z = 79) melts at 1063° C. Thus, **for the continuous spectrum, the atomic number of the target material partly determines the quantity of x rays produced.**

The relationship between atomic number and the production of characteristic radiation is quite different. **The atomic number of the target material determines the energy,** or quality, **of characteristic x rays produced.** For example, the K-shell characteristic x rays for tungsten (Z = 74) vary from 57 to 69 keV; those of tin (Z = 50) vary from 25 to 29 keV; and those of lead (Z = 81) have energies between 72 and 88 keV.

Molybdenum Target. With a high atomic number anode like tungsten, the x-ray beam consists almost entirely of bremsstrahlung radiation. The contribution from characteristic radiation varies somewhat with tube voltage, but it never makes up a large percentage of the total beam. With lower atomic number anodes, however, bremsstrahlung production is less efficient. Efficiency also diminishes as the tube voltage is decreased. The combination of a low atomic number anode and low tube voltage reduces the efficiency of bremsstrahlung production to the point at which characteristic radiation assumes greater importance. Molybdenum anode tubes are designed to take advantage of this principle for breast radiography. Maximum tube

voltage for mammography is approximately 40 kVp. At this voltage the 17.5-keV K-alpha and 19.6 keV K-beta characteristic radiation of molybdenum makes up a significant portion of the total radiation output of a molybdenum target x-ray tube. In Chapter 6 we will discuss use of a molybdenum filter to cause the characteristic radiation to make up an even larger fraction of the x-ray beam from a molybdenum tube.

To summarize, the atomic number of the target material determines the quantity (number) of bremsstrahlung produced and determines the quality (energy) of the characteristic radiation.

Voltage (kVp) Applied. We have reviewed how the energy of the photons emitted from the x-ray tube depends on the energy of the electrons in the electron stream that bombards the target of the x-ray tube. The energy of the electrons is, in turn, determined by the peak kilovoltage (kVp) used. Therefore, **the kVp determines the maximum energy** (quality) **of the x rays produced.** In addition, higher kVp techniques will also increase the quan-

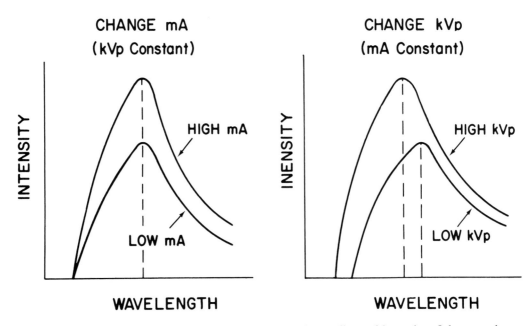

Figure 2–17   The effect of kVp and tube current on the quality and intensity of the x-ray beam

tity of x rays produced. The amount of radiation produced increases as the square of the kilovoltage:

Intensity is proportional to $(kVp)^2$

The wavelength of the characteristic radiation produced by the target is not changed by the kVp used. Of course, the applied kilovoltage must be high enough to excite the characteristic radiation. For example, using a tungsten target, at least 70 kVp must be used to cause the K-characteristic x rays to appear.

X-Ray Tube Current. The number of x rays produced obviously depends on the number of electrons that strike the target of the x-ray tube. The number of electrons depends directly on the tube current (mA) used. The greater the mA the more electrons that are produced; consequently, more x rays will be produced. This principle was reviewed earlier in this chapter.

The effect of x-ray tube potential (kVp) and mA (x-ray tube current) on the wavelength (quality) and intensity of the x-ray beam is illustrated in Figure 2–17.

SUMMARY

X rays are produced by energy conversion when a fast-moving stream of electrons is suddenly decelerated in the target of an x-ray tube. An x-ray tube is a specially designed vacuum diode tube. The target of an x-ray tube is usually tungsten or an alloy of tungsten. Heat production in the x-ray tube is minimized by using the line focus principle and a rotating anode.

X rays are generated by two different processes, resulting in (1) the production of a continuous spectrum of x rays (bremsstrahlung) and (2) characteristic x rays. The quantity (number) of the x rays generated is proportional to the atomic number of the target material (Z), the square of the kilovoltage $[(kVp)^2]$, and the milliamperes of x-ray tube current (mA). The quality (energy) of the x rays generated depends almost entirely on the x-ray tube potential (kVp).

CHAPTER

3 *X-Ray Generators*

An x-ray generator is the device that supplies electric power to the x-ray tube. It is not an electrical generator in the strict sense of the word, because by definition a generator converts mechanical energy into electrical energy. An x-ray generator begins with a source of electrical energy. In the United States, any building will have 115- or 230-V, 60-Hz alternating current available. Most radiology departments will have three-phase power available in the range of 208 to 230 V. The x-ray generator modifies this energy to meet the needs of the x-ray tube. The tube requires electrical energy to meet the needs of the x-ray tube. The tube requires electrical energy for two purposes: to boil electrons from the filament and to accelerate these electrons from the cathode to the anode. The x-ray generator has a circuit for each of these functions, and we will refer to them as the filament and high-voltage circuits. Also, the generator has a timer mechanism, a third circuit, which regulates the length of the x-ray exposure. These three circuits are all interrelated but, to simplify the discussion, we will describe them separately. We will not, however, discuss the overall design of the electric system but will leave the technical problems in the capable hands of the x-ray equipment manufacturer.

The mechanism of an x-ray generator is usually continued in two separate compartments: a control panel or console and a transformer assembly. Control panels may be very simple or quite complex, and any attempt to describe a single panel or console would be of little value. The controls allow the operator to select the appropriate kVp, mA, and exposure time for a particular radiographic examination. Meters measure the actual mA and kVp during the exposure. One exposure button (standby) readies the x-ray tube for exposure by heating the filament and rotating the anode, and the other button starts the exposure. The timing mechanism terminates the exposure.

The second component of the x-ray generator, the transformer assembly, is a grounded metal box filled with oil. It contains a low-voltage transformer for the filament circuit and a high-voltage transformer and a group of rectifiers for the high-voltage circuit. The potential differences in these circuits may be as high as 150,000 V, so the transformers and rectifiers are immersed in oil. The oil serves as an insulator and prevents sparking between the various components. By definition, **a transformer is a device that either increases or decreases the voltage in a circuit. A rectifier changes alternating current into direct current.**

TRANSFORMERS

As mentioned earlier, the x-ray generator receives 115- or 230-V, 60-Hz (cycles per second) alternating current. Filament heating requires a potential difference of approximately 10 V, whereas electron acceleration requires a potential difference that can be varied between 40,000 and 150,000 V. Transformers are used to change the potential difference of the incoming electric energy to the appropriate level.

Before we describe transformers, we

must pause briefly to discuss the meaning of potential and potential difference. Potential is a relative term. For a discussion of electrical circuits, the earth (ground state) is considered to be at zero potential. A point in a circuit with an excess of electrons has a negative potential, while a point with a deficiency of electrons has a positive potential. Both potential and potential difference are measured in volts. If one point has a negative potential of 10 V, and another point has a positive potential of 10 V, the potential difference between them is 20 V, and electrons will tend to flow toward the positive potential. Now suppose one point has a negative potential of 30 V and another point a negative potential of 10 V; the potential difference is still 20 V. Electrons will flow toward the point with a negative potential of 10 V. This flow of electrons represents a current, and is produced by a potential difference. A voltmeter is used to measure the potential difference between two points. The terms "potential difference" and "voltage" are synonymous, and will be used interchangeably.

A transformer consists of two wire coils wrapped around a closed core. The core may be a simple rectangle with the windings wound around opposite sides of the rectangle, such as is shown in Figure 3–1A. The circuit containing the first coil (which is connected to the available electric energy source) is called the **primary circuit,** and the circuit containing the second coil (from which comes the modified electric energy) is called the **secondary circuit.** Other core configurations may be used, and the secondary windings may be wrapped on top of (but insulated from) the primary windings. The core of a transformer is laminated. It is made up of thin sheets of special iron alloys separated from each other by thin insulating layers. These sheets are clamped tightly together. The purpose of the laminations is to reduce eddy currents, which waste power and appear as heat in the transformer core.

Figure 3–1 Current induction by a transformer

When current flows through the primary coil, it creates a magnetic field within the core, and this magnetic field induces a current in the secondary coil. Current only flows through the secondary circuit when the magnetic field is changing (either increasing or decreasing): no secondary current flows while the magnetic field in the core is in a steady state. We can demonstrate this principle with a simple experiment. In Figure 3–1A the primary circuit is connected to a battery and the secondary circuit to a voltmeter. When the switch in the primary circuit is closed, the battery drives current through the primary coil, which creates a magnetic field in the iron core. As the magnetic field increases, it induces a current through the secondary coil. Thus current builds up a potential difference between the two ends of the coil, and the voltmeter needles swings to one side. As soon as the magnetic field stabilizes, the potential across the secondary coil drops to zero and remains there until the switch in the primary coil is opened. When the switch is opened, the magnetic field decreases, and again this changing field induces a potential difference across the secondary coil. The polarity of the potential is reversed, and the voltmeter needle moves in the opposite direction. The voltage across the primary coil is shown in Figure 3–1B, and that across the secondary coil in Figure 3–1C. The important fact to remember is that a **current only flows in the secondary circuit when the magnetic field is increasing or decreasing.** No current flows while the magnetic field is stable. For this reason, steady direct current (like that from a battery) in the primary coil cannot be used to produce a continuous current through the secondary coil.

Alternating current is used for a transformer because it is produced by a potential difference (voltage) that changes continuously in magnitude and periodically in polarity (Fig. 3–2). Current flows in one direction while the voltage is positive and in the opposite direction while the voltage is negative. The most important characteristic of alternating current is that its voltage changes continuously, so it produces a continuously changing magnetic field. Therefore, an alternating current in the primary coil of a transfer produces an alternating current in the secondary coil.

Laws of Transformers

Two simple laws govern the behavior of a transformer.

1. **The voltage in the two circuits is proportional to the number of turns in the two coils.**

$$\frac{N_p}{N_s} = \frac{V_p}{V_s}$$

N_p = number of turns in the primary coil
N_s = number of turns in the secondary coil
V_p = voltage in the primary circuit
V_s = voltage in the secondary circuit

For example, suppose the primary coil has 100 turns and the secondary coil has 30,000 turns. If the potential difference across the primary coil is 100 V, the potential difference across the secondary coil will be

$$\frac{100}{30,000} = \frac{100}{V_s}$$

and

$$V_s = 30,000 \text{ V}$$

A transformer with more turns in the secondary coil than in the primary coil increases the voltage of the secondary circuit and, appropriately, is called a step-up transformer. One with fewer turns in the secondary coil decreases the voltage and is called a step-down transformer.

2. The second law of transformers is simply a restatement of the law of the conservation of energy. A transformer cannot create energy. An increase in voltage must be accompanied by a corresponding decrease in current. The product of the voltage and current in the two circuits must be equal.

$$V_p I_p = V_s I_s$$

V_p = voltage in the primary coil
I_p = current in the primary coil
V_s = voltage in the secondary coil
I_s = current in the secondary coil

In our previous example the voltage across the primary coil was 100 V, and that across the secondary coil 30,000 V. If the current in the primary coil is 30 A, then the current in the secondary coil will be

$$100 \times 30 = 30,000 \, I_s$$
$$I_s = 0.1 \text{ A (100 mA)}$$

Figure 3–2 Alternating current wave form

The product of voltage and current is power. If the potential difference is in volts and the current is in amperes, then power will be in watts:

$$W = V \times I$$
$$W = watts$$
$$V = volts$$
$$I = amperes$$

In the last example the power in the transformer is 3,000 W; it is the same on both the high-voltage (100 V × 30 A) and low-voltage (30,000 V × 0.1 A) sides of the transformer. The wire in the transformer must be large enough to carry the current without overheating. As a result, high-voltage transformers are both large and heavy, which also makes them very expensive.

In summary, a step-up transformer increases the voltage and decreases the current, while a step-down transformer decreases the voltage and increases the current. These laws assume 100% transformer efficiency, which cannot be achieved, but they are sufficiently accurate for our purposes.

There are two basic circuits in a diagnostic x-ray unit. One circuit contains the step-up transformer and supplies the high voltage to the x-ray tube. The other circuit contains a step-down transformer and supplies the power that heats the filament of the x-ray tube. A transformer called the "autotransformer" supplies the primary voltage for both these circuits. We must now discuss, in order:

The autotransformer
The x-ray tube filament circuit
The high-voltage circuit

The Autotransformer

The voltage supplied to the x-ray room connects to the x-ray generator through an autotransformer in most cases (we will discuss an arrangement that does not use an autotransformer when we consider medium-frequency generators). The autotransformer has several functions:

Provides voltage for the x-ray tube filament circuit
Provides voltage for the primary of the high-voltage transformer
Provides suitable voltage for subsidiary circuits, which we will not consider
Provides a convenient location for the kVp meter that indicates the voltage to be applied across the x-ray tube

An autotransformer consists of a **single winding** wound on a laminated closed core (Fig. 3–3). The autotransformer works on the principle of self-induction. An alternating current applied between the input points (A and B, Fig. 3–3) will induce a flow of magnetic flux around the core. This magnetic flux will link with all the turns forming the coil, inducing a voltage into each turn of the winding. For example, if 230 V are applied between points A and B (Fig. 3–3), and the points A and B connect to 115 turns of the autotransformer winding, the volts per turn will be 2. By a suitable selection of taps one may select the number of turns to supply the necessary

Figure 3–3 The autotransformer

voltage to the other components of the x-ray generator. In Figure 3–3, a connection between terminals O and P will tap 115 turns and supply 230 V. There are only 55 turns and 110 V between terminals O and X, while 160 turns provide 320 V. Notice that, within a very limited range, an autotransformer can function as a step-up or step-down transformer.

We will discuss the specific connections from the autotransformer (filament circuit, high tension transformer primary, kVp meter) in the following sections.

Filament Circuit

The filament circuit regulates current flow through the filament of the x-ray tube (Fig. 3–4). The filament is a coiled tungsten wire that emits electrons when it is heated by this current flow (thermionic emission, explained in Chapter 2). Not much power is needed to heat this filament to the necessary high temperature; a current flow of 3 to 5 A with an applied voltage of about 10 V are typical values. This current merely heats the filament, and does not represent the current across the x-ray tube.

The power to heat the x-ray tube filament is provided by a small step-down transformer called the "filament transformer." The filament is connected directly to the secondary winding of this transformer. The primary winding of the filament transformer obtains its voltage by tapping off an appropriate number of turns from the autotransformer (Fig. 3–5). This voltage will be around 100 to 220 V across the primary winding. To reduce this to the desired 10 V range, the step-down

transformer in the filament circuit has approximately 10 to 20 times as many turns of wire in the primary coil as in the secondary coil. The secondary winding of the filament transformer has only a very small voltage across it, and is connected to the filament of the x-ray tube. The x-ray tube, of course, has a very high voltage across it. This makes it necessary to provide high-voltage insulation between the secondary and primary windings of the filament transformer. The filament transformer is usually placed in the same oil-filled grounded metal tank as the high-voltage transformer.

Precise control of filament heating is critical, because a small variation in filament current results in a large variation in x-ray tube current. Remember that x-ray tube current is produced by the flow of electrons from their point of origin (the filament) to the anode (target) of the x-ray tube. A change is filament voltage of about 5% will result in a 20- to 30-% change in x-ray tube current. The x-ray filament current may be controlled by altering the voltage to the primary of the step-down transformer by addition of resistors connected in series in the circuit leading from the autotransformer. The resistors may be a number of separate resistors chosen by a switch or a push button on the control panel, or may be a single variable resistor as shown in Figure 3–4. If resistance is increased, more voltage must be used to push current through the resistance, making less voltage available to the filament transformer primary. For example, a current of 4 A and a resistance of 1.5 ohms (Ω) will reduce voltage by 6 V. This is the application of Ohm's Law, which states:

Volts = Current (amperes) × Resistance (ohms)

Several other components in the filament circuit are used to stabilize the voltage to the filament transformer, including a voltage stabilizer and a frequency stabilizer. There is also a circuit that automatically compensates for the space charge effect.

Figure 3–4 Filament circuit

These stabilizing and compensating circuits could be shown in Figure 3–4 as boxes in the circuit between the autotransformer and the filament transformer, but we choose to refrain from drawing them.

High-Voltage Circuit

A simplified schematic of the high-voltage (cathode-anode) circuit is shown in Figure 3–5. The circuit has two transformers, an autotransformer and a step-up transformer. We have also shown the x-ray tube filament transformer. The autotransformer is actually the kVp selector and is located in the control panel. The voltage across the primary coil of the step-up transformer can be varied by selecting the appropriate number of turns in the autotransformer. Only five selections are shown in Figure 3–5, but actually the kVp can be adjusted in steps from approximately 40 to 150 kVp.

The step-up transformer, which is sometimes called the high-voltage transformer, has many more turns in the secondary coil than in the primary coil, and it increases the voltage by a factor of approximately 600. The potential difference across the secondary coil may be as high as 150,000 V, so the step-up transformer is immersed in oil in the transformer assembly for maximum insulation.

Two meters are incorporated into the high-voltage circuit, one to measure kVp and the other to measure mA. The meters themselves are located on the control panel, but their connections are in the high-voltage circuit, as shown in Figure 3–5. They indicate the potential across the x-ray tube and the actual current flowing through the tube during an x-ray exposure. A voltmeter measures the difference in electrical potential between two points. Electrons moving through the difference in potential constitute an electric current. In a closed circuit, the same number of electrons flows through all points. An ammeter counts the number of electrons flowing past a point per unit time, and it can be placed in the circuit wherever it is most convenient.

The ratio of the voltage across the primary and secondary coils in a transformer is proportional to the number of turns in

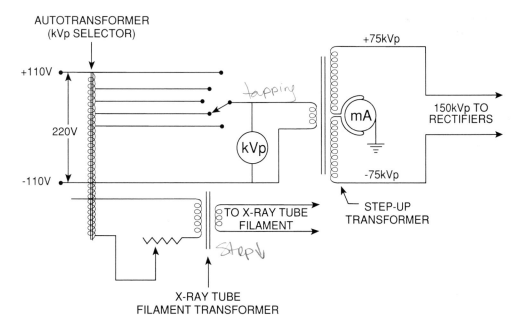

Figure 3–5 High-voltage (cathode-anode) circuit and x-ray tube filament circuit

the two coils. Some voltage is lost in the rectifier circuit, but with the appropriate calibrations the potential difference in the high-voltage side of the circuit (i.e., across the x-ray tube) can be measured indirectly on the low-voltage side of the transformer. Therefore, the kVp meter can be placed in the circuit between the autotransformer and step-up transformer, as shown in Figure 3–5. The voltage which energizes the kVp meter is the voltage from the auto-transformer that will be applied to the primary winding of the high-voltage transformer when the exposure begins. Because the kVp meter records the selected kVp before the actual exposure begins, it is usually termed the "prereading peak kilovolt-meter." The circuit for the prereading kVp meter shown in Figure 3–5 is greatly simplified. The voltage in this circuit is relatively small and the meter can be located on the control panel with a minimum of insulation, and without serious risk of electrical shock.

The connections for the mA meter must be in the secondary coil of the high-voltage transformer to record current flow accurately. Transformers are not 100% efficient, so the current through the primary coil is not an accurate representation of the current in the secondary coil. The mA meter is in a circuit with a potential difference of up to 150 kVp and, to minimize the risk of an electric shock, the connections are made at the point at which the transformer is grounded, which is the center of the coil. With a voltage across the coil of 150 kVp, the potential on one side is +75 kVp and on the other side −75 kVp. The center of the coil is at zero potential and, if the meter is connected at this point, it may be placed on the control panel without risk of shock to the operator. Remember, although the meter is remote from the x-ray tube, it measures the actual current flow across the tube, because the same number of electrons flows through all portions of a closed circuit.

Rectification

Rectification is the process of changing alternating current into direct current, and the device that produces the change is called a **rectifier.** The high-voltage transformer provides an alternating voltage for the x-ray tube. The simplest way to use this high voltage is to hook an x-ray tube directly to the secondary windings of the step-up transformer, with one side of the transformer connected to the cathode (filament) and the other to the anode (target) of the x-ray tube. Such an arrangement is shown in Figure 3–6. When the cathode is negative with respect to the anode, electrons flow at high speed from the cathode to the anode and x rays are produced. During the next half of the electrical cycle the target (anode) of the x-ray tube is negative and the filament positive, so electrons, if they are available, would flow away from the target toward the filament. It would be highly undesirable to have electrons moving from the target to the filament for two reasons: (1) such electrons would not pro-

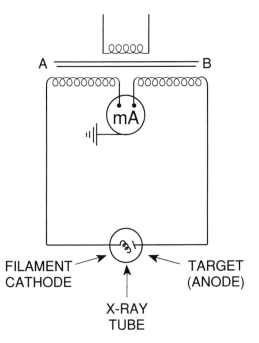

FILAMENT   CATHODE   TARGET (ANODE)

X-RAY TUBE

Figure 3–6   The circuit for self-rectification

duce useful x rays, and (2) such electrons would further heat the filament and reduce its lifetime. By blocking current flows in the inverse half of the electrical cycle, the x-ray tube changes an alternating current into a direct current, so it is, in effect, a rectifier. Because only half of the electrical wave is used to produce x rays, the wave form is called **half-wave rectification.** Figure 3–7A shows the wave form of the incoming electrical supply, Figure 3–7B shows that of half-wave rectification, and Figure 3–7C shows that of full-wave rectification for comparison. Only the upper half of each electrical cycle is used to produce x rays. When the x-ray tube itself serves as a rectifier, the circuit is called "self-rectified."

Self-rectification has two disadvantages. First, half of the available electrical cycle is not utilized to produce x rays, so exposure times must be twice as long as they would be if the whole cycle were utilized. Second, as repeated or prolonged exposures heat the anode, it may become hot enough to emit electrons and to produce a current during the inverse half-cycle. The electrons in this current would bombard the filament and eventually destroy it. Therefore, to protect the x-ray tube and to improve the efficiency of the x-ray production, special rectifiers are incorporated into the high-voltage circuit.

Rectifiers. A rectifier is a device that allows an electrical current to flow in one direction but does not allow current to flow in the other direction. Rectifiers are incorporated into the x-ray circuit in series with the x-ray tube. Exactly the same current flows through the x-ray tube and the rectifiers.

High-voltage rectifiers can be of the vacuum-tube type (often called "thermionic diode tubes") or they can be of solid-state composition. In modern equipment, tubes are no longer used and we will not discuss them. Solid-state rectifiers are smaller, more reliable, and have a longer life. Selenium was the first material used for solid-state rectifiers. In 1965 high-voltage silicon rectifiers were introduced, and today most x-ray generators use silicon rectifiers.

Semiconductor. **The heart of a solid-state rectifier is a semiconductor, which is usually a piece of crystalline silicon.** Silicon contains four valence electrons. In a solid, such as silicon, there are numerous energy levels permissible for electrons. Figure 3–8 diagrams the last-filled and the first-unfilled energy bands for any semiconductor. The valence electrons must lose or gain energy to move from one energy level to another. This sounds like the transitions of K and L electrons that produce characteristic x rays, but in this case energy differences are much smaller and the resulting radiation is either heat or light. Electrons in the

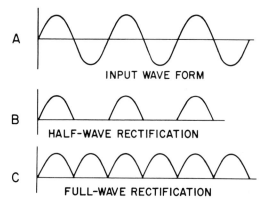

Figure 3–7   Electrical wave forms for full-wave and half-wave rectification

Figure 3–8   Outer electron energy bands in a solid

conduction band (which corresponds to unfilled energy levels) are relatively free from atomic bonding and may move freely through the semiconductor material.

In the picture of an atom that we present there are energies that are not available for electrons to reside in. Obviously, these are the energies between the allowed energy levels. As we bring numerous atoms together to make solid materials, these unallowable energies remain to form what we call the "forbidden energy gap." We can characterize three types of materials by the size of the energy gap. If there is no forbidden region at normal temperature and pressure, the material is called a "conductor." If, the forbidden region is in the order of an electron volt, the material is called a "semiconductor." If the forbidden gap is of the order of 10 eV the material is an insulator. For a semiconductor at absolute zero temperature all the electrons are in the valence band (and all the energy states in that band are filled), and there are no electrons in the conduction band. At absolute zero temperature, the semiconductor behaves as an insulator. At room temperature, some of the electrons are thermally raised to the conduction band and are available to support a current. So the word "semiconductor" describes material that at low temperatures acts like an insulator, but at normal room temperature acts like a conductor. It follows that an insulator will not have electrons in the conduction band at normal temperatures, and a conductor will always have electrons in the conduction band at normal temperatures. This concept is diagrammed in Figure 3–9.

N-type Semiconductors. Silicon contains four valence electrons. If a material with five valence electrons is added as an impurity to the silicon lattice (which means crystal), the added atoms will take the place of some silicon atoms throughout the crystal. Notice that in Figure 3–10 one of the five valence electrons of the impurity is not utilized in the bonding (this is a covalent

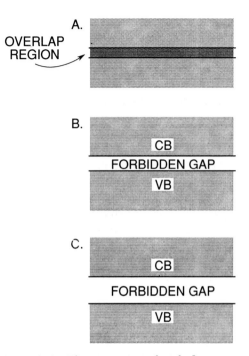

Figure 3–9 Electron energy bands for a conductor (*A*), semiconductor (*B*), and insulator (*C*)

bond) with silicon. This unbound electron can move about in the crystal much easier than one of the bound electrons. The impurity is called a **donor** since it donates an extra electron. The crystal resulting from the addition of the donor is called **N-type,** with N derived from the negative charge of the surplus electron. The most commonly used donor materials are arsenic and antimony, added in tiny amounts of about one atom of impurity for each 10^7

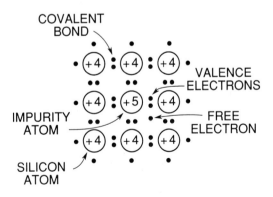

Figure 3–10 N-type silicon semiconductor

atoms of silicon. The donor electrons require only about 0.05 eV of energy to raise them to the conduction band, compared to 1.1 eV for electrons in the valence band of silicon. The .05 eV means this energy level is .05 eV below the bottom of the conduction band, and therefore in the forbidden gap. Energy levels that appear in the gap are called "traps."

P-type Semiconductors. If an impurity with only three valence electrons is added to silicon, the impurity atom will have only three electrons to share with four surrounding silicon atoms. This is diagrammmed in Figure 3–11. One silicon atom now has an electron that is looking for another electron with which to form a covalent bond. The absence of this electron is called a "hole." Since the hole is a positive "particle," as compared to the negative electron, the material is called a **P-type** semiconductor. A hole can migrate through the lattice structure by an electron from a neighboring bond filling the hole, thus leaving a hole at a new site. Note that the hole moves in a direction opposite that of the electron. This new hole may be filled by another electron, and so forth. The P-type traps are about .08 eV above the top of the valence band and in the forbidden region. The only other way to form a hole is to raise an electron from the valence band to the conduction band, requiring 1.1 eV. The P-type impurities used in semiconductors are indium, gallium, and aluminum. The trap level is a function of which impurity is used, but all trap levels have about the same energy. P-type impurities are called **acceptors.**

P-N Junctions. We will discuss a P-N junction as if it were possible to mechanically join the N-type and P-type materials. Actually, a P-N junction can be formed only by a complex process in which the P and N materials are diffused into a single crystal.

When N-type and P-type crystals are joined, a **P-N junction** is created. The N-type material is rich in electrons (solid circles in Fig. 3–12A) and the P-type is rich in holes (open circles in Fig. 3–12A). When the junction is formed, electrons diffuse across the junction, as shown in Figure 3–12B. One might expect diffusion to continue until there was uniform distribution of holes and electrons. This is not the case because an electrostatic barrier is created

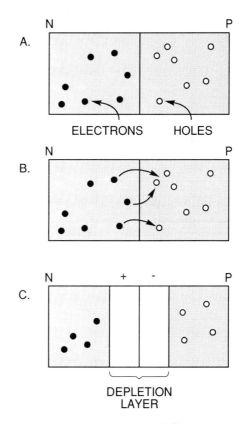

Figure 3–12 The process of forming a PN junction (diode)

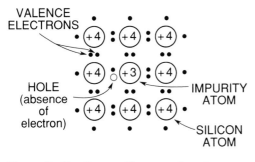

Figure 3–11 P-type silicon semiconductor

that limits diffusion. When electrons leave the N-type material, the junction area is left with a net positive charge. Similarly, the P-type material acquires a negative charge. This creates what is called a "depletion layer." The depletion layer has a junction potential that is opposite in sign to the designation of the materials (i.e., the junction potential is positive on the side of the N-type and negative on the side of the P-type material). This is diagrammed in Figure 3–12C. In silicon, the junction potential is about 0.7 V. The device formed by a P-N junction is called a **diode. Solid-state rectifiers are diodes.**

If a voltage is applied to a diode, current will flow or not flow depending on the polarity. If the polarity of the applied voltage is opposite that of the junction, electrons will flow from the N-type material across the junction barrier to the P-type material and current will flow. This is shown in Figure 3–13, in which the negative pole of a battery is connected to the N-type material and the positive pole to the P-type. This is called **forward bias.** If the polarity of the applied voltage were reversed, with the negative pole of a battery being connected to the P-type material, the junction potential would be augmented and no current would flow. This is called **reverse bias.** Since a P-N diode conducts current in a forward direction only, it meets our definition of a rectifier. Note that holes will move in opposite direction to the electrons under an applied voltage, and since they

Figure 3–14 Symbol for a solid-state rectifier (diode)

are positive they will contribute to the current flow.

Figure 3–14 shows the symbol for a solid-state rectifier. Notice that the arrow points in the direction of current flow, which by convention in physics is opposite to the flow of electrons. This is confusing, but a fact of life when one must deal with physics. Figure 3–15 diagrams a solid-state rectifier and the associated terms and symbols.

Silicon Rectifiers. A single silicon rectifier (called a cell) will resist a reverse voltage of about 1000 V, which is 10 to 20 times higher than a selenium rectifier. Silicon rectifiers can withstand a temperature of up to 392° C, considerably higher than selenium at 266° C. A silicon rectifier is made up of a number of cells, or individual diodes, connected together to form a cylin-

Figure 3–13   Forward bias of a PN diode

Figure 3–15   A solid-state rectifier

drical stack that might have dimensions of 20 to 30 cm long by 20 mm diameter. Such a rectifier can operate up to 150 kVp and 1000 mA. Modern x-ray equipment uses solid state silicon rectifiers.

Half-Wave Rectification. We have already described one form of half-wave rectification, self-rectification by the x-ray tube (see Fig. 3–6). The same wave form is produced by two rectifiers connected in series with the x-ray tube, as shown in Figure 3–16. With the voltage shown in the illustration, electrons flow through the x-ray tube from the cathode to the anode. When the voltage reverses during the inverse half of the alternating cycle, the rectifier stops current flow. When rectifiers are used in this manner they produce half-wave rectification. The only advantage of

Figure 3–17 The circuit for full-wave rectification (two pulses per cycle). Combination of the four diodes is called a diode bridge

the rectifiers is that they protect the x-ray tube from the full potential of the inverse cycle.

Full-Wave Rectification. Modern x-ray generators employ full-wave rectification, which utilizes the full potential of the electrical supply. Figure 3–7C shows the wave form produced by full-wave rectification. Both halves of the alternating voltage are used to produce x rays, so the x-ray output per unit time is twice as large as it is with half-wave rectification.

Figure 3–17 is a schematic presentation of the high-voltage circuit for full-wave rectification. The voltage across the circuit is supplied by the step-up transformer. In Figure 3–17, if side A of the step-up transformer is negative with respect to B, electrons will flow from A through rectifier R1 to the x-ray tube, and return through rectifier R2 to side B (shown as solid lines through the rectifiers). Note that electrons entering the bank of four rectifiers from side A of the transformer cannot flow

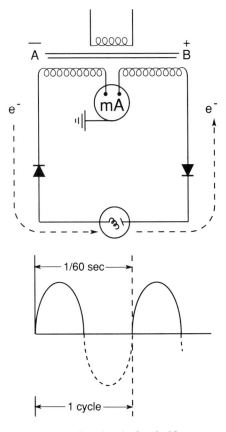

Figure 3–16 The circuit for half-wave rectification (one pulse per cycle)

through rectifier R4 to reach the target of the x-ray tube. This direction of electron flow produces a reverse bias on the rectifier and current cannot flow. In the following half-cycle, side B of the transformer becomes negative, and side A positive. Electrons will now reach the filament of the x-ray tube by flowing from B through rectifier R3 to the filament and return via rectifier R4 to side A of the transformer (shown as dashed lines through the rectifiers). In this manner, the four rectifiers produce a pulsating direct current (unidirectional) through the x-ray tube even though the transformer supplied an alternating input current. The voltage across the tube, however, still fluctuates from zero to its maximum level, and x rays are generated in 120 short bursts each second. Figure 3–18 shows the intensity of the x-ray beam superimposed on the electrical voltage of the x-ray tube during one half-cycle. As you can see, most of the x rays are generated during the central high-voltage portion of the cycle.

The principal disadvantage of pulsed radiation is that a considerable portion of the exposure time is lost while the voltage is in the valley between two pulses. The time spent bombarding the target with low-energy electrons does little except to produce heat in the target and to produce low energy x-rays, which are absorbed in the patient and raise patient dose. This disadvan-

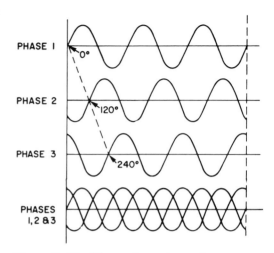

Figure 3–19   Three-phase alternating current wave forms

tage is not shared by three-phase generators, which we will discuss next.

TYPES OF GENERATORS

Three-Phase Generators

Three-phase generators produce an almost constant potential difference across the x-ray tube.

Commercial electric power is usually produced and delivered by three-phase alternating-current generators. It is easier to understand three-phase current if we think of each phase in terms of degrees rather than in terms of time. Figure 3–19 shows all three phases separately and superimposed on one another (bottom). Phase two lags 120° behind phase one, and phase three 120° behind phase two. Thus, a three-phase generator produces an almost constant voltage, because there are no deep valleys between pulses.

Three-phase generators are complex, so we will present only a simplified explanation of three basic types:

> Six pulse, six-rectifier
> Six pulse, twelve-rectifier
> Twelve-pulse

Three-Phase Transformers. A three-phase transformer has three sets of primary and secondary windings. The three

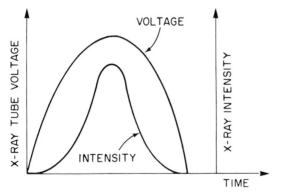

Figure 3–18   X-ray intensity superimposed on the electrical voltage

sections of copper windings in the primary or secondary are connected in one of two configurations, termed **delta** and **wye** (also called **star**). These are diagrammed in Figure 3–20. These diagrammatic representations of the wye and delta windings are not to be interpreted as the physical structure of the devices; the arrangement of the coils is suggested because of the voltage relationships. The physical appearance of a single-phase transformer may look just like a three-phase transformer except for a few more wires hanging out of the latter. If the same three-phase voltage is applied to a wye and a delta, the output voltage of the two are not the same. We find that the output voltage may have the same maximum value, but there is a 30° shift in the phase between the two. This phase shift is critical in the 12-pulse transformer to be discussed shortly. Generally, the primary windings are of the delta configuration, and the secondary more often wye or both.

Six-Pulse, Six Rectifier. This design employs a delta-wound primary transformer with a wye-wound secondary transformer. The output of the secondary windings is rectified with six solid-state rectifiers. Figure 3–21 is a diagram of a six-pulse, six-rectifier generator. The wye winding and the six rectifiers are essentially three full-wave bridges tied together. Figure 3–19 shows the relationship of three-phase out-

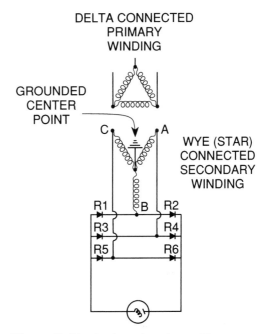

Figure 3–21 A six-pulse six-rectifier transformer

put, and the rectifier arrangement will full-wave rectify each of the voltages presented in this figure. In the drawing of Figure 3–19, there are three maximum and three minimum voltages in one complete cycle (1/60 sec). When rectified, there will be six positive maximum voltages per cycle. Thus the term "six pulse." We will follow voltage through only one set of coils in Figure 3–21 to indicate how full-wave rectification takes place. Suppose A is negative with respect to B. Electrons will then flow from A through rectifier R3 to the filament of the x-ray tube, then to the target of the tube and through rectifier R2 to coil B. During the next half-cycle, B would be negative with respect to A, and electron flow would be from B through R1 through R4 to A. By this method, full-wave rectification of all three phases will produce six pulses per cycle (360 pulses per second). Since the voltage supplied to the x-ray tube never falls to zero, the ripple factor is significantly reduced and has a theoretical value of

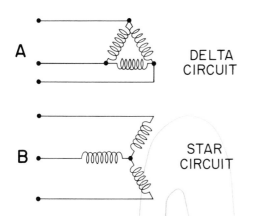

Figure 3–20 *A.* Delta winding. *B.* Wye (or star) winding

13.5%. We must now digress a moment and explain this term **ripple factor.**

The ripple factor is the variation in the voltage across the x-ray tube expressed as a percentage of the maximum value. With a single-phase circuit the ripple factor is 100% because the voltage goes from zero to a maximum value with each cycle (Fig. 3–22). A six-pulse circuit has a ripple factor of 13.5%, which means that at 100 kV the voltage fluctuates between 86.5 and 100 kV. A twelve-pulse circuit has a theoretical ripple factor of 3.5%. When three-phase generators are operated under load, the ripple factor is accentuated. This is known as the **load ripple-factor, and is always greater than the theoretical ripple.** The load ripple-factor of a twelve-pulse, three-phase system is about 5%.

Six-Pulse Twelve-Rectifier. A six pulse, twelve-rectifier transformer is diagrammed in Figure 3–23. This circuit is still a six-pulse circuit with a 13.5% theoretical ripple factor. Notice that this circuit has a fixed potential to ground, an advantage over the six-rectifier circuit. This allows a 150-kV generator to have a transformer that provides a voltage of -75 kV to $+75$ kV to the x-ray tube, simplifying insulating requirements.

Twelve-Pulse. A twelve-pulse transformer looks similar to the six-pulse,

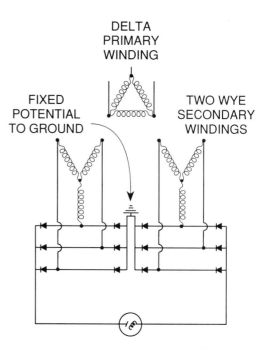

Figure 3–23 A six-pulse twelve-rectifier transformer

twelve-rectifier transformer. The difference is that the secondary is not a double wye connection; it is a wye and a delta connection (Fig. 3–24). This is the reason we previously mentioned the delta and wye types of electrical wiring configuration. When a delta and a wye winding are connected together in the secondary, the output of the delta will lag the wye by 30°. The result of this is that the output of one winding will fill in the ripple of the other, resulting in a twelve-pulse rather than a six-pulse output. The theoretical ripple is now reduced to 3.5%, with a load ripple factor of about 5%. Modern generators are designed on the principle of one-wye and one-delta configuration in the windings of the high-voltage transformer.

Compared to the 100% ripple factor of a single-phase system, three-phase generators produce a nearly constant potential. This nearly constant potential gives three-phase generators a major advantage over single-phase generators that produce a pulsating direct-current potential. Three-

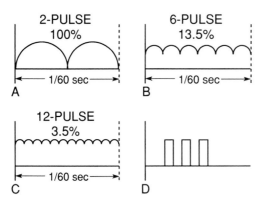

Figure 3–22 The ripple factor in single-phase two-pulse (*A*), three-phase six-pulse (*B*), and three-phase twelve-pulse (*C*) circuits. (*D*) Chopped DC

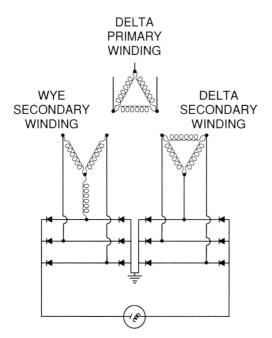

DELTA
PRIMARY
WINDING

WYE
SECONDARY
WINDING

DELTA
SECONDARY
WINDING

Figure 3–24 A twelve-pulse three-phase transformer

phase generators produce x rays efficiently throughout the exposure, and the average x-ray energy is somewhat higher because no time is spent bombarding the x-ray tube target with low-energy electrons.

A second major advantage of three-phase generators is a much higher tube rating for extremely short x-ray exposures. Three-phase generators are now being built to deliver a tube current of up to 2000 mA. They make it possible to produce radiographs with extremely short exposure times and high repetition rates, so they are excellent for angiography.

Power Storage Generators

When mobile radiographic equipment is taken to a patient's room, the available power supply is often inadequate. Power storage generators provide a means of supplying power for the x-ray tube independent of an external power supply. There are two types of power storage generators:
1. Capacitor discharge generators
2. Battery-powered generators

Capacitor-Discharge Generators. A capacitor is an electrical device for storing charge, or electrons. In a capacitor discharge generator, standard 110-V or 220-V power is fed into a step-up transformer. The output of the high-voltage transformer is rectified and used to charge a large capacitor or a bank of capacitors. Once the capacitor is charged, it can be discharged through the x-ray tube. This type of unit uses a grid-controlled x-ray tube to start and stop the x-ray exposure. You will recall from Chapter 2 that a grid-controlled x-ray tube contains its own "switch" (the grid) that allows the tube to be turned on and off. The kV across the x-ray tube is controlled by the kV across the capacitor or capacitors. The kV across the capacitor is controlled by the voltage output of the high-voltage transformer and can be varied by adjusting the kV selector on the autotransformer. Capacitor discharge units typically provide a very high milliamperage (as high as 500 mA) for very short exposure times.

These units are small and easy to move about. Each exposure starts at the same kVp even if line voltage is undependable, since the capacitors are always charged to the same potential. However, the unit has a significant limitation to its mAs output (typically limited to 30 to 50 mAs). When exposure begins, the capacitor begins to discharge, so the kV will fall during the exposure. As a general rule, there will be a drop of about 1 kV for 1 mAs. For example, an exposure of 30 mAs beginning at 90 kV would drop to 60 kV by the end of the exposure. This limits the usefulness of capacitor discharge generators for use in radiography of thick body parts such as the abdomen.

The capacitor discharge unit is not a cordless mobile unit. The capacitor must be charged immediately prior to use. It is not practical to charge the unit in the x-ray department and then take it elsewhere in the hospital for use, because the charge rapidly leaks away from the capacitor. At the end of each exposure the capacitors must be recharged, which in most units is done automatically.

Battery-Powered Generators. In battery-powered generators, a standard power supply is used to charge large capacity nickel-cadmium batteries. The fully-charged unit can then operate completely independent of connection to an outside power supply.

The direct current from the batteries does not supply the x-ray tube directly since high-voltage transformers will not operate on constant DC power. The output from the batteries is fed into a DC chopper, which interrupts the current many times each second; a typical value is 500 times per second. Figure 3–22D illustrates what a chopped DC voltage looks like. This produces a 500-Hz pulsed DC current that is supplied to the primary winding of the high-voltage transformer. The high-voltage output from the secondary of the transformer is then rectified and supplied to the x-ray tube as a 1000-pulse-per-second wave form. The 1000-pulse wave form, theoretically, has 100% ripple. At this frequency (1000), the wave form can be conveniently smoothed by relatively simple circuitry to provide nearly constant potential. (The same could be done for 120-pulse voltage, but the circuitry would be very bulky.)

A battery-powered portable unit is heavy and requires regular battery maintenance. The batteries can be recharged from any convenient power supply, with full charging requiring about 12 hours. The advantages of the battery-powered unit are its ability to (1) store considerable energy to generate x rays and (2) to make exposures independent of a power supply. A typical unit can store 10,000 mAs. Unlike a capacitor-discharge unit, the battery unit supplies a constant output of kV and mA throughout the exposure.

Medium-Frequency Generators

A new type of generator, called a "medium-frequency generator," uses the principle of high-frequency current to produce an almost constant potential voltage to the x-ray tube with a transformer of small size.

The basic principle involved is this: **in a transformer, the voltage induced in the secondary coil is proportional to the rate of change of current in the primary coil.** (Induced voltage is proportional to the time rate of change of magnetic flux. This is a statement of Faraday's Law.) Thus far, we have considered generators in which the rate of change of current in the primary coil was determined by 60-Hz power supply except for the 500 HZ of the battery-powered generator. A medium-frequency generator converts the 60-Hz power-line frequency to up to 6500 Hz before it is fed to the primary coil of the transformer.

Let us first consider an overview of a medium-frequency generator (Fig. 3–25). The incoming power supply is standard 60-Hz current. The current is rectified and smoothed. This direct current is then fed to a device, often called a chopper, which converts the smoothed DC into a chopped DC with a frequency of about 6500 Hz. (Look at Fig. 3–22D to see what we mean by chopped DC.) This 6500-Hz chopped DC supplies the primary of a step-up transformer, which steps up the voltage. The high-voltage 6500-Hz output of the transformer is rectified to produce 13,000 high-voltage pulses per second, and then smoothed by filters before being applied to the x-ray tube. This provides voltage to the x-ray tube that is nearly ripple-free.

One advantage of the medium-frequency generator is not apparent: it supplies a constant, nearly ripple-free voltage to the x-ray tube regardless of the input power. No special power supply or voltage regulators are required. Another advantage is the very small size of these generators. You may find it hard to believe that a 30-kW or 50-kW (we will explain kW ratings of generators later in this chapter) generator can be contained in a single unit with about the same dimensions and weight

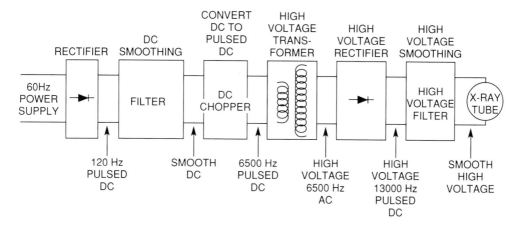

Figure 3–25 Block diagram of a medium-frequency generator

as a regular x-ray tube housing. We must explain why increasing the frequency of voltage input to the primary of a step-up transformer allows the transformer to be made smaller. First, remember that the output is determined by the rate of change of flux, and is proportional to the frequency, the number of windings in the secondary, and the cross-sectional area of the core.

$$V \sim fnA$$

V = output voltage
f = frequency
n = number of windings
A = core cross-sectional area

For a given transformer, we can maintain a constant output voltage by increasing the frequency and decreasing the number of turns or the core cross-sectional area. (This statement illustrates the point, but it is not true that one could indiscriminately increase the output of any transformer by increasing input frequency. Complex design changes are required.) The result of all this is that both the iron core and amount of wire can be reduced to make a smaller transformer. For larger generators (80 kW and 100 kW) the high-voltage transformer is not contained in the tube head, but is still reduced to about one-third the size of a conventional twelve-pulse transformer.

In summary, medium-frequency gener-

ators provide a nearly constant voltage to the x-ray tube that is not dependent on the power supply. Operation at a high frequency results in a more efficient transformer that can be made much smaller than conventional transformers. This small size is especially convenient for portable units.

TRANSFORMER RATING

The rating of a transformer states the maximum safe output of its secondary winding. If the rating is exceeded, the transformer may overheat and burn out its insulation and windings. The rating is expressed as the maximum safe output of its secondary winding in **kilowatts.** Remember that a watt is the unit of electric (as well as mechanical) power, with a kilowatt obviously being a thousand watts.

For three-phase generators, kilowatt (power) ratings are calculated according to the following formula (recall that kV × mA = watt):

$$kW = \frac{kV \times mA}{1000}$$

kW = kilowatts
kV = kilovolts
mA = milliamperes

Thus, the ratings of a three-phase generator operating at 100 kV and 500 mA is

$$\frac{100 \times 500}{1000} = 50 \text{ kW}$$

This would then be termed a 50-kW generator.

For single-phase generators the formula is modified:

$$kW = \frac{kV \times mA \times 0.7}{1000}$$

The factor 0.7 comes from the fact that in single-phase generators the voltage varies from zero to some peak value. To figure the average power we must consider the average voltage (this is usually called the root mean square, or R.M.S., voltage). In single-phase circuits, this relationship is:

$$R.M.S. = \frac{peak}{\sqrt{2}} = 0.707 \text{ peak}$$

So, the formula for single-phase-generator power rating converts the kV to R.M.S. voltage by using the factor $\frac{1}{\sqrt{2}}$, or about 0.7. Since the transformer is driving an x-ray tube, we can consider the current to be fairly constant, so an average value is not needed for current.

In most three-phase circuits, R.M.S. voltage is about 0.95 peak, which is close enough to 1 that it can be ignored. This slight difference actually serves as a safety factor.

Kilowatt ratings of x-ray generators are determined when the generator is under load, and it is convenient to test at a voltage level of **100 kVp,** because calculations are simplified. Thus, an 80-kW constant potential generator would be one that could operate at 100 kV and 800 milliamperes (mA). Be careful! Some constant potential generators are rated at 150 kVp, and are called 150-kV generators. The same generator may have the capability of producing 1000 mA. It is wrong to think of this as a 150-kW generator unless it can operate at 150 kVp and 1000 mA simultaneously. A generator might be able to operate at:

150 kVp and 500 mA (75 kW)
100 kVp and 800 mA (80 kW)
80 kVp and 1000 mA (80 kW)

This hypothetical generator has an 80-kW rating (as determined at 100 kV). The kW loading a generator can accept may vary considerably with different kV and mA settings. When comparing generators, one may find the comparison of kW ratings useful. But one must also inquire about the available kW output at the kV and mA levels at which the generators will generally be used. This is especially important when considering a unit for use at high-kV techniques.

EXPOSURE SWITCHING

A switch is the device that turns the high voltage applied to the x-ray tube on and off. Switching presents design engineers with interesting problems. These problems arise from switching off the currents in the circuits very rapidly and removing all the energy that is stored in the voltage-smoothing networks. If the current is turned off improperly, high-voltage spikes may be introduced that can damage the equipment. If the voltages in the smoothing circuits are not removed, the voltage across the x-ray tube cannot go to zero. Switching circuits, then, must solve both of these problems, but how they do this need be of little concern to the radiologist.

There are two categories of switching for modern generators. Switching may take place in the primary circuit of the high-voltage transformer where there are high currents and low voltage. Switching may also take place in the secondary circuit where there are low currents and high voltage. In most general purpose three-phase units, switching occurs in the primary circuit and is called **primary switching.** Switching in the secondary circuit is generally used in units designed for rapid, repetitive exposures or where extremely short exposure times are needed, and is called **secondary switching.**

Primary Switching

There are three types of primary switches: electromechanical contractors, thyratrons, and solid-state silicon-controlled rectifiers. Electromechanical switches and thyratrons are being phased out.

Silicon-Controlled Rectifiers. The primary switching found in most modern generators uses solid-state semiconductors called **silicon-controlled rectifiers (SCRs)** or **thyristers.** SCRs may be thought of as solid-state thyratrons. Other control rectifiers may come into common use, but we will talk only about the SCR. A control rectifier is a rectifier that can be turned on and off by a logic signal (which in reality is just a small voltage pulse).

Figure 3–26 is a schematic of an SCR; its symbol is also shown. This thyristor consists of a cathode (negative end), an anode (positive end), a gate, and three junctions. Notice that this is similar to a series of diodes in that there are NP and PN junctions. If the cathode is made negative and the anode positive, current can flow through the two NP junctions (they are forward biased), but no current can flow through the one PN junction (it is reversed biased). Remember, electrons in a diode will flow freely from N-type material to P-type material, but will not flow freely from P to N material. If a small positive voltage (about 1 V) is applied to the gate, the reverse bias at the PN junction will be overcome and electrons will flow through the thyristor. This is the way a thyristor functions: a small positive pulse (the logic signal) to the gate causes a large current to flow through the thyrister. The response of the gate is almost instantaneous, making the thyristor useful when very fast switching is necessary. Notice that a thyristor is also a rectifier (this is the "R" part of the SCR). Electrons will not flow from anode to cathode because there are two PN junctions that prevent electron flow. We will leave the way SCRs are put into circuits to the engineers.

Secondary Switching

Secondary switching takes place on the high voltage side of the transformer or at the x-ray tube itself. Remember that switches in the high-voltage circuit must prevent high-voltage breakdown, so they must be insulated to withstand high voltage. Two types of secondary switching are used today:

Triode vacuum tubes
Grid-controlled x-ray tubes

It is currently possible, but not yet practical, to replace triode vacuum tubes by stacking rectifying devices in a manner similar to silicon-controlled rectifiers. Grid-controlled x-ray tubes are described in Chapter 2. As with the SCR, we choose not to discuss the way triode tubes are designed into the circuit.

Primary Versus Secondary Switching

While the technical details of switching need not bother us, it will be of some value to consider the appropriate practical uses or advantages of primary versus secondary switching. We define "practical" to include cost and availability in today's technology.

Primary Switching. Almost all general purpose generators use primary switching. In today's technology and pricing mechanisms, it is easier and cheaper to put switching into the primary circuit. Primary switching can produce exposures as short as 1 or 2 milliseconds (ms), but it cannot produce these exposures at a high repetitive rate as well as secondary switching can.

Secondary Switching. Secondary switching is used in special-purpose generators, such as those needed for angiography and

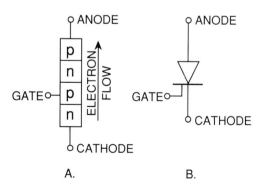

Figure 3–26 An SCR, or thyristor, shown schematically (*A*) and as its symbol (*B*)

cinefluorography. This technology makes it easier, compared to primary switching, to have sharp, crisp exposures with rapid on-and-off rates with many repeated exposures. Triode tubes will allow exposures as short as 0.5 ms at an exposure rate of up to 80 per second and a power output of up to 150 kW. The main application of grid-controlled x-ray tubes is in cinefluorography with maximum mA of about 400 to 600 mA. Exposure rates as high as 500 per second are possible. Grid controlled x-ray tubes are generally not appropriate for the high-milliampere loading required for angiography using regular rapid filming techniques.

In the final analysis, few physicists and no radiologists care how the switching is done so long as it meets the specifications of the generator.

FALLING LOAD GENERATORS

The purpose of a falling load generator is to produce an x-ray exposure in the shortest possible exposure time by operating the x-ray tube at its maximum kilowatt rating during the entire exposure. Note that falling-load generators are not used to give very short exposure times; they give shorter exposure times than would be obtained with a fixed-tube mA technique.

Let us go directly to an example to explain how this generator functions. Look at Figure 3–27, the theoretical chart for an x-ray tube operating at 70 kVp. If an exposure of 70 kVp and 200 mAs is desired, this x-ray tube could be operated at 70 kVp, 200 mA, and 1.0 sec (200 mAs) to produce such an exposure. Notice that any attempt to get a shorter exposure would fail, because the tube is limited to 0.5 sec at 300 mA (150 mAs), 0.3 sec at 400 mA (120 mAs), etc. Thus, we must accept an exposure time of at least 1.0 sec to get 200 mAs.

Now let us examine how the falling load principle allows us to use the higher mA settings to obtain 200 mAs in a shorter time

Figure 3–27   Theoretic x-ray tube rating chart at 70 kVp

(shown by the shaded areas in Fig. 3–28). The operator does not set an exposure time, but tells the generator to produce 200 mAs at 70 kVp. The exposure will begin at 600 mA, the highest mA available in this example, then will drop the tube current to 500 mA when the 70-kVp line crosses the 600-mA line. Corresponding reductions of tube current will occur at 400 and 300 mA until the required 200 mAs has been accumulated. In our hypothetical situation, the 200 mAs will be composed of

600 mA	×	.05 sec	=	30 mAs
500 mA	×	.15 sec	=	75 mAs
400 mA	×	.10 sec	=	40 mAs
300 mA	×	.20 sec	=	60 mAs
Total		0.50 sec		205 mAs

By operating the x-ray tube at its maximum tolerance, the falling load generator has

Figure 3–28   Principle of the falling load generator

produced 200 mAs in 0.5 sec, as opposed to 1.0 sec for a fixed mA technique.

There are some problems with the falling load principle. Operating the tube at high mA causes maximum focal spot blooming. Heating the anode to its maximum capacity with each exposure shortens x-ray tube life. Manufacturers generally set the tube to operate at somewhat lower than maximum loading.

One additional consideration must be mentioned. When mA is lowered, there is an automatic rise in kV if some form of kV compensation is not used. Modern falling load generators provide an almost constant kV.

Falling load generators are expensive. They find their greatest use with automatic exposure generators where simple operator controls are desired.

EXPOSURE TIMERS

A variety of ways to control the length of an x-ray exposure have been developed. We will mention these briefly, and consider only phototimers in any detail.

There are four basic types of exposure timers:
1. Mechanical timers (rarely used today)
2. Electronic timers
3. Automatic exposure control (phototimers)
4. Pulse-counting timers

Electronic Timers

Electronic timers all work on the same principle. The length of the x-ray exposure is determined by the time required to charge a capacitor through a selected resistance. The exposure button starts the exposure and also starts charging the capacitor. The exposure is terminated when the capacitor is charged to a value necessary to turn on associated electronic circuits. The exposure time is therefore determined by the length of time for the capacitor to charge, and this time can be varied by varying the value of the resistance in the charging circuit. We leave the exact details of these structures to the engineers.

Automatic Exposure Control (Phototimer)

Mechanical and electronic timers are subject to human error. The operator selects the exposure time that he believes will produce a film of the desired density. He can measure the patient's thickness, but must estimate the density of the tissues that will be included in the radiographic field. If his estimate is incorrect, the resulting radiograph will be improperly exposed. Automatic exposure controls, also called phototimers, have been developed to eliminate human error. They measure the amount of radiation required to produce the correct exposure for a radiographic examination. It is first necessary to select a kilovoltage that will produce satisfactory penetration of the part to be examined. Once the kVp is selected, either the technologist or a phototimer must select the mAs that will produce a proper exposure. The goal is to produce a satisfactory radiograph with each attempt, and to reproduce this radiograph reliably each time another examination is required.

The essential element in phototimers is a device that can detect radiation and, in response to this radiation, produce a small electric current. There are three such devices:
1. Photomultiplier detectors
2. Ionization chambers
3. Solid-state detectors

Phototimers can be located in front of the cassette, and are called **entrance** types, or behind the cassette as **exit** types.

Photomultiplier Phototimers. This is the most common type of automatic exposure control (Fig. 3–29). The detector is made of lucite, which is a material that can transmit light. The lucite is coated with one or more (commonly three) areas of a phosphor that will emit light when irradiated with x rays (these lucite detectors are usually called lucite paddles). Each phosphor

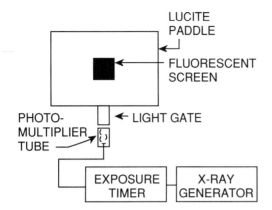

Figure 3–29 Photomultiplier automatic exposure control (phototimer)

area is about 100 square centimeters (100 cm²) in size. When a phosphor generates light, the intensity of the light is obviously proportional to the intensity of x rays that reached the phosphor. The lucite transmits this light to an output region called a "light gate." The light gate directs the light to the photocathode of a photomultiplier tube, where the light is converted to an electric current that is amplified to produce an electrical signal. The electric current generated by the photomultiplier tube may be used to charge a capacitor. When the capacitor reaches a predetermined charge it can be used to bias the gate of a thyrister in the x-ray circuit and cause the exposure to terminate. Photomultiplier phototimers may be used as entrance or exit types. The lucite paddle is almost completely radiolucent, so it will not produce a detectable image if placed in front of a cassette. The lucite serves two functions: it is the support that holds the fluorescent screen or screens, and it transmits light to the photomultiplier tube so that the photomultiplier tube may be kept out of the x-ray field (the photomultiplier tube would produce an image on the radiograph).

Photomultiplier phototimer response is a function of kVp because low energy photons are absorbed more readily in the phosphor. This presents a problem. At lower peak kilovoltage (about 60 kVp) the phos-

phor absorbs a higher percentage of the x-ray beam than it does at higher kVp. This may cause the phototimer to terminate a low kVp exposure before the film has been adequately exposed. This problem is usually handled automatically. Sensors detect the kVp being used, and the phototimer detector will be decreased in sensitivity if low kVp is being used.

A photomultiplier tube is a vacuum tube. It consists of a photocathode, several intermediate electrodes (called "dynodes"), and an anode. When light strikes the photoemissive layer on the photocathode, the photoemissive material emits photoelectrons in numbers proportional to the intensity of the light. The intermediate electrodes are coated with a material that emits secondary electrons when struck by another electron. The electrons are accelerated by a positive potential from one dynode to the next, with each dynode giving rise to more electrons. Photomultiplier tubes come in many sizes and shapes, and are used extensively in nuclear medicine and physics laboratories. The final number of electrons collected at the anode represents the output current, and this output current is proportional to the intensity of the light that struck the photocathode. Inherent in the operation of a photomultiplier tube is the requirement for a stable high-voltage supply. There is some instability in photomultiplier tubes.

Ionization Chamber Autotimers. Ionization chambers are almost always used as entrance-type autotimers. An ionization chamber is very slightly imaged on film, but the image is so faint it is lost in the images of anatomic parts.

Ionization chambers come in many shapes and sizes; the one we describe is used in automatic timers. An ionization chamber consists of two thin parallel sheets of aluminum or lead foil. Gas (usually room air) is present between the plates. The gas becomes ionized when struck by radiation, and ionization is in direct proportion to the amount of radiation. Prior to exposure a charge is placed on the parallel plates by applying a voltage across them. This is exactly like charging a capacitor. In fact, the structure we have described is a parallel plate capacitor. When the gas is ionized by radiation, the negative ion (electron) moves toward the positive plate and the positive ion (ionized gas atom) moves toward the negative plate. When the ions arrive at the plates they neutralize part of the charge that has been placed on the plates. This reduction in charge reduces the residual voltage across the plates. When the voltage has been reduced to a previously determined value, an electronic circuit is activated that will terminate the exposure.

Solid-State Autotimers. Solid-state devices are becoming more common in automatic timers. A variety of solid-state radiation detectors are on the market today that operate on the basis of radiation-producing ionization in or near a PN structure. Other devices work on the basis of photoconductivity and could also be used. Our mention of these two types is an indication of how fluid solid-state technology is. We are told by our equipment engineer that at the present time most solid-state autotimers use PN junction techniques. Solid-state devices offer the advantage of small size, almost no x-ray beam absorption, and a consistent, rapid response. An informal poll of several of our local equipment suppliers indicated that photomultiplier tubes and ionization chambers are still in the majority at this time.

Miscellaneous Autotimer Topics

Use of automatic timer devices requires attention to a number of details; we will use this section to discuss some of these.

The number, size, and position of the radiation detector(s) is important. There may be one, two, or three detectors; the three-field automatic timer is most popular. A single detector positioned in the center of the film is commonly used in fluoroscopic spot film devices. Three-field devices have three detectors, usually with the same areas (e.g., 50 cm²) but with different shapes. For example, a chest unit might have a rectangular-shaped detector in its center (in the region of the mediastinum) and two more laterally placed square detectors. The technologist can choose to use one, two, or all three detectors. Use of the central field may permit a good view of the thoracic spine but overexpose the lung fields. The lateral detectors will serve the lung fields well unless one lung happens to be opaque. Obviously, correct alignment of body parts and detector fields is important. In addition, collimation is important because scatter radiation reaching a detector may cause premature termination of an exposure.

When phototimers are used it is essential that the phototimer be adjusted for the film, intensifying screen, and cassette being used. Any variation in film or screen speed or cassette absorption will result in a change in film density. The Department of Health and Human Services requires that a phototimer show variation of no more than 10% from exposure to exposure.

Automatic timers have density control buttons that can increase or decrease the sensitivity of the detectors.

Automatic timers are equipped with a backup timer that will act as a safety factor to terminate an exposure in case of equipment failure. The Department of Health and Human Services regulations state that the generator must automatically terminate an exposure at 600 mAs for 50 kV or greater, and at 2000 mAs for kV under 50.

Pulse-Counting Timers

A technique used extensively in measuring time is to measure the occurrence of a periodic event. For example, a most accurate clock, the atomic clock, counts the very stable frequency of atomic oscillation. In the electronic world, timing is accomplished by counting pulses of a regular periodic voltage. In fact, the periodic pulse train is called the clock. When it is necessary to time exposures of a few milliseconds, a convenient way to measure such a time would be to count voltage pulses of high frequency. Obviously, the higher the frequency, the more pulses that are counted for a given exposure period. The higher frequency has a tendency to reduce the error in the time period.

Pulse-counting timers use this technique of voltage pulse counting to control the time of short exposure techniques. High frequencies can be generated by the oscillation in a quartz crystal whose frequency of oscillation is determined by the size, orientation of the cut of the crystal, and the mode of oscillation (technical details that we will not investigate further; we will, however, discuss piezoelectric oscillation in Chapter 20 on ultrasound). With a quartz crystal it is quite easy to obtain megahertz frequencies that are extremely stable. As an example, assume the crystal oscillates at 1,000,000 Hz. A 10-ms time could be measured by counting 10,000 pulses. The large number of pulses accounts for the accuracy, because a small error of plus or minus a few pulses will make no significant difference in exposure time.

SUMMARY

An x-ray generator supplies electrical energy to the x-ray tube and regulates the length of the radiographic exposure. The x-ray tube requires two sources of energy, one to heat the filament and the other to accelerate electrons between the cathode and anode. The filament circuit contains a variable resistance, which is the current selector, and a step-down transformer. The cathode-anode circuit, called the high-voltage circuit, contains an autotransformer and a step-up transformer. The autotransformer serves as the kVp selector.

The incoming electrical supply to the x-ray generator has an alternating potential. Rectifiers are devices (usually silicon diodes) that transmit a current in only one direction. Single-phase generators may have half-wave rectification (60 pulses per second). Three-phase generators may be six-pulse (360 pulses per second) with a theoretical ripple factor of 13.5%, or twelve-pulse (720 pulses per second) with a ripple factor of 3.5%. Special types of generators include capacitor-discharge generators, battery-powered generators, medium-frequency generators, and falling load generators.

Transformers are given a rating that indicates the maximum safe output of the secondary windings. Such ratings are expressed as the kilowatt rating.

Exposure switching may be primary switching or secondary switching. Almost all general purpose generators use primary switching. Secondary switching requires use of triode vacuum tubes or grid-controlled x-ray tubes, and is used for fast, repetitive exposures.

Exposure timers include mechanical timers (obsolete), electronic timers, automatic exposure controls (phototimers), and pulse-counting timers. Automatic exposure control may be achieved with photomultiplier detectors, ionization chambers, or solid-state detectors.

4 *Basic Interactions Between X Rays and Matter*

Atoms are bonded into molecules by electrons in the outermost shell. X-ray photons may interact either with orbital electrons or with the nucleus of atoms. In the diagnostic energy range, the interactions are always with orbital electrons. If these electrons happen to be the ones bonding atoms into molecules, the bonds may be disrupted and the molecular structure altered. The molecular bonding energies, however, are too small to influence the type and number of interactions. A group of oxygen atoms will stop the same number of x-ray photons, regardless of their physical state. It does not matter if the oxygen is free as a gas or is bound to hydrogen as water. The important factor is the atomic makeup of a tissue and not its molecular structure.

There are five basic ways that an x-ray photon can interact with matter. These are:
1. Coherent scattering
2. Photoelectric effect
3. Compton scattering
4. Pair production
5. Photodisintegration

As we discuss each of these interactions, you will see that at times x-ray photons are **absorbed,** while at other times they are merely **scattered.** When photons are absorbed, they are completely removed from the x-ray beam and cease to exist. When

photons are scattered they are deflected into a random course, and no longer carry useful information. Because their direction is random, they cannot portray an image, and the only thing they produce on a film is blackness. In the language of the information transfer theorist, scatter radiation adds **noise** to the system. You can gain some insight into the effect of noise with a simple analogy. Imagine yourself listening to music on your car radio as you drive past an airport. As a plane approaches the music becomes more difficult to hear until finally, when the plane is directly overhead, it becomes completely inaudible. Even though the music is still there, you cannot hear it. Radiation noise does exactly the same sort of thing. It destroys image quality. We refer to the noise created by scatter radiation as "film fog." When an x-ray film is badly fogged, the image may be completely obscured. It is still there, but we cannot see it. An understanding of the production of scatter radiation is of vital importance, so pay particular attention to it as we discuss the basic interactions between x rays and matter.

COHERENT SCATTERING

The name "coherent scattering" is given to those interactions in which radiation undergoes a change in direction without a change in wavelength. For this reason, the term "unmodified scattering" is sometimes used. There are two types of coherent scattering, Thomson scattering and Rayleigh scattering. In Thomson scattering a single electron is involved in the interaction. Rayleigh scattering results from a cooperative interaction with all the electrons of an atom. Both types of coherent scattering may be described in terms of a wave-particle interaction, and are therefore sometimes called "classical scattering." Rayleigh scattering is shown in Figure 4–1. Low-energy radiation encounters the electrons of an atom and sets them into vibration at the frequency of the radiation. A vibrating electron, because it is a charged particle, emits radiation. The process may be envisioned as the absorption of radiation, vibration of the atom, and emission of radiation as the atom returns to its undisturbed state. This is the only type of interaction between x rays and matter that does not cause ionization. To produce an ion pair, a photon must transfer energy to the atom. No energy is transferred, and no ionization occurs with coherent scattering. Its only effect is to change the direction of the incident radiation. The percentage of radiation that undergoes coherent scatter-

ing is small compared to that of the other basic interactions; in general, it is less than 5%. Some coherent scattering occurs throughout the diagnostic energy range, but it never plays a major role. Even though it produces scattered radiation, which contributes to film fog, the total quantity is too small to be important in diagnostic radiology.

PHOTOELECTRIC EFFECT

Before beginning a discussion of the photoelectric effect, we are going to digress a moment to review a few points about atomic physics. Atomic structure is extremely complex, but we can greatly simplify it and still have a fairly good idea of how these interactions occur. The atom consists of a central nucleus and orbital electrons. The nucleus is important in our present discussion only as a means of keeping the electrons in the atom. The positively charged nucleus holds the negatively charged electrons in specific orbits, or shells. The innermost shell is called the K shell, and the more peripheral shells are named consecutively L, M, N, and so forth. These shells have a limited electron capacity. The K-shell can hold only two electrons. If more electrons are present in the atom they must move out to the L shell, which has a capacity of eight electrons. Each shell has a specific binding energy. The closer the shell is to the nucleus, the tighter the electrons in that shell are bound to the nucleus. The electrons in the outermost shell are loosely bound. They are essentially free and, appropriately, are called "free electrons." The energy value of electronic shells is also determined by the atomic number of the atom. K-shell electrons are more tightly bound in elements with high atomic numbers than they are in elements with low atomic numbers. In fact, the differences are sizable. For example, the K-shell binding energy for lead is 88 keV, while the K-shell binding energy for calcium is only 4 keV. Electrons in the K shell are at a lower energy level than electrons

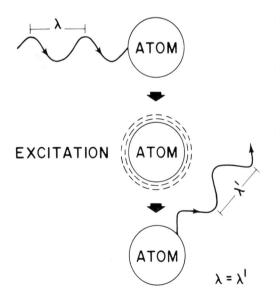

Figure 4–1   Coherent Rayleigh scattering

in the L shell. If we consider the outermost electrons as free, than inner shell electrons are all in energy debt. Their energy debt is greatest when they are close to the nucleus in an element with a high atomic number.

The photoelectric effect is shown in Figure 4–2. We will quickly run through the whole interaction and then fill in some details later. An incident photon, with a little more energy than the binding energy of a K-shell electron, encounters one of these electrons and ejects it from its orbit. The photon disappears, giving up all its energy to the electron. Most of the photon's energy is needed to overcome the binding energy of the electron, and the excess gives the electron kinetic energy. The electron, which is now free of its energy debt, flies off into space as a photoelectron. It becomes a negative ion and is absorbed almost immediately, because charged particles have little penetrating power. The atom is left with an electron void on the K shell but only for an instant, because an electron immediately drops into the void to fill the K shell. This electron usually comes from the adjacent L shell, occasionally from the M shell and, on rare occasions, from free electrons from the same, or another, atom. As an electron drops into the K shell it gives up energy in the form of an x-ray photon. The amount of energy is characteristic of each element, and the radiation produced by the movement of electrons within an atom is called "characteristic radiation." When the K-shell void is filled by an outer shell electron from the same atom, the atom is left with a deficiency of one electron, and it remains a positive ion. If a free electron from another atom fills the void, then the other atom becomes a positive ion, and the result is the same. The photoelectric effect always yields three end products: (1) characteristic radiation; (2) a negative ion (the photoelectron); and (3) a positive ion (an atom deficient one electron).

Probability of Occurrence

Three simple rules govern the probability of a photoelectric reaction.

1. **The incident photon must have sufficient energy to overcome the binding energy of the electron.** For example, the K-shell electrons of iodine have a binding energy of 33.2 keV. An x-ray photon with an energy of 33.0 keV absolutely cannot eject them from their shell. The photon may interact at the L or M shells but not at the K shell.

2. **A photoelectric reaction is most likely to occur when the photon energy and electron binding energy are nearly the same,** provided of course that the photon's energy is greater. A 34-keV photon is much more likely to react with a K-shell electron of iodine than a 100-keV photon. In fact, the probability of a photoelectric reaction drops precipitously as photon energy increases. It is inversely proportional

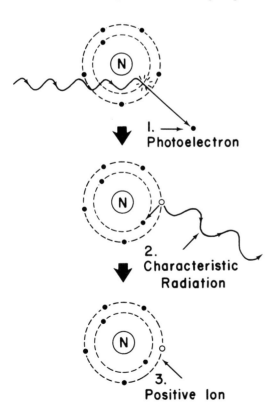

Figure 4–2 Photoelectric effect

to approximately the third power of energy, or, expressed in mathematical form:

$$\text{Photoelectric effect} \sim \frac{1}{(\text{energy})^3}$$

3. The tighter an electron is bound in its orbit, the more likely it is to be involved in a photoelectric reaction. Electrons are more tightly bound in elements with high atomic numbers than in elements with low atomic numbers, as shown in Table 4–1. Most interactions occur at the K shell in elements with low atomic numbers, because the K shell contains the most tightly bound electrons. In elements with high atomic numbers, however, the energy of the incident photons is frequently insufficient to eject a K-shell electron, and many photoelectric reactions take place at the L- and M-shell levels. Because elements with high atomic numbers bind their electrons more tightly, they are more likely to undergo photoelectric reactions. The probability of the photoelectric effect increases sharply as the atomic number increases. In fact, it is roughly proportional to the third power of the atomic number:

$$\text{Photoelectric effect} \sim (\text{atomic number})^3$$

In summary, photoelectric reactions are most likely to occur with low energy photons and elements with high atomic numbers provided the photons have sufficient energy to overcome the forces binding the electrons in their shells. In fact, the photoelectric effect cannot take place with a "free" (not bound to an atom) electron. If you like, you may call this a "forbidden" interaction.

Characteristic Radiation

We first mentioned characteristic radiation when we discussed the production of x rays in Chapter 2. Characteristic radiation generated by the photoelectric effect is exactly the same. The only difference is in the method used to eject the inner shell electron. In an x-ray tube a high-speed electron ejects the bound electron, while in a photoelectric interaction an x-ray photon does the trick. In both cases the atom is left with an excess of energy equal to the binding energy of the ejected electron. All physical systems seek the lowest possible energy state. For example, water always runs downhill. An atom with an electron deficiency in the K shell is in a higher energy state than an atom with an L-shell electron deficiency. The atom releases this excess energy in the form of photons. Usually an electron from an adjacent shell drops into an inner shell void, as shown for an iodine atom in Figure 4–3. The K-shell binding energy for iodine is 33.2 keV, while the L-shell binding energy is 4.9 keV, and more peripheral shells have even lower binding energies. When an electron from an L shell falls to the K shell, a 28.3-keV (33.2 − 4.9 = 28.3) photon is released. The void in the L shell is then filled with a photon from the M shell with the production of a 4.3-

Table 4–1. K-Shell Electron Binding Energies of Elements Important in Diagnostic Radiology

ATOMIC NUMBER	ATOM	K-SHELL BINDING ENERGY (keV)
6	Carbon	0.284
7	Nitrogen	0.400
8	Oxygen	0.532
13	Aluminum	1.56
20	Calcium	4.04
50	Tin	29.2
53	Iodine	33.2
56	Barium	37.4
74	Tungsten	69.5
82	Lead	88.0

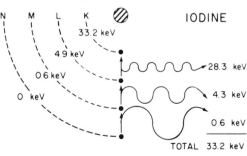

Figure 4–3 Characteristic radiation from iodine

keV photon. This process is continued until the whole 33.2 keV of energy has been converted into photons. Of course, the lower energy photons are of no importance in diagnostic radiology, because they are absorbed immediately. Occasionally an inner shell void is filled by an electron from distant peripheral shells, or even by free electrons. When a free electron moves into the K-shell void in iodine, a single photon of 33.2 keV is generated. This is the most energetic characteristic radiation that iodine can produce.

The K-shell binding energies of some elements important in diagnostic radiology are shown in Table 4–1. Calcium, which has the highest atomic number of any element found in the body in significant quantity, emits a 4-keV maximal energy characteristic photon, which is little energy by x-ray standards. It is absorbed within a few millimeters of its site of origin. The contrast agents iodine and barium are the only elements encountered in diagnostic radiology that emit characteristic radiation energetic enough to leave the patient and fog an x-ray film.

Characteristic radiation is usually referred to as "secondary radiation" to differentiate it from scatter radiation, a distinction that hardly seems necessary because the end result is the same for both, a photon that is deflected from its original path.

Applications to Diagnostic Radiology

As diagnostic radiologists we can look at the photoelectric effect in two ways, one good and the other bad. Starting with the good, it produces radiographic images of excellent quality. The quality is good for two reasons: first, the photoelectric effect does not produce scatter radiation and second, it enhances natural tissue contrast. X-ray image contrast depends on some tissues absorbing more x rays than other tissues. Contrast is greatest when the difference in absorption between adjacent tissues is large. Because the number of reactions depends on the third power of the atomic number, the photoelectric effect magnifies the difference in tissues composed of different elements, such as bone and soft tissue. So, from the point of view of film quality, the photoelectric effect is desirable. From the point of view of patient exposure, though, it is undesirable. Patients receive more radiation from photoelectric reactions than from any other type of interaction. All the energy of the incident photon is absorbed by the patient in a photoelectric reaction. Only part of the incident photon's energy is absorbed in a Compton reaction, as you will see in the next section. Because one of our primary goals is to keep patient doses at a minimum, we must keep this point in mind at all times. The importance of the photoelectric effect can be minimized by using high-energy (kVp) techniques. In general, we should use radiation of the highest energy consistent with that of diagnostic quality x-ray films to minimize patient exposure.

In summary, the likelihood of a photoelectric interaction depends on two factors: the energy of the radiation and the atomic number of the absorber. The reaction is most common with low energy photons and absorbers with high atomic numbers. Photons usually strike tightly bound K-shell electrons, and they must have more energy than the electron binding energy. Photoelectric reactions are desirable from the point of view of film quality, because they give excellent contrast without generating significant scatter radiation. Unfortunately, patient exposures are much higher than with any other type of interaction.

COMPTON SCATTERING

Almost all the scatter radiation that we encounter in diagnostic radiology comes from Compton scattering. Figure 4–4 diagrams this reaction. An incident photon with relatively high energy strikes a free outer shell electron, ejecting it from its orbit. The photon is deflected by the electron

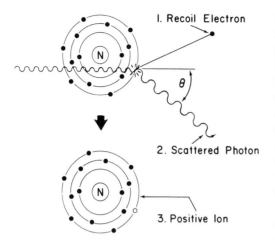

Figure 4–4   Compton scattering

so that it travels in a new direction as scatter radiation. The photon always retains part of its original energy. The reaction produces an ion pair, a positive atom and a negative electron, which is called a "recoil" electron.

The energy of the incident photon is distributed in two ways. Part of it goes to the recoil electron as kinetic energy, and the rest is retained by the deflected photon. Unlike a photoelectric reaction in which most of a photon's energy is expended freeing the photoelectron from its bond, in a Compton reaction no energy is needed for this purpose, because the recoil electron is already free. The incident photon always retains some of its original energy. Two factors determine the amount of energy the photon retains: its initial energy and its angle of deflection off the recoil electron. If you think of the Compton reaction as a collision between two billiard balls, the energy transfer is easier to understand. The cue ball is the incident photon, and the second ball is a free electron. When the cue ball strikes the second ball, they both deflect in a predictable manner. With a glancing blow the angle of deflection of the cue ball is small, and only a small quantity of energy is transferred to the second ball. The cue ball retains almost all its initial energy. With a more direct hit the

cue ball deflects at a greater angle and loses more energy. Finally, with a direct hit, maximal energy is transferred to the second ball but, unlike the cue ball in billiards, a Compton photon never gives up all its energy. The photon retains some energy and deflects back along its original path at an angle of 180°. Figure 4–5 shows the amount of energy a 75-keV photon retains as it is deflected through various angles. As you can see, more energy is lost with larger angles of deflection.

To make our comparison between a Compton reaction and billiard balls complete, we must make one last adjustment in the analogy. Billiard balls all have the same mass, but we want to compare them with photons whose energies vary. We can keep our analogy going by using cue balls of different masses. Thus, a lightweight cue ball simulates a low energy photon, and a heavy cue ball simulates a high energy photon. Now, imagine both the lightweight and the heavy cue balls striking a second ball a glancing blow at an angle of 45°. The lightweight ball has little momentum, and it will deflect at a much greater angle than the heavy ball, which has more momentum. Photons also have momentum, and the higher the energy of the photons, the more difficult they are to deflect. With x-ray energies of 1 MeV (million electron volts), most scattered photons deflect in a forward direction. In the diagnostic energy range, however, the distribution is more symmet-

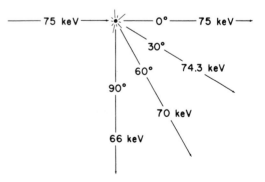

Figure 4–5   Energy of Compton-scattered photons

ric. Figure 4–6 shows the pattern of distribution of scattered photons from a 100-keV x-ray beam. The distance from the point of the interaction is used to express the percentage of scattered photons at various angles. Remember, this is a flat representation of events that are occurring in three dimensions. You can picture the three-dimensional distribution by rotating the pattern around its longitudinal axis. With lower energy radiation, fewer photons scatter forward and more scatter back at an angle of 180°. This distribution is fairly constant throughout the diagnostic energy range.

The classic formula for calculating the change in wavelength of a scattered photon is

$$\Delta\lambda = 0.024 (1 - \cos\theta)$$

$\Delta\lambda$ = change in wavelength (Å)
θ = angle of photon deflection

Most of us think in terms of kiloelectron volts and not wavelength. We can change wavelength from the above formula to kilovoltage energy with the following conversion factor:

$$keV = \frac{12.4}{\lambda}$$

λ = wavelength (Å)
keV = energy of photon

The amount of energy retained by scattered photons after a Compton reaction is shown in Table 4–2. In the diagnostic energy range up to 150 keV, the photon retains most of its original energy, and very little is transferred to the recoil electron.

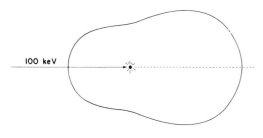

Figure 4–6 Distribution of Compton-scattered photons

Table 4–2. Energy of Compton-Scattered Photons for Various Angles of Deflection

ENERGY OF INCIDENT PHOTON (keV)	ENERGY OF SCATTERED PHOTONS (keV)			
	PHOTON DEFLECTION ANGLE			
	30°	60°	90°	180°
25	24.9	24.4	24	23
50	49.6	47.8	46	42
75	74.3	70	66	58
100	98.5	91	84	72
150	146	131	116	95

At narrow angles of deflection, scattered photons retain almost all their original energy. This creates a serious problem in diagnostic radiology, because photons that are scattered at narrow angles have an excellent chance of reaching an x-ray film and producing fog. They are exceedingly difficult to remove from the x-ray beam. In fact, they cannot be removed by filters because they are too energetic, and they cannot be removed by grids because their angle of deflection is too small. Because we have no way of removing them from the useful beam, we must accept them and tolerate an image of diminished quality.

Scatter radiation from Compton reactions is also a major safety hazard. As you can see in Table 4–2, even after a photon has been deflected 90°, it still retains most of its original energy. This means that the scatter radiation that arises in the patient during a fluoroscopic examination is almost as energetic as the primary beam. It creates a real safety hazard for the fluoroscopist and other personnel who must be in exposure rooms.

Probability of Occurrence

The probability of a Compton reaction depends on the total number of electrons in an absorber, which in turn depends on its density and the number of electrons per gram. In Chapter 5 we will show that all elements contain approximately the same number of electrons per gram, regardless of their atomic number. Therefore, the number of Compton reactions is independent of the atomic number of the absorber. The likelihood of a reaction, however, does depend on the energy of the radiation and the density of the absorber. The number of reactions gradually diminishes as photon energy increases, so that a high energy photon is more likely to pass through the body than a low energy photon.

Because Compton reactions occur with free electrons, we must define this term a little more precisely. An electron can be considered free when its binding energy is a great deal less than the energy of the incident photon. With the photon energies used in diagnostic radiology (10 to 150 keV), only the outer shell electrons are free in the elements with high atomic numbers. For the elements with low atomic numbers, those found in soft tissues, all electrons can be considered free, because even those on the K shell are bound with an energy of less than 1 keV.

PAIR PRODUCTION AND PHOTODISINTEGRATION

The last two basic interactions, pair production and photodisintegration, do not occur in the diagnostic energy range. They have no importance in diagnostic radiology, and we will only discuss them briefly. In pair production, a high energy photon interacts with the nucleus of an atom, the photon disappears, and its energy is converted into matter in the form of two particles. One is an ordinary electron and the other is a positron, a particle with the same mass as an electron but with a positive charge. Because the mass of one electron is equal to 0.51 MeV, and pair production produces two electron masses, the interaction cannot take place with photon energies less than 1.02 MeV.

In photodisintegration, part of the nucleus of an atom is ejected by a high energy photon. The ejected portion may be a neutron, a proton, an alpha particle, or a cluster of particles. The photon must have sufficient energy to overcome nuclear binding energies of the order of 7 to 15 MeV.

Because pair production does not occur with photon energies less than 1.02 MeV, and photodisintegration does not occur with energies less than 7 MeV, neither of these interactions is of any importance in diagnostic radiology, where we rarely use energies above 150 keV.

RELATIVE FREQUENCY OF BASIC INTERACTIONS

Figure 4–7 shows the percentage of each type of interaction for water, compact bone, and sodium iodide, with photon energies ranging from 20 to 100 keV. The total number of reactions is always 100%. The contribution of each interaction is represented by an area in the illustration. Thus, if coherent scattering accounts for 5% of the interactions, Compton scattering for 20%, and the photoelectric effect for 75%, the total is 100%. Water is used to illustrate the behavior of tissues with low atomic numbers, such as air, fat, and muscle. The total number of reactions is less for air than for water, but the percentage of each type is approximately the same. Compact bone contains a large amount of calcium, and it represents elements with intermediate atomic numbers. Iodine and barium are the elements with the highest atomic numbers that we encounter in diagnostic radiology, and they are represented by sodium iodide.

As you can see in Figure 4–7, coherent scattering usually contributes around 5% to the total, and plays a minor role throughout the diagnostic energy range. In water, Compton scattering is the dominant interaction, except at very low photon energies (20 to 30 keV). The contrast agents, because of their high atomic numbers, are involved almost exclusively in photoelectric reactions. Bone is intermediate between water and the contrast agents. At low energies, photoelectric reactions are more common, while at high energies, Compton scattering is dominant.

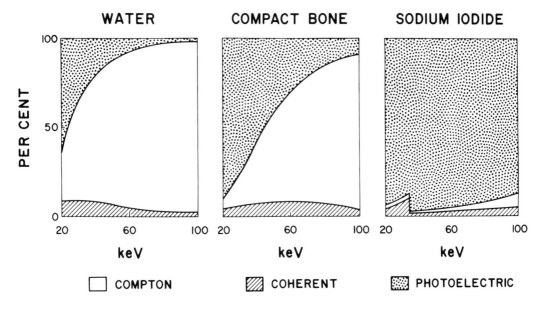

Figure 4–7 Percentage of coherent, photoelectric, and Compton reactions in water, compact bone, and sodium iodide

SUMMARY

Only two interactions are important in diagnostic radiology, the photoelectric effect and Compton scattering. Coherent scattering is numerically unimportant, and pair production and photodisintegration occur at energies above the useful energy range. The photoelectric effect is the predominant interaction with low energy radiation and with high atomic number absorbers. It generates no significant scatter radiation and produces high contrast in the x-ray image but, unfortunately, exposes the patient to a great deal of radiation. At higher diagnostic energies, Compton scattering is the most common interaction between x rays and body tissues, and is responsible for almost all scatter radiation. Radiographic image contrast is less with Compton reactions than with the photoelectric effect.

5 *Attenuation*

Quantity and quality are two terms used to express the characteristics of an x-ray beam. Quantity refers to the number of photons in the beam, and quality refers to their energies. The intensity of a beam is the product of the number and energy of the photons, so it depends on both quantity and quality. A beam of 50-keV photons has a greater intensity than a beam made up of a comparable number of 20-keV photons. **Attenuation is the reduction in the intensity of an x-ray beam as it traverses matter by either the absorption or deflection of photons from the beam.** Because it is a measure of a change in x-ray intensity, attenuation depends on both the quantity and quality of the photons in a beam. For our purpose, it would be simpler to think of attenuation only in terms of quantity. Then a reduction in intensity would merely be a reduction in the number of photons in the beam. We can do this if we limit our discussion to the attenuation of monochromatic radiation. Later in the text, we will clarify why quality does not change with monochromatic radiation. To further simplify our discussion, we will disregard the attenuation of secondary radiation resulting from coherent or Compton scattering and the characteristic radiation of the photoelectric effect. Once a photon has undergone any of these reactions, it will be considered completely attenuated—that is, totally removed from the beam.

MONOCHROMATIC RADIATION

The attenuation of a beam of monochromatic radiation is shown schematically in Figure 5–1. A beam of 1000 photons is directed at a water phantom. The intensity of the beam is decreased to 800 photons by the first centimeter of water, which is an attenuation of 20%. The second centimeter of water decreases the intensity to 640 photons, which is 20% less than had passed through the first centimeter. With each succeeding centimeter of water, 20% of the remaining photons are removed from the beam.

The quality of monochromatic radiation does not change as it passes through an absorber. Remember, we are only discussing primary photons, the photons that, at most, have only one interaction. If we begin with a group of photons with an energy of 60 keV, then the transmitted photons will all have the same energy. Their numbers will be reduced, but their quality will not be changed. So, when we talk about a change in the intensity of a monochromatic beam, we are really talking about a change

Figure 5–1 Attenuation of monochromatic radiation

in the number, or quantity, of photons in the beam. A 50% reduction in the number of photons is a 50% reduction in the intensity of the beam. The attenuation of polychromatic radiation is much more complicated, and we will not discuss it until the end of the chapter.

When the number of transmitted photons and absorber thickness are plotted on linear graph paper, a curved line results (Fig. 5–2A). The initial portion of the curve is steep, because more photons are removed from the beam by the first few centimeters of absorber. After the beam has passed through many centimeters of water, only a few photons remain. Although each centimeter continues to remove 20% of the photons, the total numbers are small, and the end of the curve is almost flat. The same numbers plot a straight line on semilogarithmic graph paper (Fig. 5–2B). When the number of photons remaining in the beam decreases by the same per-

centage with each increment of absorber, as with monochromatic radiation, the attenuation is called exponential. Exponential functions plot a straight line on semilogarithmic graph paper.

ATTENUATION COEFFICIENTS

An attenuation coefficient is a measure of the quantity of radiation attenuated by a given thickness of an absorber. The name of the coefficient is determined by the units used to measure the thickness of the absorber. Four attenuation coefficients are described in classic texts on radiologic physics but only two are important in diagnostic radiology, the linear and mass attenuation coefficients.

Linear Attenuation Coefficient

The linear attenuation coefficient is the most important coefficient for diagnostic radiology. It is a quantitative measurement of attenuation per centimeter of absorber,

Figure 5–2 Attenuation of monochromatic radiation plotted on linear (*A*) and semilogarithmic graph paper (*B*).

so it tells us how much attenuation we can expect from a certain thickness of tissue. Because we measure our patients in centimeters, it is a practical and useful attenuation coefficient. In the next section, after we have discussed the mass attenuation coefficient, you will understand why the linear coefficient is more useful. Its symbol is the Greek letter μ.

The unit of the linear attenuation coefficient is per centimeter, and thus the name **linear** attenuation coefficient, because a centimeter is a linear measurement. The expression per cm is the same as 1/cm, and is usually written cm^{-1}.

It is important to realize that **the linear attenuation coefficient (μ) is for monochromatic radiation,** and that it is specific both for the energy of the x-ray beam and for the type of absorber. Water, fat, bone, and air all have different linear attenuation coefficients, and the size of the coefficient changes as the energy of the x-ray beam changes. When the energy of the radiation is increased the number of x rays that are attenuated decreases, and so does the linear attenuation coefficient.

The mathematics involved in the derivation of the exponential equation for x-ray attenuation is beyond the scope of this book. The formula is

$$N = N_0 e^{-\mu x}$$

N = number of transmitted photons
N_0 = number of incident photons
e = base of natural logarithm
μ = linear attenuation coefficient
x = absorber thickness (in centimeters)

This is a classic equation, and it has the same format as the equation for the decay of radionuclides. In fact, most people find it easier to think in terms of radionuclide decay, so we will digress for a moment. Radionuclides decay at an exponential rate. This rate is usually measured and defined in terms of half-life, which is the time that it takes a material to decay to one half its original activity. For example, ^{131}I has a half-life ($T_{1/2}$) of 8.04 days. If we started

with 100 units of activity, at the end of 8.04 days we would have 50 units, and at the end of another 8.04 days we would only have 25 units. The equation for this exponential decay is

$$N = N_0 e^{-\lambda t}$$

N = activity of remaining radionuclide
N_0 = activity of original radionuclide
e = base of natural logarithm (2.718)
λ = decay constant (seconds $^{-1}$)
t = time (seconds).

The decay constant (λ) can be easily related to half-life ($T_{1/2}$), which is a more familiar concept. After the elapsed time of one half-life ($T_{1/2}$), the quantity of remaining activity is $N_0/2$. The exponential decay equation can be rewritten as

$$\frac{N_0}{2} = N_0 e^{-\lambda T_{1/2}}$$

Dividing both sides by N_0, the equation becomes

$$\frac{1}{2} = e^{-\lambda T_{1/2}}$$

We would then go to a table of exponential values and find the value of the exponent $\lambda T_{1/2}$, which makes $e^{-\lambda T_{1/2}}$ equal to $\frac{1}{2}$ or, more simply, we could just look up the logarithm of $\frac{1}{2}$ in a table of natural logarithms. We would find this value to be -0.693. We can now rewrite the exponential decay equation:

$$\lambda \cdot T_{1/2} = 0.693 \text{ or } \lambda = \frac{0.693}{T_{1/2}}$$

The decay constant (λ) for any radionuclide can be calculated if we know its half-life. For example, the decay constant for ^{131}I ($T_{1/2} = 8.04$ days) is

$$\lambda = \frac{0.693}{8.04 \text{ days}} = 0.086/\text{day}$$

The attenuation of monochromatic radiation is exactly the same. All we need do is substitute thickness (cm of absorber) for time (seconds). The names are changed, but the concept remains the same. The decay constant (λ) becomes the linear attenuation coefficient (μ), and half-life ($T_{1/2}$) becomes the half-value layer (HVL). The product of the linear attenuation coefficient and half-value layer is equal to 0.693:

$$\mu \times HVL = 0.693, \text{ or } HVL = \frac{0.693}{\mu}$$

The half-value layer is the absorber thickness required to reduce the intensity of the original beam by one half. It is a common method for expressing the quality of an x-ray beam. A beam with a high half-value layer is a more penetrating beam than one with a low half-value layer.

If the values from the attenuation of the x-ray beam in Figure 5–1 are used in the exponential attenuation equation, the linear attenuation coefficient can be calculated as

$$N = N_0 e^{-\mu x}$$

where N is 800 photons transmitted, N_0 is 1000 initial photons, and x is 1 cm of water.

$$800 = 1000 \, e^{-\mu(1)} = \frac{1000}{e^{\mu}}$$

$$e^{\mu} = \frac{1000}{800} = 1.25$$

$$\mu = 0.22/cm$$

The last step in the calculation requires a table of exponential values, or natural logarithms, or a calculator. After we have determined the linear attenuation coefficient, the half-value layer of the beam can be calculated as

$$HVL = \frac{0.693}{\mu} = \frac{0.693}{0.22} = 3.15 \text{ cm}$$

You can see from Figure 5–1 that the beam is reduced to one half its original intensity in the fourth 1-cm block of water, which confirms our calculations.

Calculating a linear attenuation coefficient is not of much practical value to a diagnostic radiologist, but the equation can be used for other purposes. There are tables available that list the linear attenuation coefficients for substances such as water, bone, sodium iodide, and most of the elements.[1] With the linear attenuation coefficient from these tables, we can calculate the percentage of transmitted photons for a whole variety of photon energies and for whatever thickness of tissue we may choose.

Mass Attenuation Coefficient

Another useful attenuation coefficient that is basic in the physics literature is the mass attenuation coefficient used to quantitate the attenuation of materials independent of their physical state. For example, water, ice, and water vapor, the three physical states of H_2O, all have the same mass attenuation coefficient. It is obtained by dividing the linear attenuation coefficient by the density (ρ), and has the symbol μ/ρ. The unit for the x-ray absorber is grams per square centimeter (g/cm^2), which contains a mass unit, and thus the name **mass** attenuation coefficient. Figure 5–3 illustrates the meaning of a gram per square centimeter by comparing aluminum and water. The density of water is 1 g/cm^3, so a square centimeter of water must be 1 cm thick to weigh 1 g. The density of aluminum is 2.7 g/cm^3, so a square centimeter of aluminum only has to be 0.37 cm thick to weigh 1 g. The arithmetic is simple. The thickness is merely the reciprocal of the density, or 1 divided by the density. A square centimeter of water 1 cm thick and a square centimeter of aluminum 0.37 cm thick both contain 1 g/cm^2.

The unit of the mass attenuation coefficient is per g/cm^2. It can be expressed in several ways: per g/cm^2 or $1/g/cm^2$ or cm^2/g; usually it is written cm^2/g.

A brief review should help to avoid confusion about units. When we talk about either the linear or mass attenuation coefficient, there are two separate units for each, one for the absorber and the other for the coefficient. The units for the absorber are cm for the linear attenuation coefficient and g/cm^2 for the mass attenuation coefficient. The units for the coefficients themselves are cm^{-1} for the linear and cm^2/g for

WATER   ALUMINUM

Density = 1 g/cm³   Density = 2.7 g/cm³

| Thickness of 1 g/cm² |
| $\dfrac{1\ \text{g/cm}^2}{1\ \text{g/cm}^3} = 1\ \text{cm}$ |

| Thickness of 1 g/cm² |
| $\dfrac{1\ \text{g/cm}^2}{2.7\ \text{g/cm}^3} = 0.37\ \text{cm}$ |

Figure 5–3   Thickness of 1 g/cm² of water and of aluminum

the mass attenuation coefficient. The unit of the coefficient is the reciprocal of the unit of the absorber.

A simple way to understand the relationship between the linear and mass attenuation coefficients is to compare the coefficients for water, ice, and water vapor (Fig. 5–4). The values in the illustration are for a 50-keV monochromatic beam. The linear attenuation coefficient for water is 0.214 cm⁻¹, and a 1-cm thickness of water absorbs 20% of the incidence beam. The same thickness of ice absorbs 18.5%, because ice is a little less dense than water. Water vapor has very little density, and a 1-cm thickness absorbs almost nothing. Density has a profound effect on x-ray attenuation at all energy levels.

The mass attenuation coefficient for water in Figure 5–4 is 0.214 cm²/g, which is the same as the linear attenuation coefficient. They must be the same, because the density of water is 1 g/cm³, and the mass attenuation coefficient is obtained by dividing the linear attenuation coefficient by the density (μ/ρ). The mass attenuation coefficient is the same for water, ice, and water vapor, which is logical because 1 g of all

three has exactly the same amount of mass. The thickness of 1 g/cm² of water is 1 cm, ice 1.09 cm, and water vapor 1670 cm. These thicknesses will all attenuate the same amount of x ray (i.e., 20%) because they all contain the same amount of mass. As you can see in Figure 5–4, the mass attenuation coefficient is independent of the density of the absorber. The coefficients for water, ice, and water vapor are all the same, but their densities vary considerably.

To say that a gram of water and a gram of water vapor both absorb the same amount of radiation is true, but the statement has no meaning to a diagnostic radiologist. In fact, it is misleading. We just do not deal with g/cm² of patient. We measure a patient's thickness in centimeters, and 1 cm of water absorbs a great deal more x ray than 1 cm of water vapor. When the effect of density is removed from the value of an attenuation coefficient, it is misleading in diagnostic radiology.

FACTORS AFFECTING ATTENUATION

Four factors determine the degree of attenuation of an x-ray beam as it passes

50 keV		Density (gm/cm^3)	Thickness of 1 gm/cm^2
Linear Attenuation Coefficient (cm^{-1})	Mass Attenuation Coefficient (cm^2/gm)		
0.214	0.214	1	WATER 1 cm
0.196	0.214	0.917	ICE 1.09 cm
0.000128	0.214	0.000598	WATER VAPOR 1670 cm

Figure 5–4 Comparison of linear and mass attenuation coefficients for water, ice, and water vapor

through matter. One involves the nature of the radiation, and three involve the composition of the matter:

RADIATION	MATTER
Energy	Density
	Atomic number
	Electrons per gram

Increasing the radiation energy increases the number of transmitted photons (and decreases attenuation), while increasing the density, atomic number, or electrons per gram of the absorber decreases the number of transmitted photons (and increases attenuation).

Relationships Between Density, Atomic Number, and Electrons per Gram

We will examine each of the four factors that affect attenuation separately, but first

we must digress to review the relationships between density (ρ), atomic number (Z), and electrons per gram (e/g).

Density and Atomic Number. The relationship between density and atomic number is complex, and no simple rule covers all situations. In general, elements with high atomic numbers are denser than elements with low atomic numbers, but there are exceptions. Gold and lead provide a good example:

	ATOMIC NUMBER	DENSITY (g/cm^3)
Gold	79	19.3
Lead	82	11.0

There is no relationship between atomic number and density when different physical states of matter are considered. Water has an effective atomic number of 7.4 regardless of its state (ice, liquid, or vapor), but its density is different in each of these three forms.

Density and Electrons per Gram. Whenever a factor is expressed in the units per gram, the concept of volume is eliminated. Because density depends on volume (weight per unit volume), there is no relationship between density and electrons per gram. A gram of water has the same number of electrons, regardless of whether they are compressed together in a 1-cm cube as a liquid, or spread out over 1670 cm³ as a vapor.

Atomic Number and Electrons per Gram. The number of electrons per gram is really a function of the number of neutrons in the atom. If the elements did not have neutrons, all materials would have 6.0 × 10²³ e/g. Table 5–1 shows the relationships between atomic number and electrons per gram for various substances important in diagnostic radiology. Hydrogen, which has no neutrons, has 6.0 × 10²³ e/g, which is twice as many as any other element. The elements found in soft tissue—carbon, nitrogen, and oxygen—all have 3.0 × 10²³ e/g, and the higher atomic elements have even fewer e/g. In general, elements with low atomic numbers have more electrons per gram than those with high atomic numbers.

Effects of Energy and Atomic Number

Energy and atomic number, in combination, determine the percentage of each type of basic interaction, so in this sense their effects on attenuation are insepara-

Table 5–1. Electrons Per Gram for Several Elements Important in Diagnostic Radiology

ELEMENTS	ATOMIC NUMBER	NUMBER OF ELECTRONS PER GRAM
Hydrogen	1	6.00 × 10²³
Oxygen	8	3.01 × 10²³
Calcium	20	3.00 × 10²³
Copper	29	2.75 × 10²³
Iodine	53	2.51 × 10²³
Barium	56	2.45 × 10²³
Lead	82	2.38 × 10²³

Table 5–2. Percentage of Photoelectric Reactions

RADIATION ENERGY (keV)	WATER (Z = 7.4)	COMPACT BONE (Z = 13.8)	SODIUM IODIDE (Z = 49.8)
20	65%	89%	94%
60	7%	31%	95%
100	2%	9%	88%

ble. Table 5–2 shows the percentage of photoelectric reactions for various radiation energies in water, bone, and sodium iodide. You can easily calculate the percentage of Compton reactions by subtracting the percentage of photoelectric reactions from 100 (ignoring the small contribution from coherent scattering). As the radiation energy increases, the percentage of photoelectric reactions decreases for water and bone; as the atomic number increases, the percentage of photoelectric reactions increases. With extremely low energy radiation (20 keV), photoelectric attenuation predominates, regardless of the atomic number of the absorber. As the radiation energy is increased, Compton scattering becomes more important until eventually it replaces the photoelectric effect as the predominant interaction. With high atomic number absorbers, such as sodium iodide, the photoelectric effect is the predominant interaction throughout the diagnostic energy range.

The linear attenuation coefficient is the sum of the contributions from coherent scattering, photoelectric reactions, and Compton scattering:

$$\mu = \mu_{coherent} + \mu_{PE} + \mu_{Compton}$$

For example, at 40 keV, the linear attenuation coefficient for water is 0.24 cm⁻¹. Of this total, 0.018 is from coherent scattering, 0.18 is from Compton scattering and the remaining 0.042 is from photoelectric attenuation. For water, the mass and linear attenuation coefficients are the same because the density of water is 1 g/cm³. For other materials, however, the mass and linear attenuation coefficients are different, but the principle is exactly the same.

If we know the relative percentage of each type of interaction, we can predict the total amount of attenuation (or transmission). Attenuation is always greater when the photoelectric effect predominates. Perhaps the difference between photoelectric and Compton attenuation will be easier to understand with an analogy. Suppose we take a flat stone and slide it along the ground at a high speed. If we slide the stone over a rough surface, such as a concrete sidewalk, friction will stop it in a short distance. If we slide the stone over a frozen pond, friction is reduced, and the stone will travel a much greater distance. In this analogy, the x-ray beam is the moving stone and attenuation is the friction that stops the stone. Photoelectric attenuation is like the concrete sidewalk and Compton attenuation is like the frozen pond. The photoelectric effect attenuates a beam much more rapidly than Compton scattering.

Energy. In addition to its influence on the type of basic interaction, energy has its own effect on attenuation. Even when all the basic interactions are of one type, attenuation decreases as the radiation energy increases. Table 5–3 shows the percentage of photons transmitted through a 10-cm-thick water phantom with various radiation energies. As you can see, the percentage of transmitted photons increases as the energy of the beam increases. With low energy radiation (20 keV), most of the inter-

actions are photoelectric, and few photons are transmitted. As the energy of the radiation increases, photoelectric attenuation becomes less important, and completely ceases at 100 keV. Even when all attenuation is from Compton scattering, the percentage of transmitted photons continues to increase as the radiation energy increases. A larger percentage of photons is transmitted with a 150-keV than with a 100-keV beam.

As the energy of the radiation increases, photoelectric attenuation decreases sharply, while Compton attenuation decreases only slightly. In the low energy range, a massive quantity of photoelectric attenuation is superimposed on a background of Compton attenuation. As the energy of the radiation increases, photoelectric attenuation diminishes until the background of Compton attenuation is all that is left. Once this happens, increasing the beam energy will cause only a slight decrease in attenuation (and slight increase in transmission).

As a general rule, the higher the energy of the radiation, the larger the percentage of transmitted photons, regardless of the type of basic interaction. The only exception to this rule occurs with high atomic number absorbers, which we will discuss next.

Atomic Number. Usually, as the radiation energy increases, x-ray transmission increases (and attenuation decreases) but, with high atomic number absorbers, transmission may actually decrease with increasing beam energy. This apparent paradox occurs because there is an abrupt change in the likelihood of a photoelectric reaction as the radiation energy reaches the binding energy of an inner shell electron. A photon cannot eject an electron unless it has more energy than the electron's binding energy. Thus, a lower energy photon is more likely to be transmitted than a higher energy photon, provided one has slightly less and the other slightly more energy than the binding energy of the electron.

Table 5–3. Percent Transmission of Monochromatic Radiation Through 10 cm of Water

ENERGY (keV)	TRANSMISSION (%)
20	0.04
30	2.5
40	7.0
50	10.0
60	13.0
80	16.0
100	18.0
150	22.0

Table 5–4. Percent Transmission of Monochromatic Radiation Through 1 mm of Lead

ENERGY (keV)	TRANSMISSION (%)
50	0.016
60	0.40
80	6.8
88	12.0
—K edge for lead—	
88	0.026
100	0.14
150	0.96

Table 5–4 shows the percentage transmission of monochromatic radiation through 1 mm of lead. A sudden change in transmission occurs at 88 keV, which is the binding energy of the K-shell electron. This is called the **K edge.** With a radiation energy just below the K edge, a fairly large percentage of the photons is transmitted (12%), while just above the K edge, transmission drops to nearly zero. Of course, the same thing is true for the low atomic number elements at the K edge, but the energies involved are usually less than 1 keV, far below those in the useful diagnostic energy range.

Figure 5–5 shows a plot of the mass attenuation coefficients of tin and lead over the range of energies used in diagnostic radiology. Remember, the higher the attenuation coefficient, the lower the number of transmitted photons. **Gram for gram, tin is a better absorber of x rays than lead between 29 and 88 keV.** This has a practical application. We are not usually concerned about attenuation per gram but, when we are carrying the gram on our back as a protective apron, our perspective changes. Because tin attenuates more radiation per unit weight than lead, it has recently come into use for this purpose. A lighter tin apron gives the same protection as a standard lead apron, or, if you have a strong back, you can use the same weight of tin for the apron and have more protection.

The commonly used contrast agents bar-

Figure 5–5 Comparison of the mass attenuation coefficients for tin and lead

ium and iodine were originally selected because of their low toxicities. A better choice, however, could not have been made if they were selected for their physical properties. Both have ideal K-shell binding energies (iodine, 32 keV; barium, 34 keV). These binding energies are approximately the same as the mean energy of most diagnostic x-ray beams, so many interactions occur at the K-shell level. Attenuation is more intense than it would be for a higher atomic number element, such as lead. Most photons in a polychromatic beam are less energetic than the 88-keV K-shell binding energy of lead.

Table 5–5 shows the atomic numbers and K edges of most elements important in diagnostic radiology. When maximum x-ray absorption is desired, the K edge of an absorber should be closely matched to the energy of the x-ray beam. For example, xeroradiography employs a selenium plate with a K edge of 12.7 keV as the x-ray absorber. This low K edge makes selenium

Table 5–5. Atomic Numbers and K Edges of Elements Important in Diagnostic Radiology

ELEMENT	SYMBOL	ATOMIC NUMBER (Z)	K EDGE (keV)
Hydrogen	H	1	.013
Beryllium	Be	4	.11
Carbon	C	6	.28
Nitrogen	N	7	.40
Oxygen	O	8	.53
Sodium	Na	11	1.1
Aluminum	Al	13	1.6
Silicon	Si	14	1.8
Sulfur	S	16	2.5
Chlorine	Cl	17	2.8
Potassium	K	19	3.6
Calcium	Ca	20	4.0
Iron	Fe	26	7.1
Copper	Cu	29	9.0
Zinc	Zn	30	9.7
Germanium	Ge	32	11.1
Selenium	Se	34	12.7
Bromine	Br	35	13.5
Yttrium	Y	39	17.0
Molybdenum	Mo	42	20.0
Silver	Ag	47	25.5
Cadmium	Cd	48	26.7
Tin	Sn	50	29.1
Iodine	I	53	33.2
Cesium	Cs	55	36.0
Barium	Ba	56	37.4
Lanthanum	La	57	39.0
Gadolinium	Gd	64	50.2
Tantalum	Ta	73	67.5
Tungsten	W	74	69.5
Gold	Au	79	80.7
Lead	Pb	82	88.0

an excellent absorber for the low energy radiation (30 to 35 kVp) used for mammography. Selenium would be a poor choice, however, as an absorber for a high-energy beam, such as the 350 kVp used for chest radiography with a field emission unit. For high-energy radiation, tungsten, with a K edge of 59.5 keV, is a much better absorber. As we shall see later, the success of the rare earth intensifying screens and of the cesium iodide image intensifier is in large part related to excellent matching of their K edges to beam energies.

Effect of Density on Attenuation

Tissue density is one of the most important factors in x-ray attenuation, and a difference in tissue densities is one of the primary reasons why we see an x-ray image. Density determines the number of electrons present in a given thickness, so it determines the tissue's stopping power. The relationship between density and attenuation is linear. If the density of a material is doubled, attenuation doubles. This is easiest to understand in terms of a gas whose density can be changed by compression. If a quantity of gas in a closed container is doubled, the number of electrons doubles. The same thickness of material now has twice as much mass, and it will attenuate twice as many photons.

Effect of Electrons per Gram

The number of Compton reactions depends on the number of electrons in a given thickness. Absorbers with many electrons are more impervious to radiation than absorbers with few electrons. Unfortunately, the number of electrons is usually expressed in the unit e/g (a mass unit) rather than e/cm³ (a volume unit). In order for the number of electrons per gram to have meaning, we must know the density of the material. Density determines the number of electrons that will be present in a given thickness, and this is what determines x-ray attenuation as we think of it in clinical radiology. By multiplying electrons per gram and density, we get electrons per cubic centimeter:

$$\frac{e}{g} \times \frac{g}{cm^3} = \frac{e}{cm^3}$$

Now we are talking about a unit we can understand. A cubic centimeter represents a thickness of 1 cm, and this is the unit we use to measure a patient's thickness.

Table 5–6 summarizes the relationships between density, e/g, and e/cm³ for air, fat, water, and bone.

When Compton reactions predominate, the number of e/cm³ becomes the most important factor in attenuation so, even though bone has fewer e/g than water,

Table 5–6. Comparison of Physical Characteristics of Air, Fat, Water, and Bone

	EFFECTIVE ATOMIC NUMBER	DENSITY (g/cm³)	ELECTRONS PER GRAM	ELECTRONS PER CUBIC CENTIMETER
Air	7.64	0.00129	3.01×10^{23}	0.0039×10^{23}
Fat	5.92	0.91	3.48×10^{23}	3.27×10^{23}
Water	7.42	1.00	3.34×10^{23}	3.34×10^{23}
Bone	13.8	1.85	3.0×10^{23}	5.55×10^{23}

bone still attenuates more radiation, because it has more e/cm³.

The number of electrons per gram can be calculated by the equation:

$$N_0 = \frac{NZ}{A}$$

N_0 = number of electrons per gram
N = Avogadro's number (6.02×10^{23})
Z = atomic number
A = atomic weight.

When comparing one element with another, we can disregard Avogadro's number, because it is a constant and affects all elements equally. The relative number of electrons per gram then becomes the simple ratio

$$\frac{Z}{A} \text{ or } \frac{\text{number of electrons}}{\text{weight of the atom}}$$

The weight of the atom is the sum of the weights of the protons and neutrons. The number of electrons and protons is equal, so the only factor that varies independently is the number of neutrons, which add mass without affecting the number of electrons. As the atomic number increases, the number of neutrons increases faster than the number of electrons. Hydrogen has no neutrons, and it has twice as many electrons per gram as any other element. Oxygen has one neutron per electron, and half as many electrons per gram as hydrogen. Lead has more neutrons than electrons, so it has even fewer electrons per gram than oxygen. In general, the high atomic number elements have about 20% fewer electrons per gram than the low atomic number elements. Table 5–1 shows the number of

electrons per gram for various elements important in diagnostic radiology.

POLYCHROMATIC RADIATION

The attenuation of polychromatic radiation is more complex than the attenuation of monochromatic radiation. Polychromatic beams contain a whole spectrum of photons of various energies (see Fig. 2–14), the most energetic of which are determined by the peak kilovoltage (kVp) used to generate the beam. **In general, the mean energy of polychromatic radiation is between one third and one half of its peak energy.** A 100-kVp beam has a mean energy of approximately 40 kV. This will vary somewhat depending on filtration.

As polychromatic radiation passes through an absorber, the transmitted photons undergo a change in both quantity and quality. The number of photons decreases because some are deflected and absorbed out of the beam, just as they are with monochromatic radiation. In contrast to monochromatic radiation, however, the quality of the beam also changes because the lower energy photons are more readily attenuated than the higher energy photons. As the low-energy photons are removed from the beam, the mean energy of the remaining photons increases.

The attenuation of polychromatic radiation is shown in Figure 5–6. The x-ray beam begins with 1000 photons having a mean energy of 40 kV. The first centimeter of absorber (water) reduces the number of photons by 35% and increases their mean energy to 47 kV. The second centimeter of water reduces the number of photons only 27%, because now the remaining photons

kVp = 100

Figure 5–6 Attenuation of polychromatic radiation

are a little more energetic, and increases their mean energy to 52 kV. If the process is continued long enough, eventually the mean energy of the beam will approach its peak energy.

When the percentage of transmission of polychromatic radiation is plotted on semilogarithmic graph paper, it results in a curved line (Fig. 5–7). The initial slope of the curve is steep, because many low-energy photons are attenuated by the first few centimeters of water. Eventually, the slope of the curve becomes similar to the slope for a monochromatic beam as the mean

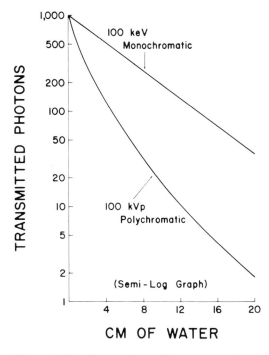

Figure 5–7 Comparison of the attenuation of polychromatic and monochromatic radiation

energy of the polychromatic radiation approaches its peak energy.

APPLICATIONS TO DIAGNOSTIC RADIOLOGY

The photons in an x-ray beam enter a patient with a uniform distribution and emerge in a specific pattern of distribution. The transmitted photons carry the x-ray image, but their pattern also carries the memory of the attenuated photons. The transmitted and attenuated photons are equally important. If all photons were transmitted, the film would be uniformly black; if all photons were attenuated, the film would be uniformly white. In neither case would there be an x-ray image. Image formation depends on a differential attenuation between tissues. Some tissues attenuate more x rays than other tissues, and the size of this differential determines the amount of contrast in the x-ray image.

To examine differential attenuation we will consider a radiograph of a hand so we only have to discuss two tissue types, bone and soft tissue. Figure 5–8 shows the linear attenuation coefficients of compact bone and water. Water is used to represent the soft tissues. Remember, the higher the linear attenuation coefficient, the greater the attenuation. As you can see, x-ray attenuation is greater in bone than in water, so the bones show up as holes in the transmitted photon pattern. We see these holes as white areas on a film. With a 20-keV x-ray beam, water has a linear attenuation coefficient of 0.77 cm^{-1} and that of bone is 4.8 cm^{-1}. Bone has a greater linear attenuation coefficient by a factor of 6. With such a large differential, the x-ray image will display a great deal of contrast. At an x-ray beam energy of 100 keV, differential attenuation is not nearly as large. Bone still attenuates more x rays than water, but now the difference is only by a factor of 0.6, so image contrast is considerably reduced.

Figure 5–8 illustrates another point. The total linear attenuation coefficient is actually made up of three separate coefficients,

Figure 5–8   Linear attenuation coefficients for water and compact bone

one for each of the basic interactions: coherent scattering, photoelectric effect, and Compton scattering. Each contributes its own component to the total linear attenuation coefficient. At low photon energies (20 keV) most of the difference in x-ray attenuation between bone and soft tisue results from a difference in the number of photoelectric reactions. More photoelectric reactions occur because bone contains calcium, which has a relatively high atomic number. At high photon energies (100 keV) the difference in x-ray attenuation between bone and soft tissues is almost entirely the result of the difference in the number of Compton reactions. Few photoelectric reactions occur in either bone or soft tissue at 100 keV. **When Compton reactions predominate, differential attenuation entirely depends on differences in density.** The reason is that denser materials have more electrons available to undergo reactions.

Figure 5–9 shows the Compton linear attenuation coefficients for water, bone,

and sodium iodide. The number of Compton reactions decreases only slightly with increasing x-ray energies. As the energy of an x-ray beam is increased from 20 to 100 keV, the Compton linear attenuation coefficient for bone decreases about 20% (while the photoelectric linear attenuation coefficient decreases more than 99%).

The shaded portion of Figure 5–9 shows the Compton mass attenuation coefficient. Remember, the mass attenuation coefficient indicates the amount of attenuation per gram, and it is not dependent on density. As you can see, a gram of water attenuates more x rays than a gram of either bone or sodium iodide by Compton reactions because water has more electrons per gram (it contains two atoms of hydrogen). Sodium iodide has even fewer electrons per gram than bone because of the high atomic number of iodine, so a gram of sodium iodide attenuates fewer photons by Compton reactions than either a gram of water or bone. Nevertheless, even when Compton scattering is the only type of basic

Compton mass attenuation coefficient ▨

Figure 5–9 Compton linear and mass attenuation coefficients for water, compact bone, and sodium iodide

interaction, there is still a difference in x-ray attenuation between water, bone, and sodium iodide in favor of the higher atomic number absorber, but the difference is entirely dependent on density.

Fat and water are always difficult to differentiate radiographically. The effective atomic number of water (7.4) is slightly greater than that of fat (5.9), so they can be differentiated by photoelectric attenuation using low energy techniques. With higher energy radiation, when Compton attenuation predominates, differentiation between fat and water depends on density and on the number of electrons per gram. Water has a greater density, but fewer electrons per gram. The net results, the number of electrons per cubic centimeter, are nearly the same for both water and fat (Table 5–6). Water has approximately 2% more e/cm^3, which is too small a difference to demonstrate with only Compton reactions. A significant difference in attenuation between fat and water can only be demonstrated effectively using low energy techniques.

SCATTER RADIATION

Our discussion of attenuation has only dealt with primary radiation, which either passes through the patient unchanged or is completely removed from the useful beam. The primary radiation carries the x-ray image. Now enters the villain, scatter radiation. It has nothing worthwhile to offer. Scatter radiation detracts from film quality and contributes no useful information.

How important is scatter radiation? How much of the density of an x-ray film is from scatter radiation? Several factors determine its importance. In most of our routine work it is important, frequently making up from 50 to 90% of the total number of photons emerging from the patient. The reason for the large number of scattered photons will be more apparent if we consider the fate of a diagnostic x-ray beam. With thick parts, such as the abdomen, only 1% of the photons in the initial beam reach the film. The rest are attenuated, the majority by Compton scattering. Fortunately, most of them do not reach the film. Nevertheless, those that reach the film make a major, and undesirable, contribution to total film blackening.

It would be more accurate to refer to all undesirable radiation as secondary radiation, which includes photons and electrons that might contribute to film fog. In actual practice, however, none of the electrons (photoelectric or recoil) have enough energy to reach the film, and the only characteristic radiation with sufficient energy to cause a problem occurs during contrast examinations with barium and iodine. The only secondary radiation of any significance comes from Compton scattering, and it has become common practice to refer to all undesirable radiation as scatter radiation, which is fairly accurate.

Factors Affecting Scatter Radiation

Three factors determine the quantity of scatter radiation. These are:
1. kilovoltage (kVp)
2. part thickness
3. field size

Scatter radiation is maximum with high-kVp techniques, large fields, and thick parts—unfortunately, this is what we usually deal with in diagnostic radiology. We rarely have any control over part thickness and frequently must use large fields. The only variable we can control is kVp, but even here we have less control than we would like because patient doses increase sharply with low-kVp techniques.

Field size is the most important factor in the production of scatter radiation. A small x-ray field (usually called a "narrow beam") irradiates only a small volume of tissue, so it generates only a small number of scattered photons. Most of them miss the film because they have a large angle of escape. Figure 5–10 shows the angle of escape for a scattered photon originating at point P. As you can see, the escape angle is much larger than the narrow angle encompassed by the primary beam. Thus, the quantity

Figure 5–10 Angle of escape for scattered photons

of scatter radiation from a narrow beam is small to begin with, and most of it never reaches the plane of the film. For this reason, narrow beam attenuation is the method used to measure the attenuation of primary radiation, and the terms **narrow beam** and **primary** radiation are used synonymously.

As the x-ray field is enlarged, the quantity of scatter radiation increases rapidly at first, and then gradually tapers off until finally it reaches a plateau, or saturation point. A further increase in field size does not change the quantity of scatter radiation that reaches the film. The total number of scattered photons in the field increases, but the number that reaches any particular point on the film remains constant. For example, consider the central point of a circular field 4 cm in diameter. Scattered photons originating from the periphery of the field can easily penetrate 2 cm of tissue to reach the field's center. If the field is increased to a 30-cm circle, however, most scatter photons do not have sufficient range to penetrate the 15 cm of tissue between the field's margin and center. So, even though more scattered photons are generated in large fields, they do not increase the quantity reaching any particular area. The saturation point for scatter radiation occurs with a field approximately 30 × 30 cm, only a 12-in. square, which is not a large field for diagnostic radiology.

The quantity of scatter radiation reaches a saturation point with increasing **part thickness,** just as it does with increasing field size. The total number of scattered photons keeps increasing as the part becomes thicker, but photons originating in the upper layers of the patient do not have sufficient energy to reach the film. Unfortunately we have little control over part thickness and, except for the occasional use of a compressed band, we must accept the patient as he is.

The effect of **kilovoltage** (kVp) on the production of scatter radiation is probably not as important as part thickness, and certainly is not as important as field size. In the low energy range (20 to 30 keV), in which the photoelectric effect predominates, extremely little scatter radiation is produced. As the radiation energy increases, the percentage of Compton reactions increases, and so does the production of scatter radiation. After Compton scattering becomes the predominant interaction, scatter radiation production tends to plateau, just as it does with increasing field size and part thickness. The energy of the point at which the plateau occurs depends on the atomic number of the tissue, but the plateau is not as well defined as it is with field size and part thickness. Even after Compton reactions predominate, the quantity of scatter radiation continues to increase with increasing beam energy because more photons scatter in the forward direction, and their greater energy allows them to penetrate greater thicknesses of tissue to reach the film.

Because we have so little control over the production of scatter radiation, we must find ways of keeping it from x-ray film after it has been generated. The most important of these is the x-ray grid, which we will discuss in Chapter 8.

SUMMARY

Attenuation is the reduction in the intensity of an x-ray beam as it traverses matter either by the absorption or deflection of photons from the beam. The attenuation of monochromatic radiation is exponential; that is, each layer of absorber attenuates the same percentage of the photons remaining in the beam. The attenuation of polychromatic radiation is not exponential. A large percentage of the low-energy photons are attenuated by the first few centimeters of absorber, so the quality (mean energy) of the remaining photons increases as the beam passes through an absorber.

The amount of attenuation depends on the energy of the radiation and three characteristics of the tissue: atomic number, density, and electrons per gram. Increasing the radiation energy increases the number of transmitted photons, while increasing the atomic number, density, or electrons per gram decreases transmission. Energy and atomic number together determine the relative percentage of photoelectric and Compton reactions. With low-energy radiation, and with high atomic number absorbers, a large amount of photoelectric attenuation is superimposed on a small background of Compton attenuation. As the energy of the radiation is increased, photoelectric attenuation diminishes, until the background of Compton attenuation is all that remains.

Density is one of the most important factors affecting attenuation, and radiographic image contrast is largely dependent on differences in tissue density. The high contrast between air and soft tissues occurs entirely because of density differences. The number of electrons per gram plays a lesser role. Generally, as the atomic number increases, the number of electrons per gram decreases, but the decrease is more than compensated by an even greater increase in density. Thus, high atomic number elements attenuate more radiation, even though they have fewer electrons per gram.

The amount of scatter radiation reaching an x-ray film increases with increasing field size, part thickness, and kilovoltage.

REFERENCE

1. Hubbell, J.H.: Photon Cross Sections, Attenuation Coefficients, and Energy Absorption Coefficients from 10 keV to 100 GeV. Washington, DC, U.S. Government Printing Office, National Bureau of Standards, Handbook 29, August 1969.

CHAPTER

6 *Filters*

Filtration is the process of shaping the x-ray beam to increase the ratio of photons useful for imaging to those photons that increase patient dose or decrease image contrast. Diagnostic x-ray beams are composed of photons that have a whole spectrum of energies; this is, they are polychromatic. Their mean energy is from one third to one half of their peak energy, so many photons fall in the lower energy range. As polychromatic radiation passes through a patient, most of the lower energy photons are absorbed in the first few centimeters of tissue, and only the higher energy photons penetrate through the patient to form the radiographic image. Because the patient's radiation dose depends on the number of absorbed photons, **the first few centimeters of tissue receive much more radiation than the rest of the patient.** This tissue can be protected by absorbing the lower energy photons from the beam before they reach the patient by interposing a filter material between the patient and the x-ray tube. Filters are usually sheets of metal, and their main function in diagnostic radiology is to reduce the patient's radiation dose. In the last part of this chapter we will discuss how heavy metal filters are also used to improve image contrast.

In a radiologic examination the x-ray beam is filtered by absorbers at three different levels. Beginning at the x-ray source, these are as follows:

1. The x-ray tube and its housing **(inherent filtration)**

2. Sheets of metal placed in the path of the beam **(added filtration)**
3. The patient

INHERENT FILTRATION

Filtration resulting from the absorption of x rays as they pass through the x-ray tube and its housing is called **inherent filtration.** The materials responsible for inherent filtration are the glass envelope enclosing the anode and cathode, the insulating oil surrounding the tube, and the window in the tube housing. Inherent filtration is measured in **aluminum equivalents,** which represent the thickness of aluminum that would produce the same degree of attenuation as the thickness of the material in question. Inherent filtration usually varies between 0.5 and 1.0 mm aluminum equivalent, and the glass envelope is responsible for most of it.

In a few special circumstances, unfiltered radiation is desirable. Because filtration increases the mean energy of an x-ray beam, it decreases tissue contrast. The decrease is insignificant in the higher energy range but with lower energy radiation, under 30 kVp, this loss of contrast may be detrimental to image quality. Beryllium window tubes are designed to produce an essentially unfiltered beam. The exit portal of the glass envelope is replaced with beryllium (atomic number 4), which is more transparent to low energy radiation than glass. The radiation from these tubes has a minimum of inherent filtration.

ADDED FILTRATION

Added filtration results from absorbers placed in the path of the x-ray beam. Ideally, a filter material should absorb all low energy photons and transmit all high energy photons. Unfortunately, no such material exists. A material can be selected, however, to absorb principally low energy radiation by utilizing the proclivity of photoelectric attenuation for low energy photons. Attenuation is most intense when the photoelectric effect is the predominant interaction and diminishes when Compton reactions predominate. The energy of the radiation filtered from the beam can be regulated by selecting a material with an appropriate atomic number. Aluminum and copper are the materials usually selected for diagnostic radiology. Aluminum, with an atomic number of 13, is an excellent filter material for low energy radiation and a good general purpose filter. Copper, with an atomic number of 29, is a better filter for high energy radiation. It is inconvenient to change filters between examinations, however, and there is a risk of forgetting to make the change. For practical reasons, most radiologists prefer to use a single filter material, usually aluminum.

Copper is never used by itself as the filter material. It is always used in combination with aluminum as a compound filter. The only reason for going to copper is to cut down on the thickness of the filter. A compound filter consists of two or more layers of different metals. The layers are arranged so that the higher atomic number element, copper, faces the x-ray tube, and the lower atomic number element, aluminum, faces the patient. Most filtration occurs in the copper, and the purpose of the aluminum is to absorb the characteristic radiation from copper. Photoelectric attenuation in copper produces characteristic radiation with an energy of about 8 keV, which is energetic enough to reach the patient and significantly increase skin doses. The aluminum layer absorbs this charac-

teristic radiation. Its own characteristic radiation has so little energy (1.5 keV) that it is absorbed in the air gap between the patient and filter.

Filter Thickness

After selecting a filter material, usually aluminum, the next step is to determine the appropriate thickness for the filter. The percentages of x-ray attenuation with 1, 2, 3, and 10 mm of aluminum for photons of various energies are shown in Table 6–1. Two millimeters of aluminum absorb nearly all photons with energies less than 20 keV, so most of the advantages of filtration are achieved by this thickness. An aluminum filter more than 3 mm thick offers no advantage; in fact, excess filtration has definite disadvantages. In Table 6–1, the column on the right shows the percentage of photons attenuated by 10 mm of aluminum, clearly excessive filtration. The effect is an overall attenuation of the beam, primarily by the absorption of high energy photons, because all the low energy photons have already been absorbed by thinner aluminum filters. The quality of the beam is not significantly altered, but its intensity is greatly diminished. This lengthens the time required to make an exposure, which increases the likelihood of the patient moving during the examination.

The National Council on Radiation Protection and Measurements has recommended the following total filtration for

Table 6–1. Percent Attenuation of Monochromatic Radiation by Various Thicknesses of Aluminum Filtration

PHOTON ENERGY (keV)	PHOTONS ATTENUATED (%)			
	1 mm	2 mm	3 mm	10 mm
10	100	100	100	100
20	58	82	92	100
30	24	42	56	93
40	12	23	32	73
50	8	16	22	57
60	6	12	18	48
80	5	10	14	48
100	4	8	12	35

diagnostic radiology.[2] The figures include both inherent and added filtration:

OPERATING kVp	TOTAL FILTRATION
Below 50 kVp	0.5 mm aluminum
50 to 70 kVp	1.5 mm aluminum
Above 70 kVp	2.5 mm aluminum

The effect of aluminum filtration on a 90-kVp polychromatic x-ray beam is shown graphically in Figure 6–1. The unfiltered beam is composed of a spectrum of photons, many of which have energies in the 10 to 20 keV range. The highest point in the curve occurs at 25 keV. Filtration reduces the total number of photons in the x-ray beam (area under the curve) but, more importantly, it selectively removes a large number of low energy photons. The intensity on the low energy side of the curve (left) is reduced considerably more than the intensity on the high energy side of the curve (right), and the highest point in the curve is shifted from 25 to 35 keV. The overall effect is an increase in the mean energy of the x-ray beam.

Effect of Filters on Patient Exposure

Trout and coworkers demonstrated the degree of patient protection afforded by filters with a series of tests, one of which is summarized in Table 6–2.[3] In this particular experiment, they made multiple radiographs of an 18-cm-thick pelvic phantom using a 60-kVp x-ray beam. The initial

Table 6–2. Exposure Dose to the Skin for Comparable Density Radiographs of a Pelvic Phantom (18 cm thick) with Various Thicknesses of Aluminum Filtration

	60-kVp BEAM	
ALUMINUM FILTRATION (mm)	EXPOSURE DOSE TO SKIN (mR)	DECREASE IN EXPOSURE DOSE (%)
None	2380	
0.5	1850	22
1.0	1270	47
3.0	465	80

radiograph was made without a filter and was then repeated with increasing thicknesses of aluminum filtration. Exposure times were adjusted to produce films of equal density, and the radiation dose to the skin over the pelvis was measured for each exposure. As you can see in Table 6–2, the decrease in patient exposure was remarkable, up to 80% with 3 mm of aluminum filtration. These percentages are for a specific examination, but they should give you some insight into the degree of protection you can expect from adequate filtration.

Effect on Exposure Factors

The major disadvantage of filtration is a reduction in the intensity of the x-ray beam. Filters absorb some photons at all energy levels, and we must compensate for the loss of higher energy photons by increasing exposure factors (mAs). Even when it is necessary to increase exposure because of filtration, the patient receives less radiation than he would from an unfiltered beam. The x-ray tube puts out more photons but the filter absorbs many of them, and the total number reaching the patient actually decreases.

Wedge Filters

Wedge filters are occasionally used in diagnostic radiology to obtain films of more uniform density when the part being examined diminishes greatly in thickness from one side of the field to the other. The filter is shaped like a wedge. The relationship between the filter and patient is shown

Figure 6–1 Energy and intensity of unfiltered and filtered polychromatic radiation

in Figure 6–2. When one side of the patient is considerably thicker than the other, the wedge compensates for the difference. Less radiation is absorbed by the thinner part of the filter, so more is available to penetrate the thicker part of the patient. Wedge filters are often used in lower-limb angiography when one images from the lower abdomen to the ankles with a single exposure.

HEAVY METAL FILTERS

(K-Edge Filters)

The development of high speed intensifying screens and high capacity x-ray tubes have made it reasonable to consider the use of heavy metal filters for general radiography. These filters make use of the K-absorption edge of elements with atomic numbers greater than 60, and may offer advantages when imaging barium or iodine. Table 6–3 lists some heavy elements that have been investigated as filters, and compares them to aluminum, iodine, and barium.

Let us begin by reviewing the absorption

Table 6–3. Atomic Numbers and K Edges Important to Heavy Metal Filters

ELEMENT	SYMBOL	ATOMIC NUMBER	K EDGE (keV)
Aluminum	Al	13	1.6
Molybdenum	Mo	42	20
Gadolinium	Gd	64	50.2
Holmium	Ho	67	55.6
Erbium	Er	68	57.5
Ytterbium	Yb	70	61.3
Tungsten	W	74	69.5
Iodine	I	53	33.17
Barium	Ba	56	37.45

characteristics of iodine and barium. The reason we use iodine and barium is to provide contrast, and contrast is greatest when the contrast agent absorbs x rays most efficiently. This maximum contrast is obtained when the photon energy of the x-ray beam is close to, but slightly above, the K-absorption edge of the absorber in question. For example, just below the K edge of iodine the mass absorption coefficient of iodine is 6.6 cm²/g. Just above the K edge the coefficient jumps to 36 cm²/g. For iodine, the K-absorption edge is at 33.17 keV. The K edge of barium is at 33.45 keV. Table 6–4 lists the mass attenuation coefficient of iodine at several keV levels, illustrating that attenuation decreases below and above the K edge and has a relative maximum immediately above the K edge.

The purpose of heavy metal filters is to produce an x-ray beam that has a high number of photons in the specific energy range that will be most useful in diagnostic imaging. An immediate question might be: what is wrong with our standard aluminum filter? The energy spectrum transmitted by

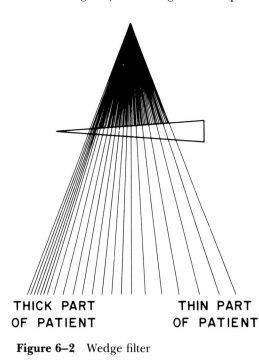

THICK PART
OF PATIENT

THIN PART
OF PATIENT

Figure 6–2 Wedge filter

Table 6–4. Approximate Mass Attenuation Coefficient (μ_p) of Iodine

keV	APPROXIMATE μ_p (cm²/g)
25	13.7
28	10.2
31	7.27
33.1	6.62
33.2	36.4
35	31.6
41	21.4

aluminum filters is too wide. The K edge of aluminum is 1.6 keV, too low to be useful as an energy selective filter for diagnostic radiology. Figure 6–3 illustrates that a 2-mm aluminum filter transmits a broad spectrum of bremsstrahlung. The same figure illustrates the effect a gadolinium filter has on the same x-ray beam. We illustrate the general concept of heavy metal filters with a gadolinium filter 0.25-mm thick because that is the most thoroughly studied of these filters. Notice that the gadolinium filter transmits increasing numbers of photons from the 25 to 50.2 keV range (i.e., the mass attenuation coefficient of Gd is decreasing from 25 to 50.2 keV). Immediately above 50.2 keV the mass attenuation coefficient of gadolinium increases dramatically and the number of transmitted photons is correspondingly diminished. The heavy metal filter transmits a significantly narrower spectrum of energies than aluminum, with decreased numbers of both low and high energy photons. The reduction in low energy photons will decrease the patient's absorbed dose. Image contrast will be improved by the reduction in higher energy photons (i.e.,

more photoelectric and less Compton attenuation). Because of increased beam filtration, increased x-ray tube loading (more mAs) is required when heavy metal filters are used. Patient dose reductions up to a factor of two, and mAs increases by a factor of two or more, have been reported. Improved contrast with a gadolinium filter has been shown maximal for thin body parts, while the need for more mAs has been minimized by use of low (about 60) kVp techniques.[1] This suggests that heavy metal filters may prove to be more useful for pediatric applications.

The usefulness of a heavy metal filter in imaging iodine is illustrated in Figure 6–4, in which the mass attenuation coefficient of iodine is compared to that of holmium.[4] The attenuation coefficient of iodine increases dramatically at the 33.17-keV K edge of iodine, and then decreases with an increase in photon energy. Conversely, the attenuation coefficient of holmium decreases steadily from 33 to 55.6 keV (the K edge of holmium), at which point attenuation by holmium increases dramatically.

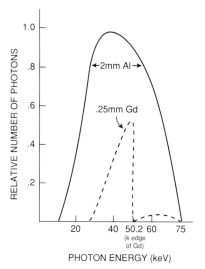

Figure 6–3 Approximate bremsstrahlung photon transmission of a 75-kVp x-ray beam through an aluminum and a gadolinium filter

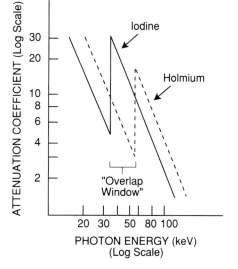

Figure 6–4 The attenuation coefficients of iodine and holmium, showing that the transmission of holmium and attenuation of iodine are simultaneously maximized in the region labeled "overlap window"

The important concept is the "window" in the 33 to 55 keV range. In this window the high transmission by the holmium filter overlaps the region of high attenuation by iodine (barium would be almost identical except its K edge is at 37.45 keV). It is this "overlap window" of about 20 keV that affords improved contrast when imaging iodine or barium when the x-ray beam filtered by a heavy metal filter is compared to that produced by an aluminum filter.

Molybdenum Filters

A special application of K edge filters is use of molybdenum filters with molybdenum target x-ray tubes used for mammography. Recall that a molybdenum target x-ray tube is often used for film-screen mammography to take advantage of the 17.5-keV K-alpha and the 19.6-keV K-beta characteristic radiation of molybdenum. When operated at 30 to 40 kVp, a molybdenum tube will also produce considerable bremsstrahlung with energies higher than 20 keV. This higher energy radiation will reduce contrast in breast soft tissue structures. To reduce the amount of higher energy radiation in the molybdenum tube spectrum, a molybdenum filter of 0.030 mm thickness is commonly used. This filter will attenuate x rays just above the 20-keV K-edge of Mo very strongly, but will transmit 57% of the 17.5 K-alpha and 67% of the 19.6 keV K-beta radiation of molybdenum.

SUMMARY

Filters are sheets of metal placed in the path of the x-ray beam near the x-ray tube housing to absorb low energy radiation before it reaches the patient. Their main function is to protect the patient from useless radiation, and they perform their func- tion remarkably well, frequently reducing skin exposures by as much as 80%. Aluminum is usually selected as the filter material for diagnostic radiology. Most high energy photons are transmitted through aluminum, while low energy photons are absorbed by photoelectric interactions. The photoelectric effect selectively absorbs low energy photons because of its dependence on energy and atomic number. The National Council on Radiation Protection and Measurement has recommended an equivalent of 2.5 mm of aluminum permanent filtration for diagnostic x-ray beams of energies greater than 70 kVp. Some higher energy useful photons are absorbed by filtration, and exposure factors must be increased to compensate for this loss. Filters are simple and inexpensive. Nowhere else in all of radiology do we gain so much for so little money. Heavy metal, or K-edge, filters are used to remove higher energy photons from the x-ray beam by taking advantage of the increase in mass attenuation coefficient at the K edge of certain elements. Except for molybdenum, these elements have atomic numbers greater than 60. Compared to aluminum, K-edge filters enhance contrast for iodine and barium, reduce patient dose, and increase tube loading.

REFERENCES

1. Burgess, A.E.: Contrast effects of a gadolinium filter. Med. Phys., 8:203, 1981.
2. National Council on Radiation Protection and Measurements: Medical X-Ray and Gamma-Ray Protection for Energies up to 10 meV. Washington, DC, U.S. Government Printing Office, Report No. 33, 1968.
3. Trout, E.D., Kelley, J.P., and Cathey, G.A.: The use of filters to control radiation exposure to the patient in diagnostic roentgenology. Am. J. Roentgen., 67:942, 1952.
4. Villagran, J.E., Hobbs, B.B., and Taylor, K.W.: Reduction of patient exposure by use of heavy elements as radiation filters in diagnostic radiology. Rad., 127:249, 1978.

7 *X-Ray Beam Restrictors*

An x-ray beam restrictor is a device that is attached to the opening in the x-ray tube housing to regulate the size and shape of an x-ray beam. Beam restrictors can be classified into three categories:

1. aperture diaphragms
2. cones and cyclinders
3. collimators

APERTURE DIAPHRAGMS

The simplest type of x-ray beam restrictor is an aperture diaphragm. It consists of a sheet of lead with a hole in the center; the size and shape of the hole determine the size and shape of the x-ray beam. Its principal advantage is its simplicity. Lead is soft, so the aperture can be easily altered to any desired size or shape. The principal disadvantage of an aperture diaphragm is that it produces a fairly large penumbra at the periphery of the x-ray beam (Fig. 7–1A). The center of the x-ray field is exposed by the entire focal spot, but the periphery of the field (P in the illustration) "sees" only a portion of the focal spot; this partially exposed area is called the **penumbra.** The width of the penumbra can be reduced by positioning the aperture diaphragm as far away from the x-ray target as possible. This is usually accomplished by attaching the diaphragm to the end of a cone.

CONES AND CYLINDERS

The second type of x-ray beam restrictor comes in two basic shapes, conical and cylindric. The flared shape of a cone would seem to be the ideal geometric configuration for an x-ray beam restrictor but the flare of the cone is usually greater than the flare of the x-ray beam, in which case the base plate that attaches the device to the tube housing is the only part that restricts the x-ray beam (Fig. 7–1B). When used in this way, it is little more than an aperture diaphragm. Beam restriction with a cylinder takes place at the far end of the barrel, so there is less penumbra (Fig. 7–1C). Cylinders may be equipped with extensions to increase their length to give even better beam restriction. A major disadvantage of aperture diaphragms, cones, and cylinders is the severe limitation they place on the number of available field sizes. Even a large assortment cannot approach the infinite variety of field sizes needed in diagnostic radiology, and changing them is inconvenient.

COLLIMATORS

The collimator is the best all around x-ray beam restrictor. It has two advantages over the other types: (1) it provides an infinite variety of rectangular x-ray fields; (2) a light beam shows the center and exact configuration of the x-ray field. Two sets of shutters (S_1 and S_2) control the beam dimensions. They move together as a unit so that the second shutter aligns with the first to "clean up" its penumbra (Fig. 7–2). The shutters function as two adjustable aperture diaphragms. Each shutter consists of four or more lead plates (Fig. 7–3). These plates move in independent pairs. One pair can be adjusted without moving the other, which permits an infinite variety of square or rectangular fields. When the

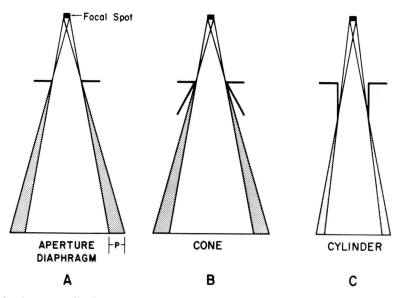

Figure 7–1   Aperture diaphragm *(A)*, cone *(B)*, and cylinder *(C)*

shutters are closed, they meet at the center of the x-ray field.

The x-ray field is illuminated by a light beam from a light bulb in the collimator. The light beam is deflected by a mirror mounted in the path of the x-ray beam at an angle of 45° (Fig. 7–4). The target of the x-ray tube and light bulb should be exactly the same distance from the center of the mirror. As the light beam passes through the second shutter opening, it is collimated to coincide with the x-ray beam. The distance from the mirror in the collimator to the target of the x-ray tube is critical. The collimator must be mounted so that the x-ray target and light bulb are exactly the same distance from the center of the mirror. If the collimator is mounted too

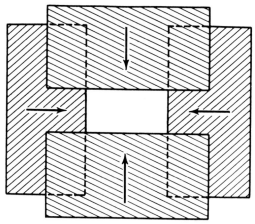

Figure 7–2   Alignment of collimator shutters   **Figure 7–3**   Collimator shutters *(top view)*

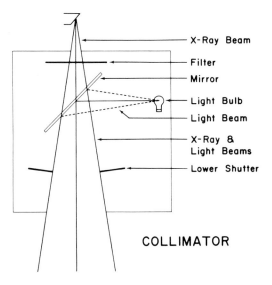

Figure 7–4 Alignment of light and x-ray beams

far from the x-ray target, the x-ray source will be further from the second shutter than the light source, and the x-ray beam will be smaller than the light beam.

A collimator can also identify the center of the x-ray field. This is accomplished by painting a cross line on a thin sheet of Plexiglas mounted on the end of the collimator. The light beam that illuminates the radiographic field also shows its center.

Collimators have a back-up system for identifying field size in case the light bulb should burn out. The x-ray field size for various target-film distances is indicated by a calibrated scale on the front of the collimator.

Today, non-mobile radiographic equipment in the United States, with a few special exceptions, must be equipped with automatic collimators. These are called **positive beam limiting (PBL)** devices.

Automatic collimators are the same as other collimators except that their shutters are motor-driven. When a cassette is loaded into the film holder (Buckey tray), sensors in the tray identify the size and alignment of the cassette. These sensors relay this information to the collimator mo-

tors, which position the shutters to exactly match the size of the film being used. A perfectly aligned collimator will leave an unexposed border on all sides of the developed film.

Positive beam limitation (PBL) devices (also called automatic light-localized variable-aperture collimators) must be accurate to within 2% of the source-to-image distance (SID). It is required that total misalignment of the edges of the light field with the respective edges of the x-ray field along either the length or width shall not be greater than 2% of the distance from the focal spot of the x-ray tube (the source of x-rays) to the center of the field. Figure 7–5 illustrates this alignment requirement. With a standard 40-in. (or 100-cm) SID, total misalignment along either the long or short sides of the true edges of the x-ray beam must not be greater than 0.8 in. (or 2 cm).

Testing X-Ray Beam and Light Beam Alignment

The alignment of the x-ray beam and light beam should be checked periodically, because the mirror tends to get out of adjustment from daily use. The only equip-

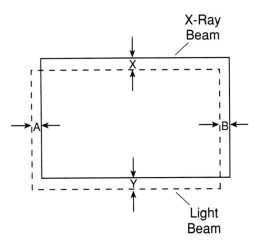

Figure 7–5 Alignment of the light beam and x-ray beam for a PBL device must be accurate to 2% of the SID. At a 40-in. SID, A + B ≤0.8 in. and x + y ≤ 0.8 in.

ment needed to test alignment includes four L-shaped wires (pieces of paper clips work nicely), a 14- to 17-in. x-ray film in a cassette, and a small lead letter "R." Place the film on the top of the x-ray table, open the collimator shutter to a convenient size (10 × 10 in.), carefully position the L-shaped wires at the corner of the light field, and place the "R" in the lower right corner. Then make an x-ray exposure (40 in., 3.3 mAs, 40 kVp) to mark the position of the x-ray field on the film. Without touching the film or wires, enlarge the field size to 12 × 12 in. and expose the film for the second time (same exposure factors).

Figure 7–6 shows a test film taken with a collimator whose mirror is out of adjustment. The dark center shows the position of the x-ray beam, and the wires indicate the position of the light beam. The second exposure (with an enlarged field) is made to ensure visibility of all the wires. The wire in the left lower corner of the illustration would not have been visible on the film without the second exposure.

To adjust a misaligned mirror, return the processed x-ray film to its original position on the x-ray table. The "R" in the lower right corner assists in orienting the film properly. Position the light beam to the images of the wires, as you did earlier for

Figure 7–6 Test film of light and x-ray beam alignment

the film exposure, and adjust the mirror in the collimator until the light beam coincides exactly with the x-ray field (dark area on the film). Then repeat the test to make sure that the mirror adjustment has correctly aligned the light and x-ray beams.

FUNCTIONS OF RESTRICTORS

Collimators and other x-ray beam restrictors have two basic functions: to protect the patient and to decrease scatter radiation.

Although patient protection is the principal reason for using collimators today, it is interesting to note that the old-time radiologists restricted x-ray beams before they knew anything about the harmful effects of low doses of radiation. They used small fields because they obtained better films with small fields. Because they had no grids, their only means of controlling scatter radiation was to limit field size, so they collimated their x-ray beams and obtained excellent films.

Patient Protection

The mechanism by which collimators protect the patient is obvious; that is, the smaller the x-ray field, the smaller the volume of the patient that is irradiated. If a 20- × 20-cm field is collimated to 10 × 10 cm, the area of the patient that is irradiated decreases from 400 to 100 cm², a fourfold decrease in area and a corresponding decrease in volume. A decrease in field size is especially significant, because area is a square function. Trimming only a few centimeters off the edge of the field significantly decreases the exposed volume of the patient.

The ideal shape for a radiographic field for maximal patient protection has never been established. Initially, all x-ray beam restrictors were round (cones) and now they are usually square or rectangular (collimators). It was argued that x-ray films are rectangular. Round fields expose portions of the patient that are not even included on the film, as shown in Figure 7–7, so x-

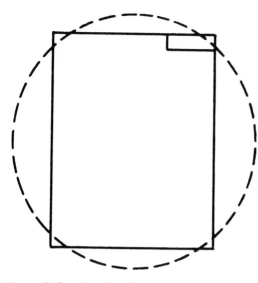

Figure 7–7 Overlap of a round field on a rectangular film

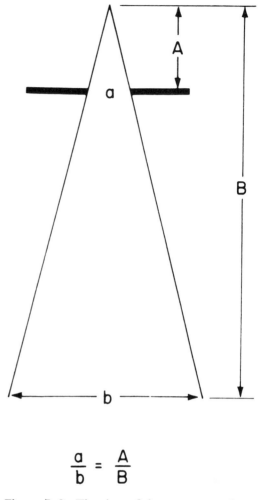

$$\frac{a}{b} = \frac{A}{B}$$

Figure 7–8 The sizes of the aperture and x-ray field are proportional to the target-aperture and target-film distances

ray beam restrictors were made square. But the ideal field shapes should be dictated by the shape of the part being examined, and not by the shape of either the film or collimator. Some parts are better examined with round fields, such as gallbladders and paranasal sinuses. Certainly a circular field that is completely encompassed by the film is the most suitable shape when a round part is being examined.

It might be interesting to look at a problem regarding beam restrictor sizes. These problems can be solved by setting up proportions between the comparable sides of similar triangles (Fig. 7–8). For example, if an aperture diaphragm (A) is 25 cm from the x-ray target, and the target film distance (B) is 100 cm, what size aperture (a) should be used to produce a 15-cm x-ray field (b) for a gallbladder examination? Using proportional triangles, the aperture hole should be

$$\frac{a}{15} = \frac{25}{100}, \text{ or } a = 15 \times \frac{25}{100} = 3.75 \text{ cm}$$

Decreased Scatter Radiation with Collimators

The quantity of scatter radiation reaching an x-ray film depends on field size; that is, the larger the field, the more scatter radiation. Figure 7–9 shows the general shape of the curves obtained when the number of transmitted primary and scattered photons are plotted against field size. The exact contribution from scatter depends on the thickness of the part being examined and on the energy (kVp) of the x-ray beam. The amount of primary radiation at the plane of the film is independent of field size. The number of transmitted primary photons, per unit area, is the same for a 1- × 1-cm field and a 30- × 30-cm field, so the number of the pri-

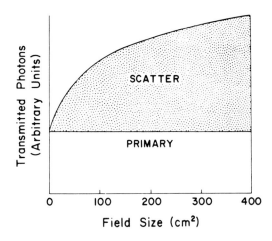

Figure 7–9   Transmitted radiation for various sizes of x-ray fields

mary photons in Figure 7–9 plots a straight line.

The number of scattered photons reaching the x-ray film depends on field size. Small x-ray fields generate little scatter radiation. As the field size is enlarged, the amount of scatter radiation increases rapidly at first, and then tapers off with larger fields. After the x-ray field reaches a size of about 30 × 30 cm, the total quantity of scatter radiation is near its maximum. Because collimators are only successful in decreasing scatter radiation with small fields, we should restrict the size of our x-ray beams as much as possible.

A final fact to remember about collima-tors is that they affect exposure factors. Small fields produce little scatter radiation, so the total quantity of blackening of the x-ray film decreases as the field size decreases. To keep film density constant, as you decrease the size of the x-ray field you must increase the exposure factors.

SUMMARY

There are three types of x-ray beam restrictors: aperture diaphragms, cones (cylinders), and collimators. Their basic function is to regulate the size and shape of the x-ray beam. Closely collimated beams have two advantages over larger beams. First, a smaller area of the patient is exposed and, because area is a square function, a decrease of one half in x-ray beam diameter effects a fourfold decrease in patient exposure. Second, well-collimated beams generate less scatter radiation and thus improve film quality. By decreasing the amount of scatter radiation, collimators also affect exposure factors. As the x-ray field size is decreased, the exposure factors must be increased to maintain a constant film density.

Collimators are the best general purpose beam restrictors. They offer two advantages over the other types: the x-ray field is illuminated, which permits accurate localization on the patient; and the x-ray field can be adjusted to an infinite variety of rectangular shapes and sizes.

CHAPTER

8 Grids

The radiographic grid consists of a series
of lead foil strips separated by x-ray-trans-
parent spacers. It was invented by Dr. Gus-
tave Bucky in 1913, and it is still the most
effective way of removing scatter radiation
from large radiographic fields. Figure 8–1
shows how a grid functions. Primary radiation is oriented in the same axis as the
lead strips and passes between them to
reach the film unaffected by the grid. Scatter radiation arises from many points
within the patient and is multidirectional,
so most of it is absorbed by the lead strips
and only a small amount passes between
them.

The interspaces of grids are filled either
with aluminum or some organic com-

pound. The main purpose of the interspace material is to support the thin lead
foil strips. Aluminum interspace grids can
probably be manufactured more precisely,
and they are structurally stronger than
grids with organic interspacers. Patient exposures are higher with aluminum because
it absorbs more primary radiation. It also
absorbs more secondary radiation, however, so contrast improvement is probably
better. At the present time both materials
are used, and there is no clear-cut differentiation as to which is better.

TERMINOLOGY

**Grid ratio is defined as the ratio between
the height of the lead strips and the distance between them.** Figure 8–2 is a cross-
sectional scale drawing of a grid with a ratio
of 8:1. The lead strips are approximately
0.05 mm thick, so that they may appropriately be considered lead foil. The interspaces are much thicker than the lead
strips. Grid ratios are usually expressed as
two numbers, such as 10:1, with the first
number the actual ratio and the second
number always 1. The grid ratio is a pa-
rameter widely used to express a grid's ability to remove scatter radiation. Ratios usually range from 4:1 to 16:1. Generally, the
higher the ratio, the better the grid functions. Grid ratios are indicated on the top
of grids by manufacturers.

Grid pattern refers to the orientation of
the lead strips in their longitudinal axis. It
is the pattern of the grid that we see from
a top view. The two basic grid patterns are
linear and crossed.

In a **linear grid** the lead strips are par-

Figure 8–1 Grid function

$$r = \frac{h}{D} = \frac{2.0}{0.25} = 8$$

r – GRID RATIO

h – HEIGHT OF LEAD STRIPS

D – DISTANCE BETWEEN
LEAD STRIPS

Figure 8–2   Cross section of a grid

allel to each other in their longitudinal axis (Fig. 8–3). Most x-ray tables are equipped with linear grids. Their major advantage is that they allow us to angle the x-ray tube along the length of the grid without loss of primary radiation from grid "cutoff."

A **crossed grid** is made up of two su-

Figure 8–3   Linear grid

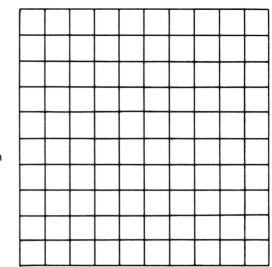

Figure 8–4   Crossed grid

perimposed linear grids that have the same focusing distance (Fig. 8–4). The grid ratio of crossed grids is equal to the sum of the ratios of the two linear grids. A crossed grid made up of two 5:1 linear grids has a ratio of 10:1, and functions about the same as a linear grid with a 10:1 ratio. Crossed grids cannot be used with oblique techniques requiring angulation of the x-ray tube, and this is their biggest disadvantage.

A **focused grid** is a grid made up of lead strips that are angled slightly so that they focus in space (Fig. 8–5). A focused grid may be either linear or crossed, because the focusing refers to the cross-sectional plane of the lead strips. Most grids are focused. Linear focused grids converge at a line in space called the **convergent line.** Crossed grids converge at a point in space called the **convergent point.** The **focal distance** is the perpendicular distance between the grid and the convergent line or point. In practice, grids have a focusing range that indicates the distance within which the grid can be used without a significant loss of primary radiation. The **focusing range** is fairly wide for a low-ratio grid and narrow for a high-ratio grid. A 5:1 grid focused at 40 in. has a focusing range of approximately 28 to 72 in., whereas a 16:1 grid

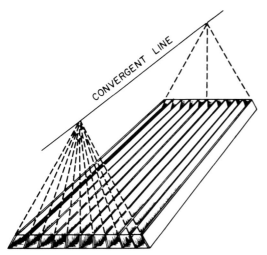

Figure 8–5 Focused linear grid

focused at 40 in. has a range of only 38 to 42 in. Focal ranges are indicated on the top of grids by manufacturers.

A **parallel grid** is one in which the lead strips are parallel when viewed in cross section. They are focused at infinity, so they do not have a convergent line. These grids can only be used effectively with either very small x-ray fields or long target-grid distances. They are frequently used in fluoroscopic spot film devices, but otherwise have little use in modern radiology.

Lines per inch is the number of lead strips per inch of grid. It can be calculated by adding the thickness of the lead strips and interspaces and dividing this sum into 1. Because the thickness of the lead strips and interspaces is usually expressed in millimeters, the answer must be multiplied by 25.4, which is the number of mm/in. The final equation is

$$\text{Lines/in.} = \frac{25.4}{D + d}$$

D = thickness of interspaces
d = thickness of lead strips
   (both in millimeters)

A grid (grid-front) cassette is a special x-ray cassette, usually used for portable radiography, with a grid built into the front of the cassette. Most grid cassettes are fo-

cused and have a fairly low grid ratio (4:1 to 8:1).

EVALUATION OF GRID PERFORMANCE

Grids are used to improve contrast by absorbing secondary radiation before it reaches the film. The "ideal grid" would absorb all secondary radiation and no primary radiation. It would give maximum film contrast without an unnecessary increase in patient exposure. The ideal grid does not exist, however, and the design of all grids is a compromise. The price of better film contrast is increased patient exposure. We must always compromise one for the other. Grids with high ratios give maximum contrast, but the improved contrast is not always worth the increased patient exposure. In every clinical situation we must weigh these two factors. To help in grid selection and design, several tests have been devised to evaluate grid performance. These tests also help us understand the way a grid functions. We will discuss three methods of evaluating performance:

1. primary transmission (Tp)
2. Bucky factor (B)
3. contrast improvement factor (K)

Primary Transmission

Primary transmission is a measurement of the percentage of primary radiation transmitted through a grid. Ideally, a grid should transmit 100% of the primary radiation, because it carries the radiographic image. The equipment for measuring primary transmission is shown in Figure 8–6. The x-ray beam is collimated to a narrow pencil of radiation, and the phantom is placed a great distance from the grid. With this arrangement, no scatter radiation reaches the grid. A small amount is produced in the phantom, but it diffuses out of the beam in the large air-gap between the phantom and the grid.

Two measurements must be made to de-

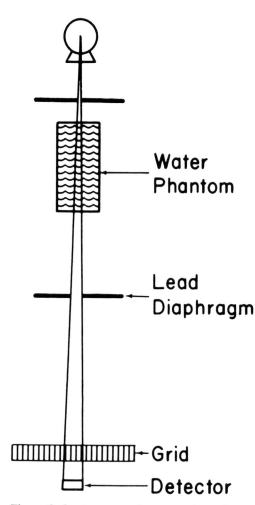

Figure 8–6 Apparatus for measuring primary transmission (Tp)

termine the percentage of primary transmission. The first measurement is made with the grid in place to determine the intensity of the radiation transmitted through the grid, and the second measurement is made after removal of the grid to determine the intensity of the radiation directed at the grid. A simple ratio of the intensity with the grid to the intensity without the grid gives the fractional transmission, which is multiplied by 100 to give the percentage of transmission:

$$T_p = \frac{I_p}{I'_p} \times 100$$

T_p = primary transmission (%)
I_p = intensity with grid
I'_p = intensity without grid

Table 8–1 shows the primary transmission for eight different grids. There is a significant loss of primary radiation with grids. For the eight grids tested, the primary transmission varied between 57 and 72.5%, and was generally lower for cross grids.

The primary transmission as measured experimentally is less than would be anticipated. If the geometric relationship between the lead strips and the x-ray target is accurate, so that there is no grid cutoff, and if no primary radiation is absorbed in the interspaces, then the percentage of the grid's surface area that is made up of interspaces will be the percentage of anticipated primary transmission. This merely determines the percentage of the grid surface area that is not lead, and is as close as we will ever come to an ideal grid. The equation for calculating the anticipated primary transmission is

$$\text{Calc. } Tp = \frac{D}{D + d} \times 100$$

Tp = anticipated primary transmission (%)
d = thickness of lead strips
D = thickness of interspaces

The measured primary transmission is always less than the calculated primary transmission.

The example in Figure 8–7 will help to demonstrate the magnitude of this difference. The dimensions are for grid number 8, shown in boldface in Table 8–1, which is a 15:1 grid with an experimentally determined primary transmission at 64%. Its lead strips are 60 μ thick and its interspaces are 390 μ wide. The calculated primary transmission is 87%, which is 23% more than the measured primary transmission. The difference is largely the result of absorption by the interspace material. Also, there is probably some loss in primary radiation because of manufacturing imperfections in the focusing of the lead strips.

Bucky Factor

The Bucky factor is the ratio of the incident radiation falling on the grid to the transmitted radiation passing through the

Table 8–1. Primary Transmission (Tp)

GRID NO.	GRID RATIO	LEAD STRIP THICKNESS, d (μ)	INTERSPACE THICKNESS, D (μ)	PRIMARY TRANSMISSIONS (μ)
1	3.4	50	320	67.5
2	2 × 3.1*	50	350	57
3	11	30	220	69
4	7	60	290	72.5
5	6	80	370	72.5
6	9	50	380	67
7	2 × 7*	50	370	72.5
8	**15**	**60**	**390**	**64**

(Modified from Hondius Boldingh.[1])
*Crossed grids

$$\text{Calc } Tp = \frac{D}{D + d} \times 100$$

$$" \quad = \frac{390}{390 + 60} \times 100$$

$$" \quad = \quad 87\%$$

Figure 8–7 Anticipated primary transmission

grid. It is a practical determination, because it indicates how much we must increase exposure factors when we change from a nongrid to a grid technique. It also tells us how much the patient's exposure dose is increased by the use of a grid. The Bucky factor is similar to primary transmission except for one difference. Primary transmission indicates only the amount of primary radiation absorbed by a grid, whereas the Bucky factor indicates the absorption of both primary and secondary radiation. It is determined with a large x-ray field and a thick phantom (Fig. 8–8). The transmitted radiation is measured with the grid in place, and the incident radiation is measured after the grid has been removed. The equation for calculating the Bucky factor (B) is

$$B = \frac{\text{incident radiation}}{\text{transmitted radiation}}$$

The Bucky factor is a measure of the total quantity of radiation absorbed from an x-ray beam by a grid so, in part, it is a

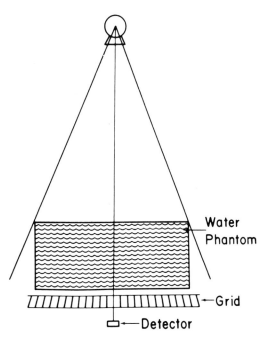

Figure 8–8 Apparatus for measuring the Bucky factor

measure of the grid's ability to absorb scatter radiation. Table 8–2 shows the Bucky factors for several different grids with two different energies of radiation. Generally, high-ratio grids absorb more scatter radiation and have larger Bucky factors than low-ratio grids. The size of the Bucky factor also depends on the energy of the x-ray beam. High-energy beams generate more scatter radiation and place a greater demand on a grid's performance than low-energy radiation. The Bucky factor for the 16:1 grid in Table 8–2 increases from 4.5 to 6 as the radiation energy increases from 70 to 120 kVp. More scatter radiation is generated by the 120-kVp beam, and the 16:1 grid successfully absorbs it. The 5:1 grid in Table 8–2, however, is not as efficient. Its Bucky factor is the same for both 70- and 120-kVp radiation. Low-ratio grids do not absorb scatter radiation from high-energy beams as well as high-ratio grids.

Although a high Bucky factor is desirable from the point of view of film quality, it is undesirable in two other respects. **The higher the Bucky factor, the greater the exposure factors and radiation dosage to the patient.** If the Bucky factor for a particular grid-energy combination is 5, then exposure factors and patient exposure both increase 5 times over what they would be for the same examination without a grid.

Contrast Improvement Factor

The contrast improvement factor (K) is the ratio of the contrast with a grid to the contrast without a grid:

$$K = \frac{\text{contrast with a grid}}{\text{contrast without a grid}}$$

This is the ultimate test of grid performance because it is a measure of a grid's ability to improve contrast, which is its primary function.

Unfortunately, the contrast improvement factor depends on kVp, field size, and phantom thickness. This is understandable, because these three factors determine the amount of scatter radiation. The larger

Table 8–2.   Bucky Factor (B)

GRID RATIO	70 kVp	120 kVp
No grid	1	1
5:1	3	3
8:1	3.5	4
12:1	4	5
16:1	4.5	6

the quantity of scatter radiation, the poorer the contrast, and the lower the contrast improvement factor. To permit comparison of different grids, the contrast improvement factor is usually determined at 100 kVp with a large field and a phantom 20 cm thick, as recommended by the International Commission on Radiologic Units and Measurements.[3] Table 8–3 shows the contrast improvement factor for eight different grids. It is more closely related to the lead content of the grid than any other factor. Generally, the higher the grid ratio, the higher the contrast improvement factor, but grid ratio is not as reliable an indicator as lead content.

Although the contrast improvement factor of a particular grid depends on kVp, field size, and part thickness, the relative quality of two grids appears to be independent of these factors. A grid that has a high contrast improvement factor at 100 kVp will have a high factor at 50 or 130 kVp. In comparing two grids, the one that performs better with low energy radiation will also perform better with high energy radiation.

Table 8–3.   Contrast Improvement Factor (K)

GRID NO.	GRID RATIO	LEAD CONTENT (mg/cm²)	CONTRAST IMPROVEMENT FACTOR (K)
1	3.4	170	1.95
2	2 × 3.1*	310	1.95
3	11	340	2.1
4	7	390	2.1
5	9	460	2.35
6	15	460	2.6
7	2 × 7*	680	2.95
8	15	900	2.95

(Modified from Hondius Boldingh.[1])
*Crossed grids.

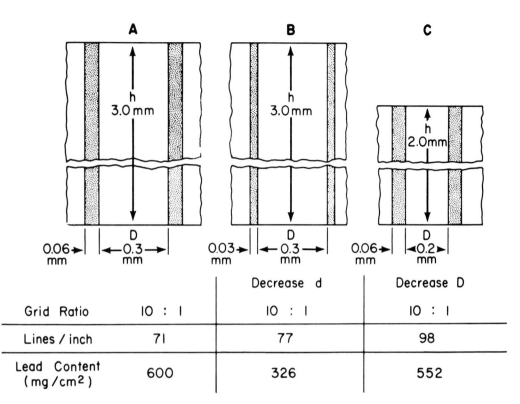

Figure 8–9 Relationship between grid ratio, lines per inch, and lead content of a grid

LEAD CONTENT

The lead content of a grid is expressed in g/cm². An easy way to understand what this means is to imagine cutting a grid up into 1-cm squares and then weighing one square. Its weight in grams is the lead content of the grid (ignoring the interspace material). The amount of lead in a grid is a good indicator of its ability to improve contrast, provided the grid is well designed. Poor design would be a solid sheet of lead.

There is a definite relationship between the grid ratio, lead content, and number of lines per inch (Fig. 8–9). If the grid ratio remains constant and the number of lines per inch is increased, the lead content must decrease. The only ways to increase the number of lines per inch is by decreasing the thickness of either the lead strips or interspaces. If the lead strips are made thinner, as in Figure 8–9B, compared to Figure 8–9A, the number of lines per inch increases without affecting grid ratio, because the thickness of lead strips is not considered in determining grid ratio. When the lead strips are made thinner, however, there is only a small increase in the number of lines per inch at a cost of a large decrease in lead content. If the number of lines per inch is increased by decreasing the width of the interspaces, as in Figure 8–9C, then the lead strips must be made shorter to keep the grid ratio constant and, again, the lead content of the grid decreases. This puts a limitation on the number of lines per inch a grid may have and still be effective. If a 10:1 grid could be constructed with 1000 lines per inch, it would be only 0.2 mm thick, and it would have too little lead to be of any real value.

In practice, when grids are constructed with many lines per inch, both the thickness and height of the lead strips are decreased. These grids are thinner, and improve contrast less than grids of comparable ratios with fewer lines per inch. A 133-line 10:1 grid improves contrast about the same as an 80-line 8:1 grid.

GRID CUTOFF

The primary disadvantage of grids is that they increase the amount of radiation that the patient receives. Another disadvantage is that they require careful centering of the x-ray tube because of the danger of grid cutoff. Grid cutoff is the loss of primary radiation that occurs when the images of the lead strips are projected wider than they would be with ordinary magnification (Fig. 8–10). It is the result of a poor geometric relationship between the primary beam and the lead foil strips of the grid. Cutoff is complete and no primary radiation reaches the film when the projected images of the lead strips are thicker than the width of the interspaces. The resultant radiograph will be light in the area in which the cutoff occurs. With linear grids there may be uniform lightening of the whole film, one edge of the

Figure 8–10 Grid cutoff

film, or both edges of the film, depending on how the cutoff is produced. The amount of cutoff is always greatest with high-ratio grids and short grid-focus distances. There are four situations that produce grid cutoff:

1. focused grids used upside down
2. lateral decentering (grid angulation)
3. focus-grid distance decentering
4. combined lateral and focus-grid distance decentering

Upside Down Focused Grid

All focused grids have a tube side, which is the side of focus of the lead strips. When a focused grid is used upside down, there is severe peripheral cutoff with a dark band of exposure in the center of the film and no exposure at the film's periphery. Figure 8–11A illustrates how cutoff occurs, and Figure 8–11B shows the resultant radiograph. The higher the grid ratio, the narrower the exposed area. When a crossed grid is used upside down, only a small square in the center of the film is exposed.

Lateral Decentering

Lateral decentering results from the x-ray tube being positioned lateral to the convergent line but at the correct focal distance (Fig. 8–12A). All the lead strips cut off the same amount of primary radiation, so there is **a uniform loss of radiation over the entire surface of the grid, producing a uniformly light radiograph.** This is probably the most common kind of grid cutoff, but it cannot be recognized by inspection of the film. All we see is a light film that is usually attributed to incorrect exposure factors. Figure 8–12B shows a series of film strips that were all taken with the same exposure factors, but with increasing amounts of lateral decentering. The x-ray tube was centered at the convergent line for the film strip on the left, and then laterally decentered 1, 2, and 3 in. for the next three strips. The films become progressively lighter as the amount of lateral decentering increases, but the exposure is

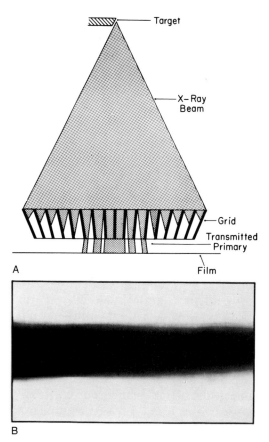

Figure 8–11 Cutoff from an upside down focused grid *(A)* and radiograph resulting from an upside down focused grid *(B)*

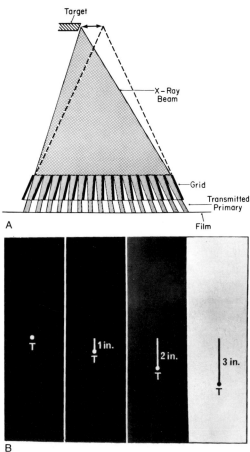

Figure 8–12 Cutoff from lateral decentering, *(A)* and series of radiographs resulting from increasing amounts of lateral decentering *(B)*

still uniform. The center and both edges of the film are equally exposed, and it's impossible to recognize the cutoff from inspection of the film.

Three factors affect the magnitude of cutoff from lateral decentering: grid ratio, focal distance, and the amount of decentering. The equation for calculating the loss of primary radiation with lateral decentering is

$$L = \frac{rb}{f_0} \times 100$$

L = loss of primary radiation (%)
r = grid ratio
b = lateral decentering distance (inches)
f_0 = focal distance of grid (inches)

The amount of cutoff increases as the grid ratio and decentering distance increase, and cutoff decreases as the focal distance increases (Tables 8–4 and 8–5). The loss of primary radiation for any given amount of lateral decentering can be minimized with low-ratio grids and a long focal distance. With a 5:1 grid focused at 72 in., there is a 14% loss of primary radiation with 2 in. of lateral decentering. If the grid ratio is increased to 16:1, the loss of primary radiation increases to 45%, and if the focal distance is then decreased to 40 in., the loss of primary radiation goes up to 80%. When exact centering is not possible, as in portable radiography, low-ratio grids and long focal distances should be used

Table 8–4. Loss of Primary Radiation from Lateral Decentering for Grids Focused at 40 Inches

GRID RATIO	LOSS OF PRIMARY RADIATION (%)					
	LATERAL DECENTERING (in.)					
	1	2	3	4	5	6
5:1	13	25	38	50	63	75
6:1	15	30	45	60	75	90
8:1	20	40	60	80	100	
10:1	25	50	75	100		
12:1	30	60	90	100		
16:1	40	80	100			

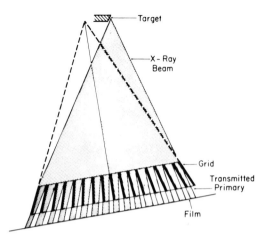

Figure 8–13 Cutoff from an off-level grid

whenever possible. It takes 8 in. of lateral decentering for 100% cutoff of primary radiation with a 5:1 grid focused at 72 in., whereas it takes only 2.5 inches of lateral decentering for complete cutoff with a 16:1 grid focused at 40 in.

Off-Level Grids. When a linear grid is tilted, as it frequently is in portable radiography, there is a uniform loss of primary radiation across the entire surface of the grid (Fig. 8–13). The effect on the film is the same as the effect of lateral decentering.

Focus-Grid Distance Decentering

In focus-grid distance decentering, the target of the x-ray tube is correctly centered to the grid, but it is positioned above or below the convergent line. If the target is above the convergent line, it is called **far** focus-grid distance decentering; if the target is below the convergent line, it is called **near** focus-grid distance decentering. The results are the same, but they differ in mag-

nitude. The cutoff is greater with near than with far focus-grid distance decentering. Figures 8–14 and 8–15 show the cutoff becoming progressively greater with increasing distance from the film center. The central portion of the film is not affected, but the periphery is light. Because the fractional loss of radiation is not uniform, it must be calculated for a point, which actually represents two parallel lines running the length of the grid on either side of the center line. The loss of primary radiation is directly proportional to the grid ratio and distance from the center line.

Table 8–5. Loss of Primary Radiation from Lateral Decentering for Grids Focused at 72 Inches

GRID RATIO	LOSS OF PRIMARY RADIATION (%)					
	LATERAL DECENTERING (in.)					
	1	2	3	4	5	6
5:1	7	14	21	28	35	42
6:1	8	17	25	33	42	50
8:1	11	22	33	45	56	67
10:1	14	28	42	56	70	83
12:1	17	33	50	67	83	100
16:1	22	45	67	90	100	

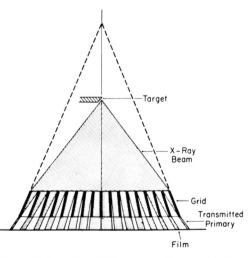

Figure 8–14 Cutoff from near focus-grid distance decentering

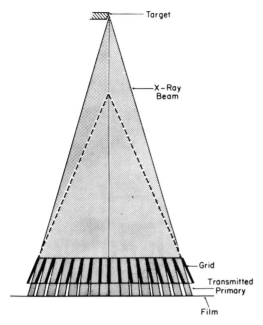

Figure 8–15 Cutoff from far focus-grid distance decentering

The equations for calculating the loss of primary radiation for near and far focus-grid distance decentering are as follows:

Near Focus-Grid Distance Decentering	Far Focus-Grid Distance Decentering

$$L = rc\left(\frac{1}{f_1} - \frac{1}{f_0}\right) \times 100 \qquad L = rc\left(\frac{1}{f_0} - \frac{1}{f_2}\right) \times 100$$

L = loss of primary radiation at point c (%)
r = grid ratio
f_0 = grid focusing distance
f_1 = target-grid distance (below convergent line; inches),
f_2 = the target-grid distance (above convergent line; inches)
c = distance from center of grid (inches)

Table 8–6 shows the extent of cutoff at various distances from the center of grids focusing at 40 in. with a 10-in. focus-grid distance decentering error. The left half of the table indicates near (30 in.) and the right half far (50 in.) focus-grid distance decentering. The loss of primary radiation increases as the grid ratio increases and as the distance from the center of the grid increases; the loss is greater with near than

with far focus-grid distance decentering. At the margin of a 14-in. wide film (7 in. from grid center), the loss of primary radiation is 35% for a 6:1 grid and 94% for a 16:1 grid with near focus-grid distance decentering. With far focus-grid distance decentering, the loss at the film margin decreases to 21% for a 6:1 grid and 64% for a 16:1 grid.

Parallel grids are focused at infinity so, of course, they are always used with near focus-grid distance decentering (Fig. 8–16). They usually have a low grid ratio to minimize cutoff. The only time there is no significant cutoff is with long target-grid distances or small fields. A film taken with a parallel grid has a dark center and light edges because of near focus-grid distance decentering.

Combined Lateral and Focus-Grid Distance Decentering

The most commonly recognized kind of grid cutoff is from combined lateral and focus-grid distance decentering. It is probably not as common as lateral decentering alone, but lateral decentering cannot be recognized as such on the resultant radiograph. Combined decentering is easy to recognize. It causes an uneven exposure, resulting in a film that is light on one side and dark on the other side. There are two kinds of combined decentering, depending on whether the tube target is above or below the convergent line. The amount of cutoff is directly proportional to the grid ratio and decentering distance, and inversely proportional to the focal distance of the grid. With high-ratio grids and large decentering errors, there is a large loss of primary radiation. With long focus-grid distances, there is less loss of primary radiation.

Combined lateral and focus-grid distance decentering above the convergent line is illustrated in Figure 8–17. The projected images of the lead strips directly below the tube target are broader than those on the opposite side, and the film is light

Table 8–6. Loss of Primary Radiation from Near and Far Focus-Grid Distance Decentering for a Grid Focused at 40 Inches

	LOSS OF PRIMARY RADIATION (%)							
	TARGET AT 30 in.				TARGET AT 50 in.			
GRID RATIO	DISTANCE FROM GRID CENTER (in.)				DISTANCE FROM GRID CENTER (in.)			
	1	3	5	7	1	3	5	7
6:1	5	15	25	35	3	9	15	21
8:1	7	20	33	47	4	12	20	28
10:1	8	25	42	58	5	15	25	35
12:1	10	30	50	70	6	18	30	42
16:1	13	40	66	94	8	32	48	64

on the near side. Cutoff is greatest on the side directly under the x-ray tube. Combined lateral and focus-grid distance decentering below the convergent line is illustrated in Figure 8–18. The projected images of the lead strips are broader on the side opposite the tube target than on the same side, and the film is light on the far side. Cutoff is least on the side under the x-ray tube. With equal decentering errors the amount of cutoff is greater with combined decentering below the convergent line than with combined decentering above the convergent line.

MOVING GRIDS

The moving grid was invented by Dr. Hollis E. Potter in 1920 and, for many years, a moving grid was called a Potter-Bucky grid. In recent years the name has been shortened to Bucky grid, which is unfortunate, because the name of the inventor is omitted. Grids are moved to blur out the shadows cast by the lead strips. Most moving grids are reciprocating, which means they continuously move 1 to 3 cm back and forth throughout the exposure. They start moving when the x-ray tube an-

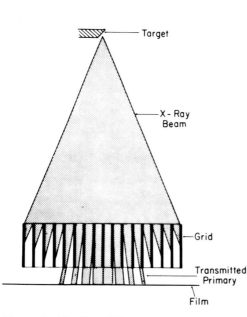

Figure 8–16 Cutoff from a parallel grid

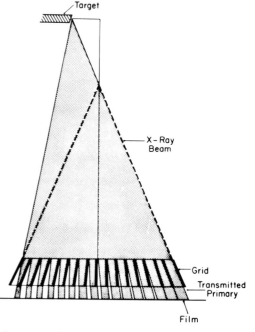

Figure 8–17 Cutoff from combined lateral and far focus-grid distance decentering

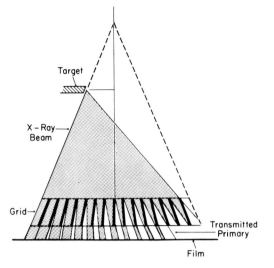

Figure 8–18 Cutoff from combined lateral and near focus-grid distance decentering

ode begins to rotate. Older grids move only in one direction and must be cocked for each exposure. They also have timers that are set for a little longer than the exposure time to avoid grid lines. These single-stroke grids are inconvenient, and are seldom used in modern equipment.

Moving grids are advantageous because they eliminate grid lines from the film. Many years ago this was important, because the lead strips were thick and unevenly spaced. With improved manufacturing methods, however, grids have improved so that grid lines are not nearly as distracting, and many radiologists now prefer stationary grids.

If you are using a moving grid and want to avoid grid lines, you must take two precautions. First, the grid must move fast enough to blur its lead strips. If it moves too slowly, you will see either the grid lines themselves or random density variations in the film that are just as distracting as the lines. Second, the transverse motion of the grid should be synchronous with the pulses of the x-ray generator. When this happens, the shadow of each lead strip is superimposed on the shadow of its neighbor. Each pulse produces a faint image of the lead

strip on the film. Between pulses, the grid moves one interspace distance so that the next lead strip is over the position of the preceding strip and, with a new pulse, the two images are superimposed. Thus, even though the grid moves, the grid lines will be distinct.

Moving grids have several disadvantages. They are costly, subject to failure, may vibrate the x-ray table, and put a limit on the minimum exposure time because they move slowly. An even more serious disadvantage is that they increase the patient's radiation dose. There are two reasons for this, the first of which is lateral decentering. Because the grid moves 1 to 3 cm during the exposure, the tube is not centered directly over the center of the grid during most of the exposure. This lateral decentering may result in a loss of as much as 20% of the primary radiation with a high-ratio grid and a short focusing distance.

The second cause of increased patient exposure is more difficult to understand. The photons are spread out uniformly on the film by a moving grid. With the identical number of photons per unit area, a film is 15% darker with a stationary grid because the photons are concentrated between the lead strips. Figure 8–19 attempts to illustrate how this happens. The total quantity of density (blackness) on the film is represented by the water level in Figure 8–19*A*. This is the amount of density that is spread out uniformly over the film by a moving grid. In Figure 8–19*B* a grid is immersed in the water to represent the grid lines on a film. Now all the water is con-

Figure 8–19 Analogy between water level and film density for moving and stationary grids

centrated between the grid lines, and the water level rises just as the amount of blackness on the film rises. The total quantity of density on the film is the same with both moving and stationary grids, but with stationary grids the film is made up of many narrow voids (grid lines) containing no density, interspersed with black lines containing all the density.

GRID SELECTION

There is no simple rule to guide the clinician in choosing a grid for any particular situation. A compromise is always involved. The price of increased "cleanup" with high-ratio grids is that patient exposure is considerably increased and that x-ray tube centering becomes more critical. You must weigh the value of a better-quality radiograph against your moral obligation to keep the patient's exposure at a minimum. There is little to be gained using high ratio grids in the low kVp range. Usually, **8:1 grids will give adequate results below 90 kVp. Above 90 kVp, 12:1 grids are preferred.** Crossed grids are only used when

there is a great deal of scatter radiation, such as in biplane cerebral angiography.

The efficiency of scatter radiation absorption by various grids is shown in Figure 8–20, which plots the fractional transmission of scatter radiation against grid ratio. There is little decrease in transmitted scatter beyond an 8:1 ratio grid, and almost no change between 12:1 and 16:1. For this reason 12:1 grids are preferable to 16:1 grids for routine radiography. The improvement in film quality in going from a 12:1 to a 16:1 grid is not worth the greater patient exposure.

AIR GAP TECHNIQUES

The x-ray grid is the most important means of reducing scatter radiation with large radiographic fields but, under certain circumstances, an alternate method, an air gap, produces comparable results with less patient exposure. The basic principle of the air gap technique is quite simple. Scatter radiation arising in the patient from Compton reactions disperses in all directions, so the patient acts like a large light bulb (Fig. 8–21A). In the illustration, scattered photons are shown radiating out from a point source, but the point actually represents a tiny block of tissue. Each ray represents a separate scattering event, and numerous scatterings within the small block produce the array shown. The closer the patient is to the film, the greater the concentration of scatter per unit area. With an air gap, the concentration decreases because more scattered photons miss the film. The name "air filtration" has been applied to air gap techniques, but this is a misnomer. **Scatter radiation decreases not from filtration but from scattered photons missing the film.** Negligible quantities of radiation are absorbed in the gap, and the beam is not appreciably hardened, so the name "air filtration" should be discarded.

There is no strong bias for forward scattering in the diagnostic energy range, so the distribution of Compton scattering is nearly random. A photon is almost as likely

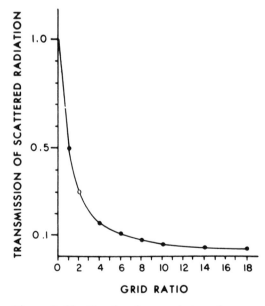

Figure 8–20   Fractional transmission of scatter radiation through grids (Courtesy of Sven Ledin and the Elema Shoenander Company)

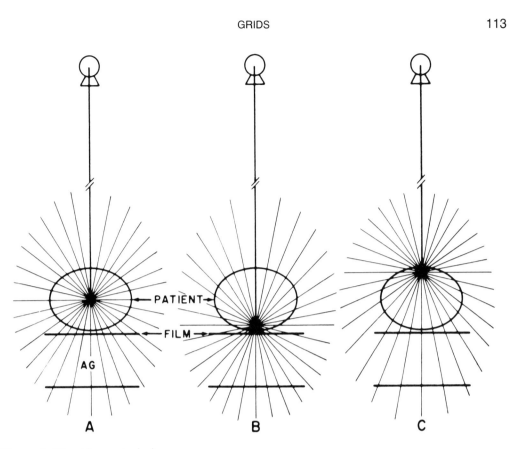

Figure 8–21 Air gap techniques

to scatter at 90° as at 45°, or 180°. With increasing energy, more photons scatter in the forward direction, but the increase is negligible in the diagnostic range. When the energy of the incident photon is increased from 10 to 140 keV, a much greater change than is likely in clinical radiology, the most probable angle of scatter only changes from 53° to 45°.[4] With a strong forward bias, as in megavoltage therapy, air gaps are ineffective as a means of controlling scatter radiation.

Figure 8–21B and C compares the distribution of scattered radiation arising from superficial tissue blocks on opposite sides of the patient. More radiation reaches the film from scattering near the exit surface (Fig. 8–21B), because the film intercepts a larger angle of the scattered "beam." The angle of interception is smaller for scattering occurring on the input side of the patient (Fig. 8–21C), be-

cause a natural "gap" separates the film from the scattering site. The difference in the contribution from the two sides is even greater than the illustration implies. Many scattered photons from the input surface (Fig. 8–21C) are absorbed during their long journey through the patient, whereas those originating near the exit surface (Fig. 8–21B) have only a short escape distance. As a result of these two factors, a greater angle of capture and less tissue attenuation, most of the scattered photons reaching the film arise in the immediately adjacent superficial tissue layers, an ideal arrangement for an air gap technique. You can see from the illustration that the air gap is most effective in removing scatter radiation when the scatter originates close to the film (Fig. 8–21B).

Optimum Gap Width

Air gap techniques are used in two clinical situations, magnification radiography and chest radiography. With magnification techniques the object-film distance is optimized for the screen-focal spot combination and the air gap reduces the scatter radiation to acceptable levels as an incidental bonus. In chest radiography the air gap is used instead of a grid and techniques are designed around the air gap. For example, image sharpness deteriorates as the gap widens, so the focal-film distance is usually lengthened from 6 to 10 ft to restore sharpness. Air gaps and grids have the same function, to remove as much scatter radiation and as little primary radiation as possible. As a measure of performance, gap width is analogous to grid ratio. A large air gap, like a higher ratio grid, removes a larger percentage of scatter radiation.

Figure 8–22 shows the ratio of scatter to primary radiation with air gap widths from ⅝ to 15 in. for three different absorber thicknesses. A ratio of 5 means that 5 scattered photons reach the film for each primary photon. At the ideal ratio of zero, all the transmitted photons are primary. As the gap increases, the ratio of secondary to primary radiation decreases, but the

change is gradual without an abrupt transition point. The optimum gap width is a matter of judgment. The following four guidelines should be used to select a gap width:

1. The thicker the part, the more advantageous a larger gap. Figure 8–22 shows that a change from a 1- to a 15-in. width produces a more marked decrease in scatter radiation for a 22-cm phantom than for a 10-cm phantom.

2. The first inch of air gap improves contrast more than any subsequent inch. The increase from a 1- to a 2-in. gap improves contrast more than an increase from a 14- to a 15-in. gap.

3. Image sharpness deteriorates with increasing gap width unless the focal-film distance is increased to compensate for the greater magnification. An increase in focal-film distance from 6 to 10 ft is customary in chest radiography to compensate for this loss of sharpness. A further increase in focal-film distance is usually not physically possible because of space limitations, or technically feasible at an acceptable exposure time because of the heat tolerance of the x-ray tube. Remember, a 50% increase in distance doubles the exposure factors.

4. If the gap is widened by moving the patient away from the film with a fixed focal-film distance, the patient is closer to the x-ray tube and his exposure increases. The increase can be corrected by a comparable increase in the focal-film distance, but this may not be a possible alternative for the reasons stated above.

Table 8–7 shows that a 5-in. air gap approaches the performance of a light (7:1)

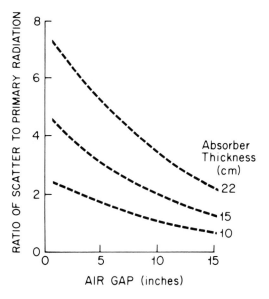

Figure 8–22 Ratio of scatter to primary radiation for various air gaps and absorber thicknesses

Table 8–7. Comparative Contrast Improvement Factors for Grid and Air Gap Techniques (100 kVp, 30- × 30-cm Field)

| ABSORBER THICKNESS (cm OF WATER) | CONTRAST IMPROVEMENT FACTOR | | | |
| | AIR GAP | | GRID | |
	5 in.	10 in.	7:1	15:1
10	1.39	1.81	1.50	1.85
20	1.37	2.21	2.10	2.85

(Data from Gould and Hale.[4])

grid for thin patients. A 10-in. gap is the same as a heavy (15:1) grid for thin patients, but not as good for thicker patients. The final decision on air gap width is usually made empirically. Changing widths from patient to patient is inconvenient. Experience has shown that a 10-in. gap and a 10-ft focal-film distance with an energy from 110 to 150 kVp produces satisfactory results.

Exposure Factors with Air Gaps

Figure 8–23 compares a 6-ft focal-film distance (FFD) with a grid to a 10-ft focal film distance with a 10-in. air gap. The exposure factor, patient exposure, and transmitted primary radiation are all assigned a value of one for the grid technique, which is used as the standard for comparison. In this example, the primary transmission of the grid is 65%, and the experimental design was chosen to produce films of equal density (same total number of photons) and contrast (same ratio of primary to secondary photons). The x-ray tube exposure

must be increased for the air gap technique because of the larger focal-film distance. Applying the inverse square law (constant KVp), exposures would have to be increased 2.8 times ($120^2 \div 72^2 = 2.8$) but the actual increase is somewhat less, because only 65% of the primary photons are transmitted through the grid. The increase is 1.8 times ($2.8 \times 0.65 = 1.8$), a substantial difference that taxes the heat capacity of the x-ray tube.

Patient exposures are usually less with air gaps than grids, because grids absorb primary photons. With the grid technique shown in Figure 8–23, 1.54 primary photons must pass through the patient for each one reaching the film ($1.0 \div 0.65 = 1.54$); the difference (35%) is absorbed in the grid. Only 1.19 primary photons need pass through the patient with the air gap technique to produce a comparable concentration per unit area of film; the difference ($1.19 - 1.0 = 0.19$ or 19%) is lost as a consequence of the inverse square law. The air gap loses less primary radiation, so the patient's exposure is less. If the patient exposure is unity with the grid, it will be 0.77 with the air gap ($1.19 \div 1.54 = 0.77$), a significant but not dramatic savings.

Magnification with Air Gaps

Two factors determine the amount of magnification, the object-film distance and the focal-film distance. Magnification is greatest with a short focal-film distance and a long object-film distance. As a general rule, image sharpness deteriorates with magnification. The objective with an air gap technique is to preserve image sharpness by lengthening the focal-film distance until magnification returns to pre-air-gap levels. Some deterioration is inevitable, however, for parts close to the film. Figure 8–24 shows that the objective is not accomplished with a 120-in. focal-film distance, at least not for a 10-in. air gap and a reasonably sized (10-in. thick) patient. Magnification is less with the 72-in. focal-film distance for all object-film distances up to

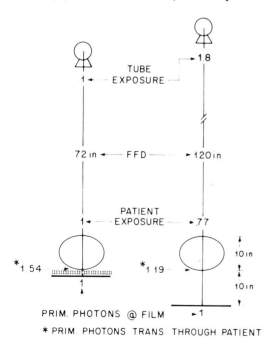

Figure 8–23 Comparison of grid and air gap techniques for chest radiography

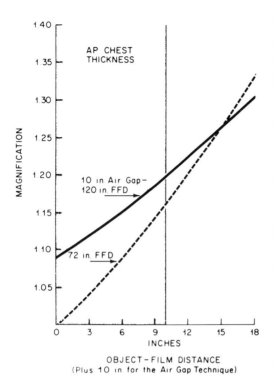

Figure 8–24 Magnification with 72-inch (no air gap) and 120-inch (air gap) focal-film distances (FFD)

15 in. The longer focal-film distance produces a more uniform magnification from the front to the back of the patient, a desirable characteristic. This uniformity is preserved with lesser air gaps. With a 5-in. gap, the curve would maintain its slope but would slide down the magnification scale to cross the 72-in. curve at a shorter object-film distance. Experienced chest radiographers do not feel that image sharpness deteriorates noticeably with air gap techniques.

SUMMARY

Radiographic grids consist of lead foil strips separated by x-ray transparent spacers. They are used to absorb scatter radiation and to improve radiographic image contrast. The grid ratio is defined as the ratio of the height of the lead strips to the distance between them, and it is the sim-

plest way of characterizing a grid. Grids come in two patterns, linear and crossed. Crossed grids consist of two superimposed linear grids; their great disadvantage is that they cannot be used with oblique techniques. Most grids are focused to a line in space called a convergent line, but they can be used over a variable range of distances called the "focal range."

Three tests have been devised to evaluate grid performance. (1) Primary transmission is a measurement of the percentage of primary radiation transmitted through a grid (usually between 60 and 70%). (2) The Bucky factor is a measurement of the total radiation (primary and scatter) absorbed by a grid. It indicates how much exposure factors must be increased because of grids, and also reveals how much more radiation the patient receives. Bucky factors range from 3 to 7, depending on the grid ratio. (3) The contrast improvement factor is a measurement of a grid's ability to improve contrast, and it is the best test of grid performance. Generally, high-ratio grids with a high lead content have the highest contrast improvement factors.

The grid ratio, lead content, and number of lines per inch are all interrelated. A grid with many lines per inch (over 100) is generally thinner and has a lower lead content than a grid of comparable ratio with fewer lines per inch.

Grid cutoff is the loss of primary radiation that occurs when the images of the lead strips are produced wider than they would be with ordinary magnification. The amount of cutoff with a particular decentering error is greatest with high-ratio grids that have a short focusing distance. Lateral decentering is the most common error, and it causes a uniform loss of primary radiation, so it is impossible to recognize on the film. With focus-grid distance decentering, the film is light on both sides, whereas with combined lateral and focus-grid distance decentering, the film is light only on one side.

Moving grids eliminate the image of the

lead strips from the film, and this is their chief advantage. Generally, exposure factors are a little greater with moving grids than with stationary grids because of a lateral decentering error during a portion of the exposure, and because the exposure is spread out over the entire surface of the film. With properly positioned stationary grids there is no decentering error, and the exposure is concentrated between the lead strips.

Grid selection involves a compromise between film quality and patient exposure. High-ratio grids produce films with better contrast at a cost of increased patient exposure. Generally, low-ratio grids are adequate for low energy radiation; 8:1 grids should be used with energies less than 90 kVp, and 12:1 grids for higher energy radiation.

Air gaps are an alternative method of eliminating scatter radiation with large radiographic fields. The intensity of scatter radiation is maximum at the patient's surface and diminishes rapidly at increasing distance from the surface. If the film is placed at a distance, the scatter simply misses the film. Focal-film distances are increased with air gap techniques in an attempt to maintain image sharpness and, as a consequence, x-ray exposure factors are greater with the air gaps than grids. Patient exposures are generally less with air gaps, however, because the grid absorbs some primary radiation.

REFERENCES

1. Hondius Boldingh, W.: Grids to reduce scattered x-ray in medical radiography. Eindhoven, Netherlands, Philips Research Laboratories, 1964, No. 1, Philips Research Reports Supplement.
2. Characteristics and Applications of X-Ray Grids, rev. ed. Liebel Flarsheim Company, 1968.
3. International Commission on Radiologic Units and Measurements: Methods of Evaluating Radiologic Equipment and Materials. Washington, DC, U.S. Government Printing Office, National Bureau of Standards, Handbook 89, August, 1963.
4. Gould, R.G., and Hale, J.: Control of scattered radiation by air gap techniques: Applications to chest radiography. Am. J. Roentgenol., *122*:109, 1974.

9 *Luminescent Screens*

The x-ray photons making up the radiographic image cannot be seen by the human eye. This information is converted into a visual image by one of two methods. A photographic emulsion can be exposed to the x rays directly. More commonly, the energy of the x rays is converted into radiation in the visible light spectrum, and this light may be used to expose x-ray film (radiography or photofluorography), or the light may be viewed directly (fluoroscopy). The sensitivity of film to direct x-ray exposure is low. Direct exposure of film would require prohibitively large patient x-ray doses for most examinations. Therefore, almost all radiographic film examinations require that the radiographic image be converted into light at some stage by a luminescent screen.

FLUORESCENCE

Luminescence refers to the emission of light by a substance. It can be caused by varying kinds of stimuli (e.g., light, chemical reactions, or ionizing radiation). The term **fluorescence** is applied to that form of luminescence produced when light is emitted instantaneously (within 10^{-8} sec of the stimulation). If the emission of light is delayed beyond 10^{-8} sec, the term **phosphorescence** is used.

Fluorescence, as used in radiology, is **the ability of crystals of certain inorganic salts** (called phosphors) **to emit light when excited by x rays.** For many years the crystals, or phosphors, of importance in radiology were calcium tungstate (the phosphor in intensifying screens) and zinc cadmium sulfide (the phosphor in fluores-cent and photofluorographic screens). Recent advances in technology have resulted in the introduction of a number of new phosphors, such as cesium iodide in image intensifier tubes and several new intensifying screen phosphors, including barium strontium sulfate, yttrium, and the rare earths gadolinium and lanthanum, and the rare earth tantalates.

INTENSIFYING SCREENS

Intensifying screens are used because they **decrease the x-ray dose** to the patient, yet still afford a properly exposed x-ray film. Also, the reduction in exposure allows use of short exposure times, which becomes important when it is necessary to minimize patient motion.

The x-ray film used with intensifying screens has photosensitive emulsion on both sides. The film is sandwiched between two intensifying screens in a cassette, so that the emulsion on each side is exposed to the light from its contiguous screen. Remember, the screen functions to absorb the energy (and information) in the x-ray beam that has penetrated the patient, and to convert this energy into a light pattern that has (as nearly as possible) the same information as the original x-ray beam. The light, then, forms a latent image on x-ray film. The transfer of information from x-ray beam to screen light to film results in some loss of information. In this and subsequent chapters we will discuss some factors involved in the degradation of information and describe what can be done to keep this to a minimum.

Construction

An intensifying screen has four layers:

1. a base, or support, made of plastic or cardboard
2. a reflecting layer (TiO$_2$)
3. a phosphor layer
4. a plastic protective coat

The total thickness of a typical intensifying screen is about 15 or 16 mils (1 mil = 0.001 in. = 0.0254 mm).

Base. The screen support, or base, may be made of high-grade cardboard or of a polyester plastic. The base of Du Pont intensifying screens is a polyester plastic (Mylar*) that is 10 mils thick (10 mils = 254 μm). Kodak X-Omatic and Lanex screens have a similar (Estar†) base 7 mils thick.

Reflecting Coat. The light produced by the interaction of x-ray photons and phosphor crystals is emitted in all directions. Much of the light is emitted from the screen in the direction of the film. Many light photons, however, are also directed toward the back of the screen (i.e., toward the base layer) and would be lost as far as photographic activity is concerned. The reflecting layer acts to reflect light back toward the front of the screen. The reflecting coat is made of a white substance, such as titanium dioxide (TiO$_2$), and is spread over the base in a thin layer, about 1 mil thick. Some screens do not have a reflecting layer (e.g., Kodak X-Omatic fine and regular).

Phosphor Layer. The phosphor layer, containing phosphor crystals, is applied over the reflecting coat or base. The crystals are suspended in a plastic (polymer) containing a substance to keep the plastic flexible. We will discuss the phosphor in more detail later. The thickness of the phosphor layer is about 4 mils for par speed screens. The thickness of the phosphor layer is increased 1 or 2 mils in high-speed screens, and is decreased slightly in detail screens.

*Mylar is a trademark of E. I. du Pont de Nemours and Company, Inc.
†Estar is a trademark of Eastman Kodak Company.

Protective Layer. The protective layer applied over the phosphor is made of a plastic, largely composed of a cellulose compound that is mixed with other polymers. It forms a layer about 0.7 to 0.8 mils thick. This layer serves three functions: it helps to prevent static electricity; it gives physical protection to the delicate phosphor layer; and it provides a surface that can be cleaned without damaging the phosphor layer.

Figure 9–1 shows a cross section of a typical par speed intensifying screen with a plastic base. Unlike the highly mechanized operation of x-ray film production, screens are largely a product of hand labor.

Phosphor

The original phosphor used in x-ray intensifying screens was **crystalline calcium tungstate** (CaWO$_4$). New (since about 1973) screen phosphor technology is being developed to increase screen speed over that available with calcium tungstate, and has resulted in the introduction of a bewildering variety of screens and corresponding films. Let us first consider calcium tungstate and then review some of the new phosphors.

Natural calcium tungstate (scheelite) is no longer used because synthetic calcium tungstate of better quality is produced by fusing sodium tungstate and calcium chloride under carefully controlled conditions. The first commercial calcium tungstate screens were made in England and Germany in 1896; they were first made in the United States in 1912. The calcium tungstate crystal must be absolutely free of any contaminant if it is to fluoresce properly. **It**

Figure 9–1 Par speed x-ray intensifying screen (cross section)

produces light primarily in the blue region of the visible spectrum, with a wavelength range of 3500 to 5800 Å (1 angstrom = 0.0001 μ = 0.00000001 cm) and a peak wavelength of about 4300 Å (430 nm), which is seen by the eye as a violet color. Although the eye is not sensitive to light of this wavelength, x-ray film emulsion exhibits maximum sensitivity to light from calcium tungstate screens. Figure 9–2 diagrams the spectrum of calcium tungstate fluorescence, the response of the eye to light of different wavelengths, and the sensitivity of x-ray film. Film sensitivity is seen to be high throughout most of the range of light emitted by the screen, a fact that ensures maximum photographic effect. Note that the film does not exhibit photosensitivity to red light, so red light can be used in the darkroom without producing any photographic effect on the film.

Intensifying Action of Screens. An intensifying screen is used because it can convert a few absorbed x-ray photons into many light photons. The **efficiency with which the phosphor converts x rays to light is termed the intrinsic conversion efficiency of the phosphor;** this is more accurately defined as the ratio of the light energy liberated by the crystal to the x-ray energy absorbed. The intrinsic conversion efficiency of calcium tungstate is about 5%. If the energy of the absorbed x-ray photon, the wavelength of the emitted light, and

the conversion efficiency of the phosphor are known, the number of light photons generated is easily calculated. For example, assume a 50-keV x-ray photon (50,000 eV) is absorbed in a calcium tungstate screen that emits most of its light at a wavelength of 4300 Å. The energy in electron volts (eV) of this light photon is calculated by

$$\lambda \text{ (wavelength)} = \frac{12.4}{\text{keV}}$$
$$4300 = \frac{12.4}{\text{keV}}$$
$$\text{keV} = \frac{12.4}{4300} \cong 0.003$$
$$\text{eV} = 3$$

The energy of a 4300 Å (430 nm) blue light photon is about 3 eV. At 100% efficiency, a 50,000 eV x-ray photon would produce about 17,000 light photons of 3 eV energy:

$$\frac{50,000}{3} \cong 17,000$$

Because the conversion efficiency of calcium tungstate is only 5%, the actual number of light photons emitted by this phosphor is about 850 (17,000 × 0.05 = 850). One reason some new intensifying screen phosphors are faster than calcium tungstate is that the new phosphor has a higher conversion efficiency (up to 20%).

The ability of light emitted by the phosphor to escape from the screen and expose the film is termed the "screen efficiency." For typical screens about half the generated light reaches the film; the rest is absorbed in the screen and is wasted. In the previous example, only half the 850 light photons generated would be able to escape from the screen and expose the film.

To examine the manner in which the screen amplifies the photographic effect of x rays, let us consider the case of a film-screen combination compared to a film alone, each irradiated by one thousand 50-keV x-ray photons. Of the 1000 photons, a high-speed calcium tungstate screen will absorb 40% (we will discuss this aspect in more detail later), or 400. Each of the 400 x-ray photons will produce 850 light pho-

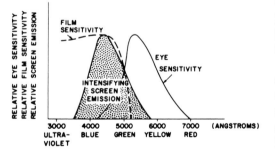

Figure 9–2   The spectral emission of a calcium tungstate x-ray intensifying screen compared to the spectral sensitivity of x-ray film and of the eye

tons, for a total of 340,000 light photons. Half of these light photons (170,000) will escape the screen and expose the film.

Let us assume that 100 light photons are needed to form one latent image center. The screen-film system in our example has caused the formation of 1700 latent image centers. (We will discuss the concept of the latent image in Chapter 10.) At this point, let us simply define a latent image center as the end product of the photographic effect of light or x rays on the film emulsion. It is possible to measure the magnitude of the photographic effect of an exposure by counting the number of latent image centers formed as a result of that exposure. In the case of x rays exposing film directly, only about 5% of the x-ray photons are absorbed by the film, so our example will cause 50 x-ray photons to react with the film emulsion. It is usually considered that one latent image center is formed for each x-ray photon absorbed by a film emulsion. The result of the same 1000 x-ray photons acting directly on film is to produce only 50 latent image centers, versus 1700 latent image centers resulting from the use of intensifying screens. In our example, the ratio of the photographic effect of screen versus nonscreen, or direct, exposure is 34:1. If kVp remains constant, direct film exposure will require 34 times as many mAs as a film-screen exposure.

A review of the example of the intensifying effect of screens is presented in Table 9–1. Stated another way, patient exposure is decreased greatly when intensifying screens are used. A measure of this decrease in exposure is termed the "intensification factor" of the screen. **The intensification factor of a screen is the ratio of the x-ray exposure needed to produce the same density on a film with and without the screen** (intensification factor is commonly determined at a film density of 1.0).

$$\text{Intensification factor} = \frac{\text{exposure required when screens are not used}}{\text{exposure required with screens}}$$

The intensification factor of $CaWO_4$ screens will increase with kVp of the x-ray beam (Fig. 9–3). The K-absorption edges of silver and bromine in the film are 26 keV and 13 keV, respectively, while the K-absorption edge of tungsten is 69.5 keV. Photoelectric absorption of low-kVp x rays will be relatively greater in film because of the low-keV K-absorption edge of silver and bromine. High-kVp x rays will be more abundantly absorbed by the photoelectric process in calcium tungstate screens. For this same reason, a heavily filtered x-ray beam will increase the screen intensification factor by removing the low-energy components of the beam. Thus, $CaWO_4$ intensifying screens are relatively faster in radiography of a thick body part, such as the lumbar spine, than when an extremity is examined. That is, only higher energy x rays can penetrate the thick part and reach the screen.

There will actually be a small number (3 or 4%) of x-ray photons directly absorbed by the film when a screen-film combination is exposed. This direct action of x rays would create so few latent image centers compared to those caused by the fluorescence of the screen that it may be ignored as having no detectable influence on total film response to the exposure.

Table 9–1. Comparison of the Photographic Effect of 1000 X-Ray Photons Used With and Without Intensifying Screens

	X-RAY PHOTONS ABSORBED BY SCREEN	X-RAY PHOTONS ABSORBED BY FILM	LIGHT PHOTONS GENERATED	LIGHT PHOTONS REACHING FILM	LATENT IMAGE CENTERS FORMED
Intensifying screen	400		340,000	170,000	1700
Direct exposure		50			50

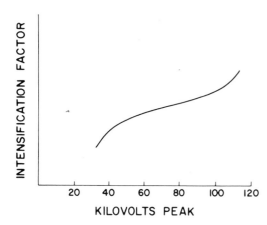

Figure 9–3 Variation of the intensification factor with kVp

Figure 9–4 Screen unsharpness is caused by light diffusion in the intensifying screen

Speed of Calcium Tungstate Intensifying Screens. Several factors determine how "fast" or "slow" a calcium tungstate screen will be. These include **thickness of the phosphor layer, size of the phosphor crystals,** presence or absence of **light-absorbing dye** in the phosphor layer, and phosphor conversion efficiency. Of course, the faster screen will allow a lower x-ray exposure to the patient, but a price for this speed must be paid. **The speed of a calcium tungstate screen and its ability to record detail are in reciprocal relationship;** that is, high speed means less detail. This statement is also true for new screen phosphors, but the subject is more complex because higher speed does not always require a thicker screen. These screens are classified as fast, medium (par speed), and slow (detail), with intensification factors in the range of 100, 50, and 25, respectively.

A thicker phosphor layer will result in a faster screen because the thick layer will absorb more x-ray photons than a thin layer. Thick screens will be faster but will cause a decrease in the clarity of the image recorded on the film. This decrease in image clarity is primarily caused by **diffusion of light** in the phosphor layer. If a thick phosphor layer is employed, an x-ray photon may be absorbed in the phosphor at some distance from the film. **The light**

photons generated by this absorbed x-ray photon are emitted in all directions. Not all the light will reach the film, but that which does will expose an area of the film that is much larger than the size of the calcium tungstate crystal that emitted the light (Fig. 9–4). In addition, some light scattering takes place in the screen, and further increases the area of illumination. The resultant light diffusion obviously causes images to have less sharp borders. Consider Figure 9–5. If an x-ray beam is directed onto a film-screen combination that has a thick lead block covering half the film, one would expect half the film to be exposed and half to be entirely unexposed, with the line between the two areas being very sharp. If the x-ray beam were to ex-

Figure 9–5 Unsharp image borders produced by light diffusion in intensifying screens

pose film alone (without screens), the line between exposed and unexposed areas would be very sharp. If the film is sandwiched between intensifying screens, however, the border is less sharp because some light will diffuse into the area under the edge of the lead block and cause exposure of film in an area that actually receives no x-ray exposure. This light, which diffused under the edge of the lead block, is not available to expose the portion of the film that is not covered by the block. The final result is the production of a more gradual change in density, which is unlike the ideal abrupt transition from black to unexposed (clear) film. (Attempts to measure the magnitude of this problem of light diffusion and scattering will lead us to consideration of the concepts of line spread function and modulation transfer function in Chapter 12).

A thin screen causes less light diffusion than a thick one because light photons are produced closer to the film. Another way to decrease light diffusion is to incorporate a substance that absorbs light in the screen. The substance is commonly a yellow dye, but the question of which color is most effective has not been resolved. The light photons that emerge from the crystal immediately adjacent to the film will obviously travel the shortest distance before leaving the phosphor layer. Scattered photons must travel longer distances in the phosphor layer, and thus they have a better chance of being absorbed by the dye. The dye will decrease the speed of the screen because it decreases the amount of light emitted. Light-absorbing dyes are included in screens designed to produce greater detail.

Resolving Power

The maximum number of line pairs per millimeter that can be resolved by the screen-film system is called the **resolving power.** A **line pair** means a line and a space. For example, two lines (or two line pairs) per mm means that there are two lines and two spaces per mm. Each line is ¼ mm wide, and each space is ¼ mm wide, thus making each line pair ½ mm wide. (A more detailed discussion of resolving power is presented in Chapter 14). X-ray film is able to record up to 100 line pairs per mm, but the slowest screens can record only a little over 10.

Screen-Film Contact

The cassette in which the intensifying screens are mounted provides a light-tight container for the film. It also serves to hold the film in tight contact with the screens over its entire surface. With good film-screen contact a dot of light produced in the screen will be recorded as a comparable dot on the film. If contact is poor, this dot of light will diffuse before it reaches the film, so that its radiographic image is unsharp.

There is a simple method for testing film-screen contact. A piece of wire screen is placed on the cassette, and a radiograph of the wire screen is made. The sharpness of the image of the wire in all regions of the film is compared, and any areas of poor film-screen contact become obvious because the image of the wire appears fuzzy. The wire screen should be made of iron, brass, or copper (aluminum and plastic screens fail to absorb enough x rays), and should have a heavier wire than that used in ordinary window screen. It is best to mount the test wire screen between two pieces of plastic, composition board, or cardboard. Poor film-screen contact will occur quickly if the cassette is handled roughly, but eventually any cassette will wear out with routine use.

Cleaning

Intensifying screens must be kept clean. Any foreign material on the screen, such as paper or blood, will block light photons and produce an area of underexposure on the film corresponding to the size and shape of the soiled area. Cleaning will eliminate the "high spots" on a screen; these high points are the major source of excessive wear. The cause of screen failure is mechanical attrition. Under normal conditions of use, x-ray photons will not damage screens. Screens are best cleaned with a solution containing an antistatic compound and a detergent; the solution should be applied gently (never rub vigorously) with a soft lint-free cloth. The cassette should never be closed after cleaning until it is absolutely dry.

NEW PHOSPHOR TECHNOLOGY

It is usually agreed that the maximum useful speed of calcium tungstate screens has been achieved. New screen phosphors have permitted greater speed, but this changing technology is complex and perplexing.

Increasing Screen Speed

We must first consider how intensifying screen speed can be increased. There are three possible ways. The phosphor layer can be made thicker to absorb more of the x-ray beam. The phosphor may have a higher conversion efficiency of x rays to light. The phosphor may be able to absorb the x-ray beam more effectively. To review, there are three possible ways to increase screen speed:

1. thicker phosphor layer
2. higher conversion efficiency phosphor
3. higher absorption phosphor

Before entering this long discussion of new phosphor technology, please review Table 9–2, which catalogs the noncalcium tungstate screens available from Du Pont and Kodak, listing phosphor composition and color of light emitted by the phosphor.

Thicker Phosphor Layer. Thick phosphor layers absorb more of the x-ray beam than thin layers. This is the major way in which the speed of calcium tungstate screens is increased. A pair of Du Pont Par Speed $CaWO_4$ screens absorbs about 20% of the x-ray beam. A pair of Du Pont Hi Plus screens absorbs about 40% of the x-ray

beam (and is twice as fast as par speed). The Hi Plus screens are not twice as thick as par screens; they are about 2.3 times as thick as the par screens. Why is this? If 100 x-ray photons struck a pair of par screens, 80 photons would be transmitted through the screens (20 are absorbed). A second set of par screens placed in the path of the 80 transmitted photons would absorb 20%, or 16 photons, allowing 64 to pass through. Thus, a double thickness of par speed screens absorbs 36% rather than 40% of the x-ray beam. It is possible to continue to increase the speed of $CaWO_4$ screens by increasing screen thickness, but unsharpness caused by light diffusion in the thick phosphor layer becomes unacceptable. In calcium tungstate screens a compromise is made between speed and sharpness.

Conversion Efficiency. In 1972, reports describing rare earth oxysulfide phosphors for use in intensifying screens were published.[10] This work was supported by a contract from the Atomic Energy Commission to the Lockheed Corporation, and this class of phosphors is sometimes referred to as the Lockheed rare earth phosphors. Rare earth intensifying screens have been commercially available since about 1973.

Chemists divide the periodic table of the elements into four basic groups: alkaline earths, rare earths, transition elements, and nonmetals. The term "rare earth" developed because these elements are difficult and expensive to separate from the earth and each other, not because the elements are scarce. The rare earth group consists of elements of atomic numbers 57 (lanthanum) through 71 (lutetium), and includes thulium (atomic number 69), terbium (atomic number 65), gadolinium (atomic number 64), and europium (atomic number 63). Because lanthanum is the first element, the rare earth group is also known as the lanthanide series. Lanthanum (La) and gadolinium (Gd) are used in the rare earth phosphors. A related phosphor, yttrium (Y), with atomic number 39, is not a

Table 9–2. Non-Calcium Tungstate Intensifying Screens Manufactured by Du Pont and Kodak

MANUFACTURER	NAME	PHOSPHOR	SPECTRAL EMISSION
Du Pont	Cronex Quanta III	Lanthanum oxybromide:thulium activated (LaOBr:Tm)	Blue
	Quanta Detail	Yttrium tantalate:thulium activated (YT$_2$O$_4$:Tm)	Ultraviolet/blue
	Quanta Fast Detail	Yttrium tantalate:niobium activated (YTaO$_4$:Nb)	Ultraviolet blue
	Cronex Quanta V	Lanthanum oxybromide:thulium activated plus gadolinium oxysulfide:terbium activated (LaOBr:Tm plus Gd$_2$O$_2$S:Tb)	Blue and green
Kodak	X-Omatic Fine	Barium lead sulfate, yellow dye (BaPbSO$_4$)	Blue
	X-Omatic Regular	Barium strontium sulfate:europium activated, neutral dye (BaSrSO$_4$:Eu)	Blue
	Lanex Fine	Gadolinium oxysulfide:terbium activated, neutral dye (Gd$_2$O$_2$S:Tb)	Green
	Lanex Medium	Gadolinium oxysulfide:terbium activated, yellow dye (Gd$_2$O$_2$S:Tb)	Green
	Lanex Regular	Gadolinium oxysulfide:terbium activated (Gd$_2$O$_2$S:Tb)	Green

rare earth but has some properties similar to those of the rare earths.

The rare earth phosphors are produced as crystalline powders of **terbium-activated gadolinium oxysulfide** (Gd$_2$O$_2$S:Tb) and **thulium-activated lanthanum oxybromide** (LaOBr:Th). Unlike CaWO$_4$, the rare earth phosphors do not fluoresce properly in the pure state. For example, maximum fluorescence of Gd$_2$O$_2$S occurs when about 0.3% of the gadolinium atoms are replaced by terbium.

The x ray to light conversion efficiency of rare earth phosphors is significantly greater than that of CaWO$_4$. It is generally correct to state that the x ray to light conversion efficiency of CaWO$_4$ is about 5%, whereas that of the rare earth phosphors is about 20%. Stated another way, one absorbed x-ray photon in a CaWO$_4$ intensifying screen will produce about 1000 light photons, and the same photon absorbed in a rare earth screen will produce about 4000 light photons. The conversion efficiency of yttrium oxysulfide screens is about the same as that of gadolinium. In the literature, actual conversion efficiency figures

quoted are CaWO$_4$ 5%, LaOBr:Th 18%, Gd$_2$O$_2$S:Tb 18%, and Y$_2$O$_2$S:Tb 18%.

A fairly new addition to the family of rare earth screens are the **rare earth tantalates,** designated by the generic formula LnTaO$_4$ where Ln is any of the lanthanide series. Tantalate phosphors can be made with most of the lanthanides, but the commercial screens that have been made use yttrium tantalate (YTaO$_4$).

Table 9–2 lists two tantalate screens of Du Pont manufacture. In the YTaO$_4$:Tm (Quanta Detail) some of the Y ions have been replaced by Tm ions. In the YTaO$_4$:Nb (Quanta Fast Detail) some of the TaO$_4$ ions have been replaced by NbO$_4$ ions. The brightest phosphor involves Nb substitution (YTaO$_4$:Nb), which has an estimated x ray to light conversion efficiency of 11%.

Higher Absorption. The fraction of the x-ray beam absorbed by a pair of par speed CaWO$_4$ screens is about 20%, high-speed CaWO$_4$ screens about 40%, and rare earth screens about 60%. The increased absorption in the faster CaWO$_4$ screens occurs because a thicker screen is used; the increased absorption in rare earth screens is a result of improvement in the absorption characteristics of the phosphor.

At diagnostic x-ray energies, absorption is almost entirely caused by the **photoelectric effect** in the high atomic number elements of the phosphor. As discussed in Chapter 4, a photoelectric reaction is most likely to occur in elements with high atomic numbers, and when the x-ray photon energy and the binding energy of the ejected K-shell electron are almost the same.

A phosphor with a higher atomic number would have higher absorption. Because the atomic numbers of tungsten (74) and lead (82) are almost at the end of the periodic table, the potential for this type of improvement is limited. It is interesting to note that the improvement in the input phosphor of image intensifier tubes involved a change from zinc sulfide (atomic numbers 30 and 16) to cesium iodide (atomic numbers 55 and 53). Actually, each of the phosphors used in the new fast intensifying screens has an atomic number lower than that of tungsten. Table 9–3 lists some of the elements found in intensifying screens, together with their atomic number (Z) and K-shell binding energy.

Figure 9–6 diagrams the approximate x-ray absorption curve of a calcium tungstate screen. Notice that the screen is less absorbing as radiation energy increases until the 70 keV K edge of tungsten is reached.

In Figure 9–7 the approximate absorption curve of Gd_2O_2S:Tb is added to the $CaWO_4$ curve. Up to 50 keV, both phosphors absorb about the same. But, at the 50.2-keV K edge of Gd, the rare earth screen develops a four- or five-fold advan-

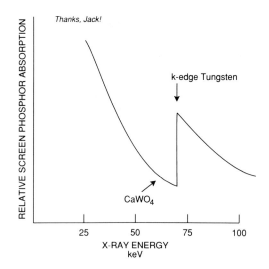

Figure 9–6 Approximate x-ray absorption as a function of x-ray photon energy in a calcium tungstate intensifying screen

tage over $CaWO_4$, which persists until the 70-keV K edge of W is reached. It is apparent that Gd, which has a lower atomic number than W, enjoys an absorption advantage over W in the x-ray energy range of 50 to 70 keV because of the differences in photoelectric absorption related to the K-shell electron binding energies of these two elements. In diagnostic radiology, however, a large percentage of x rays in the beam will have an energy less than 50

Figure 9–7 Comparison of the approximate x-ray absorption as a function of x-ray photon energy in $CaWO_4$ and Gd_2O_2S

Table 9–3. Atomic Number and K-Shell Binding Energy of Some Screen Phosphors

ELEMENT	ATOMIC NUMBER (Z)	K-SHELL BINDING ENERGY (keV)
Yttrium (Y)	39	17.05
Barium (Ba)	56	37.4
Lanthanum (La)	57	38.9
Gadolinium (Gd)	64	50.2
Tungsten (W; wolfram)	74	69.5

keV, making the advantage of gadolinium much less. This is why lanthanum is added to the phosphor of some rare earth screens (such as the Du Pont Cronex Quanta V). Lanthanum, with its K edge at 39 keV, effectively "closes the window" between 39 and 50 keV.

In Figure 9–8 the approximate x-ray absorption curves of LaOBr, Gd_2O_2S, and $CaWO_4$ are compared. By combining the two rare earth phosphors, the rare earth screen has a significant absorption advantage over $CaWO_4$ in the 39- to 70-keV range.

Figure 9–9 shows the approximate absorption of yttrium oxysulfide (Y_2O_2S:Tb is the phosphor in the GAF Rarex B Mid-speed screens) compared to that of $CaWO_4$. Notice that $CaWO_4$ and Y_2O_2S match from 17 to 70 keV. Although these two phosphors absorb about the same x-ray energy, the Y_2O_2S screen produces more light photons because of its higher x ray to light conversion efficiency (18 versus 5%).

Let us summarize this section. The K edges of Ba, La, and Gd correspond closely to the maximum intensity of x rays in the primary beam, causing much of the energy in the primary beam to decrease in the re-

Figure 9–9 Comparison of the approximate x-ray absorption curves of $CaWO_4$ and Y_2O_2S

gion of increased absorption for these phosphors. This is the principal reason that these phosphors have higher absorption of x rays used in diagnostic radiology as compared with $CaWO_4$, even though the atomic number of tungsten (74) is higher than that of barium (56), lanthanum (57), or gadolinium (64). The absorption for yttrium (39) is the same as that of tungsten from 17 to 70 keV, but yttrium is "faster" because of a higher conversion efficiency.

Emission Spectrum

This section will deal with the wavelength (color) of light emitted by the various phosphors, an important consideration because **the light output of the screen and the maximum sensitivity of the film used must be matched.**

The spectrum of light emitted by some of the new screen phosphors is quite different from that of $CaWO_4$, which produces a continuous spectrum of light in the blue region with a peak wavelength of about 4300 Å (430 nm) shown in Figure 9–2. Some phosphors other than calcium tungstate also produce light in the blue-violet range. Table 9–4 lists some of these phosphors. Natural silver halide films are

Figure 9–8 Comparison of the approximate x-ray absorption curves of $CaWO_4$, LaOBr, and Gd_2O_2S

Table 9–4. Spectral Emission of Several Screen Phosphors

PHOSPHOR	SPECTRAL EMISSION, PEAK WAVELENGTH (nm)	EXAMPLE
Tungsten	430	Du Pont Cronex family
Barium lead sulfate	360	Kodak X-Omatic Fine
		Du Pont Hi Speed
Barium strontium sulfate	380	Kodak X-Omatic Regular
Yttrium tantalate:niobium	410	Du Pont Quanta Fast Detail

maximally sensitive to light of this wavelength. Figure 9–10 shows in graphic form the approximate spectral emission of the screen phosphors listed in Table 9–5, compared to the sensitivity of natural silver halide film (such as Du Pont Cronex films and Kodak X-Omatic films). Keep in mind that the speed of these screens covers a wide range.

We must now consider the light emission of the rare earth phosphor $Gd_2O_2S:Tb$. The spectral emission of this earth phosphor is produced by the terbium ion. The terbium emission is not a continuous spectrum (as is $CaWO_4$) but is concentrated in narrow lines with a very strong peak at 544 nm, which is in the green light part of the spectrum. There are less intense emission peaks in the blue, blue-green, yellow, and red areas. Because standard x-ray silver halide film will not absorb (i.e., is not sensitive to) light in the green area, a special film must be used with these screens. Such films are Kodak Ortho G and Du Pont Cronex 8. (This subject will be explored in more detail in Chapter 11.) Figure 9–11 is a graph of the spectral emission of the Kodak Lanex regular screen (which contains $Gd_2O_2S:Tb$ in its phosphor) and the sensitivity of Kodak Ortho G film. Because the sensitivity of natural silver halide film stops at about 500 nm, use of this film with some rare earth screens would result in loss of much of the speed of these screens because the film would be insensitive to much of the light produced.

Figure 9–10 Approximate spectral emission of several different intensifying screen phosphors compared to the natural sensitivity of silver halide

Table 9–5. Speed Class of Various Intensifying Screens

MANUFACTURER	NAME	PHOSPHOR	SPECTRAL EMISSION	FILM	SPEED CLASS
Du Pont	Cronex Par Speed	$CaWO_4$	Blue	Cronex 4	100
	Cronex Hi Plus	$CaWO_4$	Blue	Cronex 4	250
	Cronex Quanta III	LaOBr:Tm	Blue	Cronex 4	800
	Cronex Quanta V	LaOBr:Tm and	Blue	Cronex 4	320
		Gd_2O_2S:Tb	Green	Cronex 8	400
	Quanta Detail	$YTaO_4$:Tm	Ultraviolet/ blue	Cronex 4	100
	Quanta Fast Detail	$YTaO_4$:Nb	Ultraviolet/ blue	Cronex 4	400
Kodak	X-Omatic Fine	$BaPbSO_4$, yellow dye	Blue	XRP	32
	X-Omatic Regular	$BaSrSO_4$:Eu, neutral dye	Blue	XRP	200
	Lanex Fine	Gd_2O_2S:Tb, neutral dye	Green	Ortho G	100
	Lanex Medium	Gd_2O_2S:Tb, yellow dye	Green	Ortho G	250
	Lanex Regular	Gd_2O_2S:Tb	Green	Ortho G	400

Note: Dupont Cronex 4 is now largely replaced by Cronex 7 and Cronex 10, and Kodak Ortho G film by T-Mat G. The older films still accurately reflect relative intensifying screen speeds, which is the purpose of this table.

The spectral emission of yttrium oxysulfide screens is similar to that of the rare earth screens in that it shows line emission, but a large fraction of the emission from a Y_2O_2S:Tb screen falls within the sensitivity range of natural silver halide films. The principal emission of the terbium at 544

Figure 9–11 Approximate spectral emission of the Kodak Lanex Regular screen (rare earth) compared to the sensitivity of Kodak Ortho G film. (This is similar to charts supplied through the courtesy of the Eastman Kodak Company)

nm, though, is still present. Yttrium oxysulfide screens may be used with natural silver halide films, but will exhibit even more speed when used with green-sensitive films.

The Du Pont Cronex Quanta V, contains two phosphors, terbium-activated gadolinium oxysulfide (Gd_2O_2S:Tb) and thulium-activated lanthanum oxybromide (LaOBr:Tm). It is interesting to note that the color of light emitted by a rare earth phosphor depends on the activator used; terbium (Tb) produces green light and thulium (Tm) blue. For example, Gd_2O_2S:Tb is a green-emitting intensifying screen phosphor, and LaOBr:Tm is a blue-emitting intensifying screen phosphor. The spectral emission of LaOBr:Tm is illustrated in Figure 9–12. The Du Pont Quanta V intensifying screen is interesting in that it contains both a blue (LaOBr:Tm) and a green (Gd_2O_2S:Tb) emitting phosphor. This "double" spectral emission allows a wider choice of suitable films, because both blue- and green-sensitive films are matched to the spectral emission of the screens.

An example of a rare earth screen with a blue-emitting phosphor is the Du Pont Cronex Quanta III, which has LaOBr:Tm at its phosphor (see Fig. 9–12). Recent advances in separating rare earths have made suitably pure supplies of lanthanum available for use in intensifying screens.

The yttrium tantalate screens emit light in the ultraviolet and blue wavelengths. Yttrium tantalate ($YTaO_4$) has an inherent broadband emission with its peak at 337 nm. Activation with thulium ($YTaO_4:Tm$) adds another peak at 463 nm. Activation with niobium ($YTaO_4:Nb$) produces a broadband emission with its peak at 410 nm. The emission spectrum of $YTaO_4:Nb$ is illustrated in Figure 9–10.

Table 9–5 is an attempt to compare roughly the relative speed (speed class) of the newer screens we have been discussing. (The term "speed class" will be discussed in more detail in Chapter 11.) It is common to express the speed of an intensifying screen relative to that of a par speed calcium tungstate screen (specifically, the Du Pont Cronex Par Speed screen). In our speed class scheme the speed of the par speed $CaWO_4$ screen is assigned a value of

100. Remember that a film that matches the spectral emission of the screen must be used. In Table 9–5 Du Pont Cronex 4 and Kodak XRP are films sensitive to blue light. Green-light-sensitive films are represented by Du Pont Cronex 8 and Kodak Ortho G films. When comparing the relative speed of various intensifying screens, the films that were used must be specified. (In Chapter 11 the characteristics of these films will be presented in more detail, and in Chapter 14 we will examine potential problems associated with very fast screens.)

Response to Kilovoltage

In the past we compared the speeds of other screens to that of $CaWO_4$ as if the $CaWO_4$ screen had a constant response to kilovoltage. The response of $CaWO_4$ to kVp is not flat, but drops down at low kVp. This is illustrated in Figure 9–13, which shows the kVp response of $CaWO_4$, LaOBr:Tm, and a combined $Gd_2O_2S:Tb$ and LaOBr:Tm phosphor. Figure 9–13 shows that the speed of the rare earth screens varies much more with kVp than

Figure 9–13 Response to kVp of a Du Pont $CaWO_4$ (Hi Plus), LaOBr:Tm (Quanta III), and dual phosphor $Gd_2O_2S:Tb$ plus LaOBr:Tm (Quanta V) screen. (Data courtesy of E.I. du Pont de Nemours & Company, Inc.)

Figure 9–12 Approximate spectral emission of LaOBr:Tm. (Data courtesy of E.I. du Pont de Nemours & Company, Inc.)

does the $CaWO_4$ screen. Note that the rare earth screens show maximum speed at about 80 kVp, with less speed at both low and high kilovoltages. The need for exposure technique adjustment because of screen speed variation with kVp is not great, and is usually of little importance unless kilovoltage lower than 70 kVp is used. It is generally advisable to establish constant kVp (with variable mAs) exposure technique charts when using noncalcium tungstate screens.

Figure 9–13 introduces two areas we will not explain until Chapter 11. Film-screen speed is often expressed as the reciprocal of the exposure in milliroentgens required to produce a net film density of 1.0. This explains the numbers used to express film-screen speed. The speed of a film-screen system depends on the speed of the screen and on the speed of the film. The films used to determine the curves in Figure 9–13 were a medium-speed and half-speed blue-sensitive film (Cronex 4 and Cronex 7) and a medium-speed green-sensitive film (Cronex 8). We will repeat Figure 9–13 in Chapter 11; don't worry if these areas are not entirely clear now.

Phototimers

Some phototimers being used today will not work well with rare earth screens. Many of these phototimers have a response time of about 30 milliseconds (i.e., it takes 30 milliseconds for the phototimer to measure the radiation and terminate the exposure). With fast screens a response time of 3 milliseconds is recommended.[3] In addition, the phototimer must be able to recognize differences in screen speed caused by variation in kVp. If a photomultiplier-type phototimer is used, the phosphor in the fluorescent screen used to convert x rays to light should be matched to the phosphor in the intensifying screen. The photomultiplier tube selected should be sensitive to the light output of the phosphor. Ionization chamber-type phototimers can be made to work satisfactorily. Use of photo-

timers with very fast screens will usually require special consideration, and one should plan for appropriate changes in advance.

Quantum Mottle

Quantum mottle, commonly called "noise," results from statistical fluctuation in the number of x-ray photons absorbed by the intensifying screens to form the light image recorded on film. With the fast screens and films now available, it is possible to use a film-screen system so fast (i.e., the screen does not have to absorb many x rays) that noise makes the resulting image unsatisfactory. (This subject will be reviewed in painful detail in Chapter 14). At this time, we only wish to emphasize that any discussion of fast screens demands careful evaluation of system noise. One pays a price for speed.

PHOTOSTIMULABLE PHOSPHOR

Conventional radiography uses an x-ray intensifying screen, x-ray film, or both as the image receptor. The exposed film is then developed and viewed. Now, a process sometimes called **computed radiography (CR)** uses a **photostimulable phosphor** as the image receptor. A phosphor that is currently used is composed of europium-activated barium fluorohalide. The phosphor crystals are coated on a screen that looks like an intensifying screen. The phosphor coated screen is contained in a cassette similar to standard film-screen cassettes. A radiographic exposure is made using conventional x-ray equipment, but here the similarity to conventional radiography ends. The photostimulable phosphor absorbs some of the energy in the x-ray beam and stores a portion of this energy as valence electrons stored in high energy traps to create a latent image. When this latent image is scanned by a laser beam, the trapped electrons return to the valence band with the emission of light. This light is viewed by a photomultiplier tube, and the output of the photomultiplier tube constitutes the signal. The signal is fed to a computer where it is processed and stored, and may be displayed in any of the normal formats. This technology is sometimes called "filmless," or "electronic," or "computed" radiography.

Luminescence

Luminescence describes the process of emission of light (optical radiation) from a material caused by some process other than heating to incandescence. Luminescent materials can absorb energy, store a fraction of it, and convert the energy into light, which is emitted.

There are two forms of luminescence that are determined by the time it takes for light to be emitted after an exciting event takes place. In fluorescence, light is emitted within 10^{-8} sec of the stimulation. This occurs when an electron is excited from one energy level, and then returns to that energy level without anything additional happening to it.

Phosphorescence is the emission of light that is delayed beyond 10^{-8} sec. This delay requires some additional interaction of the electron; normally this is described as a trapping of the electron in some localized energy state. Intensifying screens are made from fluorescent material that emits its light immediately after stimulation. This is just fine, because film is there to capture the light. However, if we would like the screen to retain the x-ray image, we would use a phosphorescent material. In radiology, there are two such applications. One is thermoluminescent dosimetry (TLD), in which the phosphor is encouraged to emit its light by heating. A thermoluscent dosimeter is a small chip of activated lithium fluoride that is exposed to radiation. The chip is then heated, and emits light in proportion to the amount of radiation it received (the term "thermoluminescence" indicates heating to liberate luminescence). The second application of phosphorescence is our current topic of photostimulable phosphors as used in computed radiography (photostimulable suggests that luminescence is going to be induced by absorption of light photons).

The material used in one commercially available photostimulable phosphor is europium-activated barium fluoride bromide (BaFBr:Eu). Europium is an activator added to BaFBr. (In the discussion of semiconductors, added materials were called "impurity atoms," but they perform the same function as activators.)

The reason for using an activator is to make traps at the activator site in the crystalline structure. Other types are produced when atoms are missing from their normal position in the lattice structure. These traps are localized energy levels at the activator or vacancy site that do not normally exist in the crystalline structure. If by chance an electron is captured in the trap, it behaves very much like an electron trapped (bound) in an atom. We remember that to remove an electron bound to an atom, we must supply it with the ionization energy of that particular atom. In doing so, we produce a positive ion (which is the atom without an electron) and an electron that is free to move away from the atom. The same is true for an electron that is trapped at an activator or vacancy site. If we want to free the electron from the trap, we must supply it with sufficient energy to free itself from the trapping mechanism. If we supply the energy, the electron is free to move through the crystalline structure, and it leaves behind an empty trap (that looks like a positive ion) ready to capture another electron. A photostimulable phosphor is a material that has activator and vacancy traps from which electrons may be removed by absorbing energy from light photons. Without looking further into the physics of trapping mechanisms, we will describe how a photostimulable phosphor plate is used in clinical radiography.

Let us acknowledge that we have not presented a complete and totally accurate picture of the physics of BaFBr:Eu. We would like to quote Hartwig Blume from the Philips PCR Technical Review, Issue No. 1, p. 3, to give a more accurate picture of the trapping of electrons and holes in the photostimulable image plates. We have no desire to get into the physics of such things as hole traps and vacancy traps.

Let me first describe a bit of the physics of the stimulable phosphor x-ray detector: The majority of x-ray photons which interact with the phosphor material interact via the photoelectric effect and create a high-energetic photoelectron. The photoelectron in turn, through a cascade process, generates a large number of low energetic electrons and holes. (A hole is a missing electron in the crystalline structure of the phosphor.) In an ordinary intensifying screen, the electrons and holes recombine with each other and create "spontaneous" luminescence which exposes the x-ray film.

In our stimulable phosphor, about half of the electron-hole-pairs recombine at europium centers during the x-ray exposure and create spontaneous, purple or near-ultraviolet luminescence characteristic for europium in BaFBr. The spontaneous luminescence is not utilized. The other half of the electrons and holes are trapped separately, holes at divalent europium sites, electrons at halogen vacancies in the crystalline lattice of the phosphor. The local concentration of trapped holes and electrons is proportional to the local x-ray exposure and represents the latent image of the x-rayed object.

By stimulation with red light, electrons can be liberated from their traps. The electrons may migrate to trapped holes and recombine with them to generate europium luminescence. To enhance the efficiency of the stimulating light, the phosphor screen is actually prepared with a very high, uniform and stable concentration of trapped electrons at halogen vacancies. Obviously, by stimulation with (red) light, the latent image is destroyed.

Photostimulable Phosphor Imaging

Let us now look at the process of photostimulable phosphor (or computed radiographic) imaging by steps as follows:

> The phosphor prior to exposure
> Formation of the latent image
> Detecting the image

To prepare a BaFBr:Eu plate for imaging, the plate is flooded with light from high intensity sodium discharge lamps. This erases any image remaining from a prior exposure.

The plate is now exposed to x rays, using standard radiographic equipment. During the exposure, electrons in the phosphor are excited into a higher energy state. About half of these electrons return to the normal energy state instantly and are no longer available for image formation. The rest of the excited electrons are trapped and form the latent image. It seems self evident that the number of trapped electrons per increment of area is directly proportional to the amount of x rays absorbed (otherwise, this would not be an imaging method). The trapped electrons may be thermally removed from the trap on a statistical basis. The thermal agitation of electrons out of the traps will degrade the latent image. In BaFBr:Eu, the image will be readable for up to about 8 hours at room temperature. We should note that the image should be retrieved as soon as possible to prevent degradation due to thermal agitation.

The image is retrieved by putting the imaging plate in a reader. The reader is made so that the plate is scanned by a small dot (about 100 microns) of light from a helium-neon laser (633-mm wavelength). The trapped electrons exposed to this small dot of laser light will absorb the laser light energy. This addition of energy will free the electrons from their traps, and they will become free to return to the lower energy state associated with the crystalline structure. Note that the crystalline state of the lattice structure has a lower energy level than the electron trap. When the electrons return to this lower energy level they will emit a light photon. Since the energy level of the normal crystalline structure is lower than the activator energy level, the light photon emitted on return to the lower energy level will have more energy (shorter wavelength) than the energy of the laser light used to excite them out of their traps. That is to say, the stimulated emission has a wavelength that is shorter than the exciting laser beam. In BaFBr:Eu, this wavelength is a narrow band in the 300 nm (ultraviolet) to 500 nm (greenish) range.

That the two lights (the laser light and stimulated emission) have different wavelengths is critical for image retrieval. After all, we have an intense red laser light and a somewhat feeble greenish light in the same vicinity, and we would like to detect the greenish light as the image signal. One way to do this is to use a filter that will absorb the red light but be transparent to the greenish light. If, after the filter, we use an optical fiber, we can conduct the signal light to a photomultiplier tube at a remote position so that the photomultiplier tube and the laser light do not interact. In reality, we would expect to have a long filter and a fiber bundle so that we would scan the laser across the image plate to produce a scan line. The entire plate can be read, a scan at a time, by moving the image plate perpendicular to the scan line of the laser beam.

In the output of the photomultiplier tube, we have a continuous point-by-point scan of the image. The output is an electrical analog signal corresponding to absorbed x rays in the image plate. This signal must be amplified, converted to a digital signal, and stored in a computer. From here on, the imaging is just like any other imaging method whose information is stored in a computer before being read by a radiologist.

Dynamic Range of Photostimulable Phosphors

When we study x-ray film in Chapter 11, we will find that high-contrast x-ray film can record exposure differences of about $100:1$ ($10^2:1$). That is, the exposure that causes the film to be developed as very black is about 100 times greater than the exposure that causes such a faint gray that it can barely be detected by the eye. It has been found that the exposure range that a photostimulable phosphor can record is about $10,000:1$ ($10^4:1$). Photostimulable phosphors are said to have a very large dynamic range compared to film. In addition, the dynamic range is linear. This means that the amount of photostimulable luminescence created by an exposure increases, or decreases, in direct proportion to the amount of x-ray exposure the phosphor receives. The actual exposure range over which this linear response is seen covers a range of about 5 microroentgens (5 $\times$ 10^{-3} mR) to about 50 milliroentgens (5 $\times$ 10^1 mR), yielding an exposure range of about $10^4:1$. Figure 9–14 is a rough graphic representation of this concept. Notice that as the exposure increases from 5 $\times$ 10^{-3} mR to 50 mR (horizontal axis of Fig. 9–14), the intensity of the resulting photostimulable luminescence increases in a linear fashion from a relative value of 1 to a value of 10^4. At this time you may want to take a glance ahead to Figure 11–5 and notice that film has a more narrow dynamic range, and a non-linear response to exposure at both the low and high ends of the exposure range. This concept of dynamic range (we will often call this "exposure latitude") will be re-examined in much more detail in Chapter 11.

What is the advantage of a system with a large, linear dynamic range? The most practical advantage deals with the technol-

Figure 9–14 The dynamic range of a photostimulable phosphor imaging plate

ogist's correct choice of exposure factors (kVp and mAs) for a radiographic examination. The wider the range of exposures the imaging system will accept, the more latitude there is in choice of kVp and mAs. A major problem in radiology departments results from the need for repeat examinations because of incorrect exposures. A wide latitude system will decrease the need for repeat exposures.

Because of this wide dynamic range, it is necessary to process photostimulable phosphor images in two steps. First, the imaging plate is scanned by a weak laser beam about 1.8 mm wide in an operation called "prereading." Only a small portion of the image stored in the plate is read out at this time. The data in this pre-reading image is analyzed to compute the exposure level and exposure range of the stored image. In this way, such things as the sensitivity of the photomultiplier tube can be adjusted to the exposure level and exposure range for any individual examination. This pre-reading thus allows examinations made with a wide range of mAs settings to be converted into diagnostically useful images. As a result, underexposed and overexposed as well as correctly exposed examinations will be processed as satisfactory images. Digital processing of these images can produce a variety of other image changes which we will consider in another chapter.

SUMMARY

Intensifying screens are used in diagnostic radiology because they reduce x-ray dose to the patient. Also, the lower exposures required (less mAs) allow the shorter exposure times needed to reduce motion unsharpness. Until about 1971, calcium tungstate was the phosphor used in most screens. New technology has resulted in very fast rare earth and other phosphors. There are three ways in which screens can be made "faster":

1. thicker phosphor layer

2. higher conversion efficiency phosphor
3. higher absorption phosphor

$CaWO_4$ screen speed is determined largely by the thickness of the phosphor layer. The newer fast phosphors exhibit a higher conversion efficiency. Higher absorption of x rays in the diagnostic range is a function of the matching of the K-absorption edge of the screen phosphor to the energy spectrum in the x-ray beam. The spectral emission of some phosphors requires that an appropriately sensitized film be used, or much of the light will be wasted. Intensifying screens are usually used in pairs, with a double-emulsion x-ray film sandwiched between the two screens in a light-tight cassette. System noise becomes important when the fastest film-screen systems are used.

Computed radiography uses a photostimulable phosphor as the image receptor. The phosphor is composed of europium activated barium fluorohalide, which is coated on an imaging plate. The phosphor temporarily stores a latent image on the imaging plate. The latent image is converted to a light image using laser stimulated luminescence. A photomultiplier tube converts the light image into an analog electrical signal. This analog signal is amplified, converted to a digital signal, and stored in a computer.

REFERENCES

1. Alves, R.V., and Buchanan, R.A.: Properties of Y_2O_2S:Tb x-ray intensifying screens. Presented at the IEEE meeting in Miami, December, 1972.
2. Balter, S., and Laughlin, J.S.: A photographic method for the evaluation of the conversion efficiency of fluoroscopic screens. Radiology, 86:145, 1966.
3. Bates, L.M.: Properties of radiographic films and intensifying screens which influence the efficacy of a film-screen combination. Contained in the syllabus of the joint BRH-ACR Conference: First Image Receptor Conference: Film/Screen Combinations, Arlington, Virginia, November 13–15, 1975. Washington, DC, U.S. Government Printing Office, HEW Publ. No. (FDA) 77-8003, 1975, p. 123.
4. Buchanan, R.A., Finkelstein, S.I., and Wickersheim, K.A.: X-ray exposure reduction using

rare-earth oxysulfide intensifying screens. Radiology, *105*:85, 1972.

5. Castle, J.W.: Sensitivity of radiographic screens to scattered radiation and its relationship to image contrast. Radiology, *122*:805, 1977.

6. Coltman, J.W., Ebbighausen, E.G., and Alter, W.: Physical properties of calcium tungstate x-ray screens. J. Appl. Physics, *18*:530, 1947.

7. Holland, R.S.: Image analysis. Contained in the syllabus of the AAPM 1975 Summer School, The Expanding Role of the Diagnostic Radiologic Physicist, Rice University, Houston, July 27–August 1, 1975, p. 103.

8. Ishida, M., Kato, H., Doi, K., Frank, P.: Development of a new digital radiographic image processing system. SPIE Vol. 347: Application of Optical Instrumentation in Medicine X, 1982, p. 42.

9. Lawrence, D.J.: Kodak X-Omatic and Lanex screens and Kodak films for medical radiography. Rochester, N.Y., Radiography Markets Division, Eastman Kodak Company File No. 5.03, June 1976.

10. Ludwig, G.W., and Prener, J.S.: Evaluation of Gd_2O_2S:Tb as a phosphor for the input screen of x-ray image intensifier. IEEE Trans. Biomed. Eng., *19*:3, 1972.

11. Meredith, W.J., and Massey, J.B.: Fundamental Physics of Radiology. Baltimore, Williams & Wilkins, 1968.

12. Meritt, C.: Computed radiography: a new approach to plain film imaging. Diagnostic Imaging. January, 1985, p. 58.

13. Morgan, R.H.: Characteristics of x-ray films and screens. Radiology, *49*:90, 1947.

14. Patterson, C.V.S.: Roentgenography: Fluoroscopic and intensifying screens. *In* Medical Physics. Vol. 2. Edited by O. Glasser. Chicago, Year Book Medical Publishers, 1950.

15. Patterson, C.V.S.: Roentgenography: Fluoroscopic and intensifying screens. *In* Medical Physics. Vol. 3. Edited by O. Glasser. Chicago, Year Book Medical Publishers, 1960.

16. Patterson X-Ray Screens: Sales Manual for Du Pont Patterson X-Ray Screen Dealers. Wilmington, Photo Products Department, E.I. du Pont de Nemours and Company, Inc., 1952.

17. Properzio, W.S., and Trout, E.D.: The deterioration of x-ray fluoroscopic screens. Radiology, *91*:439, 1968.

18. Roth, B.: X-ray intensifying screens. Contained in the syllabus of the AAPM 1975 Summer School, The Expanding Role of the Diagnostic Radiologic Physicist, Rice University, Houston, July 27–August 1, 1975, p. 120.

19. Sonoda, M., Takano, M., Miyahara, J., Kato, H.: Computed radiography utilizing scanning laser stimulated luminescence. Radiology, *148*:833, 1983.

20. Philips Medical Systems, Inc., 710 Bridgeport Avenue, Shelton, CT, 06484. PCR Technical Review, Issue No. 1.

21. Stevels, A.L.N.: New phosphors for x-ray screens. Medicamundi *20*:12, 1975.

22. Ter-Pogossian, M.: The efficiency of radiographic intensifying screens. *In* Technological Needs for Reduction of Patient Dosage from Diagnostic Radiology. Edited by M.L. Janower. Springfield, IL, Charles C Thomas, 1963.

23. Thompson, T.T., Radford, E.L., and Kirby, C.C.: A look at rare-earth and high-speed intensifying screens. Appl. Radiol., *6*:71, 1977.

10 *Physical Characteristics of X-Ray Film and Film Processing*

When an x-ray beam reaches the patient, it contains no useful medical information. After the beam passes through and interacts with the tissues in the part examined, it contains all the information that can be revealed by that particular radiographic examination. This is represented by variation in the number of x-ray photons in different areas of the emergent beam. We are unable to make direct use of the information in this form, however, and must transfer it to a medium suitable for viewing by the eye. The method of transfer might involve a magnetic tape or disc, a fluoroscopic screen, or xerography. The most important material used to "decode" the information carried by the attenuated x-ray beam is photographic film. The film may be exposed by the direct action of x rays. More commonly, the energy of the x-ray beam is converted into light by intensifying screens, and this light is used to expose the film.

It is unfortunate that the transfer of information from the x-ray beam to the screen-film combination always results in a loss of information. In reviewing x-ray film, we must examine both the film and those factors that influence the amount of information lost in the transfer process.

FILM

X-ray film is photographic film consisting of a photographically active, or radia-tion-sensitive, emulsion that is usually coated on both sides of a transparent sheet of plastic, called the base. Firm attachment between the emulsion layer and the film base is achieved by use of a thin layer of adhesive. The delicate emulsion is protected from mechanical damage by layers known as the supercoating (Fig. 10–1).

Film Base

The only function of the film base is to provide a support for the fragile photographic emulsion. Three characteristics of the base must be considered. First, it must not produce a visible pattern or absorb too much light when the radiograph is viewed. Second, the flexibility, thickness, and strength of the base must allow for ease of processing (developing) and produce a radiograph that "feels right" when handled (a film too "floppy" to "snap" under the hangers of a viewbox gets a cool reception). Third, the base must have **dimensional sta-**

Figure 10–1 Cross section of a double emulsion x-ray film

bility; that is, the shape and size of the base must not change during the developing process or during the stored life of the film. Figure 10–2 illustrates a radiograph in which the base has slowly diminished in size over a period of 22 years. Notice how shrinking of the base has thrown the unshrinking emulsion into folds, producing a wrinkled appearance.

Original x-ray "plates" consisted of a glass plate with the emulsion coated on one side. It is no longer possible to make a "flat plate of the abdomen," because x-ray plates are not available. The onset of World War I cut off the supply of photographic glass from Belgium and created a demand for a less fragile x-ray film for use by the Army. Cellulose nitrate, previously used as a base for photographic film, was adapted for use in x-ray film in 1914. Cellulose nitrate is quite flammable, however, and several fires were caused by improper handling and storage of the film. Because of this fire hazard a new "safety base" film was urgently sought and, in 1924, a "safety" film with a

Figure 10–2 Wrinkled emulsion resulting from shrinking of the film base

cellulose triacetate base was developed. In 1960 the first medical radiographic film using a polyester base was introduced. **Polyester** as a film base offers the advantage of improved dimensional stability, even when stored under conditions of varying humidity, and it is much stronger than acetate.

What is polyester? It is similar to Dacron* polyester fiber used in clothing. The raw materials, dimethyl terephthalate (DMT) and ethylene glycol, are brought together under conditions of low pressure and high temperature to form a molten polymer that is then literally stretched into sheets of appropriate size and thickness to form film base. Cronex* film is an example of a polyester-base film, and the characteristics of polyester may be appreciated by examining a piece of "cleared" Cronex film.

Triacetate and polyester bases are clear and colorless. In 1933 the first commercialized blue tint was added to x-ray film in an effort to produce a film that was "easier" to look at, causing less eyestrain. Present x-ray film is tinted blue. The blue dye may be added to the film base or to the emulsion.

Triacetate base was about 0.008 in. (8 mils) thick, and polyester base is 7 mils thick. The slightly thinner polyester base has handling properties approximately equal to those of the thicker acetate.

Photographic emulsion would not adhere to the finished base if applied directly. Therefore, a thin layer of adhesive substance is applied to the base to ensure perfect union between base and emulsion.

Emulsion

The two most important ingredients of a photographic emulsion are **gelatin** and **silver halide.** The exact composition of the various emulsions is a closely guarded industrial secret. Most x-ray film is made for use with intensifying screens, and has emulsion coated on both sides of the base. Emulsion thickness varies with film type,

*Dacron and Cronex are trademarks of E.I. du Pont de Nemours and Company, Inc.

but is usually no thicker than 0.5 mil. A thicker emulsion would not be useful because of the inability of light to penetrate to the deeper layers.

Gelatin. Photographic gelatin for x-ray film is made from bone, mostly cattle bone from India and Argentina. (Useless information: India and Argentina do not have better cows, but they have a lot of them. They also have inexpensive labor to process the bones.) Gelatin satisfies several exacting requirements better than any other suspension medium. It keeps the silver halide grains well dispersed and prevents the clumping of grains. Processing (developing and fixing) solutions can penetrate gelatin rapidly without destroying its strength or permanence, and gelatin is available in a reasonably large quantity and uniform quality.

Silver Halide. Silver halide is the light-sensitive material in the emulsion. The halide in medical x-ray film is about 90 to 99% silver bromide and about 1 to 10% silver iodide (the presence of AgI produces an emulsion of much higher sensitivity than a pure AgBr emulsion). The silver iodobromide crystals are precipitated and emulsified in the gelatin under exacting conditions of concentration and temperature, as well as the sequence and the rate at which these chemicals are added. The method of precipitation determines crystal size, structural perfection, and concentration of iodine. In general, the precipitation reaction involves the addition of silver nitrate to a soluble halide to form the slightly soluble silver halide:

$$AgNO_3 + KBr \rightarrow AgBr + KNO_3$$

The silver halide in a photographic emulsion is in the form of small **crystals** suspended in the gelatin. The crystal is formed from ions of silver (Ag^+), ions of bromine (Br^-), and ions of iodine (I^-) arranged in a cubic lattice (Fig. 10–3). These grains, or crystals, in a medical x-ray film emulsion are small but still relatively large compared to fine-grain photographic

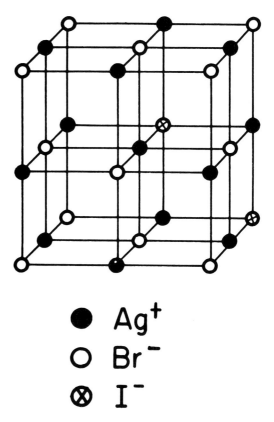

● Ag^+

○ Br^-

⊗ I^-

Figure 10–3 The silver iodobromide crystal lattice

emulsions. Crystal size might average 1.0 to 1.5 microns (1 micron = 0.001 millimeter) in diameter with about 6.3×10^9 grains per cubic centimeter of emulsion, and each grain contains an average of 1,000,000 to 10,000,000 silver ions.

The silver iodobromide grain is not a perfect crystal because a perfect crystal has almost no photographic sensitivity. There are several types of crystal defects. A point defect consists of a silver ion that has moved out of its normal position in the crystal lattice; these interstitial silver ions may move in the crystal (Fig. 10–4). A dislocation is a line imperfection in the crystal, and may be thought of as a brick wall that contains one row in which the bricks are not the same size as all the other bricks, thus causing a strain in the wall structure.

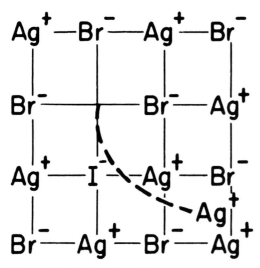

Figure 10–4 A point defect

This may be the way in which the iodine ion strains the crystal.

Chemical sensitization of a crystal takes several forms. It is commonly produced by adding a sulfur-containing compound, such as allylthiourea, to the emulsion, which reacts with silver halide to form silver sulfide. The silver sulfide is usually located on the surface of the crystal and is referred to as the **sensitivity speck.** It is the sensitivity speck that traps electrons to begin formation of the latent image centers.

Latent Image

Metallic silver is black. It is silver that produces the dark areas seen on a developed radiograph. We must explain how exposure of the sensitized silver iodobromide grains in the film emulsion to light (from x-ray intensifying screens), or to the direct action of x rays, initiates the formation of atomic silver to form a pattern. The energy absorbed from a light photon gives an electron in the bromine ion enough energy to escape. The electron can move in the crystal for relatively large distances as long as it does not encounter a region of impurity or fault in the crystal.

$$Br^- + light\ photon \rightarrow Br + electron$$

A site of crystal imperfection, such as a dislocation defect, or an AgS sensitivity speck, may act as an electron trap where the electron is captured and temporarily fixed. The electron gives the sensitivity speck a negative charge, and this attracts the mobile interstitial Ag^+ ions in the crystal. At the speck, the silver ion is neutralized by the electron to form a single silver atom:

$$Ag^+ + electron \rightarrow Ag$$

This single atom of silver then acts as an electron trap for a second electron. The negative charge causes a second silver ion to migrate to the trap to form a two-atom silver nucleus. Growth of silver atoms at the site of the original sensitivity speck continues by repeated trapping of electrons, followed by their neutralization with interstitial silver ions. The negative bromine ions that have lost electrons are converted into neutral bromine atoms, which leave the crystal and are taken up by the gelatin of the emulsion. Figure 10–5 diagrams the development of a two-atom latent image according to the Gurney-Mott hypothesis.[6]

A single silver halide crystal may have one or many of these centers in which atomic silver atoms are concentrated. The presence of atomic silver is a direct result of the response of the grain to light exposure, but no visible change has occurred in the grain. These small clumps of silver can, however, be seen with electron microscopy. These clumps of silver atoms are termed **latent image centers,** and are the sites at which the developing process will cause visible amounts of metallic silver to be deposited. The difference between an emulsion grain that will react with the developing solution and thus become a visible silver deposit and a grain that will not be "developed" is the presence of one or more latent image centers in the exposed grain. At least two atoms of silver must be present at a latent image center to make a grain developable (i.e., to become a visible deposit of silver). In practical terms the minimum number to produce developability is

Figure 10–5 Formation of the latent image

probably between three and six. The more silver atoms that exist at a latent image center, the greater the probability that the grain will be developed. Some centers will contain several hundred silver atoms. Under the usual conditions, the absorption of one quantum of light by a silver halide grain will produce one atom of silver and one of bromine.

Direct X-Ray Exposure

The photographic effect of direct absorption of x rays by the emulsion is not caused by electromagnetic radiation itself but by electrons emitted when the x-ray photon interacts with the silver halide in the emulsion. These electrons come from

photoelectric absorption or Compton scattering, and have rather long ranges in the emulsion. In fact, an electron produced in this way may react with many grains in an emulsion. The manner in which the energy of the electrons is imparted to the photographic emulsion is complex and will not be considered in detail. The final result is freeing of electrons from the bromide ion, producing bromine atoms and an electron that can move to a trapping site and begin the process of latent image formation. The energy of one absorbed x-ray photon can produce thousands of silver atoms at latent image sites in one or several grains. Even this large number of silver atoms is low, considering the energy of the absorbed photon. Most of the energy of the absorbed photon is lost in processes that do not produce any photographic effect (such as losses to gelatin). Only 3 to 10% of the photon energy is used to produce photolytic silver. The photographic effect of direct x-ray exposure on an emulsion can be increased by a factor of almost 100 by proper chemical sensitization of the emulsion.

The sensitivity of film to direct x-ray exposure varies significantly (by a factor of 20 to 50) with the energy (kVp) of the x-ray beam. This x-ray spectral sensitivity is most important when considering use of film to measure x-ray exposure dose (i.e., film badge monitoring). Above 50 kVp, the efficiency with which absorbed x-ray photons are utilized to produce a photographic effect decreases significantly with increasing photon energy. At about 50 kVp the average keV of the x rays produced will be close to the K-shell binding energy of silver (25.5 keV) and bromine (13.5 keV). This will cause the film to exhibit maximum photoelectric absorption of 50-kVp x rays. Figure 10–6 shows, in a rough graphic form, the way in which the x-ray sensitivity of film varies with kVp.

The sensitivity also varies greatly with the way in which the film is developed. The amount of blackening (density) on the de-

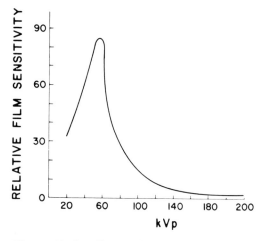

Figure 10–6 Film sensitivity varies with radiation quality

veloped film may be used as an indication of how much x-ray exposure (i.e., how many milliroentgens) the film has received. Because the sensitivity of the film varies greatly with the energy (kVp) of the x rays, however, blackening of a piece of film does not give an accurate estimation of the exposure to which the film has been subjected. For example, a film subjected to an exposure of 50 mR at an x-ray energy of 50 kVp will, after development, exhibit a much higher density (amount of blackening) than an identical film subjected to an exposure of 50 mR by 200-kVp x rays. The problem of variation of film sensitivity with radiation energy is partially solved by placing various metal filters in front of the film in an attempt to control the energy (kVp) of the x rays that reach different areas of the film. The accuracy of film badge monitoring of x-ray exposure is about ±20%. Film badge monitoring of personnel exposure offers several advantages over other methods, such as ionization chambers. The film badge provides a permanent record, and is small in size and weight, rugged, and inexpensive.

Supercoating

Covering the emulsion is a thin layer, commonly gelatin, that serves to protect the emulsion from mechanical damage. In special types of film this supercoat, or anti-abrasive coating, may contain substances that make the film surface smooth and slick. This is a desirable quality in film that must be transported through a cut film rapid film changer.

FILM PROCESSING
Development

Development is a chemical process that amplifies the latent image by a factor of millions (about 100,000,000) to form a visible silver pattern. The basic reaction is reduction (addition of an electron) of the silver ion, which changes it into black metallic silver:

$$Ag^+ + electron \rightarrow Ag$$

The developer is the reducing agent. Development is generally an all-or-none phenomenon, because an entire grain is developed (reduced) once the process begins. The process is usually initiated at the site of a latent image speck (commonly on the surface of the grain). It is believed that the action of the silver atoms in the latent image is to accelerate (catalyze) the reduction of the silver ions in the grain by the developing chemicals. The silver in a grain that does not contain a latent image can be reduced by the developer, but at a much slower rate. Thus, **time is a fundamental factor in the developing process.** Development should be discontinued when the differential between exposed developed grains and unexposed undeveloped grains is at a maximum.

Modern developing solutions contain two developing agents, hydroquinone plus phenidone or metol. Hydroquinone was discovered to be a developing agent in 1880. Hydroquinone requires a strong alkali to activate it. Developers made of hydroquinone are characterized by high contrast. Metol developers became available in 1891, and are characterized by high speed, low contrast, and fine grain. Phenidone was discovered in 1940, and is similar to metol. Both metol and phenidone are used mainly in combination with hydroquinone. This statement is usually expressed the other way around by stating that hydroquinone is used mainly in combination with metol or phenidone. Two agents are used because of the phenomenon of **synergism,** or superadditivity. The mixture results in a development rate greater than the sum of the developing rate of each developing agent. The reasons for development synergism are complex and not fully understood, so we will not explore the details.

The chemistry of developing is not our chief interest, but the formulas for the basic reactions help in gaining a good understanding of the process. As shown in Figure 10–7, the developing agent reduces silver ions to metallic silver, causing oxidation and inactivation of the developing agent and the liberation of hydrogen ions. Note that the reaction must proceed in an alkaline solution. When hydroquinone is oxidized to quinone, two electrons are liberated to combine with the two silver ions to form metallic silver (Fig. 10–7A). The reaction of phenidone is similar (Fig. 10–7B).

The silver thus formed is deposited at the latent image site, gradually enlarging this initially microscopic black spot into a single visible black speck of silver in the emulsion.

In addition to **developing agents,** the developing solution contains (1) an **alkali** to adjust the pH, (2) a **preservative** (sodium sulfite), and (3) **restrainers,** or antifoggants. The **alkali** adjusts the hydrogen ion concentration (pH), which greatly affects the developing power of the developing agents, especially hydroquinone. In addition, the alkali serves as a buffer to control the hydrogen ions liberated during the development reaction. Most radiographic developers function at a pH range of 10 to 11.5. Typical alkalies include sodium hydroxide, sodium carbonate, and borates (sodium metaborate and sodium tetraborate).

Sodium sulfite is added for two reasons. The oxidation products of the developing agents decompose in alkaline solution and form colored materials that can stain the emulsion. These products react rapidly with sodium sulfite to form colorless soluble sulfonates. In addition, sodium sulfite acts as a preservative. In alkaline solution the developing agent will react with oxygen from the air. The sulfite acts as a preservative by decreasing the rate of oxidation, especially that of hydroquinone. Sulfite removes oxygen from the air dissolved in the solution, or at the surface of the solution, before it has time to oxidize the developing agent.

Fog is the **development of unexposed silver halide grains** that do not contain a latent image. In a complex manner, dilute concentrations of soluble bromide (potas-

Figure 10–7   Basic chemical reactions involved in the development process. Hydroquinone (A) or phenidone (B) may be used as the developer

sium bromide) decrease the rate of fog formation. To a lesser degree the bromide also decreases the rate of development of the latent image. Soluble bromide produced as a byproduct of the development process also affects the activity of the developer. The development reaction in a 90-sec x-ray processor must be completed in about 20 sec. This rapid rate of development requires that the temperature of the developing solution be quite high, usually between 90 and 95° F. This rapid, high-temperature rate of developing requires that modern x-ray developers contain additional antifoggants to permit rapid development of exposed grains but minimize fog development. The most significant dif-

ference in commercial x-ray developing solutions is in the antifoggants present.

Developer formulas also contain other ingredients designed to influence swelling of the x-ray film emulsion, development rate, and physical properties. All developers contain the same basic functional components: developer (reducing agent), alkali, preservatives, and bromide. Differences in antifoggants and other ingredients are often proprietary, so we cannot give specific examples.

The bromide ions released by the reduction of silver ions to silver atoms pass into the developing solution. It is mainly this increase in bromide concentration that limits the life of developing solutions.

Replenishment

We have seen that, during use, developing solutions consume developing agents and preservatives, but acquire hydrogen ions and bromide. Each time a film is processed in an automatic processor a small portion (about 60 ml in a 10-L tank) of the developing solution is removed and replaced with a replenishment solution. The purpose of this replenishment is to maintain developing agent concentration, preservative concentration, bromide concentration, and pH at a constant level for the lifetime of the developer solution. Almost all radiographs are now processed in automatic film processors with automatic developer replenishment. Traditional replenishment was developed for high volume operations where many films are processed each day. However, many automatic processors operate in small installations where few films are developed each day. Under these circumstances, oxidation of developer is more important than the consequences of the development process. We will discuss replenishment requirements for both **high volume (developing reaction dependent)** and **low volume (oxidation reaction dependent)** situations.

The development reaction may be written:

$$2\ AgBr\ +\ H_2Q\ +\ Na_2SO_3$$
(silver bromide + hydroquinone + sodium sulfite)
|
Development
↓
$$2\ Ag\ +\ HBr\ +\ HQSO_3Na\ +\ NaBr$$
(Silver + hydrobromic acid +
hydroquinonemonosulfonate + sodium bromide)

Notice that each time a film is processed, **bromide and acid are formed** and some **developer is consumed.** Replenishment of developer must compensate for these changes by being free of bromide, by containing alkaline agents and buffers and, to a lesser extent, restoring depleted preservative and developing agents. With normal use in a busy department, the lifetime of a tank of developer in an automatic film processor is about 2 to 3 months. A typical replenishment rate is to replace 60 ml of developer with replenisher for each 14- × 17-in. film processed.

Now, let us consider a tank of developer that sits for long periods of time with few films being processed. In this situation, oxidation of the developer becomes more important than the development reaction. The **oxidation** reaction may be written:

$$H_2Q\ +\ Na_2SO_3\ +\ O_2$$
(hydroquinone + sodium sulfite + oxygen)
|
Oxidation
↓
$$HQSO_3Na\ +\ NaOH\ +\ Na_2SO_4$$
(hydroquinonemonosulfonate +
sodium hydroxide + sodium sulfate)

Notice that the oxidation reaction **raises the pH** of the developer by forming sodium hydroxide. This is just the opposite of the development reaction in which the acid formed lowers developer pH. Also, the **oxidation reaction produces no bromide.** Since few films are processed, replenishment is infrequent. Also, since standard replenisher has a higher pH than developer and no bromide, routine replenishment will maintain the high pH and dilute bromide. Bromide concentration drops rapidly, and this has an adverse effect on film sensitometry.

Developer and replenisher formulas are modified for low volume applications. Developers have a lower pH and higher sulfite concentration to retard oxidation, and a high buffering capacity to minimize the pH effects of oxidation. Replenishers compensate mostly for oxidation rather than development. The replenisher has a lower pH than developer and contains bromide. Replenishment rate is usually higher (about 90 ml per 14- × 17-in. film) to increase developer turnover rate.

The main consequence of an abnormal composition of developer ingredients is to produce films with a sharp decrease in toe gradient (we will discuss the terms "toe" and "gradient" in Chapter 14). Such a change makes it hard to detect low contrast images in the lighter (lower density) areas of a radiograph.

In summary, the chemical composition of the developer and replenisher, and the replenishment rate, must provide a constant composition of solution in the developer tank of an automatic processor. The most important parameters are pH and bromide concentration. Restoration of consumed preservatives and developing agents is also required.

Fixing

Only part of the silver halide in the emulsion is reduced to silver during developing. The remaining silver halide impairs both the immediate usefulness and permanence of the developed radiograph. Therefore it must be removed, but the fixing solution must remove silver halide without damaging the image formed by metallic silver.

The solubility of silver halide (we will use silver bromide as an example) in a water solution is controlled by the concentration of silver and halide ions. Silver bromide is only slightly soluble in water. The product of the silver and bromide ions in solution is always constant for any given temperature, and may be expressed by the equation

Silver ion × bromide ion = constant

If the concentration of silver ions could be reduced, the concentration of bromide ions would have to increase, which means that more silver bromide would have to dissolve from the emulsion. Thus, the solubility of silver halide would increase. The function of the fixing agent is to form water-soluble complexes in which silver ions are tightly bound. The soluble complex thus formed effectively removes silver ions from the solution.

Two agents form satisfactory stable complexes with silver ions, cyanides and thiosulfates. Cyanides are poisonous and are not generally used. **Thiosulfate** in the form of the sodium or ammonium salt is the common fixing agent, or "hypo." Why is it called hypo? In earlier chemical nomenclature, the compound we call sodium thiosulfate ($Na_2S_2O_3$) was given the name hyposulfite of soda, and "hypo" it remains to photographers. At least three silver thiosulfate complexes are formed in the fixing solution; their identities need not concern us. A typical reaction might be

Silver bromide + sodium thiosulfate →

silver thiosulfate complex + sodium bromide

The ammonium thiosulfate salt is more active, and is used in fixer supplied in the form of a liquid concentrate.

In addition to thiosulfate, the fixing solution contains a substance to harden the gelatin. Hardening results in a decrease in the swelling of gelatin, making it tougher and more resistant to abrasion. The hardener is usually a chromium or aluminum compound. The fixing bath also contains an acid, stabilizers, and a buffer to maintain the acidic pH level.

An incompletely fixed film is easily recognized because it has a "milky" or cloudy appearance. This is a result of the dispersion of transmitted light by the very small silver iodobromide crystals that have not been dissolved from the emulsion.

Washing

After developing and fixing, the film must be well washed with water. Washing serves primarily to remove the fixing-bath chemicals. Everyone has seen an x-ray film that has turned brown with age. This is the result of incomplete washing. Retained hypo will react with the silver image to form brown silver sulfide, just as silverware acquires a brown tarnish when exposed to the hydrogen sulfide produced by cooking gas. The general reaction is

Hypo + silver → Silver sulfide (brown)
+ Sodium sulfite

SUMMARY

X-ray film is a photographic film coated with emulsion on both sides of the film base. The light-sensitive material in the emulsion is a silver iodobromide crystal. X-ray film is only slightly sensitive to direct x-ray exposure. Impurities in the silver halide crystal structure increase the light sensitivity of the film emulsion. Light, or x-ray, exposure causes the grains in the emulsion to develop an invisible latent image. The developing process magnifies the latent image to produce a visible pattern of black metallic silver.

The sensitivity of x-ray film to direct x-ray exposure varies with the kVp of the x-ray beam.

REFERENCES

1. Baines, H., and Bomback, E.S.: The Science of Photography. 2nd Ed. London, Fountain Press, 1967.
2. Fuchs, A.W.: Evolution of roentgen film. Am. J. Roentgenol., 75:30, 1956.
3. James, T.H., and Higgins, G.C.: Fundamentals of Photographic Theory. 2nd Ed. New York, Morgan and Morgan, 1968.
4. Martin, F.C., and Fuchs, A.W.: The historical evolution of roentgen-ray plates and films. Am. J. Roentgenol., 26:540, 1931.
5. Mees, C.E.K., and James, T.H.: The Theory of the Photographic Process. 3rd Ed. New York, Macmillan, 1969.
6. Neblette, C.B.: Photography, Its Materials and Processes. 6th Ed. New York, Van Nostrand, 1962.
7. Wayrynen, R.E., Holland, R.S., and Trinkle, R.J.: Chemical Manufacturing Considerations and Constraints in Manufacturing Film, Chemicals and Processing. Proceedings of the Second Image Receptor Conference: Radiographic Film Processing, Washington, DC, March 31–April 2, 1977, pp. 89–96. Washington, DC, U.S. Government Printing Office, 1977, Stock No. 017-015-00134-2.
8. Wuelfing, P.: High stability developer for medical x-ray processing. SPIE Vol. 555 Medical Imaging and Instrumentation, 1985, p. 91.

11 *Photographic Characteristics of X-Ray Film*

The diagnostic accuracy of a radiographic film examination depends, in part, on the visibility of diagnostically important information on the film. Understanding the relationship between the exposure a film receives and the way the film responds to the exposure is essential to intelligent selection of proper exposure factors and type of film to provide maximum information content of the radiograph.

What is meant by the term "exposure" of an x-ray film or film-screen combination? Exposure is proportional to the product of the milliamperes of x-ray tube current and the exposure time. Thus, an exposure of 100 milliamperes for 1 second is expressed as 100 milliampere-seconds, usually written 100 mAs. An exposure of 100 mAs could also be produced by using 50-mA tube current for 2 sec, 200 mA for 0.5 sec, 500 mA for 0.2 sec, and so forth. In this chapter, film exposure is assumed to mean exposure of the x-ray film by light from x-ray intensifying screens, unless otherwise stated.

Exposure (mAs) of the x-ray film produces film blackening, or density. The quality of the x-ray beam (kVp) has more effect on image contrast. Two general but not completely accurate statements should be kept in mind:

1. mAs controls film density
2. kVp controls image contrast

This chapter will discuss the response of the x-ray film to exposure.

PHOTOGRAPHIC DENSITY

When the x-ray beam passes through body tissues, variable fractions of the beam will be absorbed, depending on the composition and thickness of the tissues and on the quality (kVp) of the beam. The magnitude of this variation in beam intensity is the mechanism by which the x-ray beam acquires the information transmitted to the film. This pattern of varying x-ray intensity has been called the x-ray image. Webster's Collegiate Dictionary defines an image as "a mental representation of anything not actually present to the senses." This definition is particularly applicable to the idea of the x-ray image. The x-ray image actually exists in space, but it cannot be seen or otherwise detected by the natural senses. The x-ray image is the pattern of information that the x-ray beam acquires as it passes through and interacts with the patient; that is, the beam is attenuated by the patient. The x-ray image is present in the space between the patient and the x-ray film (or x-ray intensifying screen). The information content of the x-ray image must be transformed into a visible image on the x-ray film with as little loss of information as possible. We have seen how the energy of the x-ray beam may be used to produce a visible pattern of black metallic silver on the x-ray film; the degree of film blackening is directly related to the intensity of radiation reaching the film or intensifying screen. The measurement of film blackness is called "photographic density"; usually, only the word **density** is used. Density is expressed as a number that is actually a **logarithm,** using the common base 10. Photographic density is defined by

$$D = \log \frac{I_0}{I_t}$$

D = density
I_0 = light incident on a film
I_t = light transmitted by the film

Refer to Figure 11–1. If ten arrows (photons) of light strike the back of the film, and only one photon passes through the film, then $I_0 = 10$ and $I_t = 1$:

$$\text{Density} = \log \frac{10}{1} = \log 10 = 1$$

Note that $\dfrac{I_0}{I_t}$ measures the **opacity** of the film (the ability of film to stop light). The reciprocal of density, $\dfrac{I_t}{I_0}$, measures the fraction of light transmitted by the film, and is

called **transmittance.** Useful densities in diagnostic radiology range from about 0.3 (50% of light transmitted) to about 2 (1% of light transmitted). A density of 2 means that $\log \dfrac{I_0}{I_t} = 2$. Because the log of 100 = 2, $\dfrac{I_0}{I_t} = 100$. Thus, for every 100 light photons incident on the film, only 1 photon, or 1%, will be transmitted. Table 11–1 lists some common values for opacity $\left(\dfrac{I_0}{I_t}\right)$, density $\left(\log \dfrac{I_0}{I_t}\right)$, and percentage of light transmission. Note that an increase in film density of 0.3 decreases transmitted light to 50% of its previous value. For example, an increase in density from 0.6 to 0.9 decreases the amount of transmitted light from 25 to 12.5%. This emphasizes the fact that the number used to signify a certain density has no units, but is a logarithm. The number 0.3 is the logarithm of 2. Thus, an increase in density of 0.3 $\left(\log \dfrac{I_0}{I_t}\right)$ means an increase in opacity $\left(\dfrac{I_0}{I_t}\right)$ of 2; opacity is doubled by a density increase of 0.3.

Higher density means a blacker film (less light transmission). In routine x-ray work, a density of 2 (1% of light transmitted) is black when viewed on a standard viewbox, and a density of 0.25 to 0.3 (50% of light transmitted) is very light.

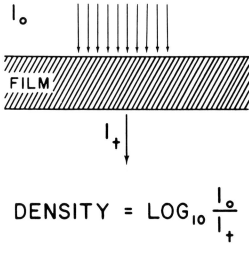

DENSITY = LOG$_{10}$ $\dfrac{I_0}{I_t}$

Figure 11–1   Photographic density

Table 11–1.   Percentage of Light Transmitted by X-Ray Films of Various Densities

OPACITY $\left(\dfrac{I_0}{I_t}\right)$	DENSITY $\left(\log \dfrac{I_0}{I_t}\right)$	LIGHT TRANSMITTED (%)
1	0	100
2	0.3	50
4	0.6	25
8	0.9	12.5
10	1.0	10
30	1.5	3.2
100	2	1
1,000	3	0.1
10,000	4	0.01

If an unexposed x-ray film is processed, it will demonstrate a density of about 0.12. This density consists of base density and fog. The plastic material used to make the film base absorbs a small amount of light. Also, the blue dye used to color some film bases adds slightly to base density. Total base density will average about 0.07. A few of the silver halide grains in an x-ray film emulsion develop without exposure. These unexposed but developed grains compose the density known as fog. Fog density of a fresh x-ray film averages about 0.05. We will refer to the subject of base and fog density several times in this chapter and in Chapter 14.

Why is density expressed as a logarithm? There are three primary reasons. First, logarithms conveniently express large differences in numbers on a small scale. For example, the difference in the light transmission represented by going from a density of 1 (10% of light transmitted) to a density of 2 (1% of light transmitted) is a factor of 10.

Second, the physiologic response of the eye to differences in light intensities is logarithmic (Fig. 11–2). Assume that a film having regions of density that equal 0.3, 0.6, and 0.9 is transilluminated by a light source of 1000 photons. The number of light photons transmitted will be 500, 250, and 125, respectively. The difference in

transmitted light photons between density 0.3 and density 0.6 is 250 (500 to 250), but between density 0.6 and density 0.9 it is only 125 photons (250 to 125). The eye will interpret density 0.3 as being exactly as much brighter than density 0.6 as density 0.6 is brighter than density 0.9. The eye has "seen" the equal differences in density rather than the unequal differences in the number of light photons transmitted.

The third reason for expressing density as a logarithm deals with the addition or superimposition of densities. If films are superimposed, the resulting density is equal to the sum of the density of each film. Consider two films, one of density 2 and one of density 1, which are superimposed and put in the path of a light source with an intensity of 1000 units (Fig. 11–3). The film of density 1 absorbs 90% of the light (100 units are transmitted) and the film of density 2 absorbs 99% of these 100 units, to allow final transmission of 1 unit of light. We started with 1000 units (I_0 = 1000) and ended with 1 unit of light (I_t = 1), so we may calculate density:

$$D = \log \frac{I_0}{I_t} = \log \frac{1000}{1} = 3$$

Figure 11–2   The reduction in intensity caused by three films having densities of 0.3, 0.6, and 0.9

Figure 11–3   The density of superimposed films is the sum of the density of the individual films

The effect of superimposing films with a density of 2 and 1 is the same as using a single film of density 3. Almost all the film used in radiology has two emulsions, one on each side of the base. The total density exhibited by the radiograph is the sum of the density of each emulsion.

CHARACTERISTIC CURVE

It is necessary to understand the relationship between the exposure a film receives and the density produced by the exposure. The relationship between exposure and density is plotted as a curve, known as the "characteristic curve" or "H and D curve" (named after F. Hurter and V.C. Driffield, who first published such a curve in England in 1890). The concept of the characteristic curve of an x-ray film exposed by light from x-ray intensifying screens is illustrated in Figure 11–4. Film density is plotted on the vertical axis and film exposure on the horizontal axis. The shape and location of this curve on the graph are important and will, we hope, take on some meaning as this chapter progresses.

Characteristic curves are derived by giving a film a series of exposures, developing the film, and plotting the resulting density against the known exposure. The actual exposure the film received may be measured in the laboratory, but such measurements are not important to use and understand the characteristic curve. (Using medium-speed intensifying screens and 80-kVp x rays, a density of 1.0 on the x-ray film requires that about 3×10^4 x-ray photons hit each square mm of the screen.) By **film exposure** we refer to the product of the intensity of the exposure (milliamperes of x-ray tube current) and time of exposure (expressed in seconds). Exposure is expressed in terms of milliampere-seconds, usually abbreviated mAs. One way to produce a characteristic curve is to expose different areas of a film with constant kilovoltage and milliamperage while varying the time of exposure (e.g., with constant

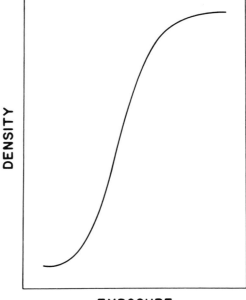

Figure 11–4 Typical characteristic curve of a screen-type x-ray film, exposed with x-ray intensifying screens

kVp and mA, doubling the time of exposure will double the mAs). The exposure is recorded as the relative exposure.

The term **relative exposure** tends to create confusion. Actually, the radiologist and technologist think in terms of relative exposure when evaluating radiographs. For example, if a radiograph of the abdomen exposed with factors of 70 kVp and 75 mAs is judged to be underexposed, the correction might involve increasing the mAs to 150. In other words, the correction involves doubling the exposure. The actual exposure (such as the number of milliroentgens or the number of x-ray photons per square mm) is not known, and does not have to be. The relationship between the two exposures, however, is important. One function of the characteristic curve is to allow the amount of change necessary to correct an exposure error to be predicted. For example, if a film with the characteristic curve shown in Figure 11–5 is underexposed so that its average density is 0.35, the corresponding relative exposure is 4. If the exposure (mAs) is doubled (relative exposure is increased to 8), it can be predicted that the average density will increase to about 0.8. The exposure is also recorded as the logarithm of the relative exposure, mainly for two reasons. First, use of a logarithmic scale allows a very wide range of exposures to be expressed in a compact graph. Second, use of log relative exposure makes analysis of the curve easier. Two exposures whose ratio is constant (e.g., one is twice the other) will always be separated by the same distance on the exposure scale, regardless of their absolute value. Refer to Figure 11–5, in which both the relative exposure and the log relative exposure are indicated, and note that **an increase in the log relative exposure of 0.3 always represents a doubling of the relative exposure.**

Analysis of the characteristic curve of a particular x-ray film provides information about the contrast, speed (sensitivity), and latitude of the film. Please refer to Figure

Figure 11–6 The regions of the characteristic curve

11–6. Even at 0 exposure the film density is not 0 but will usually be 0.2, or less. This density is made up of fog (development of unexposed grains of silver halide in the emulsion) and base densities (opacity of the film base), which have been previously discussed. Therefore, total density on an exposed and developed film will include base and fog densities. The minimum density caused by base and fog in a "fresh" film is about 0.12. To evaluate density produced by the exposure alone, base and fog densities must be subtracted from the total density. Second, note that at low density (toe) and high density (shoulder), the film shows little change in density despite a relatively large change in log relative exposure (Fig. 11–6). The important part of the characteristic curve is between the toe and shoulder, and in this region the curve is almost a straight line. In this "straight line" portion the density is approximately proportional to the log relative exposure. For example, if log relative exposure 1.1 produces a density of 1.0, and log relative exposure 1.3 produces a density of 2.0, we

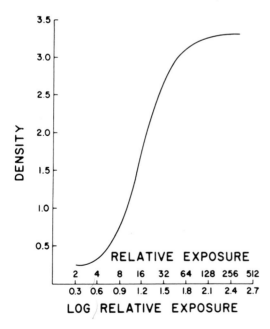

Figure 11–5 The relationship between relative exposure and the corresponding log relative exposure

can predict that a density of about 1.5 will be produced by a log relative exposure of 1.2 (these figures correspond roughly to the characteristic curve of Figure 11–6).

Film Contrast

The information content of the invisible x-ray image is "decoded" by the x-ray film into a pattern of variations in optical density, known as "radiographic contrast." Radiographic contrast is the density difference between image areas in the radiograph. There are many definitions of contrast, but we will use the simple definition that contrast is the difference in density existing between various regions on the film. Radiographic contrast depends on subject contrast and on film contrast. Subject contrast depends on the differential attenuation of the x-ray beam as it passes through the patient. The discussion of attenuation in Chapter 5 has already introduced the important aspects of subject contrast. Subject contrast was seen to be affected by the thickness, density, and atomic differences of the subject, the radiation energy (kVp), contrast material, and scatter radiation. The major theme of the remainder of this chapter will be film contrast.

The information content of the x-ray image is the pattern of varying intensity of the x-ray beam caused by differential attenuation of x rays by the subject. Few x rays reach the film through areas of bone or opaque contrast material, while many photons are transmitted through soft tissue, and the air around the patient stops almost no x-ray photons. The kVp must be selected with care so that the numbers of photons attenuated by bone and soft tissue are in the proper proportion to produce an x-ray image of high information content for the film intensifying screen to "decode." The correct kVp is tremendously important in producing proper subject contrast. This relationship (kVp and contrast) will be examined in detail in Chapter 14. Using the correct mAs causes the total

number of x rays in each part of the attenuated x-ray beam to be sufficient to produce correct overall density in the processed film. Because exposure (mAs) determines the total number of x rays in the beam, mAs may be considered analogous to light in producing an ordinary photograph. Too little, or too much, mAs results in an underexposed or overexposed radiograph.

Subject contrast may be thought of as one factor that controls the log relative exposure that reaches the film. That is, film directly under a bone receives a low exposure, whereas a high exposure reaches the film under soft tissue areas of the subject. A consideration of film contrast must examine how the film responds to the difference in exposure produced by subject contrast. Film contrast depends on four factors:

1. characteristic curve of the film
2. film density
3. screen or direct x-ray exposure
4. film processing

Shape of the Characteristic Curve. The shape of the characteristic curve tells us how much change in film density will occur as film exposure changes. The slope, or gradient, of the curve may be measured and expressed numerically. One such measurement is called **film gamma.** The gamma of a film is defined as the maximum slope of the characteristic curve, and is described by the formula

$$\text{Gamma} = \frac{D_2 - D_1}{\log E_2 - \log E_1}$$

where D_2 and D_1 are the densities on the steepest part of the curve resulting from log relative exposures E_2 and E_1. Figure 11–7 shows an example of how film gamma is calculated. The gamma of x-ray films exposed with intensifying screens ranges from 2.0 to 3.5.

In radiology the concept of film gamma is of little value because, as illustrated in Figure 11–7, the maximum slope (steepest)

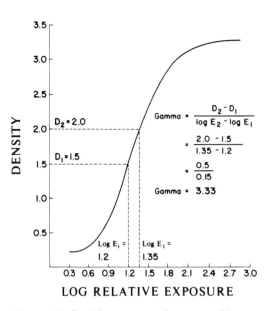

Figure 11-7   The gamma of an x-ray film

Figure 11-8   The average gradient of an x-ray film

portion of the characteristic curve is usually very short. We are interested in the slope of the curve over the entire range of useful radiographic densities (0.25 to 2.0). The slope (gradient) of a straight line joining two points of specified density on the characteristic curve is called the **average gradient.** The average gradient is usually calculated between density 0.25 and 2.0 above base and fog for radiographic films. Such a calculation is shown in Figure 11-8, which is the same curve from which gamma was calculated in Figure 11-7. In calculating average gradient, D_1 is always 0.25 and D_2 is 2.0; therefore, $D_2 - D_1$ is always 1.75. In Figure 11-8, log E_2 and E_1 are 1.4 and 0.85, respectively.

If the average gradient of the film used is greater than 1, the film will exaggerate subject contrast and, the higher the average gradient, the greater this exaggeration will be. A film with average gradient of 1 will not change subject contrast; a film with an average gradient of less than 1 will decrease subject contrast. Because contrast is very important in radiology, x-ray films all have an average gradient of greater than 1. For example, consider a radiograph of

the hand (exposed with a screen-film combination) made with an x-ray beam of proper energy (kVp) to cause the bones to absorb four times as many photons as the soft tissue. This means that four times as many x-ray photons will reach the film under soft tissues as will reach the film under bone. The difference in log relative exposure between bone and soft tissue reaching the film under the hand is 0.6 (log 4 = 0.6). If we assign a value of 1.5 as the log relative exposure in the soft tissue area (E_S), then the log relative exposure corresponding to the bones (E_B) is 0.9 (Fig. 11-9). These two exposures will produce film densities of 0.8 (bone density) and 2.8 (soft tissue density) on the hypothetical film's characteristic curve depicted in Figure 11-9. This is a density range of 2.0, corresponding to an overall brightness range of 100:1 when the film is transilluminated and viewed (100 is the antilog of 2.0). Thus, subject contrast resulting in an exposure range to the x-ray film of 4:1 has been exaggerated, or amplified, in the viewed radiograph into a brightness range (radiographic contrast) of 100:1.

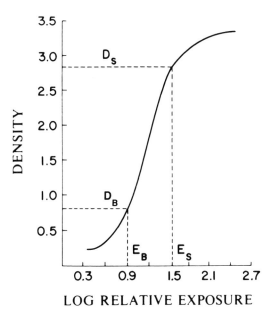

Figure 11–9 Film contrast amplifies subject contrast if the average gradient is greater than one

Film Density. The slope of the characteristic curve (i.e., film contrast) changes with density. This is especially true in the toe and shoulder regions (see Fig. 11–5). Let us emphasize that the ratio of the difference in log relative exposure is determined by the kVp selected (such as the 4:1 ratio between soft tissue and bone in the example of the hand). If the kVp remains constant, this ratio will remain constant for any one examination despite change in exposure time, milliamperes, or focus-film distance. All these last mentioned factors, however, will determine the actual value of the exposure, thereby determining the location of the exposure on the log relative exposure axis of the characteristic curve of the film.

Let us consider an x-ray study of the abdomen in which the kVp chosen results in one area transmitting about 1.6 times more radiation than another. This means a log relative exposure difference of 0.2 (log 1.6 = 0.2). We will assume that the film used for this study has the characteristic curve

depicted in Figure 11–10. If the factors of time, milliamperes, and focus-film distance (the inverse square law) are correct, the log relative exposures will produce film density falling along the steep portion of the characteristic curve. This will produce a density difference (radiographic contrast) of 0.6, or a difference in light transmission of 4:1 (antilog 0.6 = 4). If the exposure puts the developed densities on the toe of the curve, however, the film is underexposed (not enough mAs), and the density difference will fall to 0.13, or a difference in light transmission of 1.35:1 (antilog 0.13 = 1.35). Note that the exposure ratio has remained the same (i.e., log relative exposure difference of 0.2) because the kVp has not been changed. Similarly, overexposure, or too many mAs, will result in densities in the shoulder region of the characteristic curve of our hypothetic film-screen combination. As shown in Figure 11–10, this will result in a density difference (contrast) of 0.2, corresponding to a difference in

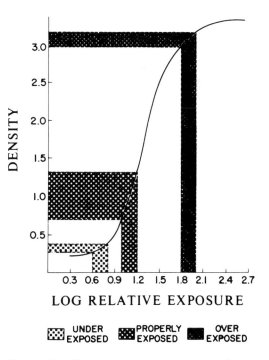

Figure 11–10 Incorrect exposures result in loss of contrast

light transmission of 1.59:1 (antilog 0.2 = 1.59). Exposures producing density at the level of 3 (0.1% of light transmitted) also produce less visible contrast under ordinary viewing conditions, because the human eye has low sensitivity to contrast at low brightness levels. This is why a spotlight must be used to aid in viewing regions of high density.

Screen or Direct X-Ray Exposure. If a film designed for exposure by light from intensifying screens is exposed to x rays directly, its characteristic curve has a considerably different shape than the curve obtained from exposure with screens. Remember, considerably more exposure (mAs) is required if no screens are used, because the intensification factor of screens may range from about 15 to 50 or more. Films exposed with par speed intensifying screens will require an x-ray exposure of approximately 1 mR to produce a density of 1; this value will rise to 30 mR or more with direct x-ray exposure.

At the same density, contrast is always lower for a film exposed to x rays only than for the same film exposed by light from intensifying screens. The reason for this difference in contrast is not precisely known. It probably is related to the complex manner in which the film emulsion responds to the energy of absorbed x-ray photons.

In addition, intensifying screens are relatively more sensitive than film to higher energy x rays. The primary x-ray beam transmitted through the patient is of higher energy than the secondary, or scatter, radiation. Scatter radiation decreases contrast, as will be discussed in detail in Chapter 14. Because intensifying screens are relatively less sensitive to the lower energy of the scatter radiation, decrease in contrast will be minimized by screens. X-ray film, because it is more sensitive to lower kVp x rays, may record the scatter radiation better than the higher energy, information-containing primary beam. The variation in film sensitivity to x rays between 50 and 100 kVp is not very great, however, and can usually be ignored in clinical radiology.

Stated another way, the average gradient of a double-emulsion x-ray film will be greatest when the film is exposed with intensifying screens. Direct x-ray exposure will produce a lower average gradient. The photochemical reasons for this phenomenon are unknown.

Film Processing (Development). Increasing the time or temperature of development (or both) will, up to a point, increase the average gradient of a film (film speed is also increased). If development time is only 40% of normal, the gradient will be reduced to about 60% of maximum. Fog will also be increased with increased development time or temperature, though, and fog decreases contrast. Therefore, it is important to adhere to the manufacturer's standards in processing film. Automatic film processing equipment has eliminated some problems associated with temperature of solutions and development time. To summarize, increasing the time or temperature of development will

1. increase average gradient (increase film contrast)
2. increase film speed (increase density for a given exposure)
3. increase fog (decrease film contrast)

Figure 11–11 shows the effect of development time (or temperature) on average gradient, film speed, and fog.

Speed

The speed of a film-screen system is defined as the reciprocal of the exposure in roentgens required to produce a density of 1.0 above base plus fog density:

$$\text{Speed} = \frac{1}{\text{Roentgens}}$$

As an example we will consider the speed of a commonly used film-screen system, Du Pont Cronex 4 film combined with Du Pont Cronex Hi Plus ($CaWO_4$) screens. Analysis

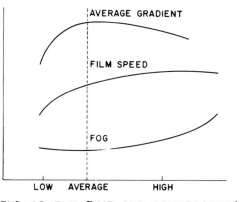

Figure 11–11 Development time influences average gradient, speed, and fog

of the curve in Figure 11–12 shows that an exposure of 0.57 mR (0.00057 R) was required to produce a net density of 1.0 above base and fog. Therefore, the speed (S) of the film-screen system for this kVp is

$$S = \frac{1}{0.00057 \text{ R}} = 1750 \text{ R}^{-1}$$

The shape of the characteristic curve is controlled by film contrast; the film speed determines the location of the curve on the log exposure scale.

Figure 11–13 shows the curves of two films that are identical except that film B is 0.3 log relative exposure units to the right of film A. Both films will show identical film contrast, but film B will require twice (antilog 0.3 = 2) as much exposure (mAs) as film A. Because the gradient of a characteristic curve varies with density, the relative speed between two films will be found to vary with the density at which speed is measured. For example, if a low-contrast and a high-contrast film are compared for speed, as in Figure 11–14, the relative speed between the two films might actually reverse with change in density. In our example, speed calculated at a density of 1.0 will show the low-contrast film (film B) to be the fastest (i.e., film B requires a lower log relative exposure to produce a

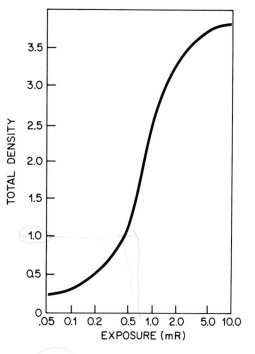

Figure 11–12 A Cronex 4 sensitometric curve (70-kVp exposure, Hi Plus screens) shows that 0.57 mR is used to reach a 1.0 net density. The system speed for 70 kVp is

$$\frac{1}{0.00057} = 1750 \text{ R}^{-1}$$

(Modified from the Cronex 4 medical x-ray film data sheet available from E.I. du Pont de Nemours Company, Inc. Modified with the help of Russell S. Holland, Ph.D.)

density of 1.0 than film A). At a density of 1.5 both films have the same speed, and above density 1.5 the higher contrast film A is faster than film B. For medical x-ray films, relative film speed is usually compared at a density of 1.0 above base and fog.

Speed Class System

The measured speed of a film-screen system depends on a number of variables, such as the kVp, amount of scatter radiation, x-ray absorption by the cassette or x-ray table top, and the way in which the film is processed. The American National Standards Institute (ANSI) has attempted

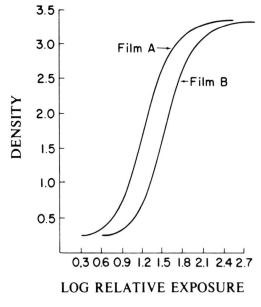

LOG RELATIVE EXPOSURE

Figure 11–13 Film speed

to standardize the way in which speed (and contrast) of medical x-ray film-screen systems is measured.[1] This standard defines test objects that are used to simulate radiography of the chest, the skull or pelvis, and the extremities. Various exposures are made at four kilovoltages, approximately

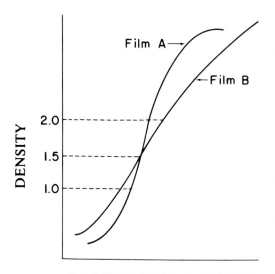

LOG RELATIVE EXPOSURE

Figure 11–14 Relative film speed varies with the density at which speed is measured

125, 80, 70, and 60 kVp. Film processing is strictly controlled. If all manufacturers followed such a rigid standard to determine speed, direct comparison of products would be easy and meaningful. As things exist now, however, published measurements of speed must be used as approximations only. For this reason, we suggest that the "speed class system" concept be used to assign relative speeds to various film-screen systems.

Refer to Table 11–2, which is the same as Table 9–5. Notice that film-screen speed is listed as speed class.* The numbers in the speed class system make up a sequence in which the logarithm of each number differs from the next number by 0.1 (i.e., this is a 0.1 log system). Table 11–3 lists the sequence from 100 to 1000 and gives the logarithm of each number. Note that the log of each number increases or decreases by 0.1 (this makes each number approximately 25% greater or less than its neighbor). Thus, the ratio between numbers in the sequence is a constant. Because log 2 = 0.3, addition of 0.3 to the log of a number multiplies the number by 2 (e.g., log 160 = 2.2, log 320 = 2.5, etc.). All of us who use a camera have used this 0.1 log system, usually without realizing it. Consider the speed of the film you use in your camera. Don't the numbers ASA 25, 32, 64, 125, 200, and 400 sound familiar? Table 11–3 does not list the sequence below 100, but simply divide by 10 to go on down (i.e., 100, 80, 64, 50, 40, 32, 25, 20, 16, and so forth).

Why propose this speed class system? First, it is a handy number sequence. It is easy to multiply or divide by 10, the numbers increase or decrease by an easily defined ratio, and a change in log of 0.3 doubles or halves a number. The other reason is that the currently available measurements of film-screen system speed are not

*This idea was proposed to us by Robert Wayrynen, Ph.D.: Reid Kellogg, Ph.D.; and Russell Holland, Ph.D., of the photo products department of E.I. du Pont de Nemours & Company, Inc.

Table 11–2. Speed Class of Various Intensifying Screens

MANUFACTURER	NAME	PHOSPHOR	SPECTRAL EMISSION	FILM	SPEED CLASS
Du Pont	Cronex Par Speed	CaWO$_4$	Blue	Cronex 4	100
	Cronex Hi Plus	CaWO$_4$	Blue	Cronex 4	250
	Cronex Quanta III	LaOBr:Tm	Blue	Cronex 4	800
	Cronex Quanta V	LaOBr:Tm and	Blue	Cronex 4	320
		Gd$_2$O$_2$S:Tb	Green	Cronex 8	400
	Quanta Detail	YTaO$_4$:Tm	Ultraviolet/ Blue	Cronex 4	100
	Quanta Fast Detail	YTaO$_4$:Nb	Ultraviolet/ Blue	Cronex 4	400
Kodak	X-Omatic Fine	BaPbSO$_4$, yellow dye	Blue	XRP	32
	X-Omatic Regular	BaSrSO$_4$:Eu, neutral dye	Blue	Ortho G	200
	Lanex Fine	Gd$_2$O$_2$S:Tb, neutral dye	Green	Ortho G	100
	Lanex Medium	Gd$_2$O$_2$S:Tb, yellow dye	Green	Ortho G	250
	Lanex Regular	Gd$_2$O$_2$S:Tb	Green	Ortho G	400

Note: Dupont Cronex 4 film is now largely replaced by Cronex 7 and Cronex 10, and Kodak Ortho G film by T-Mat G. The older films still accurately reflect relative intensifying screen speeds, which is the purpose of this table.

Table 11–3. Speed Class System of Numbers from 100 to 1000

Number	100	125	160	200	250	320	400	500	640	800	1000
Logarithm	2	2.1	2.2	2.3	2.4	2.5	2.6	2.7	2.8	2.9	3.0

standardized. Published values are accurate for the conditions under which they were determined, but such conditions vary. Until rigid standards (such as the ANSI method[1]) are adopted by industry, assigning a particular film-screen system speed to one of the numbers in the 0.1 log system appears reasonable. There are more than 1000 film-screen combinations on the market today, so some "lumping" of an otherwise enormous variety of expressions of speed seems necessary. Some of you may have also noticed that the mAs stations of some x-ray generators now use an 0.1 log sequence of steps.

Latitude

Unlike average gradient and speed, film latitude is not expressed in numeric terms. Latitude refers to the range of log relative exposure (mAs) that will produce density within the accepted range for diagnostic radiology (usually considered to be density 0.25 to 2.0). Let us consider two hypothetical films (Fig. 11–15), one a high-contrast film (film A) and one a lower contrast film (film B). If the density recorded on the film is to remain in the range of 0.25 to 2.0, film A will be limited to a log relative exposure

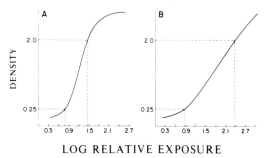

LOG RELATIVE EXPOSURE

Figure 11–15 Film B has greater latitude than film A

range of 0.75 to 1.42, or a difference in log relative exposure of 0.67 corresponding to an actual ratio of 4.68 to 1 (antilog 0.67 = 4.68). Film B will remain in the designated density values over a range of log relative exposure from 0.85 to 2.35, or a difference in log exposure of 1.50 corresponding to an actual ratio of 31.6:1. Film B is said to have greater latitude than film A in that it will accept a wider range of exposures. Note that film B has greater latitude but less film contrast. Generally speaking, **the latitude of a film varies inversely with film contrast.** There are two practical aspects to this concept of film latitude. For the technologist exposing a film, the film with more latitude makes the exposure less critical; if he has picked the proper kVp for adequate penetration, he has more room for error in his choice of exposure (mAs). Generally, the radiologist is interested in high contrast, which means films of less latitude. But there may be situations in which a wide range of subject contrast (such as in the chest) must be recorded, and in such cases the film with the lower contrast but higher latitude may produce a radiograph in which many small changes in film exposures (i.e., subject contrast) can be recorded. Such lower contrast but higher latitude films are available to the radiologist. (We will discuss another aspect of exposure latitude as it pertains to kVp and subject contrast in Chapter 14).

Double-Emulsion Film

Films used for routine radiography have photosensitive emulsion coated on both sides of the base support. There is a physical and photographic reason for this. The emulsion is applied to the base in liquid form. When the emulsion dries, it shrinks to about one tenth of its original volume. Most of the decrease in volume causes a decrease in thickness of the emulsion, but there is also a slight tendency to shrink in area. If emulsion were put on only one side of the base, shrinking of the emulsion would cause the film to curl toward the

emulsion side. An identical emulsion on each side of the base prevents this curling. The photographic advantage of a double emulsion is important only when the film is exposed with intensifying screens. We may assume that each emulsion receives an identical exposure from each screen, because any filtering action of the front screen that might act to decrease the intensity of x rays reaching the back screen is small.

Consider the case of a single-emulsion film in a cassette, which receives two exposures, $\log E_1$ and E_2, and responds with densities D_1 and D_2. Film contrast for this exposure difference may be expressed as

$$\text{Contrast} = \frac{D_2 - D_1}{\log E_2 - \log E_1}$$

If this same exposure is now used to expose a double-emulsion film with light from intensifying screens, each emulsion will respond with densities D_1 and D_2. When two films are superimposed, the resulting density is the sum of the densities of each film. Therefore, when the double-emulsion film is viewed, the densities of each emulsion are added, and the resulting total density will now be $D_1 + D_1 = 2D_1$ and $D_2 + D_2 = 2D_2$. The exposures E_2 and E_1 have not changed, but we have allowed two emulsions to respond to the exposure. The contrast that the eye now sees is

$$\text{Contrast} = \frac{2D_2 - 2D_1}{\log E_2 - \log E_1} = \frac{2(D_2 - D_1)}{\log E_2 - \log E_1}$$

Because $\log E_2 - \log E_1$ is the same for each exposure, we may compare contrast without the $\log E_2 - \log E_1$ term:

$$\text{Single emulsion contrast} = D_2 - D_1$$

$$\text{Double emulsion contrast} = 2(D_2 - D_1)$$

The double-emulsion film has produced twice the contrast of a single-emulsion film. Obviously, the overall density of the double-emulsion film is increased, resulting in increased film speed. For a film being exposed to x rays directly, a similar effect could be produced by making a single-emulsion film with a thicker emulsion. Because light photons are easily absorbed by the emulsion, however, only the outer layer of the emulsion is affected by light from intensifying screens. This is one reason why x-ray film designed for exposure by light from two intensifying screens (in a cassette) has a thin emulsion on each side of the base, rather than a single thick emulsion.

EMULSION ABSORPTION

To expose an x-ray film with intensifying screens, it is necessary for the silver halide grains in the film to absorb the light emitted by the screen phosphor. The ability of the film grains to absorb light depends on the wavelength, or color, of the light. **Standard silver halide films absorb light in the ultraviolet, violet, and blue regions of the visible spectrum.** Used with calcium tungstate or barium lead sulfate screens, such films worked well because these phosphors emitted light that was absorbed by natural silver halide (Fig. 11–16). Note that natural silver halide film does not absorb in the green and yellow portions of the visible spectrum, where much of the light from some rare earth phosphors is emitted (see Fig. 11–18). You will recall that the peak wavelengths from some rare earth screens, such as Kodak Lanex screens, are produced by the terbium ion with about 60% of its energy at about 544 nm (green light). It is possible to extend the sensitivity of film to the green wavelengths by coating the silver halide grains with a thin layer of dye that absorbs the green light and then transfers this absorbed energy to the grain. Such green-sensitive film is called **ortho** film. Similarly, the silver halide grain can be coated with a dye that absorbs red light, and this is called a **pan** film (panchromatic: sensitive to light of all colors). This is illustrated in Figure 11–17. When rare earth screens are used, an appropriate film should be used if one is to take advantage of all the light emitted by the screen. Such a combination is the Kodak Lanex screen and Ortho G film (Fig. 11–18).

Please look back at Figure 9–12, which shows the spectral emission of LaOBr:Tm (found in Du Pont Cronex Quanta III and Quanta V screens). Remember that this rare earth, activated by thulium, produces light to which natural silver halide film is sensitive. Compare the twin peaks of 374 nm and 463 nm in Figure 9–12 to the sensitivity of silver halide as shown in Figure 11–17. The more recently introduced yttrium tantalate intensifying screens also emit light in the ultraviolet and blue wavelengths to which natural silver halide films exhibit maximum sensitivity. Some rare earth phosphor screens use green-sensitive

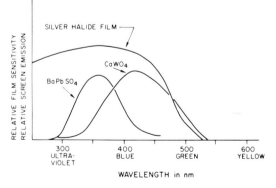

Figure 11–16 The spectral emission of barium lead sulfate and calcium tungstate intensifying screens compared to the spectral sensitivity of natural silver halide (not drawn to scale)

Figure 11–17 Relative spectral sensitivity of natural silver halide, ortho, and pan films

Figure 11–18 Spectral emission of Kodak Lanex Regular screens and the spectral sensitivity of Kodak Ortho G film (the bars and curve are approximations used for illustration only, and no attempt to achieve accuracy was made)

Figure 11–19 Spectral sensitivity of natural silver halide and ortho film compared to the transmission of an amber and a red safelight filter

film, some use blue-sensitive film, and some (e.g., Cronex Quanta V) may use either.

Darkroom Safelight

The use of ortho films requires that the correct darkroom safelight be used. For many years an amber safelight (such as the Kodak Type 6B filter) has been used with blue-sensitive films. The amber safelight emits light to which ortho film is sensitive, however, and will produce "safelight fog" if used with such film. With ortho films a safelight filter shifted more toward the red is required (this removes the green light to which ortho film is sensitive). Such a red safelight filter is the Kodak GBX-2 filter. Figure 11–19 illustrates the approximate sensitivity of regular silver halide film and ortho film as compared to the transmission of an amber (6B) and a red (GBX-2) safelight filter.

Crossover Exposure

Crossover exposure, also called "print-through exposure," occurs when a double-emulsion x-ray film is exposed in a cassette containing two intensifying screens. Ideally, each film emulsion would receive light only from the screen in contact with the emulsion. Crossover is the exposure of a film emulsion to light emitted by the screen opposite the emulsion. The main cause of this crossover is incomplete absorption of light by the adjacent emulsion. This unabsorbed light passes through the film base to reach the opposite emulsion. The crossover light is spread because of diffusion, scattering, and reflection caused by the film base and interfaces between the emulsions and film base. Crossover exposure is a significant contributing factor to unsharpness in film-screen systems.

How important is this crossover light in terms of total film exposure? With green-sensitive films, up to 40% of the total exposure is attributed to print-through. Blue-sensitive emulsions (natural silver halide) are slightly more efficient light absorbers and, with blue light systems, crossover is responsible for less than one third of the total exposure (about 30 to 32% with $CaWO_4$ screens, and only 23% with $BaSrSO_4$ screens).

The ideal way to reduce print-through is to increase light absorption in the silver halide grains of the film emulsion. This would improve image quality without reducing system speed. The original film designed to reduce print-through had a light-absorbing dye coated on both sides of the film base. This anticrossover dye absorbed light attempting to diffuse through the base into the opposite emulsion, and decreased crossover exposure to only about

13% of the total exposure. System speed was decreased by about 40% with this film.

At present, two technologies attempt to reduce crossover exposure by increasing light absorption in the film emulsion. These technologies involve:

1. Matching screen light emission to silver halide natural sensitivity
2. Changing the shape of the silver halide grains

In Chapter 9, we discussed yttrium tantalate phosphor intensifying screens. The ultraviolet/blue light emission of this phosphor is an excellent match for the natural light-absorbing sensitivity of silver halide. For example, Du Pont reports a reduction in print-through from 33% using calcium tungstate screens to 19% using the same film with yttrium tantalate screens. Print-through can be decreased even more when a dye, matched to the light emission of the screens, is added to the emulsion. Using a film that incorporates this dye technology reduces print-through to only 14% of total exposure. The film incorporating dye in the emulsion is a higher speed film, the result being no loss of system speed.

A different approach to increasing light absorption in the film emulsion was introduced by Kodak: tabular silver halide grains. Tabular grains of silver halide have a thickness that is less than one tenth their diameter. This results in flat film emulsion grains that present a much larger surface area to incident light photons when compared to an equal mass of conventionally shaped grains. This large surface-area-to-volume ratio allows tabular grains to absorb significantly more light photons when compared to an emulsion containing an equal mass per unit area of conventional grains. Reduction in crossover is due to increased absorption in the tabular silver halide grains. The reduction in the crossover exposure fraction for conventional versus tabular grain film is in the range of 29 to 30%, versus 15 to 19%. We must emphasize that these percentages are only useful as approximate indications of decrease in crossover. There are different ways of determining the fraction of crossover, and significantly different answers result with different methods. One must not use the actual numbers to compare products. We report some figures from the literature to illustrate the concept of reduction in print-through, not as a means of deciding which type of film or screen does the best job.

TRANSPARENCY VERSUS PRINT

Why is a radiograph viewed as a transparency rather than as a print, like an ordinary photograph? The density of a print is related to the amount of light reflected or absorbed by the paper. The density of the maximum black of most photographic printing papers is between 1.3 and 1.7. A few papers give density values as high as 2.0 (glossy-surfaced paper gives the highest maximum black). Obviously, such a limitation on maximum density would be intolerable in radiology, in which densities up to 2.0, and occasionally greater, are commonly encountered. This limitation is overcome by viewing the radiograph as a transparency, which permits use of density ranges up to a maximum of 3.0 or more for diagnostic radiology films and up to 6.0 for industrial x-ray use.

SUMMARY

The amount of blackening of an x-ray film is expressed by the term "photographic density." The most useful range of density in diagnostic radiology is 0.25 to 2.0, although densities up to 3.0 are sometimes used.

Analysis of the characteristic curve of a film provides information about the contrast, speed, and latitude of the film. Film contrast amplifies subject contrast if the average gradient of the film is greater than 1. Film contrast will vary with the amount of exposure (density), the way the film is exposed (intensifying screens or direct action of x rays), and the way the film is developed.

Double-emulsion films produce greater contrast than single-emulsion films (assuming light is used to expose the film).

X-ray film is viewed as a transparency because of the greater range of density available.

The film must be able to absorb the wavelength of light emitted by the intensifying screen.

REFERENCES

1. American National Standards Institute: American National Standard Method for the Sensitometry of Medical X-Ray Screen-Film-Processing Systems. New York, American National Standards Institute, 1982. (Available as ANSI PH2.43-1982 from the American National Standards Institute, 1430 Broadway, New York, NY 10018.)
2. Bates, L.M.: Some Physical Factors Affecting Radiographic Image Quality: Their Theoretical Basis and Measurement. Washington, DC, U.S. Government Printing Office, 1969, Public Health Service Pub. No. 999-RH-38.
3. Brixner, L., Holland, R.S., Kellog, R.E., Mickish, D., Patten, S.H., Zegarski, W.: Low print-through technology with rare earth tantalate phosphors. SPIE Vol. 555 Medical Imaging and Instrumentation, 1985, p. 84.
4. Doi, K., Loo, L.N., Anderson, T.M., and Frank, P.H.: Effect of crossover exposure on radiographic image quality of screen-film systems. Radiology, 139:707, 1981.
5. Huff, K.E., and Wagner, P.W.: Eastman Kodak Company Report: Crossover and MTF characteristics of a tabular-grain x-ray film. Eastman Kodak Company, Rochester, New York 14650.
6. Lawrence, D.J.: Kodak X-Omatic and Lanex screens and Kodak films for medical radiography. Rochester, NY, Eastman Kodak Company, Radiography Markets Division, File No. 5.03, June 1976.
7. Meredith, W.J., and Massey, J.B.: Fundamental Physics of Radiology. Baltimore, Williams & Wilkins, 1968.
8. Ostrum, B.J., Becker, W., and Isard, H.J.: Low-dose mammography. Radiology, 109:323, 1973.
9. Presentation Script: New Screen Technology. Prepared by Photo Products Department. Wilmington, Del., E.I. du Pont de Nemours & Company.
10. Rao, G.U.V., Fatouros, P.P., and James, A.E.: Physical characteristics of modern radiographic screen-film systems. Invest. Radiol., 13:460, 1978.
11. Seeman, H.E.: Physical and Photographic Principles of Medical Radiography. New York, John Wiley and Sons, 1968.
12. Sensitometric Properties of X-Ray Films. Rochester, NY, Eastman Kodak Company, Radiography Markets Division.
13. Thompson, T.T.: Selecting medical x-ray film. Part 1. Appl. Radiol., 4:47, 1974.
14. Thompson, T.T.: Selecting medical x-ray film. Part II. Appl. Radiol., 4:51, 1974.
15. Wayrynen, R.E.: Radiographic film. Contained in the syllabus of the 1975 AAPM Summer School: The Expanding Role of the Diagnostic Radiologic Physicist, Rice University, Houston, July 27–August 1, 1975, p. 112.
16. Wayrynen, R.E.: Fundamental aspects of mammographic receptors film process. In Reduced Dose Mammography. Edited by W.W. Logan and E.P. Muntz. New York, Masson Publishing USA, 1979, pp. 521–528.
17. Weiss, J.P., and Wayrynen, R.E.: Imaging system for low-dose mammography. J. Appl. Photogr. Eng., 2:7, 1976.

12 *Fluoroscopic Imaging*

X rays were discovered because of their ability to cause fluorescence, and the first x-ray image of a human part was observed fluoroscopically. Dr. Glasser, in his book, **Dr. W. C. Röntgen,** recounted:

> To test further the ability of lead to stop the rays, he selected a small lead piece, and in bringing it into position observed to his amazement, not only that the round dark shadow of the disc appeared on the screen, but that he actually could distinguish the outline of his thumb and finger, within which appeared darker shadows—the bones of his hands.[1]

THE FLUOROSCOPE

The first generation fluoroscopes consisted of an x-ray tube, an x-ray table, and a fluoroscopic screen (Fig. 12–1). The fluorescent material in the screen was copper-activated zinc cadmium sulfide that emitted light in the yellow-green spectrum (giving rise to the term "green screen" as a syno-nym for fluoroscopy in the good old days). A sheet of lead glass covered the screen, so the radiologist could stare directly into the screen without having the x-ray beam strike his eyes. Screen fluorescence was so faint that fluoroscopic examinations were carried out in a dark room by a radiologist who had dark-adapted his eyes by wearing red goggles for 20 to 30 minutes prior to the examination.

Residents trying to learn fluoroscopic techniques were at an enormous disadvantage because it was impossible to see what the professor claimed he was seeing on the dim screen. The days of red goggles and green screens are gone forever.

Visual Physiology

In 1941, at a meeting of the Radiologic Society of North America in Chicago, Dr. W. Edward Chamberlain startled his audience when he announced that the light

Figure 12–1 Fluoroscope

reflected from the piece of paper he was holding in his hand was 30,000 times brighter than the illumination of a fluoroscopic screen.[3] Radiologists had always known that the fluoroscopic screen was poorly illuminated, but no one before Chamberlain had ever bothered to measure it. How can we see anything with so little light? The answer is found in the eye's amazing ability to adapt to low levels of illumination.

The retina contains two different types of light receptors, rods and cones. Cones (central vision) function most efficiently in bright light, while rods (peripheral vision) function best with low levels of illumination. Daylight (cone) vision is called photopic vision, and night (rod) vision is called scotopic vision. The differences between day and night vision are so great that humans can be considered to have two almost totally separate vision systems.

The cones are concentrated very densely in the fovea at the center of the retina, and are sparsely scattered over the rest of the retina. The dense concentration of cones gives high visual acuity for direct vision, and the sparse population in the remainder of the retina contributes to daylight peripheral vision. The cones are almost completely blind to low levels of illumination.

There are no rods in the fovea, so scotopic vision is entirely peripheral vision. Also, the density of rods (and the interconnecting network of nerves) is less over the remainder of the retina than the density of cones in the fovea. The result is that scotopic (rod) vision is less acute than photopic (cone) vision. Rods can be extremely sensitive to low levels of illumination. Rods are most sensitive to blue-green light, and daylight levels of these wavelengths of light greatly reduce the sensitivity of rods to low (night) illumination levels. Fluoroscopists had to "dark adapt" by wearing red goggles to filter out blue-green wavelengths for periods of over half an hour to allow the rods to recover peak sensitivity before fluoroscopy.

The dim fluoroscopic images required use of rod vision, with its poor visual acuity and poor ability to detect shades of gray (contrast). What was needed was a way to produce an image bright enough to allow cone vision without giving the patient an excessive radiation exposure. The solution came in the form of the x-ray image intensifier, developed in the 1950s.

IMAGE INTENSIFIER DESIGN

The components of an x-ray image intensifier are shown in Figure 12–2. The tube itself is an evacuated glass envelope, a vacuum tube, which contains four basic elements:

1. input phosphor and photocathode
2. electrostatic focusing lens
3. accelerating anode
4. output phosphor

After an x-ray beam passes through the patient, it enters the image intensifier tube. The input fluorescent screen absorbs x-ray photons and converts their energy into light photons. The light photons strike the photocathode, causing it to emit photoelectrons. These electrons are immediately drawn away from the photocathode by the high potential difference between it and the accelerating anode. As the electrons flow from the cathode toward the anode, they are focused by an electrostatic lens, which guides them to the output fluorescent screen without distorting their geometric configuration. The electrons strike the output screen, which emits the light photons that carry the fluoroscopic image to the eye of the observer. In the intensifier tube, the image is carried first by x-ray photons, then by light photons, next by electrons, and finally by light photons.

Input Phosphor and Photocathode

The input fluorescent screen in image intensifiers is **cesium iodide** (CsI). The input phosphor of older image intensifiers was silver-activated zinc-cadmium sulfide. CsI is deposited on a thin aluminum sub-

INPUT PHOSPHOR
and
PHOTOCATHODE

OUTPUT PHOSPHOR

Figure 12–2   Input phosphor and photocathode (*A*) and output phosphor of an image intensifier (*B*)

strate by a process called "vapor deposition." An interesting and useful characteristic of CsI is that during the deposition process the crystals of CsI grow in tiny needles perpendicular to the substrate. This is useful because the phosphor layer exhibits minimal lateral light diffusion. When one of these needle-shaped crystals absorbs an x-ray photon and produces light, the light will be transmitted to the photocathode with little scattering.

Image quality is dramatically better with cesium iodide input screens than it was with the older zinc-cadmium sulfide screens. Three physical characteristics of cesium iodide make it superior; the vertical orientation of the crystals, a greater packing density, and a more favorable effective atomic number. Since cesium iodide can be vacuum-deposited, it requires no inert binder, so more active material can be packed into a given space. The packing density of cesium iodide is three times greater than that of zinc-cadmium sulfide. Phosphor thicknesses have been reduced comparably from approximately 0.3 mm

with zinc-cadmium sulfide to 0.1 mm with cesium iodide. The principal advantage of the thinner phosphor layer combined with needle-shaped crystals is improved resolution. The resolution of a CsI image intensifier will be about 4 line pairs per millimeter (with a range of 3 to 5 lp/mm).

Ideally, for maximum photoelectric absorption, the K-absorption edge of a phosphor should be as close to the energy of the x-ray beam as possible, provided the energy of the edge does not exceed that of the beam. An obvious problem arises in attempting to accomplish this ideal. Beam energy is a spectrum, a whole array of energies, whereas the K edge is a single energy or, at most, several energies, depending on the number of different absorbers in the phosphor. The mean energy of an x-ray beam is approximately one third of its peak energy, depending somewhat on the kVp and filtration. Most fluoroscopy on adults is done at a peak energy of from 80 to 120 kVp, which is a mean energy between 30 and 40 keV. Table 12–1 shows the K edges of some elements used in phos-

Table 12–1. Atomic Number and
K-Absorption Edge

ELEMENT	ATOMIC NUMBER	K-ABSORPTION EDGE (keV)
Sulfur	16	2.5
Zinc	30	9.7
Cadmium	48	26.7
Iodine	53	33.2
Cesium	55	36.0

phors. The energy of the K edge of cadmium (26.7 keV) is quite good, but its chemical mates, zinc (9.7 keV) and sulfur (2.5 keV), are far from ideal. The K edges of cesium (36 keV) and iodine (33.2 keV) are almost perfect. The more appropriate atomic numbers of cesium and iodine give these screens a substantial advantage over those made of zinc-cadmium sulfide. Cesium iodide input screens absorb approximately two thirds of the incident beam as opposed to less than one third for zinc-cadmium sulfide, even though the cesium iodide screen is only one third as thick.

The **photocathode** is a photoemissive metal (commonly a combination of antimony and cesium compounds). When light from the fluorescent screen strikes the photocathode, photoelectrons are emitted in numbers proportional to the brightness of the screen. The photocathode is applied directly to the CsI input phosphor. Light from the CsI passes directly into the photocathode. Older tubes had a thin light transparent barrier between the input phosphor and the photocathode. Light diffusion in this barrier reduced resolution.

Let us review the process to this point. A uniform beam of x rays has passed through a patient and been attenuated by the patient. This attenuated beam of x rays passes through the glass front of the image intensifier tube and the thin aluminum substrate of the input phosphor layer (CsI). The CsI crystals produce light in proportion to the intensity of the incident x-ray beam. The light photons react with the photocathode. Photoelectrons are emitted from the photocathode. The numbers of

electrons produced are proportional to the intensity of the light (Fig. 12–3A).

Now we have to get the electrons to the other end of the image intensifier tube and make them maintain their relative position. We do this using an electrostatic focusing lens and an accelerating anode.

Electrostratic Focusing Lens

The lens is made up of a series of positively charged electrodes that are usually plated onto the inside surface of the glass envelope. These electrodes focus the electron beam as it flows from the photocathode toward the output phosphor. Electron focusing inverts and reverses the image. This is called a point inversion because all the electrons pass through a common focal point on their way to the output phosphor (Fig. 12–2). Each point on the input phosphor is focused to a specific point on the opposite side of the output phosphor. For undistorted focusing, all photoelectrons must travel the same distance. The input phosphor is curved to ensure that electrons emitted at the peripheral regions of the photocathode travel the same distance as those emitted from the central region. The image on the output phosphor is reduced in size, which is one of the principal reasons

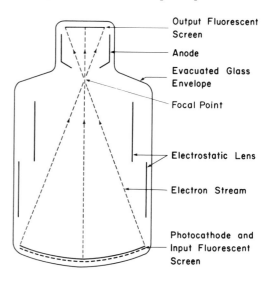

Figure 12–3   X-ray image intensifier tube

why it is brighter, a point to which we will return later.

Accelerating Anode. The anode is located in the neck of the image tube (Fig. 12–2). Its function is to accelerate electrons emitted from the photocathode toward the output screen. The anode has a positive potential of 25 to 35 kV relative to the photocathode, so it accelerates electrons to a tremendous velocity.

Output Phosphor. The output fluorescent screen of image intensifiers is silver-activated zinc-cadmium sulfide, the same material used in first-generation input phosphors. Crystal size and layer thickness are reduced to maintain resolution in the minified image. The diameter of most output screens ranges from about ½ to 1 in. Because the electrons are greatly accelerated, they emit more light photons from the output screen than were originally present at the input screen. The number of light photons is increased approximately 50-fold.

A thin layer of aluminum is plated onto the fluorescent screen (Fig. 12–3B) to prevent light from moving retrograde through the tube and activating the photocathode. The aluminum layer is very thin, and high-energy photoelectrons easily pass through it en route to the output screen.

The glass tube of the image intensifier is about 2 to 4 mm thick, and is enclosed in a lead-lined metal container. The lead lining protects the operator from stray radiation.

The output phosphor image is viewed either directly through a series of lenses and mirrors, or indirectly through closed-circuit television. A mirror optical system is shown in Figure 12–4. As you can see, light travels a long distance, and it is reflected and focused several times. This can be done with only minimal loss of brightness. The mirror image is only visible in a small viewing angle. If the operator moves his head a few degrees to one side, the image is lost. His freedom of movement is

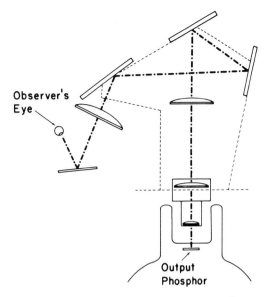

Figure 12–4 Mirror optical system of an image intensifier

limited by the mirror, making it difficult, if not impossible, to palpate the patient. Also, only one observer can view the image, which is a serious disadvantage in training beginning fluoroscopists.

Viewing the output of an image intensifier (II) is done via a closed circuit television chain in modern systems. But we would also like to be able to record the image on photospot or cine film when appropriate. We could record the film image from the TV camera signal, but the resulting image would be degraded by the television chain. It is better to expose the film directly to the output phosphor of the image intensifier tube. To maintain continuous TV viewing while exposing the film means that we must split the light from the II output into two paths at the time of film exposure. During routine fluoroscopy, all the light output of the II is directed to the TV camera. When film mode is selected, a semitransparent (often termed "partially silvered") mirror is positioned in the light beam, as shown in Figure 12–5. With this arrangement, most of the light (about 90%) goes to the film camera, but enough can pass through the mirror to form a TV pic-

Figure 12–5 Optical coupling between an image intensifier and viewing system

ture. Since the exposure level has been increased, 10% of the available light will still produce a satisfactory TV image. In the filming mode, the exposure is not continuous so the TV picture comes on only during the exposure time and shows the actual image being recorded by the film. We will return to the topic of photospot and cine cameras in the next chapter.

In some systems, the image is coupled to the TV camera by a fiberoptic bundle (fiber face plate). Fiberoptic coupling precludes filming directly from the output phosphor of the image intensifier tube. A fiber face plate is a bundle of fine optically shielded glass fibers (several thousand per mm²) that is a few millimeters thick. In the future it may be possible to obtain films that are acceptable from the TV signal, and we predict that all image tubes will be coupled directly to TV cameras.

BRIGHTNESS GAIN

Two methods are used to evaluate the brightness gain of image intensifiers. The first compares the luminance of an intensifier output screen to that of a Patterson-type B-2 fluoroscopy screen when both are exposed to the same quantity of radiation.

The brightness gain is the ratio of the two illuminations:

$$\text{Brightness gain} = \frac{\text{intensifier luminance}}{\text{Patterson B-2 luminance}}$$

If the image intensifier is 6000 times brighter, the brightness gain is 6000. The concept is easy to understand, and was readily accepted by radiologists. Patterson-type B-2 fluoroscopic screens, however, vary from one batch to another, and deteriorate at an unpredictable rate with time so brightness gain measurements are not reproducible. Because of this lack of reproducibility, the International Commission on Radiologic Units and Measurements (ICRU) has recommended a second method of evaluation, called the "conversion factor," to supersede the older brightness gain method. The **conversion factor** is a ratio of the luminance of the output phosphor to the input exposure rate:

$$\text{Conversion factor} = \frac{\text{cd/m}^2}{\text{mR/sec}}$$

Output screen luminance is measured in candelas (abbreviated cd, and defined as the luminous intensity, in the perpendicular direction, of a surface of a 1/600,000 m² of a black body at the temperature of freezing platinum under a pressure of

101,325 Nt/m² . . . ridiculous to remember). Radiation quality and output luminance are explicitly defined, so the method is accurate and reproducible.

The brightness gain, often called "intensification factor," of modern image intensifiers can easily reach 10,000 (values of 20,000 are possible). The conversion factor usually equals about 1% of the brightness gain, so a conversion factor of 100 is about the same as brightness gain of 10,000. Most specifications for image intensifiers will quote the conversion factor.

The brightness gain tends to deteriorate as an image intensifier ages. This means that the patient dose with an old image intensifier tends to be higher than that with a new intensifier of the same type. Because the deterioration can proceed at a rate of about 10% per year, a periodic check of image intensifier brightness can be valuable. Unfortunately, an accurate check is somewhat complicated. Some indication of image intensifier aging can be obtained by comparing the input dose level required for automatic brightness control operation with the dose level under the same conditions as when the intensifier was new.

The brightness gain of an image intensifier comes from two completely unrelated sources, called "minification gain" and "flux gain." We will discuss them separately.

Minification Gain

The brightness gain from minification is produced by a reduction in image size. The quantity of the gain depends on the relative areas of the input and output screens. Because the size of an intensifier is usually indicated by its diameter, it is more convenient to express minification gain in terms of diameter:

$$\text{Minification gain} = \left(\frac{d_i}{d_0}\right)^2$$

where d_i is the diameter of input screen, and d_0 is the diameter of output screen. Most x-ray image intensifiers have an input screen from 5 to 9 in. in diameter and an output screen approximately 1 in. in diameter. Image intensifiers with 12- to 16-in. diameter input screens are available. We will briefly consider these big tubes shortly. With a 1-in. output screen, the minification gain is simply the square of the diameter of the input screen; that is, a 9-in. intensifier has a gain of 81.

The brightness gain from minification does not improve the statistical quality of the fluoroscopic image. The same number of light photons make up the image regardless of the size of the output screen. For example, a 6-in. intensifier with a 2-in. output phosphor has a minification gain of 9 ($6^2 \div 2^2 = 36 \div 4 = 9$), whereas the same intensifier with a 1-in. output phosphor has a gain of 36. The total light output of both units is exactly the same, however, so the same number of photons make up both images. The photons are compressed together on the smaller screen and the image is brighter, but its statistical quality is not improved.

Theoretically, brightness can be increased indefinitely by minification. A 9-in. intensifier with a $1/16$-in. output screen would have a brightness gain from minification alone of over 20,000. Excess minification produces a very small image, though, which has a definite disadvantage. Before the image can be viewed it must be greatly magnified, which not only reduces the brightness but also magnifies the fluoroscopic crystals in the output screen, resulting in a precipitous drop in resolution.

Flux Gain

Flux gain increases the brightness of the fluoroscopic image by a factor of approximately 50. For each light photon from the input screen, 50 light photons are emitted by the output screen. In simplified terms, you may think of one light photon from the input screen as ejecting one electron from the photocathode. The electron is accelerated to the opposite end of the tube, gaining enough energy to produce 50 light photons at the output screen.

The total brightness gain of an image intensifier is the product of the minification and flux gains:

Brightness gain = minification gain × flux gain

For example, with a flux gain of 50 and a minification gain of 81 (9-in. intensifier with a 1-in. output screen), the total brightness gain is 4050 (50 × 81).

IMAGING CHARACTERISTICS

Contrast

Contrast can be determined in various ways, and there is no universal agreement as to which is best. The following is a description of the simplest method. A $\frac{1}{4}$-in. thick lead disc is placed over the center of the input screen. Disc size is selected to cover 10% of the screen; that is, a 0.9-in. diameter disc is used for a 9-in. image intensifier. The input phosphor, with the disc in place, is exposed to a specified quantity of radiation, and brightness is measured at the output phosphor. Contrast is the brightness ratio of the periphery to the center of the output screen. Defined in this way, contrast ratios range from approximately 10:1 to better than 20:1, depending on the manufacturer and intended use.

Two factors tend to diminish contrast in image intensifiers. First, the input screen does not absorb all the photons in the x-ray beam. Some are transmitted through the intensifier tube, and a few are eventually absorbed by the output screen. These transmitted photons contribute to the illumination of the output phosphor but not to image formation. They produce a background of fog that reduces image contrast in the same way that scattered x-ray photons produce fog and reduce contrast in a radiographic image. The second reason for reduced contrast in an image intensifier is retrograde light flow from the output screen. Most retrograde light flow is blocked by a thin layer of aluminum on the back of the screen. The aluminum layer must be extremely thin, however, or it would absorb the electrons that convey the fluoroscopic image. Some light photons penetrate through the aluminum, pass back through the image tube, and activate the photocathode. The cathode emits photoelectrons, and their distribution bears no relationship to the principal image. These electrons produce "fog" and further reduce image contrast. Contrast tends to deteriorate as an image intensifier ages.

Lag

Applied to image intensifiers, lag is defined as persistence of luminescence after x-ray stimulation has been terminated. With older image tubes, lag times were 30 to 40 ms. With CsI tubes, lag times are about 1 ms. The lag associated with vidicon television tubes is now more of a concern than image intensifier lag times.

Distortion

The electric fields that accurately control electrons in the center of the image are not capable of the same degree of control for peripheral electrons. Peripheral electrons do not strike the output phosphor where they ideally should, nor are they focused as well. Peripheral electrons tend to flare out from an ideal course. The result is unequal magnification, which produces peripheral distortion. The amount of distortion is always greater with large intensifiers because the further an electron is from the center of the intensifier, the more difficult it is to control. Figure 12–6 shows a cine image of a coarse wire screen taken with a 9-in. intensifier. As you can see, the wires curve out at the periphery; this effect is most noticeable at the corners. This same effect has been observed in optical lenses and termed the "pincushion effect," and the term is carried over to image tubes. The distortion looked like a pincushion to the guy who named it. Generally this distortion does not hamper routine fluoroscopy, but it may make it difficult to evaluate straight lines (for example, in the reduction of a fracture).

Unequal magnification also causes un-

Figure 12–6 Test film of a wire screen (35 mm cine frame) from a 9-in. image intensifier

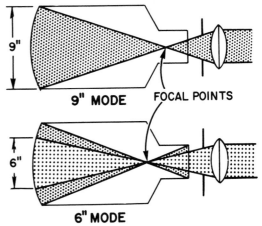

Figure 12–7 Dual-field image intensifier

equal illumination. The center of the output screen is brighter than the periphery (Fig. 12–6). The peripheral image is displayed over a larger area of the output screen, and thus its brightness gain from minification is less than that in the center. A fall-off in brightness at the periphery of an image is called **vignetting.** Unequal focusing has another effect on image quality; that is, resolution is better in the center of the screen.

In summary, the center of the image intensifier screen has better resolution, a brighter image, and less geometric distortion.

MULTIPLE-FIELD IMAGE INTENSIFIERS

Dual-field or triple-field image intensifiers attempt to resolve the conflicts between image size and quality. They can be operated in several modes, including a 4.5-in., a 6-in., or 9-in. mode. The 9-in. mode is used when it is necessary to view large anatomic areas. When size is unimportant, the 4.5- or 6-in. mode is used because of better resultant image quality. Larger image intensifiers (12- to 16-in.) frequently have triple-field capability.

Field size is changed by applying a simple electronic principle: the higher the voltage on the electrostatic focusing lens, the more the electron beam is focused. Figure 12–7

shows this principle applied to a dual-field image intensifier. In the 9-in. mode, the electrostatic focusing voltage is decreased. The electrons focus to a point, or cross, close to the output phosphor, and the final image is actually smaller than the phosphor. In the 6-in. mode the electrostatic focusing voltage is increased, and the electrons focus farther away from the output phosphor. After the electrons cross, they diverge, so the image on the output phosphor is larger than in the 9-in. mode. The optical system is preset to cover only the format, or size, of the smaller image of the 9-in. mode. In the 6-in. mode, the optical system "sees" only the central portion of the image, the part derived from the central 6 in. of the input phosphor. Because this image is less minified, it appears to be magnified when viewed through a television monitor. The physical size of the input and output screens is the same in both modes; the only thing that changes is the size of the output image. Obviously, the 6- and 9-in. modes have different minification gains. Exposure factors are automatically increased when the unit is used in the 6-in. mode to compensate for the decreased brightness from minification.

While we are discussing intensifier size, there is another point to consider. A 9-in. image intensifier does not encompass a

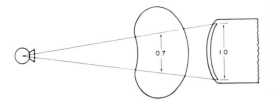

Figure 12–8 Reduction of fluoroscopic field size by an image intensifier

9-in. field in the patient. The x-ray image is magnified by divergence of the beam (Fig. 12–8). The intensifier sees a much smaller field than its size would imply, an important point to consider when ordering a unit to perform a particular function.

Large Field of View Image Intensifier Tubes

The development of digital angiography was associated with a need for large image intensifier tubes that could image a large area of the patient. This is especially true in abdominal angiography. Image intensifier tubes with diameters of 12, 14, and 16 in. are now available to meet this need.

Conventionally sized image intensifier tubes (up to about 10 in.) are made with a glass envelope with a glass convex input window. Use of a glass input window on the new large tubes became impractical because the glass would be so thick it would absorb a significant fraction of the x-ray beam (remember that these tubes are under a high vacuum). These larger tubes may have an all-metal envelope with a lightweight, non-magnetic metal (aluminum, titanium, or stainless steel) input window. These big tubes usually allow triple-field imaging, such as a 6-in., 9-in., and 14-in. mode with a 14-in. diameter tube. The magnification factor with the small field can be helpful when fluoroscopy is used to guide delicate invasive procedures such as percutaneous biliary and nephrostomy

procedures. Remember that there is an automatic increase in exposure rate in the magnified viewing mode. Contrast and resolution will be improved when only the central area of these large tubes is used, and distortion will be minimized. These tubes are large, somewhat bulky to use, and very expensive.

SUMMARY

Early fluoroscopy was accomplished by radiologists looking directly at a fluoroscopic screen. The image on the screen was only .0001 as bright as the image of a routinely viewed radiograph, so dark adaptation of the eyes was required.

In the 1950s the image intensifier alleviated this situation by producing an image bright enough to be viewed with cone vision. The input phosphor of modern image intensifiers is cesium iodide; the output phosphor is zinc cadmium sulfide (green light). Brightness gain is the product of minification gain and flux gain. Imaging characteristics important in the evaluation of image intensified fluoroscopy include contrast, lag, and distortion. Large field of view image intensifier tubes are available to fill special needs, such as digital and spot-film angiography. Most image intensifiers allow dual-field or triple-field imaging.

REFERENCES

1. Glasser, O.: Dr. W.C. Röntgen. Springfield, IL, Charles C Thomas, 1945.
2. Medical X-Ray and Gamma-Ray Protection for Energies up to 10 MeV. Washington, DC, National Council on Radiation Protection and Measurements, 1968, Report No. 33.
3. Chamberlain, W.E.: Fluoroscopes and fluoroscopy. Radiology, *38*:383, 1942.
4. Sturm, R.E., and Morgan, R.H.: Screen intensification systems and their limitations. Am. J. Roentgenol., *62*:613, 1949.
5. Thompson, T.T.: A Practical Approach to Modern Imaging Equipment. Boston, MA, Little, Brown and Co., 1985, pp. 81–126.

13 *Viewing and Recording the Fluoroscopic Image*

Before the invention of the x-ray image intensifier, attempts at displaying the fluoroscopic image on television were only partially successful. The large fluoroscopic screen required an elaborate optical system, and suboptimal screen brightness produced a weak video signal. The development of the image intensifier solved both these problems. Its small output phosphor simplifies optical coupling, and its bright image produces a strong video signal.

CLOSED-CIRCUIT TELEVISION

The components of a television system are a camera, camera control unit, and monitor (Fig. 13–1). To avoid confusion in nomenclature, we will use the terms "television" and "video" interchangeably. Fluoroscopic television systems are always closed-circuit systems; that is, the video signal is transmitted from one component to the next through cables rather than through the air, as in broadcast television. A lens system or a fiberoptic system conveys the fluoroscopic image from the output phosphor of the image intensifier to the

video camera, where it is converted into a series of electrical pulses called the **video signal.** This signal is transmitted through a cable to the camera control unit, where it is amplified and then forwarded through another cable to the television monitor. The monitor converts the video signal back into the original image for direct viewing.

Before discussing the individual components of a television system, we will move a little ahead of ourselves and describe the nature of the video picture. An appreciation of this will make the design of both the camera and monitor easier to understand. The television image is similar to the screened print shown in Figure 13–2. It is made up of a mosaic of hundreds of thousands of tiny dots of different brightness, each contributing a minute bit to the total picture. When viewed from a distance the individual dots disappear, but at close range, or with magnification, they are clearly visible. The dot distribution is not random or haphazard in a television picture. Instead, the dots are arranged in a specific pattern along horizontal lines, called **horizontal scan lines.** The number of lines varies from one television system to another but, in the United States, most fluoroscopy and all commercial television systems use 525 scan lines. To avoid confusion we must clarify the meaning of television lines. When a radiologist thinks of lines, it is usually in terms of lines per unit length. For example, if a grid has 80 lines, the unit is "lines per inch." Television lines

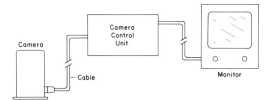

Figure 13–1 Components of a television system

Figure 13–2 Dot picture and enlargement of a screened print

have only the unit of "lines," and no unit of length. The 525 lines in most television systems represent the total number in the entire picture, regardless of its size. The lines are close together in a small picture tube and spread apart in a large tube, but in both the total number is the same.

Television Camera

The vidicon camera is the one usually employed for fluoroscopy, and is the only one that we will discuss in any detail. There are several types of vidicons; one is the plumbicon, which we will mention. The vidicon camera is a relatively inexpensive, compact unit. The essential parts of a vidicon camera are shown in Figure 13–3. The most important part is the vidicon tube, a small electronic vacuum tube that measures only 1 in. in diameter and 6 in. in length (larger tubes are sometimes used). The tube is surrounded by coils, an electromagnetic focusing coil, and two pairs of electrostatic deflecting coils.

The fluoroscopic image from the image intensifier is focused onto the target assembly, which consists of three layers: (1) a glass face plate; (2) a signal plate; and (3) a target. The only function of the glass face plate is to maintain the vacuum in the tube (remember, an electron beam must travel in a vacuum). Light merely passes through the face plate on its way to the target. The signal plate is a thin transparent film of graphite located on the inner surface of the face plate. It is an electrical conductor with a positive potential of approximately 25 V.

The vidicon target is functionally the most important element in the tube. It is a thin film of photoconductive material, usually antimony sulfide (Sb_2S_3) suspended as globules in a mica matrix. In a plumbicon the photoconductive material is lead monoxide (PbO). Each globule is about 0.001 in. in diameter and is insulated from its neighbors and from the signal plate by the mica matrix. The function of the globules is complex, but they behave like tiny capacitors. After reviewing the other elements in the camera, we will return to these globules and discuss them in more detail.

The cathode is located at the opposite end of the vidicon tube from the target and is heated indirectly by an internal electric coil. The heating coil boils electrons from the cathode (thermionic emission), creating an electron cloud. These electrons are immediately formed into a beam by the control grid, which also initiates their acceleration toward the target. The cathode-heating coil assembly with the control grid is called an "electron gun" because it shoots electrons out of the end of the control grid. As the electron beam progresses down the

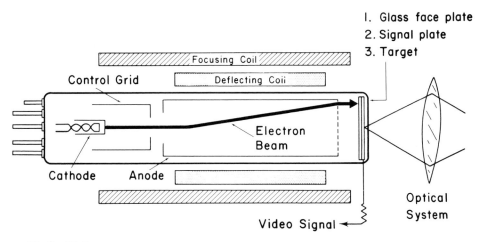

1. Glass face plate
2. Signal plate
3. Target

Figure 13–3 Vidicon camera

tube, it moves beyond the influence of the control grid and into the electrostatic field of the anode. The anode has a positive potential of approximately 250 V with respect to the cathode. The electrons are accelerated to a relatively high velocity, but they are still low energy electrons (about 250 eV). The anode extends across the target end of the tube as a fine wire mesh. The wire mesh and signal plate form a uniform decelerating field adjacent to the target. The signal plate ($+25$ V) has a potential of 225 V less than that of the wire mesh ($+250$ V), so electrons should flow from the signal plate to the wire mesh. The electrons from the cathode are accelerated to relatively high velocities, however, and they coast through the decelerating field like a roller coaster going uphill. By the time they reach the target, they have been slowed to a near standstill (they are now 25-eV electrons). The decelerating field also performs a second function: it straightens the final path of the electron beam so that it strikes the target perpendicularly.

Because the electron beam scans a fine mosaic of photoconductive globules, it is critical that the electron beam not spread out as it goes through the tube. This is accomplished by an electromagnetic focusing coil that wraps around the vidicon tube.

This coil extends almost the entire length of the tube and creates a constant magnetic field parallel to the long axis of the tube; this field keeps the beam of electrons in a narrow bundle. The electrons progress down the tube in a series of oscillating spirals, and strike the target as a finely focused beam (Fig. 13–4A).

The electron beam is steered by variable electrostatic fields produced by two pairs of deflecting coils that wrap around the vidicon tube. Vertical deflecting coils are

A

ELECTRON BEAM

Spiral Path

Magnetic Field

FOCUSING COIL

B

ELECTRON BEAM

Electric Field

DEFLECTING COIL

Figure 13–4 Focusing and deflecting coils

shown in Figure 13–4*B*. By alternating the voltage on the coils, the focused electron beam is moved up and down to scan the target. The other pair of coils moves the beam from side to side along a horizontal line. All four coils, working together, move the electron beam over the target in a repetitive scanning motion.

Video Signal

Now that we have discussed the physical makeup of the camera, we can return to the critical target end of the tube and the formation of the video signal (Fig. 13–5*A*).

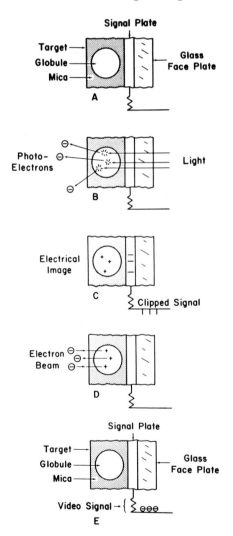

Figure 13–5 Formation of the video signal

When a globule absorbs light, photoelectrons are emitted (Fig. 13–5*B*). The electrons are immediately attracted to the anode and removed from the tube. The globule, having lost electrons, becomes positively charged. Since the globule is insulated from its surroundings it behaves like half of a tiny capacitor, and draws a current onto the conductive signal plate. The current that flows onto the signal plate is ignored, or clipped, and is not recorded (Fig. 13–5*C*). Similar events occur over the entire surface of the target. A brighter area in the light image emits more photoelectrons than a dim area, and produces a stronger charge on the tiny capacitors. The result is a mosaic of charged globules that store an electrical image that is an exact replica of the light image focused onto the target.

The electron beam scans the electrical image stored on the target and fills in the holes left by the emitted photoelectrons, thus discharging the tiny globule capacitors. After the capacitors are fully discharged (no more positive charges are left), no additional electrons can be deposited in the globules. It was indicated earlier that the electrons in the electron beam were reduced to low energy electrons before they entered the target. There are two reasons for this. Reason one is that we want no electrons to enter the target after the positive charge has been neutralized. The second reason is that the electrons should not have sufficient energy to produce secondary electrons when they do enter the globules. Of course, high energy secondary electrons would be able to neutralize the positive charge in other globules and degrade the image. Excess electrons from the scanning beam drift back to the anode and are removed from the tube. When the electrons in the scan beam neutralize the positive charge in the globules, the electrons on the signal plate (Fig. 13–5*D*) no longer have an electrostatic force to hold them on the plate. They will leave the plate via the resistor. These moving electrons form a current flowing through a resistor, and therefore a voltage appears across the resistor. This voltage, when collected for each neutralized globule, constitutes the video signal (Fig. 13–5E). The globules are not all discharged at the same time. Only a small cluster, a dot, is discharged each instant in time. Then the electron beam moves on to the next dot in an orderly sequence, discharging all the globules on the target. The result is a series of video pulses, all originating from the same signal plate but separated in time. Each pulse corresponds to an exact location on the target. Reassembling these pulses back into a visible image is done by the camera control unit and the television monitor.

Charge-Coupled Device TV Camera

A charge-coupled device is usually written and spoken of as a **CCD.** A CCD is a semiconductor device that can store charge in local areas and, on an appropriate signal from the outside, transfer that charge to a readout point. In conjunction with a photoelectric cathode, the CCD makes a very nice TV camera (or video camera). The CCD camera forms a picture in much the same way as a vidicon: the light photons from the scene to be imaged are focused on the photoelectric cathode where electrons are liberated in proportion to the light intensity. These electrons are captured in little charge buckets (potential wells) built into the CCD device. So the distribution of captured (stored) electrons in the charge buckets represents the stored image. This is exactly the same as the stored image in the vidicon, except the vidicon stores positive charge whereas the CCD stores negative charge. The difference between the vidicon and the CCD camera is in the readout process. The vidicon is read out by an electronic beam. The CCD is read out by the charge in the charge buckets being moved from one bucket to the next until the charge reaches the edge of the CCD where it forms an electrical signal. The total readout is accomplished

one line at a time, so here, too, we have scan lines.

The readout process reminds us of a fire brigade with water buckets. The brigade passes the buckets along a line of men until the water reaches the end of the line. This comparison is pretty good, but we would have to make one small change. Instead of the buckets being passed along, we would have to dump the water from one bucket into the next. A problem comes up because there is already water in all the buckets. In the fire brigade then, we would need empty buckets between each bucket containing water. So in the CCD, there are empty spaces into which the charge may move. The motion of the charge is controlled by changing the depth of the charge buckets. To collect charge, the buckets must have a deeper potential well (bucket), than the next well position. The charge may be passed to the next well position by making that position have a deeper potential well than the bucket containing the charge. It is important to realize that electrons from one bucket can never mix with electrons from another bucket.

CCD cameras need no readout electron beam (or controlling coils), and can be made shorter than the vidicon tube. In addition to small size, the readout process is amenable to digital systems, so the CCD camera would fit nicely in a digital imaging system (enhanced by digital control of the device readout). However, resolution is still controlled by the same things that control resolution from a vidicon. We might expect the use of CCD cameras to increase in radiology because it is an emerging technology, not because of improved resolution. The CCD finds application in information processing as well as imaging, and may be more important in memory applications than in imaging application. We will give you the information from a Fairchild publication.[2] A Fairchild CCD 211 is a 244 × 190 element array, which is a 4 to 3 ratio for TV presentation. This device dissipates 100 mW at a 7 MHz data rate. It operates at voltages from 12 to 15 V (note that there are no extremely high voltages, as in vidicon). All this on a chip that is .245 by .245 in. The TV camera you buy for home use today will be a CCD camera.

Television Monitor

The last link in the television chain is the monitor. It contains the picture tube and the controls for regulating brightness and contrast.

A picture tube is similar to a vidicon camera tube (Fig. 13–6). Both are vacuum tubes and both contain an electron gun, control grid, anode, focusing coil, and deflecting coils. A picture tube, however, is much larger. The focusing and deflecting coils are wrapped around the neck of the tube, and they control the electron beam in exact synchrony with the camera tube. The brightness of the individual dots in the picture is regulated by the control grid. The control grid receives the video signal from the camera control unit, and uses this signal to regulate the number of electrons in the electron beam. To produce a bright area in the television picture, the grid allows a large number of electrons to reach the fluorescent screen. To produce a dark area, the grid cuts off the electron flow almost completely.

The anode is plated onto the inside surface of the picture tube near the fluorescent screen. It carries a much higher positive potential (10,000 V) than the anode of the camera tube (250 V), so it accelerates the electron beam to a much higher velocity. The electrons strike the fluorescent screen at the flared end of the tube, which makes the screen emit a large number of light photons. The generation of light photons over the entire surface of the tube is the visible television image. Many secondary electrons are set free by the impact of the electron beam with the screen, and they are attracted to the anode and conducted out of the picture tube.

A large tube, like a television picture tube, can never be completely evacuated. Some residual gas is always present, and "outgassing" (release of absorbed gas) from the components of the monitor adds to the problem. These gas molecules are eventually ionized and removed from the tube by an ion trap located in the end of the monitor (Fig. 13–6).

Color monitors are slightly different in two respects. First, three electron guns are required, one for each of the colors red, blue, and yellow. The second difference is that the fluorescent screen must be composed of three different fluorescent materials, one for each of the three colors. The screen is not made up of continuous fluorescent material, but rather is made up of alternating dots of the three colors. The controls must allow the yellow electron gun to send electrons only to the yellow phosphor. Of course, the same is true for the red and blue electron guns. With this arrangement, a red image can be obtained by only the red electron gun emitting electrons, but orange requires both the red gun and the yellow gun to emit electrons. With appropriate combination of the three colors, the entire color spectrum from black to white can be covered. In radiology, we do not need color TV cameras because the images to be recorded are produced by a single color phosphor. But if we were to use color cameras, we would find that they must have photoconducting targets for

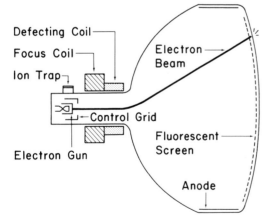

Defecting Coil

Focus Coil

Ion Trap

Control Grid

Electron Gun

Electron Beam

Fluorescent Screen

Anode

Figure 13–6 Television monitor

each of the three colors and some filtering system to assure that the right color interacts with the right phosphor. Today, color television pictures that appear in various radiologic procedures are really nothing more than computer-generated color images (e.g., color Doppler, SPECT, and nuclear medicine).

TELEVISION SCANNING

The television image is stored as an electrical image on the target of the vidicon tube, and it is scanned along 525 lines by a narrow electron beam 30 times per second. Each scan of the entire target is called a "frame." The electron beam scans the target in much the same manner that we read a page in a book. Beginning at the top left corner, it drifts across a line, sending out a video signal as it moves, and then rapidly returns to the left margin and repeats the process over and over until all 525 lines have been read. When we reach the last line of a page, we move on to the top line of the next page and continue reading. The electron beam does exactly the same thing, only it does not have to turn pages. Instead, as the beam reads, it also erases. As the electron beam discharges the globule capacitors, it erases their image. As soon as a line is read and erased, it is ready to record a new image, and it begins immediately. When the electron beam returns it sees a different image than it saw the time before. Because the electron beam scans the target 30 times each second, the change in the image from one scan to the next is slight, and our eyes perceive a continuous motion in exactly the same way that we see motion in a cine film.

The eye can detect individual flashes of light, or flicker, up to 50 pulses per second. A television monitor only displays 30 frames per second, so an electronic trick, called **interlaced horizontal scanning,** is employed to avoid flicker. Instead of scanning all 525 lines consequently, only the even-numbered lines are scanned in the first half of the frame, and only the odd-numbered lines are scanned during the second half (Fig. 13–7). Each pass of the electron beam over the video target is called a field, and consists of $262\frac{1}{2}$ lines. Although only 30 frames are displayed each second, they are displayed in 60 flashes of light (fields), and flicker disappears.

We have used a 525-line system to illustrate scanning. Systems with a larger (two or four times) number of vertical lines are available and desirable, but are not yet economically practical for routine use.

Video Signal Frequency (Bandpass)

Bandpass, also called "bandwidth," is the frequency range that the electronic components of the video system must be designed to transmit. An analogy with sound will simplify the explanation. Sound is audible at frequencies from about 16 Hz to 30,000 Hz. Sound equipment (e.g., recorders, amplifiers, and speakers) is designed to transmit this range of frequencies. The range from the lowest to the highest frequency is called the bandpass (Fig. 13–8). The electronic components are engineered to transmit all the frequencies in this range as accurately as possible. The cutoffs are not sharply defined at the two frequency extremes, and not all frequencies are transmitted with the same quality. Thinking in terms of music, bandpass is the frequency range that the electronic components must "pass" from the "band" to the listener. A video signal is exactly the same as an audio signal, except that the video signal covers a wider range of frequencies.

As the electron beam moves along a horizontal scan line, a video signal is transmitted to the camera control unit and then forwarded to the TV monitor. The frequency of the video signal will fluctuate from moment to moment, depending on the nature of the television image. Figure 13–9 shows one scan line of an image containing four equally spaced black-and-white lines, or four line pairs (4 lp). As the electron beam moves across the image, the video signal increases and decreases in volt-

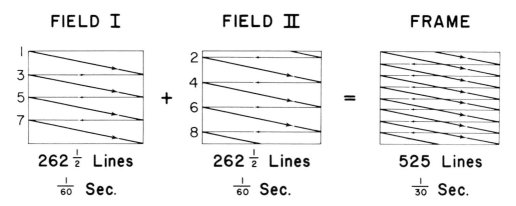

Figure 13–7   Interlaced horizontal scanning

age in a cyclic fashion. Like alternating current, one cycle (the shaded area in the illustration) includes one up-limb and one down-limb and represents two lines, or one line pair. The scanning process is repeated over and over, 525 times per frame and 30 frames per second. We can calculate the frequency, or number of cycles per second, of the video signal generated by the four-line-pair image by multiplying the number of cycles per scan line (four in this case) by the number of scan lines per frame by the number of frames per second:

$$\frac{\text{cycles}}{\text{scan line}} \times \frac{\text{scan lines}}{\text{frame}} \times \frac{\text{frames}}{\text{seconds}} = \text{cycles/sec}$$

$$4 \quad \times \quad 525 \quad \times \quad 30 \quad = 63{,}000$$

When the number of line pairs in the image changes, the frequency of the video signal also changes. The lowest frequency signal occurs with an image of one line pair (i.e., a screen that is half black and half white). The highest frequency signal is determined by the amount of money that one is willing to pay for electronic equipment.

Vertical resolution is determined only by the number of vertical scan lines (525 in our illustration). Suppose we would like to image a test object that has 2000 black-and-white line pairs (4000 lines total). What would we see with our 525-line camera? The 2000 line pairs might be recorded in the photocathode, but our scan electron beam, which covers the full area of the TV monitor in 525 lines, would see on each line scan four black lines and four white lines. The output video for that scan line would be an average of the four line pairs, or a gray line. The next scan would see the same. The total output would be a nice uniform gray image (no line-pair resolution). What we need to image line pairs is a dark line for one scan line and a light line for the next scan line. This is the most that we can do. For a 525-vertical-line system, the maximum line-pair structure that can be resolved on the TV monitor is 262½ line pairs. Notice that there are no units of line pairs (not 262½ lines per inch or meter or mile), just 262½ line pairs per TV monitor image. These 262½ line pairs of a 525-line system displayed on a 6-in. monitor will look better than the same 525 lines displayed on a 13- or 19-in. monitor. A system

Figure 13–8   Frequency range of audible sound and the bandpass required for accurate transmission

TV CAMERA

Figure 13–9   The video signal from one scan line of a line pair phantom

with more scan lines would give better vertical resolution. Our task now is to match horizontal resolution to vertical resolution, a more difficult concept to explain, since horizontal resolution is not determined by the number of scan lines.

A reasonable compromise is a system with equal vertical and horizontal resolution. For the horizontal resolution to be equal to the vertical resolution in a 525-line system, the horizontal resolution must be $262\frac{1}{2}$ line pairs. The horizontal resolution is determined by the bandpass of the TV system. The bandpass must be able to transmit sufficient information to produce this resolution. For a 525-line system, the lowest and highest frequency signals will be as follows:

$$\frac{cycles}{scan\ line} \times \frac{scan\ lines}{frame} \times \frac{frames}{second} = cycles/sec$$

Minimum:
$$1 \quad \times \quad 525 \quad \times \quad 30 \quad = 15{,}750$$

Maximum:
$$262\frac{1}{4} \times \quad 525 \quad \times \quad 30 \quad = 4{,}130{,}000$$

The frequency of the video signal will fluctuate between a minimum of 15,750 Hz and a maximum of 4,130,000 Hz. To transmit the signal accurately, the electronic components should have a bandpass of 4.13 to 0.016 MHz, or approximately 4.1 MHz. Actually, a somewhat higher bandpass is required. About 10% of the scan time is lost in retracing from one line to another. This additional 10% increases the required bandpass to approximately 4.5 MHz for a 525-line system. At this bandpass, vertical and horizontal resolution are equal.

Remember, **vertical resolution depends on the number of vertical lines** (such as 525), **whereas horizontal resolution is determined by the bandpass.** Most x-ray television systems today have a bandpass (also called bandwidth) of 5 MHz with a 525-line system. Higher vertical-line systems are available, such as 875 and 1024 lines with a bandpass of up to 20 MHz. These systems are expensive and not yet used routinely.

For the purpose of illustrating concepts our discussion thus far has assumed that a 525-line TV system actually uses all 525 lines to form an image. In fact, significantly fewer than 525 lines are available for image formation. This is a technical problem that we will not discuss in depth.

Synchronization

It is necessary to synchronize or coordinate the video signal between the camera and monitor; that is, to keep them in phase with each other. The camera control unit adds synchronization pulses to the video signal at the end of each scan line and scan field. Appropriately, they are called "horizontal and vertical synchronization pulses." They are generated during the retrace time of the electron beam, while no video signal is being transmitted. First, the picture screen is blackened by a blanking pulse, and the synchronization signal is added to the blanking pulse. If the synchronization pulses were added to the video signal while the screen was white, they would generate noise in the form of white streaks, but no visible noise is produced by synchronization on a black screen.

TELEVISION IMAGE QUALITY

Resolution

As we have stated, the number of scan lines available for image formation in a 525-line TV camera is significantly less than 525 lines. Some lines are lost to prevent the retrace and blanking signals from showing on the TV screen. We have been discussing absolute maximum resolution. In no system do we ever attain maximum values, and in the final analysis the resolution of a system must be measured. Usually this determination is made by the manufacturer, and may appear in the specifications as vertical lines and bandpass. Resolution of 370 lines (185 line pairs) may be typical in a 525-line system, and this is the value we will use in the following discussion.

The overall resolution of the imaging system (i.e., the image-intensifier/lines/TV system) depends on the size of the input image. If the TV monitor resolution of 185 lp is used to show a large picture, resolution will be poor. For example, suppose we use television to display the image from a 9-in. image intensifier. Converting to millimeters, a 9-in. image intensifier is 229 mm in diameter (9 in. × 25.4 mm/in.). The system resolution in lp/mm is as follows:

$$\frac{185 \text{ lp}}{229 \text{ mm}} = 0.8 \text{ lp/mm}$$

Table 13–1 shows resolutions for three different-sized image intensifiers. The same numbers would apply to a triple-model (4.5-, 6-, and 9-in.) image intensifier. The television monitor always displays the same 185 lp but, when supplied with the image from a 4.5-in. image intensifier, this 185 lp represents a resolution of 1.6 lp/mm, twice as good as the 0.8 lp/mm of the 9-in. image intensifier. Even though a resolution of 1.6 lp/mm is a considerable improvement, it falls far short of displaying the entire resolution of cesium iodide image intensifiers. These tubes have a resolution of up to 1 lp/mm, and some are available in 12- to 16-in. sizes. The only way that this resolution can be adequately displayed at the present time is with a film system such as a 35 mm cine, or spot film cameras.

The 370 vertical lines must be displayed as 370 lines on the TV monitor. A 10-in. (diagonal diameter) TV monitor has a vertical height of about 6 in., and 370 lines distributed over 6 in. will produce a good image. If the same 370 lines are displayed on a larger TV monitor, individual lines might become visible. At the same normal

Table 13–1. Resolution of a TV Imaging System for Various-Sized Image Intensifiers

SIZE OF IMAGE INTENSIFIER		TELEVISION RESOLUTION
in.	mm	(lp/mm)
4.5	114	1.6
6	152	1.2
9	229	0.8

*Based on a 525-line TV system with a total resolution of 185 lp.

viewing distance, the image on a small TV screen will look better than that on a large screen.

Contrast

Both the camera and monitor affect the contrast of a television image. A vidicon camera reduces contrast by a factor of approximately 0.8, and the monitor enhances contrast by a factor of 2. The lead monoxide target vidicon (plumbicon) tube does not cause any decrease in image contrast. The net result is a definite improvement in contrast beyond that of the image intensifier alone. Furthermore, both the brightness and contrast levels can be regulated with the monitor, so the optimum combination can be selected to best show a point of interest. There is a correct way to adjust contrast and brightness of the television monitor. Turn up the contrast control knob until background noise becomes visible, then reduce the contrast level slightly. Then turn down the brightness control level until the darkest part of the picture is black. Increasing the brightness level alone will decrease contrast, so the brightness and contrast control knobs should always be adjusted together.

Lag

An undesirable property of most vidicon tubes is lag, or stickiness, which becomes apparent when the camera is moved rapidly during fluoroscopy (i.e., the image blurs). Lag occurs because it takes a certain amount of time for the image to build up and decay on the vidicon target. In one respect a certain amount of lag is actually advantageous. It averages out the statistical fluctuations that normally occur with low-dose fluoroscopy, and minimizes the annoying effects of quantum mottle. Plumbicon (lead monoxide) television camera tubes demonstrate significantly less lag than do standard vidicon tubes. The lag of a vidicon is usually not a problem with routine fluoroscopy, but may become a problem in cardiovascular fluoroscopy. The image generated by a plumbicon tube will show more quantum mottle than a standard vidicon image.

Automatic Brightness Control

The brightness of the image changes constantly in all fluoroscopic systems as the fluoroscope is moved from one area of the patient to another. Usually this does not cause any serious problem, and both the chest and abdomen can be examined with preset exposure factors. With television fluoroscopy, however, changes in image brightness seriously affect image quality. As the fluoroscope is moved from the abdomen to the chest a sudden surge of brightness floods the system, the image becomes chalky, and all detail is lost. Therefore, the brightness level of the television monitor must be controlled within rather narrow limits. This may be accomplished by varying the x-ray exposure factors or varying the sensitivity of the television system. A photocell located between the image intensifier and television camera measures the brightness of the fluoroscopic image, and it transmits a signal back to the x-ray control unit to adjust the exposure factors. If brightness is controlled by varying sensitivity of the TV system the term **automatic gain control** is sometimes used. **Automatic brightness control** refers to control of x-ray exposure levels.

AUTOMATIC GAIN CONTROL

One way to control brightness of the image on the TV monitor is to vary the sensitivity of the television system by varying the sensitivity of the television cameras or varying the gain of the television amplification system. Automatic gain control is a fairly simple and inexpensive way to control image brightness. However, it does not change the x-ray dose rate to the patient. This can result in unnecessary patient exposure, because brightness may be reduced by reducing TV system sensitivity rather than decreasing patient exposure. Also, increasing sensitivity of the system without increasing radiation exposure will not improve quantum mottle and will increase electronic noise.

Automatic Brightness Control. There are three ways to change the radiation input to the image intensifier input phosphor:

> kVp variability
> mA variability
> pulse width variability

kVp Variability. For kVp variability, kVp will vary while mA stays constant. This method offers fast response times, as opposed to variable mA techniques. Also, variable kVp units produce satisfactory images over a wide range of viewing conditions (a wide dynamic range).

mA Variability. An mA-variable brightness control allows the operator to choose a fixed kVp. The automatic brightness control varies the mA as needed. The response time of this type of control is slow since changes in mA require that the temperature of the x-ray tube filament change in order to change mA. This method is relatively simple and inexpensive, and offers the operator control of kVp. The dynamic range of this control is less than the kVp-variable units, so the operator must choose a kVp appropriate for the examination being done. It has been suggested than an mA-variable system, with a convenient kVp control, is the best general purpose automatic brightness control system.

Combined Control. A number of systems vary both kVp and mA to control brightness. This technique offers a wide dynamic range. Many of these units offer the option of manual selection of either kVp or mA, making them in effect either a kVp- or mA-variable unit.

Pulse Width Variability. This type of brightness control system is used with cine cameras, or with video disc storage systems. Both kVp and mA are constant for one examination. The length of each exposure is controlled with a grid-controlled x-ray tube or a constant potential generator with secondary switching. This method offers

the advantage of very fast response times and a very broad dynamic range, and allows the operator to choose the mA and kVp levels best suited for the examination. One obvious disadvantage is the complexity and expense associated with switching in the secondary circuit.

FLUOROSCOPIC IMAGE RECORDERS

There are two modes of recording the fluoroscopic image. First, the light image from the output phosphor of the image intensifier may be recorded on film with a photospot camera or cine camera. Routine spot films are made directly with x rays, but since they are recorded on film we discuss them with cine and photospot cameras. The second group of recorders makes use of the electrical signal generated by the TV camera. This group of recorders includes magnetic tape, magnetic discs, and optical discs. The three recorders may employ either analog or digital signals.

Light Image Recorders

Spot Film Recorder. Spot film devices are old friends of radiologists and technologists of all ages. These devices interpose an x-ray film cassette between the x-ray beam and the image intensifier tube. The standard 9½-in. square cassette may now be replaced with cassettes of several sizes in some fluoroscopic units. The technique of using a spot film device should be familiar to anyone reading this text.

During fluoroscopy, the radiologist may at any time elect to move the cassette from its park position (where it is shielded by lead) to a position ready for exposure. There is a delay of about ¾ to 1 sec before a film can be moved into position and an exposure made. Several factors make this delay necessary. First, the cassette is rather heavy, and some time is required to move it into position and bring it to a completely motionless position prior to exposure. Some changes at the x-ray tube are also required. Fluoroscopy is conducted at about 80–90 kVp (sometimes higher) and 1 to 3 mA of tube current. Exposure of the spot film uses fluoroscopic kVp, but requires much higher mA settings in the 300 to 400 mA range. Some time is required to increase x-ray tube filament heating, and the x-ray tube anode rotation speed is usually increased. A phototimer controls the length of exposure.

Spot Film Cameras

A spot film (often called "photospot") camera is a camera that records the image output of an image intensifier on a film. Typically, the film is roll film of size 70 or 105 mm, or cut film 100 mm in size.

Recall that the light from the output phosphor of the image intensifier is converted into a parallel beam image by a lens placed close to the output phosphor (refer back to Fig. 12–5). A semitransparent mirror placed in this parallel beam will allow about 15% of the light to travel on to the TV camera, and reflect the remainder to a photospot camera or a cine camera. Originally confined to gastrointestinal fluoroscopy, spot film cameras are now used to record all types of fluoroscopic images, including angiography. This has been made possible by the improved resolution of cesium iodide image intensifier tubes. Large field of view image intensifier tubes with input phosphor diameters of up to 16 in. allow large areas of the body to be imaged without moving the image intensifier. Therefore, we can take a single photospot film that covers almost the entire abdomen (this could not be done with a 9-in. tube). A significant advantage of spot film cameras over any direct filming methods is a substantial reduction in patient exposure. The recommended per-frame exposure for photospot film cameras is 100 micro-Roentgens (μR). The exposure for a comparable spot film is 300 μR, three times as much. The disadvantages and other advantages of spot film cameras relate to convenience, economics, and the clinical setting. For gastroenterology, cameras are

more convenient than conventional spot films. The film does not have to be changed between exposures, and the delay between initiation and completion of an exposure is shorter, because no cassette has to be moved into position for a spot film camera. Exposure times are shorter (in the 50-ms range), so motion is less likely to be a problem. In addition, films can be taken more rapidly. Most commercial units are designed to function at a maximum framing frequency of 12 frames/second. Since the camera is recording directly from the output phosphor of the image intensifier tube, it is possible to record and view the image at the same time. The resolution of the resulting films is that of the image intensifier, about 4 line pairs per mm (a range of 3 to 5 lp/mm). Resolution of routine spot films is theoretically greater than that of spot film camera films, but longer exposure times required for spot films may degrade the image because of motion unsharpness.

Many observers feel that angiography recorded on 100- or 105-mm spot film cameras is the equal of that recorded on standard x-ray film exposed in rapid film changers. This is largely a reflection of the very short exposure times with spot film cameras. Other advantages of spot film cameras include reduction in dose to only 30% or less of that of routine filming, and a savings in film costs of greater than 80%. One must admit that the little films are a nuisance to process and store, and it takes some practice to feel comfortable looking at angiograms on such a small format.

Framing with Spot Film Cameras. The output phosphor of the image intensifier tube is round, but the shape of the film used in spot film cameras is square. Matching the output to the film means that either part of the image or part of the film cannot be used. The term "framing" refers to the utilization of the available area on the film. Four framing formats may be used with spot film cameras. These are illustrated in Figure 13–10, and we will briefly describe each.

FRAMING MODE	EXACT FRAMING	EQUAL AREA FRAMING	MEAN DIAMETER FRAMING	TOTAL OVERFRAMING
ILLUSTRATION				
FILM AREA USED	79 %	91 %	96 %	100 %
IMAGE AREA UNUSED	0 %	9 %	16 %	36 %
RELATIVE IMAGE SIZE	1.0	1.13	1.21	1.41

Figure 13–10 Framing formats for spot film cameras

Exact Framing. The entire circular intensifier image is included in the useable square film frame. The word "useable" refers to the fact that part of the film is lost to the transport system (i.e., perforations along the edge of the film). The exact amount lost depends on the film size and design of the transport system, and varies somewhat from one manufacturer to another. With exact framing, no part of the image is lost but 21% of the film is wasted.

Equal Area Framing. The area of the intensifier image is equal to the useable square film area. Approximately 9% of both the image and film are lost.

Mean Diameter Framing. The diameter of the intensifier image is equal to the mean of the transverse and diagonal dimensions of the useful square film area; 16% of the image is lost but only 4% of the film is unused.

Total Overframing. The diameter of the intensifier image is equal to the diagonal dimensions of the useful square film area. The entire film is used, but 36% of the image is unused.

The optimum frame format depends on several factors: (1) the size of the image intensifier, (2) the size of the film, and (3) the clinical application for which the imaging system is intended. For any given system, the size of the recorded image enlarges as the diameter of the framing format increases (Fig. 13–10). Note in the illustration that the arrow increases in size as the framing format increases. For this reason, more overframing is recommended for small films (70 mm) than for larger films (105 mm). In general, exact framing is not recommended for any clinical application. It is especially undesirable for 70 mm film, because the final image is too small. Total overframing is not recommended, except possibly for 70 mm film in which maximum magnification is desirable. Either equal area or mean diameter framing is recommended for most clinical situations. Total overframing is impractical with larger film sizes (100 mm and 105 mm).

The film for spot film cameras should have a relatively low contrast. An average gradient between 1.0 and 1.6 has been recommended by the Inter-Society Commission for Heart Disease Resources.[4] A minimum exposure of 100 μR/film is required to minimize quantum mottle. This is the exposure at the input phosphor of the image tube after the x-ray beam has traversed the patient and grid. Remember that quantum mottle originates in the fluorescent screen, so it is not affected by the size of the recorded image. Therefore, the same exposures are recommended for both 70 mm and 105 mm films.

Cinefluorography

Cinefluorography is the process of recording fluoroscopic images on movie (cine) film. The cine camera records from the output phosphor of the image intensifier through a series of lenses and mirrors. In this edition we will eliminate the detailed discussion of lens systems found in previous editions. A beam splitting mirror allows simultaneous cine recording and television viewing, just as with spot film camera recording.

Two film sizes are currently being used for cinefluorography, 16 mm and 35 mm. In the United States, 98% of all cine is done on 35 mm film, and 95% of all cine studies involve the heart. Therefore, our major emphasis will be on 35 mm cardiac cinefluorography.

Cine Camera. Cinefluorography is married to the motion picture industry. We are stuck with their horizontal rectangular format, even though it is not well suited to our needs. All cine cameras are commercial movie cameras with a few minor modifications. Two film sizes are available, 16 mm and 35 mm. The basic components of the camera are a lens, iris diaphragm, shutter, aperture, pressure plate, pulldown arm, and film transport mechanism.

Light enters the camera through the lens and is restricted by the aperture, a rectangular opening in the front of the camera. The size and shape of the aperture define the configuration of the image reaching the film. Figure 13–11 shows the image sizes as defined by the apertures of 16-mm and 35-mm cameras. Apertures for 35 mm film are usually 18 × 24 mm.

The shutter is a rotating disc with a sector cut out of its periphery (Fig. 13–12). It is located in front of the aperture. As the shutter rotates, it interrupts light flow into the camera. The size of the shutter opening is expressed as the number of degrees in the cutout portion of the sector. Openings

Figure 13–11 Film formats as defined by the apertures of 16 mm and 35 mm cameras

of 160° are usually employed for cinefluorography. While the shutter is closed, the pulldown arm advances the film to the correct position for the next exposure (Fig. 13–13). The pressure plate holds the film against the camera aperture so that it is located in the proper image plane.

An electric drive motor advances the film from the supply reel past the aperture to the takeup reel. A meter attached to the supply reel indicates the amount of unexposed film in the camera. The x-ray pulses and shutter opening are synchronized by an electrical signal from the drive motor. The framing frequency, or number of frames per second, is usually 60, divided or multiplied by a whole number (e.g., 7½, 15, 30, 60, or 120).

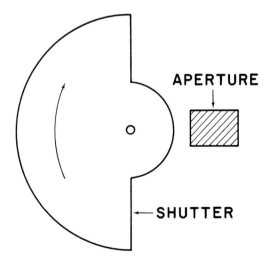

Figure 13–12 Cine camera shutter

Figure 13–13   Cine camera

The combination of the framing frequency and shutter opening determines the amount of time available for both the exposure and pulldown. For example, with a 180° shutter opening and 60 frames per second, the time available for both the exposure and pulldown is 1/120 sec. At slower framing frequencies, both are longer. With a smaller shutter opening, the available exposure time is shorter than the pulldown time.

Framing. The concept of framing is presented in the spot film camera section of this chapter. The term **overframing** is important to understand. Framing is controlled by the lens of the cine camera. Exact framing means that the entire image (the output phosphor of the II) just fits on the cine film (refer back to Fig. 13–10). Overframing means that only a portion of the image is recorded on the film. The film image with overframing is larger than the film image for exact framing, and this increased size is usually desirable. Overfram-

ing means that some of the output image is not recorded. Extremes of overframing are generally avoided because patient exposure in areas not recorded is undesirable. Framing characteristics are established when the cine system is installed.

X-Ray Exposure. The timing and intensity of the x-ray exposure are controlled during cinefluorography by two electrical signals that originate from within the cine system. One signal coordinates the x-ray exposure with the open time of the camera shutter (synchronization), and the other maintains a constant level of intensifier illumination by varying the exposure factors for areas of different thickness or density (automatic brightness control).

Synchronization. When cinefluorographic equipment was in the embryonic stages of its development, x rays were generated continuously throughout a filming sequence, and the patient was needlessly irradiated when the camera shutter was closed. These continuous exposures had two serious disadvantages: large patient exposures and decreased life expectancy of the x-ray tube. In all modern cinefluorographic systems the x-ray output is intermittent, and the exposure is synchronized with the open time of the camera shutter. The shutter of the camera is timed by 60 Hz power and permits shutter speeds that are fractions or multiples of the number 60 (e.g., 7½, 15, 30, 60, and 120 frames exposed per second). The x-ray beam is usually synchronized with shutter opening either by switching in the secondary circuit of a constant potential generator or by use of a grid-controlled x-ray tube. We have already discussed the topic of automatic brightness control with image intensified fluoroscopy.

To conduct a cine examination, the radiologist must be able to monitor the cine image. The beam-splitting mirror reflects approximately 10% of the light from the image intensifier for monitoring purposes. Although this percentage is small, it must be remembered that the exposure factors and brightness of the intensifier phosphor are greatly increased during cinefluorography, and that the monitoring image brightness is not much different from that used for routine fluoroscopy. At low framing frequencies the image flickers because the x rays are pulsed, but flicker does not interfere with monitoring.

TV IMAGE RECORDERS

We have just discussed methods of recording the image from the light output of the image intensifier. The second method of recording the fluoroscopic image involves recording the electrical signal from the TV camera. We will discuss magnetic tape, magnetic disc, and optional disc recorders.

Tape Recorders

A tape recorder is used for both recording and playback. As a recorder, it receives a video signal from the camera control unit and, for playback, transmits the signal to one or several television monitors. Both these transmissions are conducted through cables, so it is a closed-circuit television system. The image is stored on ½-, ¾-, 1-, or 2-in. wide polyester base tape, coated on one side with a magnetic film. Two-inch video tape records a better quality image. Both open-reel (reel-to-reel) and cassette tapes are available.

A schematic presentation of a tape recorder is shown in Figure 13–14. The three essential components, besides the electronic circuitry, are a magnetic tape, a writing head, and a tape transport system. These requirements are the same for either open-reel or cassette tape recorders. Really, the only difference in the two types is the format in which the tape is stored and handled. The same type of head is used for both recording and playback, and we will call it a "writing head." The writing head converts an electrical signal into a fluctuating magnetic field for recording, and converts a magnetic signal into an electrical signal for replay. Some recorders have separate recording and playback heads, whereas in others one head performs both functions. The drive spindle moves the tape past the writing head at a constant velocity. The tape is kept in physical contact with the writing head at all times during both recording and playback.

The writing head of a tape recorder is shown in Figure 13–15. The head is similar to a transformer in that it consists of a magnetic core, such as an iron-nickel alloy wrapped with two coils of wire, but the writing head is different in two ways. First, a narrow segment, or gap, is cut from the core, as shown in Figure 13–15. Second, the two coils are wired together so that their magnetic fields reinforce each other. As a changing electric current moves through the coils, a changing magnetic field is produced in the gap. When the current in the illustration moves from left to right, the magnetic field is in the direction of the arrows. The field reverses when the current changes direction. The magnetic

Figure 13–14   Components of a tape recorder

field extends out beyond the gap in the writing head (Fig. 13–16). This extended magnetic field is the critical portion that interacts with the magnetic tape.

The magnetic layer of tape is composed of oxides of magnetic materials. The molecules of this material behave like tiny bar magnets, called "dipoles." Each dipole aligns itself in a magnetic field like the needle of a compass. They are randomly arranged on unrecorded tape (Fig. 13–16A). As the tape moves past the writing head gap, the alignment of the dipoles is changed to coincide with the magnetic field impressed on them while they are passing the gap (Fig. 13–16B). When the video signal (sine curve in Fig. 13–16) is negative, the dipoles are aligned toward the left; when the signal is positive, alignment is in the opposite direction. At the zero points in the video signal, no magnetic field exists in the gap, and dipole alignment is random. The degree of alignment is exaggerated in the illustration to demonstrate the

point. The actual alignment is proportional to the strength of the magnetic field. Complete alignment is prevented by the neighboring molecules, which offer some resistance to dipole movement, and by the inertia of the dipoles themselves. Once the tiny magnetic particles leave the magnetic field in the gap, they retain their orientation until some other magnetic force causes them to change.

Playback is exactly the reverse of the recording process, except that the magnetic dipoles are not unaligned in playback. The partially aligned magnetic dipoles have a magnetic field of their own. As this field moves past the gap in the writing head, it induces a magnetic field in the core, which in turn induces an electrical signal in the wire coils. This is the video signal that is forwarded to the display monitor.

Every component of the video signal must be recorded on a different portion of the magnetic tape. The transport system must move fast enough to keep a fresh supply of tape at the writing heads. If the tape moves too slowly, the dipole alignment of one cycle is unaligned by the magnetic field of the next cycle. To record a frequency of several million cycles per second, the tape must move at a very high velocity. This is accomplished by moving both the tape and writing heads (Fig. 13–17). The tape moves diagonally past paired writing heads mounted on either side of a rapidly revolving drum. The tape moves in one di-

Figure 13–15   Writing head

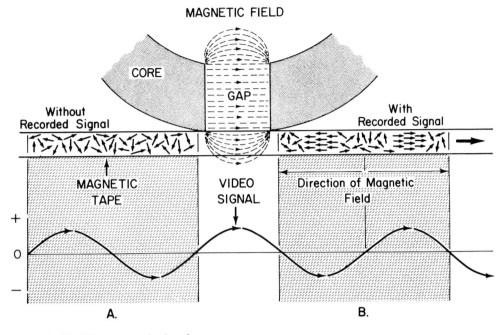

Figure 13–16 The magnetic signal on tape

rection and the writing heads move in the opposite direction. While one head is recording the other is away from the tape, so only one writing head is recording at any particular time. Each writing head records one video frame as it passes diagonally across the tape. The signal is laid down in separate tracks (Fig. 13–18). The tape moves just fast enough to separate the tracks of the two heads. Consecutive lines are always written by different heads. Video tracks are separated by a narrow guard band.

Cassette tape recorders are now increas-ing in popularity. They have only one advantage over other systems, ease of loading and unloading the tape. Otherwise cassette recorders are exactly the same as other tape recorders.

Magnetic tape is low in cost and widely used. But it has significant limitations. The rate at which data can be recorded is limited by the speed of tape movement. Retrieving a stored image from a tape can lead to long access times if the exam is stored far from the start of the tape. Magnetic tape is not a good permanent recording medium because the direct contact between the head and the tape causes tape wear and degradation of the recorded

Figure 13–17 Tape recorder

Figure 13–18 Video tracks on tape

data. The polyester base of the tape must be properly stored or distortion will result. Shelf life of magnetic tape is about 2 years.

Magnetic Disc Recorders

Magnetic disc and tape recorders operate on similar physical principles, but they have different functions. Tape recorders are designed to show motion, comparable to a movie camera. Disc recorders are designed to show stationary images, more like a spot film camera. A tape recorder can be used to show a single frame by stopping the tape against the revolving drum, but this subjects the tape to considerable physical wear. Disc recorders are designed to stop action. The discs themselves look like phonograph records. The video tracks are laid down in preset grooves. Each groove in a disc is a completely separate track. The tracks are not continuous from groove to groove. One picture frame is recorded in each track. When a particular frame is selected for replay, the same picture is shown over and over 30 times a second for as long as the operator desires.

Discs have several advantages over tape. **The most important one is random access.** The video grooves are numbered, and the recorder can go directly to any desired number, without playing the intervening numbers. This instantaneous access (as short as 30 ms) is considerably different than a tape recorder, which may take several minutes to reach a specific frame, even with a rapid wind mode. Another advantage of discs is that they are not subjected to physical wear in the stop action mode. Actually, they are designed to operate in this mode. One use of this "stop action" or "freeze frame" mode is to record a fluoroscopic image, then review that image while planning the proper approach for a variety of invasive procedures (rather than use continuous fluoroscopic viewing). Typical clinical applications include angioplasty, arterial embolizations, and hip pinnings. Dose reductions to patient and physician greater than 50% (as high as 90%) may be obtained. Wear is reduced because the writing head does not touch the disc. In a clinical setting, disc recorders may be used as a substitute for spot films, and the x-ray exposure factors are frequently increased, just as they would be for spot films. This exposure increase improves the quality of the disc image by decreasing quantum mottle. Primarily because of this exposure increase, image quality is generally better with discs than with tapes. Resolution is best with the smallest image intensifier mode consistent with the clinical situation.

Magnetic disc or tape may be used to record either digital or analog signals. The images recorded from a TV camera are normally recorded as analog signals. With the increasing interest in digital imaging, more images undoubtedly will be stored in the digital format. Digital interest is a product of computer technology, since computers use the digital format. Nearly every computer in the world has a magnetic disc recorder associated with it.

Magnetic disc recorders used in radiology now have a bandpass limitation of about 5 MHz. However, enormous information storage capabilities are available. Information can now be stored at a rate of 2.5 megabytes per second, and it is anticipated that storage of 1.8 gigabytes (a gigabyte = 10^9 bytes) on an 8-in. disc will soon be available. Magnetic discs find wide application in computer science.

Optical Discs

It is anticipated that laser optical discs will begin to replace magnetic hard discs. Current technology centers on the optical WORM (Write Once Read Many Times) discs, but erasable optical discs are now becoming commercially available. WORM discs begin with a rigid substrate such as glass, plastic, or aluminum. A photoactive recording medium is coated on the substrate. Recording is accomplished by marking or burning an indentation on the photoactive layer using a laser source. Readout depends on reflection or scattering of light by these defects in the photoactive layer. The storage capability of the disc is determined by the size of the focused laser beam and the ability to space adjacent tracks close to each other. Storage capabilities of optical discs range from 10 to 50 times that of a comparably sized magnetic disc. Standardization of optical discs is not yet developed. Currently, disc sizes vary from 3.5 to 14 inches in diameter, with storage capabilities ranging from 50 megabytes to 6.8 gigabytes. The shelf life of an optical disc is at least 10 years, and probably much longer. It is anticipated that optical discs will replace magnetic discs, both for use with image intensified fluoroscopy and for digital archiving (data storage) applications.

SUMMARY

Once the image is formed by the x-ray beam it is necessary to get the information to the radiologist. With fluoroscopy, this is done by displaying the image on a TV monitor. To make such a display, the image is processed by a television camera tube. The tube may be a standard vidicon, a plumbicon, or a CCD. The image is displayed on a TV monitor. Standard x-ray closed-circuit television uses a 525×525 format with a 5-MHz bandpass. Vertical resolution is limited by the scan line format (number of vertical lines), whereas horizontal resolution is a function of the bandpass. Display formats using more vertical lines and a higher bandpass are available and desirable, but currently limited in clinical use because of higher cost.

It is often necessary to record the fluoroscopic image. Either the light image from the II output phosphor or the electronic signal from the TV camera may be recorded. The light image is recorded by a photospot camera or a cine camera. We have included routine spot films in this category because we did not know where else to put them. The electronic signal from the TV camera may be recorded in analog or digital format on magnetic tape, magnetic disc, or optical disc.

REFERENCES

1. International Commission on Radiation Units and Measurements: Cameras for image intensifier fluoroscopy. Washington, DC, International Commission on Radiation Units and Measurements, 1969, Report 15.
2. Fairchild Weston. The solid state imaging technology. CCD imaging division. 810 West Maude Ave., Sunnyvale, CA 94086.
3. Jost, R.G., and Mankovich, N.J. Digital archiving requirements and technology. Investigative Radiology, 23:803, 1988.
4. Judkins, M.P., Abrams, H.L., Bristow, J.D., et al.: Report of the Inter-Society Commission for Heart Disease Resources. Circulation, 53:No. 2, February, 1976.
5. Thompson, T.T., editor. A Practical Approach to Modern Imaging Equipment. Little, Brown and Co., Boston/Toronto, 1985.

CHAPTER

14 *The Radiographic Image*

The basic tool of diagnostic radiology is the radiographic image. The radiologist must be thoroughly familiar with the factors that govern the information content of these images. R. E. Wayrynen* has suggested that the term **image clarity** be used to describe the visibility of diagnostically important detail in the radiograph.[21] Two basic factors determine the clarity of the radiographic image: contrast and image quality.

Image clarity
↙ ↘
Contrast   Image quality

A discussion of image clarity is difficult because there are so many subjective factors involved. Many problems concerning image visibility are the result of the physiologic and psychologic reactions of the observer rather than of the physical properties of the image. There is no well defined relationship between the amount of information on a film and the accuracy of interpretation of the film. Many overlooked lesions are large and easy to see in retrospect. In this chapter the physical properties of contrast and image quality will be considered.

CONTRAST

The term **radiographic contrast** refers to the difference in density between areas in the radiograph. Differing degrees of grayness, or contrast, allow us to "see" the information contained in the x-ray image.

*Technical Manager, X-ray Markets, E.I. du Pont de Nemours & Company, now retired.

Radiographic contrast depends on three factors:

1. subject contrast
2. film contrast
3. fog and scatter

Subject Contrast

Subject contrast, sometimes called **radiation contrast,** is the difference in x-ray intensity transmitted through one part of the subject as compared to that transmitted through another part. In Figure 14–1, assume that a uniform beam of x rays strikes an object made up of a block of muscle (A) and a block of bone (B) of equal thickness. Few x rays are transmitted through the bone, but most go through the muscle. The attenuated x-ray beam now contains many x rays in the area beneath muscle and few beneath bone; this difference of intensity in the beam caused by the object is subject contrast.

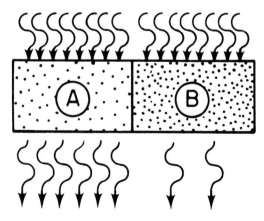

Figure 14–1 Equal thickness of muscle (A) and bone (B) do not equally attenuate an x-ray beam

Obviously, the effect of subject contrast on the x-ray beam cannot be seen directly. Because the x-ray beam exposes the film, however, anything that attenuates the x-ray beam will similarly affect the radiographic image on the film. As has been previously discussed, variations in the intensity of the x-ray beam caused by subject contrast are greatly amplified by the film. Subject contrast is the result of the attenuation of the x-ray beam by the patient, and attenuation has been discussed in detail in Chapter 5. A brief review will emphasize the pertinent points.

Subject contrast depends on

1. thickness difference
2. density difference
3. atomic number difference
4. radiation quality (kVp)

Thickness Difference. If an x-ray beam is directed at two different thicknesses of the same material, the number of x rays transmitted through the thin part will be greater than the number transmitted through the thick part. This is a relatively simple but important factor contributing to subject contrast. If I_S is the intensity of the x-ray beam (I) transmitted through the thin (small) segment, and I_L is the intensity transmitted through the thick (large) segment, subject contrast may be defined in the following way (Fig. 14–2):

$$\text{Subject contrast} = \frac{I_S}{I_L}$$

Another less obvious cause of difference in tissue thickness is the presence of a gas-filled cavity. Because gas attenuates almost no x rays, the presence of a pocket of gas in a soft tissue mass has the same effect on the x-ray beam as decreasing the thickness of the soft tissue mass. In ventriculography the brain ventricles are visible because they are filled with air. The x-ray beam then "sees" the cross section of brain containing a gas-filled ventricle as being "thinner" than that of the adjacent solid brain substance.

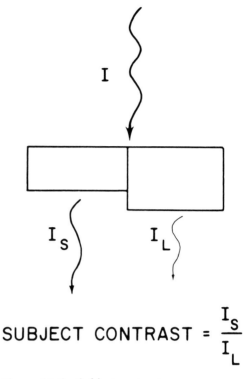

$$\text{SUBJECT CONTRAST} = \frac{I_S}{I_L}$$

Figure 14–2 Subject contrast

Density Difference. The difference in density between body tissues is one of the most important factors in causing subject contrast. The greater the density (i.e., mass per unit volume) of a tissue, the greater is its ability to attenuate x rays. Consider ice and water. Because ice floats in water, it is less dense than water. Water is about 9% more dense than ice. Equal thicknesses of ice and water will demonstrate subject contrast to an x-ray beam because the water attenuates 9% more of the beam than does the ice.

Atomic Number Difference. Subject contrast depends on the relative difference in attenuation of the x-ray beam by different tissues in the body. In diagnostic radiology, attenuation of the x-ray beam by the photoelectric effect makes the most important contribution to subject contrast. Photoelectric absorption is increased in substances with high atomic numbers, especially when low-kVp x rays are used. The effective atomic numbers of bone, muscle (water), and fat are

Bone	13.8
Muscle	7.4
Fat	5.9

Bone will attenuate many more x rays than muscle or fat, assuming equal thicknesses. Subject contrast between bone and muscle is high. Muscle and fat, with little difference in atomic number, show little difference in their ability to attenuate x rays by the photoelectric absorption process, and less difference by Compton reactions. Use of low-kVp (below 30) x rays produces the greatest possible difference in photoelectric x-ray absorption between muscle and fat. Soft-tissue radiography, such as mammography, requires the use of low-kVp x rays because the small differences in atomic number between breast tissues produce no subject contrast unless maximum photoelectric effect is used.

Contrast Media. The use of contrast materials with high atomic numbers (53 for iodine and 56 for barium) gives high subject contrast. Photoelectric absorption of x rays in barium and iodine will be proportionally much greater than that in bone and tissue because of the large differences in atomic number.

Radiation Quality. The ability of an x-ray photon to penetrate tissue depends on its energy; high-kVp x rays have greater energy. Selecting the proper kVp is one of the most important matters to consider in choosing the proper exposure technique. If the kVp is too low, almost all the x rays are attenuated in the patient and never reach the film.

The kilovoltage selected has a great effect on subject contrast. Low kVp will produce high subject contrast, provided the kVp is high enough to penetrate the part being examined adequately.

In general terms, the reason low kVp produces greater subject (or radiation) contrast than high kVp can be explained by a simple example. In Figure 14–2, subject contrast was defined as $\frac{I_S}{I_L}$. Assume that 100 x rays of low kVp (such as 50 kVp) strike the object (Fig. 14–3A). Most of these low-energy x rays are attenuated by the thick part, but quite a few can penetrate the thin part. Assume the numbers to be 25 (thick) and 40 (thin). By the definition of subject contrast,

$$\text{Subject contrast} = \frac{40}{25} = 1.60,$$

which states that the thin part transmits 60% more x rays than the thick part at 50 kVp. If the kVp is then increased to 80 (Fig. 14–3B), more x rays will get through both the thick and thin parts. Both I_S and I_L will increase, but I_S will increase more than I_L, so $\frac{I_S}{I_L}$ becomes smaller, and subject contrast is decreased. Figure 14–3B assumes values of $I_S = 80$ and $I_L = 60$, giving subject contrast of $\frac{80}{60} = 1.33$, or only 33% difference in transmitted radiation intensity.

As a general rule, low kVp gives high subject contrast. This is often called **short-scale contrast** because everything is black or white on the film, with fewer shades of gray in between. High kVp gives lower subject contrast, called **long-scale contrast,** because there is a long scale of shades of gray between the lightest and darkest portions of the image.

Exposure Latitude. A low-contrast film (shallow slope of the characteristic curve) has greater exposure latitude. That is, a wider range of mAs settings will produce proper film density if the kVp is satisfactory. Similarly, kVp will also have an effect on exposure latitude. High-kVp techniques will allow a wider range of mAs settings (wide exposure latitude) but will result in relatively less contrast. **Low-kVp techniques produce high subject contrast** because there is a large variation in the in-

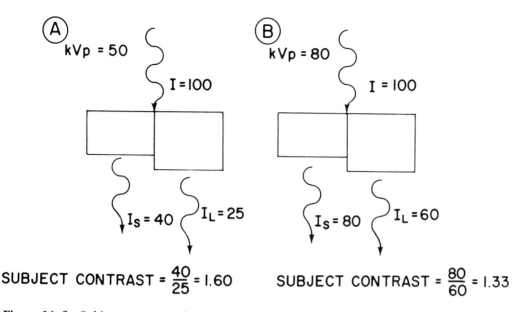

Figure 14–3 Subject contrast varies with the kVp of the x-ray beam

tensity of the transmitted x-ray beam in different parts of the patient. The x-ray film must then "decode" a range of exposure from low to high. This wide range of exposure (log relative exposure) must fall within the steep portion of the characteristic curve (Fig. 14–4A). When a low kVp is used, the mAs must be carefully selected.

Figure 14–4A shows that if the exposure (mAs) is only a little too low, the low-exposure areas (i.e., under bone) will produce exposures in the toe area of the curve. Likewise, excessive mAs will rapidly move high-density exposures onto the shoulder of the curve. Both these mistakes will decrease film contrast. High-kVp exposures

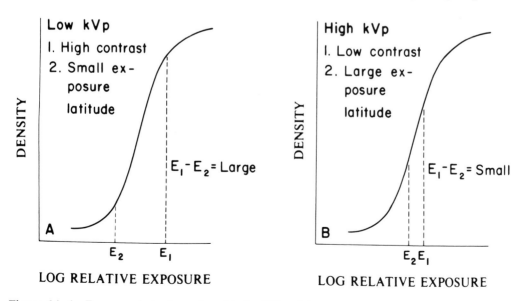

Figure 14–4 Exposure latitude varies with the kVp of the x-ray beam

produce less difference in intensity between areas of the attenuated x-ray beam; this is why **high kVp gives less subject contrast.** With a high-kVp technique, the film has to "decode" a smaller difference in log relative exposure between the low- and high-exposure areas.

Figure 14–4*B* diagrams how a high-kVp technique (using the same object and film-screen system) will "use up" a much shorter portion of the steep portion of the film's characteristic curve. Using high kVp, the technologist has considerable room for error in the choice of mAs, because the exposure range can move up or down on the curve and still fall within the steep portion of the curve.

To review, **kVp influences subject contrast** (exposure differences) **and exposure latitude; mAs controls film blackening** (density). Consider a specific example. A chest film (par speed film-screen combination, 6-ft distance, no grid, exposed with factors of 70 kVp and 6.6 mAs [400 mA, 1/60 sec]) would result in a radiograph with high contrast. The exposure of 6.6 mAs, however, is critical at 70 kVp. An error of ±50% would probably produce a radiograph with a great deal of its density on the toe or shoulder of the film curve, resulting in an unacceptable loss of contrast. Another chest examination exposed at 100 kVp and about 3 mAs would result in a low-contrast radiograph, but changing the exposure (3 mAs) by a factor of ±100% would probably not reduce radiographic contrast. Obviously, fewer mAs or more mAs produces a lighter (less density) or darker (more density) radiograph, but the density range still falls on the steep portion of the film curve. At 100 kVp the exposure can be varied considerably; this is termed **large exposure latitude.** At 70 kVp, the exposure must fall within a narrow range (i.e., there is small exposure latitude).

To make matters more complicated, kVp does have an effect on film blackening. This effect is approximately equal to the fourth power of the kVp. For example, if kVp is increased from 50 to 60 the change in film density (if mAs remains constant) will be about

$$\frac{60^4}{50^4} = 2.07$$

Because kVp has doubled film density, mAs would have to be cut in half. An old rule says: "If you add 10 kVp, cut mAs in half." This holds true around 50 to 60 kVp, but kVp change has less effect on film density at higher ranges. For example, at 85 kVp, an increase of 15 kVp is required to double the film blackening power of the beam.

Subject contrast thus is seen to vary with the makeup of the subject (thickness, density, atomic number), the use of contrast material, and the kVp of the x-ray beam.

Film Contrast

Film contrast has been discussed as a photographic property of x-ray film (see Chap. 11). **X-ray film will significantly amplify subject contrast** provided the exposure (mAs) is correct (keep away from the toe and shoulder of the characteristic curve). Under good viewing conditions, a density difference of about 0.04 (difference in light transmission of 10%) can be seen.

Fog and Scatter

The effect of fog and scatter is to reduce radiographic contrast.

Scattered radiation is produced mainly as a result of **Compton** scattering. The amount of scatter radiation increases with increasing part thickness, field size, and energy of the x-ray beam (higher kVp). Scatter is minimized by collimation of the x-ray beam (use as small a field size as possible) and the use of grids or air gaps. **Scatter radiation that reaches the x-ray film or film-screen combination produces unwanted density.**

Fog is strictly defined as those silver halide grains in the film emulsion that are developed even though they were not exposed by light or x rays. The amount of fog in an unexposed x-ray film can be demonstrated easily. Cut the unexposed film in half. Develop (fully process) one-half of the film and clear (fix, wash, and dry only) the other. The density difference between the two film halves represents the amount of fog present. **Fog produces unwanted film density, which lowers radiographic contrast.**

Another type of unwanted film density may result from accidental exposure of film to light or x rays. This is usually also called "fog" or "exposure fog" and, although the term is not absolutely correct, it has established itself by common usage. These two types of "fog" are different in origin, but both lower film contrast in the same manner.

True fog is increased by the following conditions:

1. Improper film storage (high temperature or humidity)
2. Contaminated or exhausted developer solution
3. Excessive time or temperature of development
4. Use of high-speed film (highly sensitized grains)

Fog, "exposure fog," and scatter add density to the film. By knowing the magnitude of this density and the characteristic curve of the film, it is possible to calculate the effect of the added density on radiographic contrast accurately. Figure 14–5 shows how fog and scatter change the slope of the characteristic curve of a film. Note that the slope of the curve is decreased (contrast is decreased) most at lower levels of density. These are the densities used most frequently in diagnostic radiology. In Figure 14–5 the gamma of the normal film, at a density of 0.9, is 2.4. When fog and scatter are added, the gamma drops to 1.8. At a density of 2.5, fog and scatter have no significant effect on the shape of the curve, but densities as high as 2.5 are seldom used in diagnostic radiology.

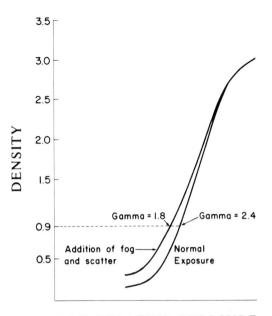

Figure 14–5 Fog and scatter decrease radiographic contrast. (Courtesy of R. E. Wayrynen[21])

To repeat, fog and scatter are undesirable because they decrease radiographic contrast by decreasing film contrast.

Image Quality

The second basic factor determining image clarity is image quality. The quality of the radiographic image may be defined as the ability of the film to record each point in the object as a point on the film. In radiology this point-for-point reproduction is never perfect, largely because of the diffusion of light by intensifying screens. There is no general agreement as to what should be included in a discussion of image quality. Our approach will involve almost no mathematics.

Image quality is influenced by

1. radiographic mottle
2. sharpness
3. resolution

Radiographic Mottle

If an x-ray film is mounted between intensifying screens and exposed to a uniform x-ray beam to produce a density of about 1.0, the resulting film will not show uniform density but will have an irregular mottled appearance. This mottled appearance (caused by small density differences) is easily detected by the unaided eye, and may be seen, if looked for, in any area of "uniform" density in a radiograph exposed with screens (e.g., the area of a chest film not covered by the patient). This uneven texture, or mottle, seen on a film that "should" show perfectly uniform density is called **radiographic mottle.** Radiographic mottle has three components:

Only **quantum mottle** is of any importance in diagnostic radiology.

Film Graininess. Film graininess makes no contribution to the radiographic mottle observed in clinical radiology. Film graininess can be seen when the film is examined with a lens producing magnification of 5 to 10 ×. With this magnification, the image is seen to be made up of a nonhomogeneous arrangement of silver grains in gelatin. Because a radiograph is almost never viewed at an enlargement of 5 ×, film graininess is not seen.

Screen Mottle. Screen mottle has two components, **structure mottle** (unimportant) and **quantum mottle** (important). Structure mottle is caused by defects in the intensifying screen, such as varying thickness or physical imperfections in the phosphor layer. Such screen irregularities can occur, but the quality control used in screen manufacturing is so good that structure mottle may be dismissed as making no contribution to radiographic mottle.

Quantum mottle is the only important cause of radiographic mottle. **Quantum** refers to a discrete unit of energy and, in this discussion, it may be considered as the energy carried by one x-ray photon. An x-ray beam may be thought of as containing a certain number of x-ray photons, or an equivalent number of quanta.

By showing a pattern of mottle, or nonuniform density, the x-ray film is telling us that it has "seen" a nonuniform pattern of light on the surface of the intensifying screen. The nonuniform pattern of light on the screen is caused by fluctuations in the number of photons (or quanta) per square millimeter in the beam that arrived at the screen. What this means is that a "uniform" beam of x rays is not uniform at all. Suppose a "uniform" x-ray beam could be frozen in space and cut into cross sections. If the number of x-ray photons per square millimeter were counted, it would be unlikely that any two square mm would contain exactly the same number of photons. The "uniform" beam is not uniform.

The actual number of x-ray photons per mm^2 obeys the law of probability, because the emission of x rays by the x-ray tube is a random event. The average number of photons per mm^2 can be calculated by adding the number in each mm^2 and dividing by the number of squares. It will then be found that the actual number in any square will almost never be the average value, but that all numbers will fall within a certain range (percent fluctuation) of the average. The law of probability says that the magnitude of this fluctuation is plus or minus the square root of the average number of photons per mm^2. (The square root of the average number of photons is usually referred to as the standard deviation.) For example, if an x-ray beam contains an average of 10,000 photons per mm^2, the number in any one square mm will fall in the range

$$10,000 \pm \sqrt{10,000} = 10,000 \pm 100$$

or any mm^2 may be expected to contain between 9900 and 10,100 photons. In some of the squares (32%) the variation will be even greater than this.

The percent fluctuation in the actual number of photons per mm² becomes greater as the average number becomes smaller. If 100 photons are used, fluctuations will be $\pm \sqrt{100}$, or ± 10, giving a percent fluctuation of $\frac{10}{100}$, or 10%. Using 10,000 photons, fluctuation is ± 100, or a percent fluctuation of $\frac{100}{10,000}$ or 1%.

Quantum mottle is caused by the statistical fluctuation in the number of quanta per unit area absorbed by the intensifying screen. The fewer quanta (x-ray photons) used, the greater will be the quantum mottle (more statistical fluctuation). Intensifying screens are used because they decrease the x-ray exposure (number of photons) needed to expose the x-ray film. Quantum mottle is seen when intensifying screens are used. Quantum mottle will be greater with high-kVp x rays because they produce a higher screen intensification factor.

The concept of quantum mottle is illustrated in Figure 14–6. The model consists of the cardboard top of a hatbox; small cardboard figures in the shape of a circle, square, and triangle placed in the hatbox top; and 1000 pennies. The pennies represent x-ray quanta, and were dropped into the hatbox top in a completely random manner. Radiographs of the model were made after 10, 100, 500, and 1000 pennies had been dropped into the hatbox top. Notice that the radiograph of 10 pennies shows no information about the makeup of the model; 100 pennies show that the hatbox top is probably round; 500 pennies show three filling defects in the hatbox top, which is definitely round; and all 1000 pennies clearly define the shape of each filling defect. In other words, a lot of pennies (quanta) provided a lot of information about the model, fewer pennies provided less information, and too few pennies provided no useful information.

Quantum mottle is difficult to see unless a high-quality radiograph is produced. A film of high contrast and good quality will show visible quantum mottle. If film con-

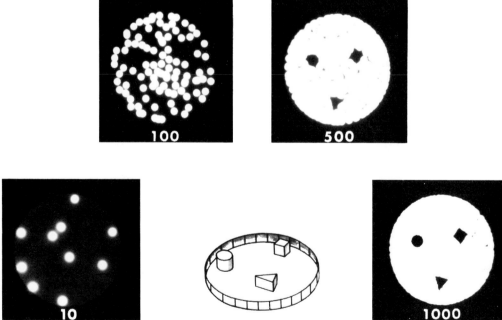

Figure 14–6 The "pennies-in-the-hatbox" model illustrating the concept of quantum mottle

trast and quality are poor, such as produced by poor film-screen contact, quantum mottle will not be visible. Thick intensifying screens may show less visible mottle on the film because of greater diffusion of light. A radiograph with poor visibility of image detail will also exhibit poor visibility of quantum mottle.

In summary, let us define radiographic mottle as the radiographic recording of the statistical fluctuations in a beam of x-ray photons.

Speed Versus Noise. Radiographic mottle is often called **noise.** Allow us to repeat an important but poorly understood fact: **noise (quantum mottle) results from statistical fluctuation in the number of x-ray photons used (absorbed) by the intensifying screens to form the image.** With currently available films and screens it is possible to obtain a film-screen system so fast that noise makes the resulting image unsatisfactory except for a few special applications such as pelvimetry. Two basic premises must be remembered:

1. High-contrast images are **SHARP-NESS**-limited
2. Low-contrast images are **NOISE**-limited

Because low-contrast images comprise most diagnostically important information, noise may seriously compromise a radiograph.

The two ways to increase the speed of a film-screen radiographic system are obvious:
1. Use a faster screen
2. Use a faster film

The way the increase in speed affects system noise (quantum mottle) is not so obvious or easy to understand. Let us illustrate this difficulty by posing a question that experience has shown almost everyone answers incorrectly. Assume that two radiographs of an abdomen are made. Both exposures use the same medium-speed x-ray film. The first exposure is made using

par speed calcium tungstate screens. The second exposure is made using high-speed calcium tungstate screens, which are exactly twice as fast (i.e., require only half the mAs) as the par speed screens. Now for the question. Which exposure (par speed or high-speed screens) will produce the radiograph with the most noise (quantum mottle)? If you answer "the high-speed system," you are wrong, in company with most of your colleagues. The correct answer is that the noise is the same for both radiographs (the noise will be more difficult to see when the thick fast screen is used because of more light diffusion, which causes decreased visibility of image detail).

The rest of this section will attempt to explain this relationship between noise and system speed, a concept made important in film-screen radiography by the introduction of noncalcium tungstate high-speed intensifying screens and fast x-ray film.

Let us try to simplify the problem by stating that, with regard to noise, there are two ways to increase the speed (i.e., lower the

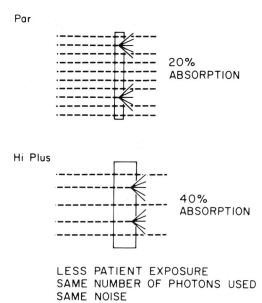

LESS PATIENT EXPOSURE
SAME NUMBER OF PHOTONS USED
SAME NOISE

Figure 14–7 Increasing speed by increasing the stopping power of the intensifying screen will not change noise x-ray dose to the patient) of a film-screen radiographic system:

1. Increase speed with no change in noise
2. Increase speed and increase noise

We need to examine each of these two methods in some detail.

1. **Increased speed with no change in noise can be done in two ways:**
   a. Increase phosphor layer thickness
   b. Use a phosphor with a higher absorption coefficient for x rays

Both these methods will increase the stopping power of the intensifying screen. Refer to Figure 14–7, which diagrams a par speed and a Du Pont Hi Plus (twice the speed of par) calcium tungstate screen. If 10 x-ray photons arrive at the par speed screen, 2 photons are absorbed (assume 20% absorption). If a Hi Plus $CaWO_4$ screen is used, the screen will absorb 40% of the x-ray beam because it is thicker than a par speed screen. Thus, to cause the high-speed screen to absorb 2 photons, we need only cause 5 photons to arrive at the screen (the amount of light produced per absorbed photon is the same in each screen). Because only half as many photons are required, exposure to the patient is cut in half and we speak of the Hi Plus screen as being twice as "fast" because we were able to decrease patient exposure by half (i.e., we cut the mAs in half). The only factor determining noise, however, is **THE NUMBER OF PHOTONS USED BY THE SCREEN.** Both the par and Hi Plus $CaWO_4$ screens have **USED** the same number of photons. The faster screen has a thicker phosphor layer, which absorbs a higher percentage of the x-ray beam. Stated another way, if the screen phosphor is the same, changes in screen speed will not result in any change in noise. This last statement has an exception. Addition of a light-absorbing dye to the screen phosphor layer will prevent some light from reaching the film. Because some light is lost, more photons must be absorbed by the screen to produce

enough light to expose the film (i.e., use of dye in slow screens decreases noise).

The price that must be paid for increased speed in $CaWO_4$ screens is more **unsharpness** caused by light diffusion in the thicker phosphor layer. Thus, the choice of which $CaWO_4$ screen to use is a compromise between

SHARPNESS vs. SPEED.

A phosphor with higher inherent absorption of x rays could give more speed without an increase in unsharpness (thicker screen not required) or noise (same x ray to light conversion efficiency as $CaWO_4$). The potential for this type of improvement is limited. Lead (atomic number 82) is the highest atomic number nonradioactive element. Tungsten (atomic number 74) is so close to lead that there is little room in the periodic table to discover phosphors with a higher atomic number. We have previously discussed how some of the new phosphors do gain some of their speed through higher inherent absorption of x rays by use of a favorably located K-absorption edge. Screen speed obtained in this manner is desirable because patient exposure is then decreased without any increase in noise or unsharpness.

2. **Increased speed with increased noise can be done in two ways:**
   a. Use a phosphor with a higher x ray-to-light conversion efficiency
   b. Use a faster film

Both these processes will have identical effects on the noise content of the finished radiograph. The system cannot distinguish between a phosphor having a higher conversion efficiency and the use of a faster film. In each case the faster system will provide an image produced by use (absorption) of fewer photons in the screen, with a corresponding increase in noise. This is illustrated in Figure 14–8, in which a par speed calcium tungstate screen (20% absorption of the x-ray beam) is compared to a rare earth screen (such as gadolinium oxysulfide), which also absorbs 20% of the x-ray beam but produces twice as much

Calcium Tungstate

20%
ABSORPTION

Rare Earth

MORE LIGHT
PER
ABSORBED PHOTON

LESS PATIENT EXPOSURE
SMALLER NUMBER OF PHOTONS USED
MORE NOISE

Figure 14–8 Increasing speed by increasing the x ray-to-light conversion efficiency of the phosphor will increase noise

light per absorbed photon (in this example). Note that the rare earth screen, by absorbing only one x-ray photon, has produced as much light as the $CaWO_4$ screen produced by absorbing two x-ray photons. It is this difference in photons absorbed by the screen that causes a change in the quantum noise (mottle). Similarly, if one uses identical screens but a film that is twice as fast, the faster film will be properly exposed with half as much light, which the screen produces by absorbing half as many photons.

The new fast screen phosphors are faster than calcium tungstate because they:
1. Absorb (use) a larger percentage of the x-ray beam (no change in quantum noise)
2. Have a higher x ray-to-light conversion efficiency (with an increase in quantum noise)

It is possible to use a film-screen combination in which system quantum mottle (noise) will produce a perceptible decrease in the visibility of low contrast images on the radiograph. In choosing one of the

noncalcium tungstate, very fast screens a compromise must thus be reached between

SPEED vs. NOISE.

Another way to look at quantum noise is to examine a terribly complex function called the **Wiener spectrum.** This may be thought of as the modulation transfer function (MTF) of the noise of an image, and we will briefly examine this concept after the discussion of MTF later in this chapter.

We will summarize the concept of quantum noise in film-screen radiography in outline form:

1. Increase speed with no change in noise
   a. Increase phosphor layer thickness
   b. Use a phosphor with a higher absorption coefficient for x rays
2. Increase speed with increased noise
   a. Use a phosphor with a higher x ray-to-light conversion efficiency
   b. Use a faster film

Sharpness

Sharpness is the ability of the x-ray film or film-screen system to define an edge. The inability of a film-screen system to record a sharp edge because of light diffusion in the intensifying screen has been previously discussed. Sharpness and contrast are closely related in the subjective response they produce. An unsharp edge can be easily seen if contrast is high, but a sharp edge may be poorly visible if contrast is low.

Unsharpness will be discussed in more detail in Chapter 15. We will review the subject briefly.

Geometric Unsharpness. Penumbra is minimized by using a small focal spot and by keeping magnification as small as possible. If you understand why the term "edge gradient" (rather than penumbra) is now preferred, you really understand what geometric unsharpness means.

Motion Unsharpness. Subject motion can be minimized by using a short exposure time. Motion of the x-ray tube during the exposure will cause unsharpness, but it is not as important as motion of the object.

Absorption Unsharpness. Absorption unsharpness results because a patient is not made up of objects that have nice sharp edges. Absorption unsharpness is greatest for round or oval objects.

Screen Unsharpness. X-ray intensifying screens cause unsharp borders because of **light diffusion** in the screen phosphor layer. Good screen-film contact is essential.

Parallax Unsharpness. Parallax unsharpness is seen only with double-emulsion films. There is an image on each emulsion, and the images are separated by the width of the film base (0.007 or 0.008 inches). When viewed from an angle, these two image edges will not overlap exactly. Parallax makes a negligible contribution to image unsharpness.

Total Unsharpness. In a radiographic image, all types of unsharpness are present. The proper method of calculating the total unsharpness is not known, but it is known that simple addition does not give the correct result. For example, assume that total unsharpness is given by

$$U_T = \sqrt{U_g^2 + U_a^2 + U_m^2 + U_s^2}$$

where U_T = total unsharpness
U_g = geometric unsharpness
U_a = absorption unsharpness
U_m = motion unsharpness
U_s = screen unsharpness

This formula is probably incorrect, but will illustrate an important point. Assume an examination in which U_g = 0.5 mm, U_a = 4 mm, U_m = 1 mm, and U_s = 0.6 mm. What is total unsharpness?

$$U_T = \sqrt{(0.5)^2 + 4^2 + 1^1 + (0.6)^2} = 4.2 \text{ mm}$$

Note that total unsharpness of 4.2 mm is largely determined by the single largest cause of unsharpness, which is 4 mm of absorption unsharpness in this example. If any unsharpness is significantly larger than the others, the largest cause of unsharpness almost completely controls total unsharpness. In our example absorption unsharpness of 4 mm is the most important. Decreasing U_g (smaller focal spot), U_m (shorter exposure time), or U_s (detail screens) would not significantly improve image sharpness. Attempts to improve the image must be directed toward the factor most responsible for a poor image. Absorption unsharpness cannot be changed, but the unsharp image edge may be made more easily visible by increasing contrast. Therefore, by increasing contrast with a lower kVp technique, it is possible that actually increasing U_g (geometric unsharpness) and U_m (motion unsharpness) by using higher mAs (larger focal spot and longer exposure time) will produce a radiograph with better visibility of fine detail. The infinite variety of boundaries encountered in the patient compounds the problem of absorption unsharpness. No matter how good the geometric conditions, absorption unsharpness may make exact delineation of the borders of small objects (such as opacified blood vessels) all but impossible.

Resolution

Imagine a photograph of a pastoral scene in which a barn and a windmill are depicted against the background of a dark blue sky. If the top edge of the roof of the barn is sharply outlined against the sky, the photograph has good sharpness. The term **sharpness** is used to describe the subjective response of crisp, or abrupt, edges (the objective correlate of sharpness is termed acutance). If each vane of the windmill is easily counted, the photograph has good resolution, or resolving power. Sharpness is the ability of an imaging system to record sharply defined margins, or abrupt edges. **Resolving power is the ability to record separate images of small objects that are placed very close together.** An imaging system may have the ability to record sharp edges but be unable to resolve fine details. Another system may yield fuzzy unsharp edges but still be able to show much fine detail. Sharpness and resolving power are different, but they are related in the subjective response they produce.

Until recently, x-ray imaging systems were evaluated by their resolving power. For example, a par speed intensifying screen might be described as having a resolving power of 8 lines per mm. Several methods of determining resolving power are used. One method uses a resolving power target made up of a series of parallel wires or lead strips, placed so that the space between each lead strip is equal to the width of the strip (Fig. 14–9). In this system, a "line" actually means a line and a space, more appropriately termed a "line pair." For example, 4 lines per mm means that there are 4 lead strips or wires per mm, with each line $\frac{1}{8}$ mm wide and each space $\frac{1}{8}$ mm wide, so that each line pair is $\frac{1}{4}$ mm wide. A commonly used resolving power target is the Buckbee-Meers resolution plate, which consists of line pairs varying from 1.0 to 9.6 per mm in 18 steps.[1]

A film-screen system is evaluated by how many line pairs per mm can be clearly seen in the developed radiograph. Another testing device uses a slit of adjustable width between two blocks of lead. After each x-ray exposure, this apparatus is moved across the film or film-screen combination a distance equal to the width of the slit, producing in this way a series of lines and spaces on the developed film.[6] All these systems depend on an observer determining how many line pairs per mm he can see, and the number will vary among observers.

Figure 14–9 A resolving power target consists of a series of lines and spaces

It is argued that these measurements only evaluate the ability of the system to depict the image of a wire, or lead strip or slit, and do not necessarily pertain to the complex shapes and varying contrasts presented to a film-screen system (or fluoroscopic system) in clinical practice. Also, the resolving power only measures a limit. Knowing that a film-screen system will resolve 8 line pairs per mm tells us that it will not produce an image of 10 line pairs per mm, but says nothing about how good or bad a job it does at 2, 4, or 6 line pairs per mm.

The basic question to consider is this. When the information in the x-ray image is transferred to the x-ray film (usually with light from intensifying screens), how much information is lost? The answer is now being sought by evaluation of the line spread function and the modulation transfer function. The physics and mathematics involved in these determinations are highly complex. We hope to present the basic concepts in an understandable form without the use of any mathematics.

LINE SPREAD FUNCTION

The fact that light diffusion by intensifying screens causes blurred, or unsharp, image edges has been discussed. The line spread function provides a way to measure this effect.

The line spread function is determined as follows. A narrow slit is formed between two jaws made of metal highly opaque to x rays, such as platinum. The width of the slit is usually 10 microns, and the metal jaws are about 2 mm thick. X rays passing through this slit are so severely collimated that they may be considered as a "line source" x-ray beam. The slit apparatus is placed in intimate contact with a film-screen system, and an exposure is made. Only the x rays passing through the 10-micron slit reach the intensifying screens. A perfect imaging system would produce an image of a line 10 microns wide on the developed film. Because of light diffusion in the screens, however, the developed film will actually show density extending out for several hundred microns on each side. The photographic effect of the x-ray beam is spread over a total distance of 800 or more microns (0.8 mm).[11] This technique provides a way to express the line spread function (LSF) numerically. Figure 14–10 shows line spread function graphs in which the relative density is shown to decrease with distance away from the 10-micron line source of x rays. Measuring film density over such a small area requires the use of a microdensitometer, which reads the density of an extremely small area of the film.

Notice on the hypothetic curves of Figure 14–10 (based on the work of Rossmann and Lubberts[13]) that the tailing off of image density is much more marked when high-speed screens are used than when medium-speed screens are used to produce the same density in the center. The shape of the curves in Figure 14–10 allows us to predict accurately that image boundaries will be less faithfully recorded when the image resulting from the use of high-speed screens is compared to that resulting from the use of slower screens. The less light diffusion, the sharper, or more abrupt, will be image edges. Sharper image edges allow imaging of finer detail in the radiograph.

The line spread function can also be used to measure the influence of factors on the image other than that of intensifying screens. These factors include x-ray film, fluoroscopic screens, focal spots of x-ray tubes, x-ray image intensifiers, motion unsharpness, and scatter radiation.

The LSF of x-ray film exposed without screens (direct x-ray exposure) is difficult to measure. There is almost no diffusion of x rays and secondary electrons in the film, so the LSF is narrow. The grain size of an x-ray film may be as large as 2.0 microns. If an x-ray photon were to pass between two grains that were side by side, it might cause both grains to be developed, producing an image 4 μ wide. The image of a line source x-ray beam exposing a film directly will be slightly broadened because of slight radiation diffusion and the finite size of the developed silver halide grains. Image diffusion is so small, however, that the LSF of film exposed to x rays is difficult to measure.

Is the determination of the line spread function of a screen-film system of any practical value? Through a series of complex mathematical manipulations the modulation transfer function of the screen-film system can be calculated from the line spread function, and the modulation trans-

Figure 14–10 Line spread function of medium-speed and fast screens. (Modified from Rossman and Lubberts[13])

fer providing a way to measure the image quality that can be produced.

MODULATION TRANSFER FUNCTION

We have discussed how the clarity of the x-ray image is influenced by **contrast, sharpness,** and **resolution.** Each of these terms may be defined separately, but their complex interrelationships that ultimately determine image clarity are much more difficult to evaluate. The modulation transfer function (MTF) is a concept that has been formulated to provide an objective measurement of the combined effects of sharpness and resolution. Let us consider that modulation means a change in the amplitude (or intensity, or amount) of an information-carrying signal. Imagine a can that contains an unknown amount of thick oil. The oil is measured by pouring it into a graduated beaker. Some of the oil will stick to the sides of the can and escape detection. The information signal seen is the oil in the beaker. The amount of information (oil) seen is less than the total amount of information in the can; the signal has been modulated (changed) because some information was lost in the transfer of oil from the can to the beaker. If careful laboratory measurements determine that the can holds 500 ml of oil, but only 400 ml is measured, the information-detecting system used will detect $\frac{400}{500}$, or 0.8, of the total information. Similarly, the MTF is an attempt to measure the amount of information transferred from the invisible x-ray image to the detecting system (x-ray film, television image, etc.). The MTF represents a ratio between the information recorded and the total amount of information available, or

$$MTF = \frac{\text{information recorded}}{\text{information available}}$$

Because recorded information can never be greater than available information, the MTF can never be greater than 1.

The MTF of a screen-film system is usually calculated from the corresponding line spread function by a complex mathematical operation known as a Fourier transformation. In practice, a computer may do the calculations from information it receives from the microdensitometer used to measure the densities making up the line spread function. A complete discussion of the specialized physics and mathematics involved in developing an MTF curve is far beyond the scope of this text, and most radiologists lack the specialized background necessary to understand such a treatment of the subject. We are indebted to R. E. Wayrynen for developing the following discussion of what the modulation transfer means, expressed in simple examples.[21]

Consider a resolving power target (Fig. 14–11). A radiograph of the target should produce a film with "square wave" changes in density, completely black in the area corresponding to the spaces and completely unexposed in areas corresponding to the metal strips, with abrupt density changes (i.e., sharp margins). Using a screen-film combination, the blackest black will have a density of about 3.0, and unexposed film will have a density of about 0.2 (base and fog densities). Because of light scattering by the screens, the actual radiograph will not show square waves. The maximum density will be less than expected, "unexposed" areas of the film will react as if they had received exposure, and the transition from minimum to maximum density will be gradual, producing the sine wave density pattern expressed graphically in Figure 14–11. Light scattering causes density to be "shoveled off" the density peaks and "poured into" the valleys, causing a **decrease in image sharpness** (less abrupt image borders) and a **decrease in contrast** (density difference between the peaks and valleys).

Now consider a resolving power target in which the widths of the opaque metal strips and the spaces become progressively smaller. The more line pairs per unit

Figure 14–11 Information is lost when the x-ray image of a resolving power target is recorded by a screen-film combination

length, the greater the amount of information presented to the screen-film system. The amount of information is usually expressed as a certain number of line pairs per mm, or a certain number of cycles per mm, both being the same. Figure 14–12 is a diagram of what happens to the image of the resolving power target recorded by the screen-film combination as information content increases. The difference in density (contrast) on the developed film between areas of maximum exposure (under the spaces) and minimum exposure becomes less as information content increases. This is caused almost entirely by light scattering in the intensifying screens. Eventually, the screen-film system becomes unable to show any density difference between lines and spaces. This represents the limit of the resolving power of the system— that is, the ability to record lines and spaces.

When an x-ray beam is directed onto a resolving power target, most x rays that encounter a space pass through the space, while those that encounter a metal strip are absorbed. In the laboratory it is possible to measure the intensity of the x-ray beam under spaces (maximum exposure) and

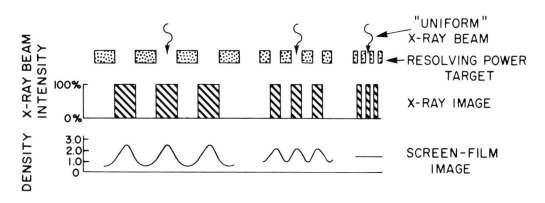

Figure 14–12 As the information content of a resolving power target increases, the ability of the screen-film system to record the x-ray image of the target decreases

lead strips (minimum exposure). The intensity may be expressed in milliroentgens, and represents the exposure received by the screen-film combination. A characteristic curve may be prepared in which the logarithm of the actual exposure (rather than relative exposure) is used to prepare the density-log E curve. On such a curve (Fig. 14–13) the measured maximum (E_{max}) and minimum (E_{min}) exposures reaching the film are recorded. Then the exposed film is processed, and the developed maximum and minimum densities are carefully measured and plotted on the curve, shown as the obtained densities D'_{max} and D'_{min} in Figure 14–13. Note that the maximum and minimum densities ac-

tually produced by the exposure are not the same as the densities expected from the measured exposures. The observed maximum density is less than predicted, and the observed minimum density is more than predicted. This is another way of graphically representing the effect of light scattering by the intensifying screens. Expressed another way, the film has acted as if it received a lower maximum exposure and a higher minimum exposure, as shown by the dotted lines in Figure 14–13.

The amplitude of the exposure input ($E_{max} - E_{min}$) to the film is known from actual measurement. The amplitude of the exposure "equivalent" output ($E'_{max} - E'_{min}$) has been calculated by knowing the char-

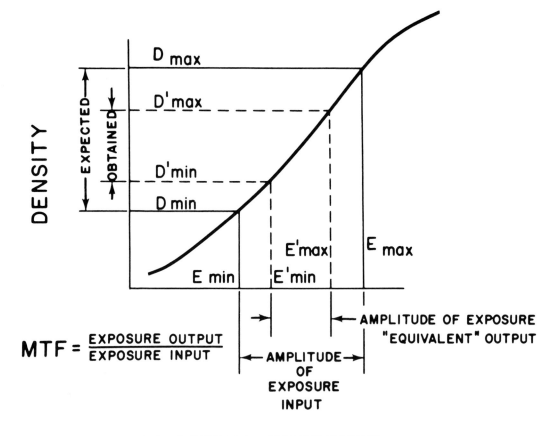

Figure 14–13 The modulation transfer function of a screen-film system may be calculated by using a resolving power target

acteristic curve of the film and by measuring film density produced by the exposure. In addition, the width of the lines and spaces of the resolving power target are obviously known. Therefore, we may now calculate the modulation transfer function (MTF) of the screen-film system at a known frequency (lines per mm) as follows (Fig. 14–13):

$$MTF = \frac{\text{exposure amplitude output}}{\text{exposure amplitude input}}$$

Using this rather laborious procedure, the MTF of a screen-film system could be calculated for 1, 2, 4, 6, 8, etc., line pairs per mm by using the appropriate resolving power target, measuring exposure input, and calculating the exposure "equivalent" output. A curve similar to that shown in Figure 14–14 would be developed, and this is the MTF curve of our hypothetical screen-film system. This curve tells us that, at 1 line pair per mm, the $\frac{\text{output}}{\text{input}}$ = about 0.8 (or 80%), which is good. At 4 line pairs per mm $\frac{\text{output}}{\text{input}}$ = about 0.3, and at 8 line pairs per mm it is about 0.1, or 10%. Remember, MTF curves are usually calculated from the line spread function, but the

meaning of the MTF curve is easier to understand if it is discussed in terms of its derivation based on the use of resolving power targets.

How is an MTF curve useful? There are no "units" of MTF. It does not measure contrast or sharpness or resolution. For the clinical radiologist, MTF curves may be useful as a more accurate way to compare the imaging qualities of competing systems, to help choose the system that best suits his needs. Consider intensifying screens again. We have discussed the fact that resolving power measures only a limit. Assume that Figure 14–14 is the MTF curve for a par speed intensifying screen. The 10% response on the MTF curve corresponds roughly to the resolving power of the imaging system. In Figure 14–14 the 10% response is about 8 line pairs per mm, so this screen would have a resolving power of 8 lines (or line pairs) per mm. But the curve also allows us to compare the relative imaging properties of the screen at frequencies lower than the resolving power.

Now consider Figure 14–15, in which hypothetic MTF curves for two x-ray intensifying screens are shown; the differences in the curves are exaggerated for the purposes of illustration. Screen A has a resolving power (10% MTF) of 6 lines per mm, while the resolving power of screen B is 14 line pairs per mm. From resolving power figures, screen B is apparently a much better screen. However, the MTF curves show that, at 4 lines per mm, screen

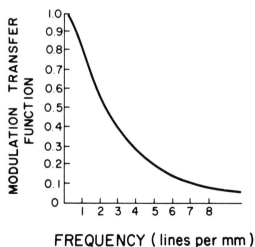

Figure 14–14 The modulation transfer function curve of a hypothetical screen-film system

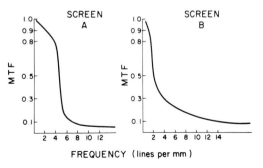

Figure 14–15 Hypothetical MTF curves of two x-ray intensifying screens

A has a response of 80%, while screen B has fallen to 30%, and at 2 lines per mm the values are 90% and 50%, respectively. Under normal viewing conditions the eye usually sees structures of a size corresponding to an information content between 2 and 4 line pairs per mm. For routine radiography, the information recorded by screen A will probably produce radiographs of greater diagnostic accuracy than those produced by screen B. On the other hand, an attempt to record very small structures would require the use of screen B. Obviously, the true difference in the characteristics and clinical applications of these screens can be appreciated only from a comparison of the respective MTF curves. Resolving power may be thought of as a single point on the MTF curves.

Modulation transfer function curves are being developed for all the imaging systems used in radiology, including screen-film systems, x-ray image amplifiers, cine and 70 mm, 90 mm, and 105 mm systems, and television viewing, including tape and disc image storage systems.

The MTF plays an important role in the evaluation of a complex imaging system. Consider, for example, a film-screen system that has a front screen, first film emulsion, film base, second film emulsion, and back screen. In optical terms this is called a "cascaded system," or a series of cascaded imaging processes. In Chapter 15, dealing with magnification radiography, we will consider the film, the x-ray tube focal spot, the x-ray intensifying screens, and the motion of the object being radiographed as four components in a cascaded system. Each component of a cascaded system has its own imaging properties, and it is often possible to express these properties in terms of the MTF of the particular component. Once the MTFs of the components of a complex system are known, the total MTF of the entire system may be obtained by multiplying the MTFs of each of the components.

As an example, if one knows that, at an object frequency of 2 line pairs per mm, the MTF of x-ray film is 1.0 (i.e., the film is perfect), the MTF of the intensifying screens is 0.7, and the MTF of the focal spot of the x-ray tube is 0.8, then total system MTF will be $1.0 \times 0.7 \times 0.8 = 0.56$. The MTF concept allows each component of an imaging system to be studied so that the optimum system may be designed. Unfortunately, in diagnostic radiology it is difficult to define the "optimum system" objectively because the elements in a radiograph that allow one to arrive at a correct diagnosis are not easily defined. It is not correct to assume that by measuring the MTF for different imaging systems radiologists can compare and decide which system to buy. The ultimate practical use of MTF measurements to both radiologists and industry is still being evaluated.

NOISE AND THE WIENER SPECTRUM

We previously introduced the concept of quantum mottle (or noise) caused by the fact that film-screen radiography is quantum-limited (i.e., the radiograph may be formed with a relatively small number of x-ray photons). This noise may be apparent visually, and it can also be measured in the laboratory. The radiologist generally considers a radiograph made with average speed film and par speed screens as being pretty good. Such radiographs require that about 50,000 x-ray photons per square millimeter be absorbed by the screen to produce an average density of 1.0. In photography this would not be considered a good image, because a typical aerial photography film will use about 20 times as many photons to form its image.

One way to describe noise objectively is by the Wiener spectrum, sometimes called the "power spectrum" of noise. The mechanics of measuring radiographic mottle (noise) present difficult problems. In one method the radiographic mottle is scanned by a microdensitometer, and the sampled density fluctuation is analyzed by a computer. Another method involves putting the "noisy" film into a type of microdensitometer in which it can be spun in a circle and illuminated from one side. The transmitted light is collected by a photomultiplier behind a scanning aperture. The fluctuation in transmitted light intensity caused by radiographic mottle is converted to a voltage fluctuation in the photomultiplier tube. Electronic analysis of this voltage fluctuation performs what amounts to a Fourier analysis, which can determine the frequency content in the noise pattern.

Let us consider for a moment what noise looks like on a microdensitometer scan. In previous discussions we assumed that such a scan across the image of a small object would produce a nice smooth scan of density change versus distance, as shown in Figure 14–11. This is not a true picture of the situation. In Figure 14–16 we show how a real microdensitometer scan across an image will appear. Assume that identical screens are used, but in Figure 14–16*A* a slow film (low noise) and in Figure 14–16*B* a fast film (high noise) is used. The small square aperture of the microdensitometer (e.g., 5 to 10 microns) will "see" the small irregular density variations that constitute radiographic mottle superimposed on the larger density change caused by the image of the object being radiographed. In fact, it is difficult to make accurate microden-

A. LOW NOISE

B. HIGH NOISE

Figure 14–16 Schematic depiction of a microdensitometer scan of the image of a blood vessel made with a low-noise (*A*) and a high-noise (*B*) imaging system

sitometer scans of noisy and unsharp images because of the presence of quantum mottle. Nice smooth microdensitometer scans of objects such as opacified blood vessels simply do not exist.

We must retreat for a moment and review the components of radiographic mottle. You will recall that there is both screen mottle (for practical purposes this is quantum mottle) and film graininess. Although the eye does not normally see film grain, the microdensitometer is able to "see" the nonhomogeneous arrangement of clumps of silver in the gelatin. Thus, a microdensitometer will detect noise of two types:

1. Quantum mottle (statistical fluctuation of x-ray quanta absorbed in the screen)
2. Film grain (noise caused by the inherent grain distribution in the film)

The Wiener spectrum is a measure of the total noise recorded by the film, **the sum of the grain noise and the quantum noise.** How does one distinguish film grain from screen mottle (quantum mottle)? This requires that two "flash" exposures of a film-screen system be made. The film in its cassette is simply placed under an x-ray tube and exposed at a reasonable kVp (one author uses 80 kVp) and low milliampere-seconds to produce a density on the processed film of about 0.7. If the film and screen (or screens) are in intimate contact, the film will record quantum mottle resulting from the nonuniform absorption of x-ray quanta (and thus nonuniform production of light) in the screen, so the resulting noise will be made up of recorded quantum noise superimposed on the inherent film grain. To measure film grain alone a specially designed cassette is used. This cassette holds the screen (or screens) 13 or 14 mm away from the film, causing the individual light flashes (scintillations) from the screen to be blurred into a pattern of completely uniform illumination before the light reaches the film. In such a circumstance the film has been exposed with a truly uniform light source (i.e., quantum mottle has become undetectable in the light pattern by the time it reaches the film), so any noise in the processed film must originate from inherent film grain. In all these experiments we assume (virtually always correctly) that the screens used are free of any structural defects that could produce noise.

Schematic representation of the Wiener spectrum of a film-screen system will depict

1. total system noise (quantum plus grain noise)
2. film grain noise (grain noise)
3. ability of the system to record the noise at increasing spatial frequency (recorded noise) (Fig. 14–17)

Note in Figure 14–17 that the lines depicting total (quantum plus grain) noise and grain noise are straight lines. This means that the amount of noise is the same at all spatial frequencies; this is termed "white noise." Considering only noise, we may consider quantum mottle as the information input that we have asked the film-screen system to record. If the system were perfect, the amount of recorded quantum noise would be the same (white noise input) at all spatial frequencies. The MTF of the film-screen system limits the ability of the system to record information

input, however, whether that information is the image of a skull, opacified blood vessel, or quantum mottle. The ability of the film-screen system to record noise decreases as the spatial frequency (line pairs per mm) increases, exactly as the ability of the system to record any image decreases with increasing spatial frequency. Depending on the MTF of the screen being used, a point is reached at which quantum noise is no longer imaged, and at this point only inherent film grain remains for the microdensitometer to detect (this might occur at about 6 to 10 line pairs per mm with typical screens). Let us not concern ourselves with a unit for measuring the Wiener spectrum, but be content to compare the position of a curve along the vertical axis to indicate more noise or less noise.

Some examples may make this topic easier to understand. Figure 14–18 shows the Wiener spectrum of radiographic mottle for two film-screen systems. System A uses a sharp (thin) screen combined with a fast

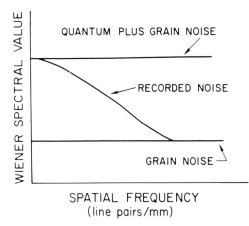

Figure 14–17 Schematic representation of the Wiener spectrum of a film-screen system

Figure 14–18 Schematic representation of the Wiener spectrum of a sharp screen combined with a fast film (*A*), and a less sharp screen combined with a slower film (*B*)

film. System B uses a less sharp (thicker) screen combined with a slower film. Note that the inherent film grain white noise is greater for the fast film (i.e., larger clumps of silver are more unevenly distributed in the gelatin) than for the slow film. System A has an increased Wiener spectral noise value because fewer x-ray quanta were absorbed (i.e., the fast film required less light). The point at which the total recorded noise curve merges with the film grain noise level indicates the relative MTF of each screen. The screen used in system A has the better MTF because it is able to record noise out to higher frequencies than system B. Without assigning any value units to the Wiener spectrum, a lot of information may still be derived from these two curves (i.e., compare total noise, film graininess, and system MTF).

Now consider Figure 14–19, which shows the Wiener spectral curves of three different screens used with the same film. Because systems A and B have the same total system noise at very low spatial frequency we can conclude that these two screens use the same number of x-ray quanta to expose the film. Likewise, because system A records noise at higher spatial frequencies, we know that screen A has a better MTF than screen B (probably because it is thinner). In fact, these two curves are similar to curves obtained with two par speed calcium tungstate screens made by different manufacturers.[20] Curve C represents a screen with significantly less total noise than that of the other two systems. This might be accomplished by using a less efficient screen phosphor (requiring absorption of more x-ray quanta to make an equal amount of light), or by using the same phosphor and including a light-absorbing dye in the phosphor layer. System C has a better MTF than that of the other systems because it records noise at a higher spatial frequency. This improved MTF might result from a thinner screen or from use of a dye in the screen to minimize light diffusion (acutance dye). This curve (C) is similar to a published Wiener spectral value curve of a detail calcium tungstate screen containing a yellow acutance dye to minimize light diffusion in the phosphor layer.[20]

As is true with MTF measurements, it is difficult to define the ultimate use of Wiener spectral curves in diagnostic radiology. It is clear that new developments in design regarding system optics, noise, and speed are offering the radiologist great flexibility in choice of an imaging system. Unfortunately, this greater flexibility creates a problem that requires greater understanding of the relation between system speed, noise, and detail visibility.

SUMMARY

Image clarity is defined as the visibility of diagnostically important detail in the radiographic image. Image clarity is determined by contrast and image quality. Radiographic contrast depends on three factors: subject contrast, film contrast, and scatter radiation plus fog. Image quality is a difficult subject to discuss because there is no good definition of what actually constitutes diagnostically important detail. Quantum mottle interferes with the smallest perceptible contrast, and is inversely proportional to the number of photons

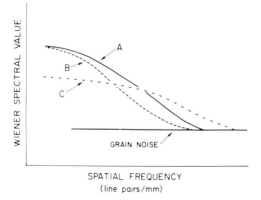

Figure 14–19 Schematic representation of the Wiener spectral curves of three different calcium tungstate intensifying screens used with the same film (see text)

used to form an image. Sharpness is the ability of an imaging system to define a sharp edge. Resolving power is the ability of an imaging system to record separate images of small objects that are placed very close together. Use of the line spread function, modulation transfer function, and Wiener spectrum concepts help to develop a better understanding of the physical factors that control the information content of the radiographic image. We have attempted to introduce the fundamentals of the LSF, MTF, and Wiener spectrum in simple terms. The bibliography lists a number of excellent articles that explore these concepts in more detail.

REFERENCES

1. Bookstein, J.J., and Steck, W.: Effective focal spot size. Radiology, *98*:31, 1971.
2. Cleare, H.M., Splettstosser, H.R., and Seeman, H.E.: An experimental study of the mottle produced by x-ray intensifying screens. Am. J. Roentgenol., *88*:168, 1962.
3. Doi, K., and Rossman, K.: Measurement of optical and noise properties of screen-film systems in radiography. SPIE Medical X-Ray Photo-Optical Systems Evaluation, *56*:45, 1975.
4. Gopala Rao, U.V., and Bates, L.M.: The modulation transfer function of x-ray focal spots. Phys. Med. Biol., *14*:93, 1968.
5. Holm, T.: Some aspects of radiographic information. Radiology, *83*:319, 1964.
6. Morgan, R.H.: The frequency response function. Am. J. Roentgenol., *88*:175, 1962.
7. Morgan, R.H., Bates, L.M., Gopala Rao, U.V., and Marinaro, A.: The frequency response characteristics of x-ray films and screens. Am. J. Roentgenol., *92*:426, 1964.
8. Roesch, W.C., Mellins, H.Z., and Gregg, E.C.: Improvements in the radiological image: A report from the Radiation Study Section of the National Institutes of Health. Radiology, *97*:442, 1970.
9. Rossman, K.: Image-forming quality of radiographic screen-film systems: The line spread-function. Am. J. Roentgenol., *90*:178, 1963.
10. Rossman, K.: Image quality. Contained in the syllabus of the proceedings of the AAPM 1971 Summer School. Physics of Diagnostic Radiology, Trinity University, San Antonio, July 12–17, 1971, pp. 220–281.
11. Rossman, K.: Image quality. Radiol. Clin. North Am., *7*:419, 1969.
12. Rossman, K.: Point spread-function, line spread-function and modulation transfer function. Radiology, *93*:257, 1969.
13. Rossman, K., and Lubberts, G.: Some characteristics of the line spread-function and modulation transfer function of medical radiographic films and screen-film systems. Radiology, *86*:235, 1966.
14. Rossman, K., and Sanderson, G.: Validity of the modulation transfer function of radiographic screen-film systems measured by the slit method. Phys. Med. Biol., *13*:259, 1968.
15. Seeman, H.E.: Factors which influence image quality and speed of film-screen combinations. *In* Technological Needs for Reduction of Patient Dosage from Diagnostic Radiology. Edited by M. L. Janower. Springfield, IL, Charles C Thomas, 1963.
16. Seeman, H.E.: Physical and Photographic Principles of Medical Radiography. New York, John Wiley and Sons, 1968.
17. Seeman, H.E.: Physical factors which determine roentgenographic contrast. Am. J. Roentgenol., *80*:112, 1958.
18. Strum, R.E., and Morgan, R.H.: Screen intensification systems and their limitations. Am. J. Roentgenol., *62*:617, 1949.
19. Wagner, R.F., and Denny, E.W.: A primer on physical parameters affecting radiographic image quality. Contained in the syllabus of the joint BRH-ACR conference, First Image Receptor Conference: Film/Screen Combinations, Arlington, VA, November 13–15, 1975, pp. 35–58.
20. Wagner, R.F., and Weaver, K.E.: Prospects for x-ray exposure reduction using rare earth intensifying screens. Radiology, *118*:183, 1976.
21. Wayrynen, R.E.: Personal communication.

15 *Geometry of the Radiographic Image*

We must briefly consider some geometric and trigonometric factors that influence the quality of the image of a radiograph. We will only consider examples of x rays originating at the x-ray tube and directed at the patient (or test object) and an x-ray film. We will assume that any object placed in the x-ray beam will absorb all the x-ray photons that hit the object. This is a very unlikely situation, but it makes examples easier to draw and understand. Because x rays travel in straight lines, the x-ray beam can be drawn as a straight line that hits the object or the film. The fact that x rays are emitted in all directions from the target of the x-ray tube has been previously discussed. In our examples we will assume the ideal situation, in which proper collimation has produced a beam that is perfectly cone-shaped, and the object is placed in the x-ray beam at a varying distance from the film. We will observe the beam from one side so its shape can be drawn as a triangle, with the focal spot of the x-ray tube as the apex (origin of x rays) and the object or the film as the base of the triangle (Fig. 15–1). In Figure 15–1, h represents the focal spot-object distance, and H is the focal spot-film distance. This type of diagram will allow us to consider two triangles, one with the object as its base and the other with the film as its base (Fig. 15–2). The two triangles have the same shape but are of different sizes, and are known as **similar triangles. The sides and altitudes of sim-** ilar triangles are proportional. This means that, in Figure 15–2,

$$\frac{a}{A} = \frac{b}{B} = \frac{c}{C} = \frac{h}{H}$$

The altitude of a triangle is a perpendicular dropped from a vertex to the opposite side or to an extension of the opposite side.

By using simple line drawings to represent the conditions of our idealized x-ray object-film conditions, and by applying the rule of similar triangles, it is possible to develop an understanding of the basic principles of magnification, distortion, and penumbra.

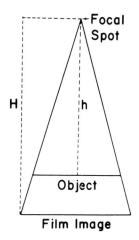

Figure 15–1 Schematic drawing of the relationship between an x-ray beam, the object being examined, and the image of the object on film

219

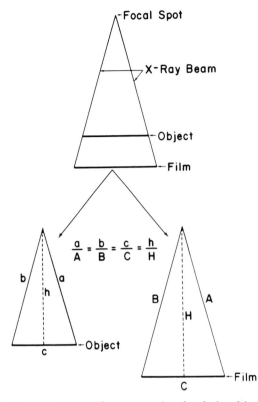

Figure 15–2 The proportional relationships of similar triangles

MAGNIFICATION

When an object is placed in the x-ray beam, it will cast a "shadow" on the film that will show some degree of enlargement. Because it is assumed that the object absorbs all the x rays that hit it, the developed film will show a clear area corresponding to the shape of the object, surrounded by blackened (exposed) film. If the object is round and flat, shaped like a coin, its magnified image will be round but larger than the coin. The image has been magnified, and the amount of magnification (M) can be defined as

$$M = \frac{\text{size of the image}}{\text{size of the object}}$$

In the clinical situation the object may be a structure or foreign body within the patient that is not available for measurement. It is usually possible to determine the x-ray

source (focal spot) to film distance and the object-film distance. The image size can be measured directly. By determining the degree of magnification, the true size of the object can be calculated. Refer to Figure 15–1, which shows a simple line drawing of an object placed some distance from the x-ray film, causing its image to be magnified by the diverging x-ray beam. The altitude of the large triangle (H) represents the distance from the focal spot of the x-ray tube to the film, often termed **focus-film distance** or **target-film distance.** The altitude of the smaller triangle (h) represents the distance from the focal spot to the object, or the **focus-object distance** or **target-object distance.** Because the sides and altitudes of similar triangles are proportional,

$$\frac{h}{H} = \frac{\text{object size}}{\text{image size}}$$

Because focus-film distance, image size, and focus-object distance can be measured directly, object size is easy to calculate. Notice that calculating simple magnification problems does not require that any formulas be learned. Consider a simple example. Using a 40-in. focus-film distance, the image of an object that is known to be 8 in. from the film measures 10 cm in length. What is the true length of the object, and how much magnification is present? Using Figure 15–1, we see that H = 40, h = 32 (40 − 8 = 32), and image size = 10 cm. Setting up the proportion:

$$\frac{40}{32} = \frac{10 \text{ cm}}{\text{object size}}$$

Solving for object size:

$$\text{Object size} = \frac{(32)\,(10)}{40} = 8 \text{ cm}$$

$$M = \frac{\text{size of the image}}{\text{size of the object}} = \frac{10}{8} = 1.25$$

What if the object is not placed directly beneath the focal spot, but is displaced to one side so that the more oblique x rays are used to form an image? If the object is flat, and remains parallel to the film, magnification will be exactly the same for the object whether central or oblique x rays are used. Consider Figure 15–3, in which the coin object is not directly beneath the x-ray tube but is still parallel to the film. The altitudes of the two triangles are exactly the same as they were when the object was directly under the focal spot (see Fig. 15–1), so the ratio of object to image size will be the same in each circumstance. In Figure 15–4 the three coins in the object plane are parallel to, and the same distance above, the film. The image of each coin will be a circle, and all the circles will be the same size.

Under usual radiographic situations, magnification should be kept to a minimum. Two rules apply: (1) **Keep the object as close to the film as possible,** and (2) **Keep the focus-film distance as large as possible.**

Consider Figure 15–1 again. Because magnification is determined by the ratio of the altitude of the two triangles, we may write

$$M = \frac{H}{h}$$

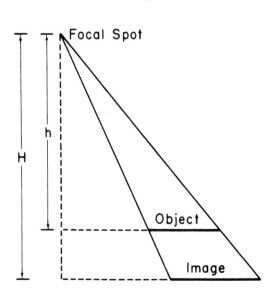

Figure 15–3 Magnification of an object by oblique rays

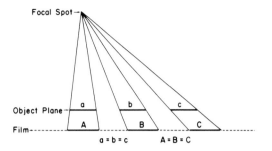

Figure 15–4 The magnification of three coins (a, b, c) all parallel to the film and the same distance above the film produces three round images (A, B, C) of equal size

If H:h = 1.0, there is no magnification. The closer the object is to the film, the closer the magnitude of altitude h will approach the value of altitude H. An increase in focus-film distance (increasing H while leaving object-film distance unchanged) will also bring the ratio H:h closer to 1. To illustrate, assume an object is 6 in. from the film. What will be the magnification if the focus-film distance is (1) 40 in., and (2) 72 in.? At 40 in. focus-film distance:

$$M = \frac{H}{h} = \frac{40}{34} = 1.18$$

At 72 in. focus-film distance:

$$M = \frac{H}{h} = \frac{72}{66} = 1.09$$

To review, magnification depends on two factors: **object-film distance** and **focus-film distance.**

DISTORTION

Distortion results from unequal magnification of different parts of the same object. Consider Figure 15–5, in which one coin (*dashed line*) is parallel to the film and the other coin (*solid line*, AB) is tilted with respect to the plane of the film. The tilted coin undergoes distortion because of unequal magnification (side A is closer to the film than side B). The image of the tilted coin will have an elliptical shape. The size and shape will vary with the amount of tilting.

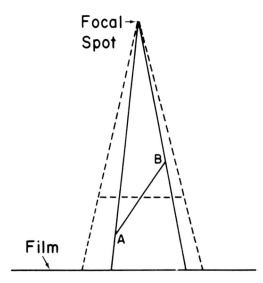

Figure 15–5   Distortion of an object (line AB) that is not parallel to the film

Distortion of the image of an object will be different in different parts of the x-ray beam. Figure 15–6 shows how distortion of the shape and size of three equally tilted coins will vary in different parts of the x-ray beam.

Distortion of thick objects occurs if they are not directly in the central part of the x-ray beam. Because different parts of thick objects are different distances from the x-ray film, each part will be magnified by a different amount. This will cause the shape of the image of most thick objects to be distorted. Only the part of a thick object that is parallel to the film will be undistorted. Figure 15–7 illustrates the relative size and shape of the image of three spheres (such as steel ball bearings) that are in different parts of the x-ray beam. The sphere that lies in the center of the beam will exhibit a round (undistorted) magnified image. The image of each of the two laterally placed spheres will be an ellipse because the x-ray beam "sees" a diameter of each of these spheres that is not parallel to the film. The x-ray beam "sees" a laterally placed spherical object in the same way it "sees" a round flat object (a coin) that is tilted with respect to the plane of the film. Notice the similarity between Figures 15–6 and 15–7.

Distortion of the relative position of the image of two objects may occur if the objects are at different distances from the film. For example, in Figure 15–8 two opaque objects, A and B, are present inside a circle. Object A is more medial than B, but A is farther from the film. The film image of object A will be lateral to the image of object B. This is because the distance between A and the midline (line a) has been magnified much more than has the distance between B and the central beam (line b). Distortion of position is minimal when the object is near the central part of the x-ray beam, and the object is placed as close to the film as possible.

PENUMBRA

Penumbra (from the Latin *pene,* meaning almost, and *umbra,* meaning shadow),

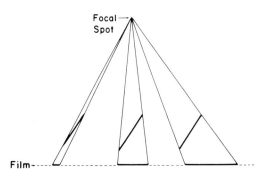

Figure 15–6   Distortion of the shape and size of the image of a tilted object depends on the position of the object in the x-ray beam

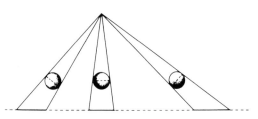

Figure 15–7   The size and shape of the image of a spherical object depends on the position of the object in relation to the central part of the x-ray beam

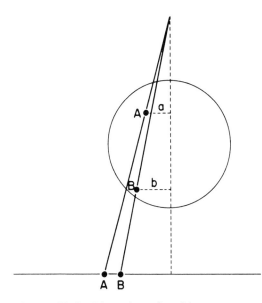

Figure 15–8 Distortion of position

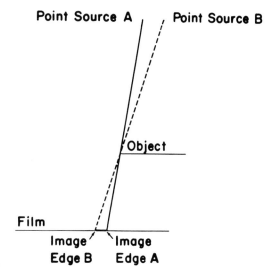

Figure 15–9 The focal spot acts as if it were composed of many point sources of x rays

often termed **edge gradient,** is defined as the region of partial illumination that surrounds the umbra, or complete shadow. In the discussion of magnification and distortion, it was assumed that the source of x rays (focal spot) was a point source. Actually, the focal spot is not a point. It has finite dimensions, usually ranging from 0.3 to 2.0 mm square. The focal spot acts as if it were composed of many point sources of x rays, with each point source forming its own image of an object. The edges of each of these images will not be in exactly the same spot on the film. Figure 15–9 shows the edge of an object formed by two x-ray sources (A and B), which represent the opposite ends of a focal spot. If A and B were the only sources of x rays, there would be two overlapping images recorded on the film. But A and B are only the opposite ends of the focal spot, a continuous line of x-ray sources. Therefore, the object edge is imaged many times between Edge B and Edge A (Fig. 15–9). The image formed by the line (focal spot) of x rays is not sharp at the edge, and varies in density. This zone of unsharpness is called **geometric unsharpness, penumbra,** or **edge gradient,** and represents the area at which the mar-

gins caused by the many "point sources" of x rays in the focal spot overlap. Figure 15–10 shows how the zone of penumbra is formed from an angled rotating anode; focal spot size has been exaggerated. The region of complete image is called the **umbra.** These terms are used in astronomy to describe a solar eclipse, in which the umbra is the area of complete shadow within which a spectator can see no portion of the sun's disc, and the penumbra is the zone of partial shadow between the umbra and the full light. Note that, as shown in Figure 15–11, the width of the penumbra is less on the anode side than on the cathode side of the x-ray tube. This effect can be used to achieve maximum sharpness by placing the object of greatest interest toward the anode side of the x-ray tube.

The width of blurring caused by penumbra can be calculated. Figure 15–11 shows the penumbra (P) caused by focal spot F (dimensions are exaggerated for illustration). Note that two similar triangles are again formed, with the apex of each triangle at the object (labeled point X), the base of the upper triangle being the width of the focal spot and the base of the lower triangle being the width of the penumbra.

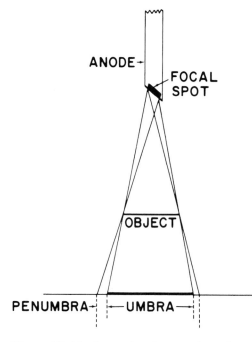

Figure 15–10   Penumbra (geometric unsharpness)

Because the sides and altitudes (H and h) of similar triangles are proportional, a simple proportion can be established between focal spot size (F), penumbra (P), focus-object distance (H), and object-film distance (h):

$$\frac{P}{F} = \frac{h}{H}$$

Using a 2-mm focal spot and a focus-film distance of 40 in., calculate the penumbra if the object is (1) 4 in. above the film and (2) 10 in. above the film. In case (1) focus-object distance (H) = 40 − 4 = 36 in.:

$$\frac{P}{2} = \frac{4}{36}$$

$$P = \frac{(4)\,(2)}{36}$$

$$P = 0.22 \text{ mm}$$

In case (2) H = 40 − 10 = 30 in.:

$$\frac{P}{2} = \frac{10}{30}$$

$$P = \frac{(2)\,(10)}{30}$$

$$P = 0.67 \text{ mm}$$

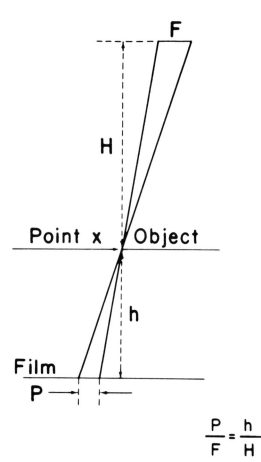

$$\frac{P}{F} = \frac{h}{H}$$

Figure 15–11   Calculation of the width of the zone of geometric unsharpness (penumbra)

In case (2), if object-film distance remains 10 in., but focus-film distance is increased to 72 in., what will be the penumbra?

$$\frac{P}{2} = \frac{10}{62}$$

$$P = \frac{(2)\,(10)}{62}$$

$$P = 0.32 \text{ mm}$$

The importance of focal spot size may be appreciated by substituting a focal spot size of 1 mm in each of the preceding examples. The width of the penumbra will be half of that caused by a 2-mm focal spot. These situations illustrate the factors that will decrease penumbra:

1. Put the object as close to the film as possible (make h small)
2. Use as large a focus-object distance as possible (make H large)
3. Use as small a focal spot as possible

Keeping the object as close to the film as possible and using a long focus-film distance also decreases magnification. The use of the magnification technique causes an increase in geometric unsharpness.

MOTION UNSHARPNESS

This term is used to describe image unsharpness caused by motion of the examined object during the exposure. Object motion will produce the same type of image unsharpness as penumbra. Object motion may be minimized by immobilizing the patient or by using a short exposure time. Similar motion unsharpness will result if the focal spot moves during the exposure. X-ray tube motion is much less important than object motion, unless considerable magnification is present. (The relationship between motion and magnification will be discussed in more detail.)

ABSORPTION UNSHARPNESS

Absorption unsharpness is caused by the way in which x rays are absorbed in the subject. This type of unsharpness arises from the gradual change in x-ray absorption across the boundary, or edge, of an object. To illustrate the meaning of absorption unsharpness, let us again assume that x rays originate from a point source (F). Figure 15–12 shows a truncated cone, cube, and sphere, which all have the same thickness and are assumed to be made of the same material. The cone will show little absorption unsharpness because its edges are parallel to the diverging beam, and its edge will be sharply defined on the film. It is apparent in Figure 15–12 that the absorption of x rays by the cube will vary along the outer edge of its upper surface, with fewer x rays being absorbed along the sides, and more in the region of the lower

Figure 15–12 The origin of absorption unsharpness

corners. With the sphere, absorption unsharpness occurs across the entire image, with maximum x-ray absorption occurring only in the center.

Absorption unsharpness produces a poorly defined margin in the image of most solid objects because there is a gradual change in film density along the image edge. The cone shows high contrast (density difference) along its edge because there is a well defined line on the film at which x-ray exposure changes from high (no absorption by the object) to low (high absorption by the object). In the case of the cube and the sphere, however, there is no abrupt change in the film exposure, only a gradual change, the magnitude of which depends on the shape of the object.

The effect of absorption unsharpness is particularly important when the accurate measurement of small round or oval structures is necessary, as in coronary angiography. Because absorption unsharpness is caused by the shape of the object being examined, it will occur no matter how exacting the conditions of generating and recording the radiographic image. Perhaps the term "subject unsharpness" would be more accurate.

INVERSE SQUARE LAW

X rays obey the physical laws of light. There is a well-known law of light propagation that states that the intensity of light falling on a flat surface from a point source is inversely proportional to the square of the distance from the point source. The principle is illustrated in Figure 15–13.

The number of x-ray photons emitted at the anode remains constant. At a distance of 1 ft, the diverging x-ray beam covers an area (A) represented by the square with each side of dimension x, or an area of $x \cdot x = x^2$. At 2 ft the diverging beam covers a square (B) in which each side is now twice as long as it was at 1 ft. The area covered by the beam at 2 ft is therefore $2x \cdot 2x = 4x^2$, which is four times the area at 1 ft. Because the intensity of the beam originating at the anode is constant, the intensity falling on square A must spread out over an area four times as large by the time it reaches square B. For example, assume that an x-ray tube has an output such that the intensity 1 ft from the tube is 144 units per square inch. At 2 ft, the 144 units are now divided between 4 square inches, or 36 units per square inch. Likewise, the intensity per square inch at 3 ft is

$$\frac{144}{3^2} = \frac{144}{9} = 16 \text{ units/in.}^2$$

and so forth. At 4 feet the intensity will be $(\frac{1}{4})^2$ or $\frac{1}{16}$ that at 1 ft.

A practical example will illustrate use of the inverse square law. Assume that an exposure of 100 mAs (100 mA for 1 sec) is needed for a film of the abdomen using a 40-in. focus-film distance. Employing portable equipment, the maximum focus-film distance that can be obtained at the bedside is 30 inches. What mAs must be used to maintain the same radiographic density as that obtained at a 40-in. distance (kVp remains constant)? Because the intensities (mAs) of the x-ray beam at 40 and 30 in. are proportional to the squares of these distances,

$$\frac{100 \text{ mAs}}{X \text{ mAs}} = \frac{40^2}{30^2} = \frac{1600}{900}$$

$$X = \frac{(100)\,(900)}{1600} = 56.25 \text{ mAs}$$

The distance from the x-ray tube to the film should be kept as large as practical to minimize the geometric unsharpness caused by penumbra. This greater distance will increase the exposure (mAs) needed to maintain proper film density. Older techniques called for a 36-in. focus-film distance but, with x-ray tubes capable of increased output, a 40-in. distance is now routine. The increased exposure required in going from 36 to 40 in. is

$$\frac{40^2}{36^2} = \frac{1600}{1296} = 1.23$$

or a 23% increase in mAs. As the output of x-ray tubes increases, techniques using up to 60-in. focus-film distance may become routine.

TRUE VERSUS GEOMETRIC MAGNIFICATION

If x rays were emitted from a point source, the magnification could indeed be determined by a simple ratio of target-film distance divided by the target-object distance. We call such a ratio the **geometric magnification (m). X rays are, in reality, emitted from an area, the focal spot.** The magnification that results with x rays from the focal spot, we call the **true magnification (M).** We would like to discuss the relation between geometric magnification (m) and true magnification (M).

Figure 15–14 illustrates magnification from a point source, in which case both magnifications are the same (m = M). If *a* represents focus-object and *b* represents object-film distance, then the equation for both true (sometimes termed "total") magnification and geometric (sometimes

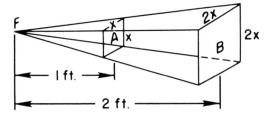

Figure 15–13   The inverse square law

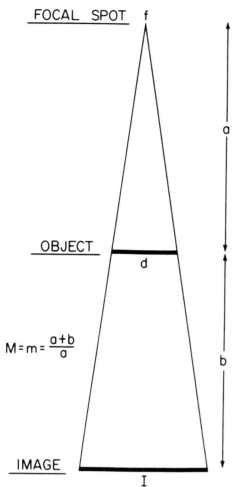

FOCAL SPOT f

OBJECT
d

$$M = m = \frac{a+b}{a}$$

IMAGE
I

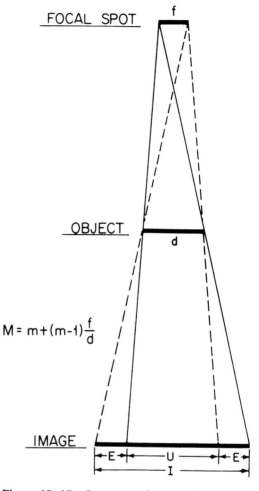

FOCAL SPOT f

OBJECT
d

$$M = m + (m-1)\frac{f}{d}$$

IMAGE
E | U | E
I

Figure 15–14 Geometry of a magnified image produced by a point source focal spot

Figure 15–15 Geometry of a magnified image produced by a focal spot with finite size

termed "nominal") magnification is the same (i.e., we are using a point source focal spot):

$$M = m = \frac{a + b}{a}$$

Unfortunately, real focal spots have a finite size. If we assume that x-ray production is of uniform intensity across the focal spot (that this is often untrue will be emphasized subsequently), and that the object is about the same size as the focal spot, the image of the object will be formed as diagrammed in Figure 15–15. Notice that the total image size (I) now contains a central region (U) and two areas of edge gradient (E).

(The term "edge gradient," rather than "penumbra," is preferred.) Derivation of the equation that must be used to calculate true magnification in this situation is an interesting exercise, but we will be content to record the equation that relates total magnification (M) to geometric magnification (m).

$$M = m + (m - 1) \left(\frac{f}{d}\right)$$

M = true magnification
m = geometric magnification

$$\left(\text{calculated from } m = \frac{a + b}{a} \right)$$

d = object size
f = focal spot size

Note that as objects become smaller than the focal spot, the term $\dfrac{f}{d}$ becomes large, and true magnification becomes much greater than geometric magnification. Conversely, if an object is large compared to focal spot size (i.e., radiography of the femur with a 1.2-mm focal spot tube), the term $\dfrac{f}{d}$ becomes small and, for practical purposes, we may conclude that M and m are identical.

To summarize, **true magnification (M) is a function of the ratio of focal spot size to object size $\left(\dfrac{f}{d}\right)$.**

An example will help in understanding this concept of true versus geometric magnification. Assume you are filming a renal angiogram using a 40-in. target-film distance and an 0.6-mm focal spot. What will be the size of the image of a 200-micron (0.2 mm) renal artery located 4 in. from the film? First we must calculate geometric magnification (m). Refer to Figure 15–16.

$$m = \frac{a + b}{a} = \frac{36 + 4}{36}$$
$$m = 1.11$$

With a punctiform focal spot image size would be 0.222 mm or 222 microns (200 × 1.11 = 222). But, because the object is small compared to the focal spot (0.2 mm vs. 0.6 mm), the term $\dfrac{f}{d}$ will be large and we must calculate how the term $(m - 1)\dfrac{f}{d}$ will affect true image size (Fig. 15–3B):

$$M = m + (m - 1)\frac{f}{d}$$
$$M = (1.11) + (1.11 - 1)\frac{0.6}{0.2}$$
$$M = 1.11 + (0.11)\,(3) = 1.44$$

Thus, true magnification is 44% versus geometric magnification of only 11%, and true image size will be 0.288 mm or 288

microns (200 × 1.44 = 288). Keep in mind that the various causes of unsharpness (i.e., screen, geometric, absorption, and motion) will make the precise boundaries of the image of our hypothetical vessel difficult to identify.

X-Ray Tube Focal Spots

Magnification radiography demands use of the smallest practical focal spot because geometric unsharpness must be reduced as much as possible. A focal spot size of 0.3 mm or less is required for magnification, but simply purchasing a standard 0.3-mm focal spot tube may not get the job done. We must examine the following:

1. What does focal spot size mean?
2. How is focal spot size measured, and how are the measurements useful?
3. How does focal spot size vary with change in tube operating conditions (mA and kVp)?

Focal Spot Size

In the United States, the National Electrical Manufacturers Association (NEMA) has established standard methods for evaluating specific aspects characterizing the focal spot.* The 1984 standards differ from previous ones. The 1984 standard specifies that the method for measuring focal spot size shall be based on use of a slit camera. A slit camera is used to measure the size of all focal spots. A slit camera is also used to measure focal spot blooming (we will discuss blooming in a few pages) and modulation transfer function (MTF). Focal spot orientation and intensity distribution are still measured with a pinhole camera. Limit of resolution is measured with a star test pattern. Six focal spot characteristics are discussed in the 1984 NEMA standard. Table 15–1 lists the characteristics and the method of measurement.

---

*NEMA Standards Publication No. XR5–1984. Measurement of Dimensions and Properties of Focal Spots of Diagnostic X-ray Tubes. National Electrical Manufacturers Association. 2101 L Street, N.W., Washington, D.C. 20037.

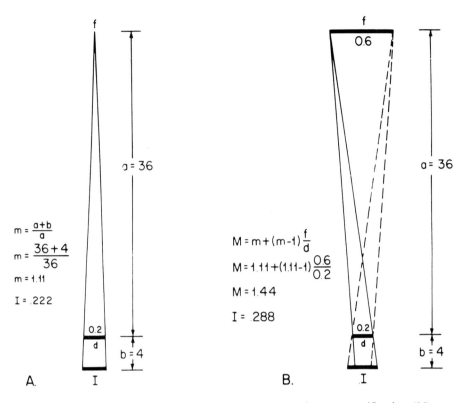

Figure 15–16   Calculation of geometric magnification *(m)* and true magnification *(M)*

Measurement. Details of construction of a slit camera need not concern us. Basically, the device consists of a .01-mm-wide slit in a piece of metal (such as tungsten) that is at least 1.5 mm thick and 5 cm long. The slit is positioned between the x-ray tube and an x-ray film (no intensifying screen), at least 100 mm from the focal spot. This produces a magnified image of the focal spot (at least 2 × magnification is required to measure a focal spot 0.4 mm to 1.0 mm in

Table 15–1.   1984 NEMA Standards of Methods for Evaluating Specific Aspects Characterizing the Focal Spot

PARAMETER	METHOD OF MEASUREMENT
Focal spot size	Slit camera
MTF	Slit camera
Blooming	Slit camera
Orientation	Pinhole
Intensity distribution	Pinhole
Limit of resolution	Star test

size). Two exposures are made. With the slit aligned with the long axis of the x-ray tube, a measure of the length of the focal spot is made. The slit is then rotated 90°, and the width of the focal spot is measured. Exposures are made at 75 kVp. Exceptions to 75 kVp exist for tubes that can not operate at 75 kVp (then use maximum kVp), and tubes that can operate at greater than 150 kVp (use 50% of the maximum kVp). The mA is the maximum mA the x-ray tube can accept for a 75-kVp, 0.1-sec exposure at the highest anode speed for which the tube is rated. Exposure time must be chosen to produce a film density of 0.8 to 1.2. Focal spot size is measured by eye, using a magnifying glass with a built-in graticule of 0.1 mm divisions and 5 × to 10 × magnification.

The NEMA standard defines the tolerance limits by which a focal spot size can vary from its stated size. The standard lists focal spots by size, starting at 0.05 mm and going to 2.0 mm in approximately 0.1-mm increments. The tolerance limit is stated, in mm, for the length and width of each focal spot size. Several examples are shown in Table 15–2. The NEMA standard lists 23 focal spot sizes. A glance at Table 15–2 indicates that a nominal 0.3-mm focal spot can actually measure 0.45 mm in width and 0.65 mm in length. When purchasing a small focal spot tube for use with exacting procedures, such as magnification radiography, one should consider specifying a true 0.3-mm (or smaller) focal spot in the contract. Expect to pay significantly more for this special consideration. For routine radiography the tolerance standards are considered acceptable.

Focal spot size measured by the slit camera is used to calculate anode heat-loading characteristics of the x-ray tube, and is the measurement (f) used in the formula to calculate true radiographic magnification (M).

The modulation transfer function of a focal spot is also determined from a slit camera image of a focal spot. A discussion of technical details of such measurements is not our purpose. Practical considerations of using focal spot MTF values will be discussed later in this chapter. Likewise, focal spot blooming will be discussed under a separate heading.

Pinhole Camera. The pinhole technique measures the intensity distribution of radiation from the focal spot. The pinhole consists of a small hole in a sheet of metal (such as tungsten or tantalum). The pinhole assembly is placed between the x-ray

tube and a sheet (no intensifying screens) of x-ray film, and an exposure is made that produces a density of 0.8 to 1.2 on the film (Fig. 15–17). If the pinhole is placed exactly halfway between the focal spot and film, as in Figure 15–17, the image of the focal spot will be the same size as the actual physical dimensions of the focal spot. However, an enlargement factor of 2 is specified for all focal spots less than 2.5 mm. This enlargement may be accomplished by making the pinhole-film distance twice the pinhole-focal spot distance. The pinhole technique will also demonstrate orientation of the focal spot.

Figure 15–18 is a photographically mag-

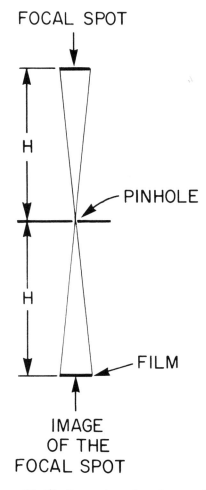

FOCAL SPOT

H

PINHOLE

H

FILM

IMAGE
OF THE
FOCAL SPOT

Figure 15–17 Formation of an image of the focal spot by a pinhole camera

Table 15–2. NEMA Tolerance Limits for Focal Spot Variation Using the Slit Camera Method

NOMINAL FOCAL SPOT DESIGNATION IN mm	MAXIMUM FOCAL SPOT DIMENSIONS IN mm	
	WIDTH	LENGTH
0.3	0.45	0.65
0.6	0.90	1.3
1.0	1.4	2.0
1.2	1.7	2.4

Figure 15–18   Pinhole image of a focal spot with edge band distribution

nified pinhole image of a focal spot showing that x-ray intensity is much greater along the edges of a focal spot than in its central area. This is termed **edge-band distribution,** and, although it is the most common type of intensity distribution, it is the least desirable. There are several problems with the pinhole technique of measuring focal spots:

1. The size of the pinhole must be small with respect to the size of the focal spot. Recommended pinhole diameters are 0.03 mm for focal spots below 1.2 mm and 0.075 mm for focal spots from 1.2 to 2.5 mm

   The 0.03-mm pinhole transmits so little radiation that producing a film image of the focal spot requires multiple exposures.

2. It is important to align the pinhole to the central beam of the x-ray tube accurately. This location is difficult to determine. Similar difficulties are encountered with the slit camera.

Limit of Resolution. A star pattern is used to determine the limit of resolution of a focal spot. Figure 15–19 shows a photograph of a star pattern. This pattern consists of a circular sheet of lead .03 to .05 mm thick, with a diameter of 45 mm, divided into 180 spokes, of which 90 are lead and 90 are blank. Each spoke subtends an angle of 2°. A star test pattern can be viewed as consisting of many line-pair test patterns, with each diameter of the star corresponding to a line pair of a different size. To determine focal spot resolution, the star test pattern is positioned about midway between the focal spot and film (do not use screens), exactly parallel to the film, and in the central axis of the x-ray beam. Figure 15–20 is a diagram of this technique, and Figure 15–21 is a picture of an actual star test pattern. As one moves toward the center of the image, an area is encountered at which the image of the rays of the star gradually disappears (D, Fig. 15–20). This is termed the "area of failure of resolution." The diameter (D) of the blurred image is measured both parallel and perpendicular to the cathode-anode axis of the tube. It must be noted that D is measured perpendicularly to the desired dimension of the focal spot (in Fig. 15–20 one would measure D for the cathode-anode axis of the focal spot in the dimension perpendic-

Figure 15–19 Photograph of a star resolution pattern. Notice inability of the camera lens to record the inner spokes

ular to the cathode-anode alignment of the tube when the exposure was made).

Resolution of the focal spot is a function of the distance D, the true magnification factor (m), and the angle subtended by each spoke in the star pattern measured in radians (2° = .035 radians). The formula is:

$$R \text{ (lp/mm)} = \frac{M}{D\,\Theta}$$

R = resolution lp/mm
M = magnification (true)
D = diameter of the blurred image of the star phantom parallel or perpendicular to the tube axis (cathode-anode axis)
Θ = angle of one of the lead spokes (radians)

M is easily measured. The diameter of the star pattern is always known (the one illustrated has a diameter of 45 mm) and the diameter of the image of the pattern is quickly measured. Magnification is calculated:

$$M = \frac{\text{image size}}{\text{object size}}$$

Note in Figure 15–20 that continuing inward from the region of failure of resolution the image of the test pattern reappears, but the light and dark lines will have shifted 180° in their alignment (called a phase shift). This is the area of spurious resolution that results from focal spots with edge band intensity distribution, and corresponds to spatial frequencies where the modulation transfer function (MTF) of the focal spot is negative. Milne has described this phenomenon in detail, so we will not further consider phase shift and spurious resolution.[10] Focal spot measurements with a star phantom depend on two characteristics of the focal spot:

1. focal spot size
2. radiation intensity distribution within the focal spot

This technique measures the resolving capacity of the focal spot, which is a function of both size and radiation intensity distribution.

The effect of the intensity distribution of a focal spot has been discussed by Milne.[9]

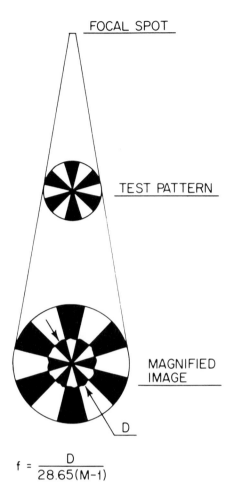

FOCAL SPOT

TEST PATTERN

MAGNIFIED
IMAGE

D

$$f = \frac{D}{28.65(M-1)}$$

Figure 15–20 Using a star resolution pattern to determine focal spot size (not drawn with correct perspective)

There are three types of intensity distribution encountered in focal spots:

1. Edge band distribution (Fig. 15–18)
2. Homogeneous distribution, in which radiation intensity is uniform throughout the focal spot
3. Centrally peaked distribution, in which radiation intensity is peaked in the central portion of the focal spot and tapers toward the margin (i.e., the "opposite" of the edge band distribution), also termed "Gaussian distribution"

The type of intensity distribution has an important influence on the resolving capacity of a focal spot. The focal spot with the best resolving power has a peaked intensity distribution, next best is homogeneous, and worst is edge band distribution.

Let us digress a moment to emphasize that the star pattern gives information about resolving power, which is the ability of the focal spot to record separate images of small objects placed closed together (i.e., a series of 100-μ interlobular vessels in the renal cortex). The ability of the focal spot to image a single, isolated 100-μ vessel is determined by the physical size of the focal spot (slit camera size), although the intensity distribution will influence the shape of the edge gradient (i.e., how sharp the edge of the vessel will appear). If one wishes to calculate true magnification (M) of a small object, the focal spot size (f) used in the equation must be that determined by the slit camera. If one wishes to determine the resolving power of a particular focal spot, the resolution determined from a star pattern is used.

Variation of Focal Spot Size with Changes in Tube Operating Conditions (Focal Spot Blooming). Two articles by Chaney and Hendee have nicely documented the fact that focal spot size varies with tube operating conditions.[5,7]

Focal spot size increases in direct proportion to tube current. This is called **blooming** of the focal spot, and is much more marked at low kVp and high mAs techniques. Weaver has reported the effect of the current on focal spot bloom at 40 and 80 kVp to be as shown in Table 15–3.[14] Focal spot bloom is much more marked parallel to the tube axis. Focal spot bloom perpendicular to the cathode-anode tube axis depends on the accuracy of the focusing of the electron beam; measurements with a star pattern show wide variation between identical models of tubes.

Focal spot size will decrease slightly with increasing kVp. As measured by Chaney and Hendee, this change was approximately proportional to $\frac{1}{f_0 V^{3/2}}$, where $f_0 =$

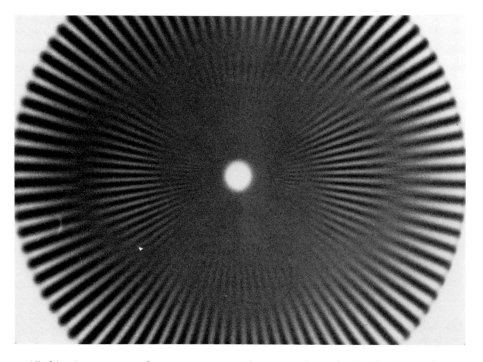

Figure 15–21   Appearance of a star test pattern image used to calculate focal spot size

focal spot size for a low tube mA and V = tube kVp.[5] Weaver has illustrated decreasing focal spot size with increasing kVp, as shown in Table 15–4.[14] There is no industry standard for focal spot blooming. Because blooming will vary significantly between supposedly identical tubes, the acceptable amount of focal spot blooming may have to be specified when purchasing a tube to be used for magnification radiography. As an alternate approach, the tube mA and kVp that must be used to produce a star pattern equivalent to a 0.3-mm focal spot in both parallel and perpendicular dimensions relative to the tube axis may have to be specified.

Off-Axis Variation. Focal spot measurements must be made in the central part of the x-ray beam. As one moves away from the central ray, the apparent size of the focal spot will change. **The projected focal spot length is much shorter in the heel (anode side) of the beam than at the cathode side.** Figure 15–22 illustrates the marked variation in focal spot length as one moves from the beam center to 10° toward the anode and 10° toward the cathode on the cathode-anode tube axis. Focal spot changes are less significant in the cross-axis direction, where focal spot shape may become more diamond-shaped but the width and length remain almost constant.

Table 15–3. Measured Sizes of a Typical Focal Spot at Various Exposure Factors

TUBE (kVp)	TUBE (mA)	FOCAL SPOT SIZE
40 kVp	100 mA	2.0 mm
40	300	2.3
80	100	1.7
80	300	1.8

Table 15–4. Measured Size of a Typical Focal Spot at Various kVp Settings, mAs Constant

TUBE (kVp)	TUBE (mA)	FOCAL SPOT SIZE
40 kVp	100 mA	2.0 mm
60	100	1.8
80	100	1.7
150	100	1.7

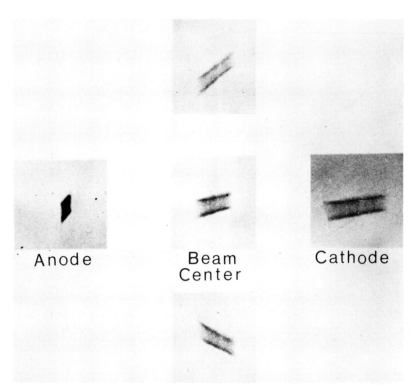

Figure 15–22 Pinhole images showing variation of focal spot size and shape at various positions in the x-ray beam

Let us conclude this short review of focal spots by emphasizing what is now an obvious fact: the radiologist who hopes to make successful use of magnification radiography must use great care in selecting an appropriate x-ray tube.

QUANTITATIVE EVALUATION OF RESOLUTION

With magnification techniques it is necessary to combine the most appropriate film-screen combination with the correct focal spot, and then to determine which amount of magnification is optimum. The serious problem of object motion must also be considered. In this respect, it is useful to study the resolution properties of the components of the entire radiographic system with the aid of the modulation transfer function (MTF) of the individual and combined components. To review briefly, an MTF is a curve that describes the ability of

an imaging system, or any part of the system, to reproduce (or record) information. An MTF of 1.0 is perfect, indicating that the system can record all the information it has received. An MTF of 0 indicates that none of the information has been reproduced. We shall use the MTF curves to compare various system components. Precise data about how the curves are derived and detailed analyses will not be considered, but these are available in the literature.[11,12]

Figure 15–23 depicts the MTF curves of three imaginary x-ray tube focal spots up to an object frequency of 10 line pairs per mm. Focal spot 1 images perfectly (MTF = 1) at all frequencies. Focal spot 2 is not nearly as good, with its MTF dropping to 0.5 at 5 line pairs per mm, and focal spot 3 is lousy, with an MTF of 0 at 6 line pairs/ mm. Obviously, one need not know much about MTF curves to be able to glance at

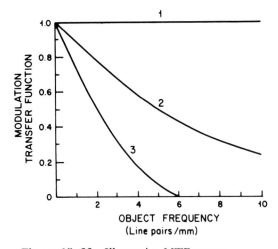

Figure 15–23　Illustrative MTF curves

Figure 15–23 and determine that curve 1 is the best, 2 is next best, and 3 is the worst. We will use the following MTF curves to make quick graphic comparisons.

There is one additional use we must make of the MTF. If one knows the MTF of each of several components of an imaging system (i.e., film, intensifying screen and focal spot), the MTF of the entire system is calculated by multiplying the MTF of each component. We will now briefly consider the MTF of

　　　Film
　　　Focal spots
　　　High-speed intensifying screens
　　　Object motion

and show how magnification influences the MTF of film, focal spots, and screens.

Film

The ability of x-ray film to image objects with a frequency of 10 to 20 line pairs per mm is so good that we may consider film to have an MTF of 1.0 for all clinical applications of magnification radiography.

Focal Spots

We will assume focal spots of uniform intensity distribution. Figure 15–24A is a set of calculated MTF curves of a 0.3-mm focal spot for magnification factors of 1.0

(contact radiography, not possible clinically), 1.2, and 2.0. **Notice how rapidly the MTF deteriorates as the magnification factor increases,** even in the case of this small focal spot. Figure 15–24B shows similar data for a 1.0-mm focal spot, emphasizing that the larger the focal spot the more drastic the deterioration of MTF produced by magnification. **Focal spot MTF is adversely affected by magnification.**

Intensifying Screens

We will consider only high-speed screens, because they are the ones usually employed for magnification angiography. Figure 15–25 diagrams the approximate MTF curves of the Du Pont Quanta II (barium fluorochloride) screens at magnifications of 1.0, 1.2, and 2.0. (Quanta II screens are no longer made, but the illustrated principle remains valid.) It is clear from Figure 15–25 that **screen MTF improves with magnification.** In fact, the worse the MTF curve of the screen, the more improvement one sees with magnification, which is fortunate because we are usually using high-speed screens in clinical situations in which magnification is attempted. It is quite easy to understand why screen MTF improves with magnification when one considers what magnification does to the frequency (line pairs per mm) of information in the image presented to the intensifying screen. Assume that a test object has a frequency of 4 line pairs/mm (Fig. 15–26). When the object is magnified by a factor of 2, the 4 line pairs are presented to the intensifying screens over an area of 2 mm, thus reducing the frequency of the image presented to the screen to 2 line pairs per mm. The frequency of the image is less than the frequency of the object, and is calculated by dividing object frequency by the magnification factor. For example, assume a test object has 6 line pairs per mm. When the object is magnified by a factor of 1.5, the 6 lines will cover 1.5 mm at the level of the intensifying screens,

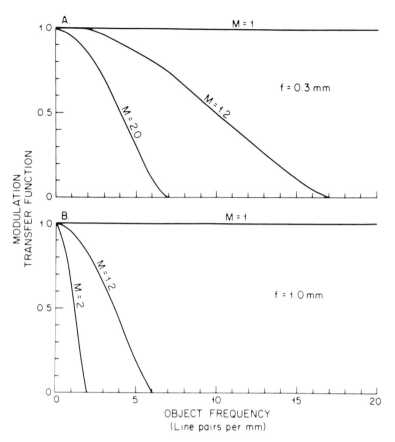

Figure 15–24 Calculated MTF curves for a 0.3-mm (A), and 1.0-mm (B) focal spot (f) at magnifications of 1, 1.2, and 2

corresponding to an image frequency of $\frac{6}{1.5}$, or 4 line pairs per mm. Similarly, at a magnification factor of 2, the object frequency of 6 line pairs/mm is reduced to an image frequency of 3 line pairs per mm. Because magnification reduces the frequency (i.e., line pairs per mm) of information that must be resolved by the intensifying screen, the screen is able to do a better job.

Focal Spot and Screens

Because focal spot MTF gets worse with magnification, and screen MTF improves, what degree of magnification is best when only focal spot and screen are considered (assume film MTF of 1.0 in all situations)? Under these conditions (no object motion),

the best resolution (MTF) is obtained by using detail screens and as little magnification as possible. In the clinical situation object motion must be considered, and this changes all the answers.

Object Motion

The amount of unsharpness caused by motion of an object is independent of the amount of magnification. Motion unsharpness depends only on

Velocity of motion
Exposure time

Velocity (v) is expressed in mm per second, and exposure time (t) is expressed in seconds. The product vt can be used to determine the MTF caused by object motion. For example, if an object is moving at a

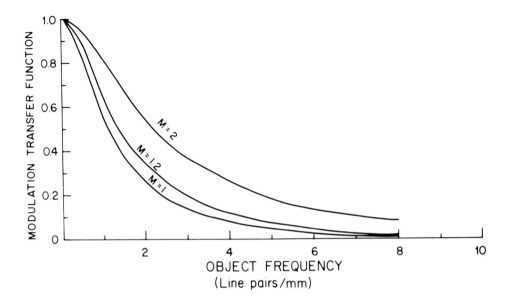

Figure 15–25 Approximate MTF curve of a Quanta II intensifying screen at magnifications of 1.0, 1.2, and 2.0. (Courtesy of E.I. du Pont de Nemours and Company, Inc.)

rate of 10 mm per second (such as a pulmonary artery), and an exposure time of 0.025 sec is used, the product vt will be 10 × 0.025 = 0.25. Assume an object frequency of 2 line pairs/mm (i.e., an opacified pulmonary artery 0.250 mm in diameter, giving two arteries and two spaces of 0.250 mm each per 1 mm). Table 15–5 shows that the MTF caused by motion will be 0.64. Table 15–5 lists the MTF caused by object motion for an object frequency of 2, 3, 5,

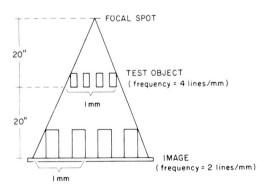

Figure 15–26 Resolution demanded at the level of the screen decreases as magnification increases

8, and 10 line pairs per mm at vt values of 0.1, 0.25, 0.5, and 1.0. The equation used to calculate these MTF values is terrifying, but is available to those able to deal with such matters.[12] From Table 15–5 it can be appreciated that knowledge of object motion is required if the optimal exposure factors in the case of moving objects are to be evaluated seriously.

As a general rule, if it is determined that the product of object motion (v) and exposure time (t) is less than 0.1, motion unsharpness will be minimal. If the value of vt is large (1.0 or greater), motion unsharpness becomes the dominant factor in total imaging system MTF. One will sacrifice any other component of the imaging system to make the exposure time shorter (i.e., use the fastest available film and screen regardless of quantum mottle and screen unsharpness). If the product of vt is greater than 0.1 but less than 0.5, a compromise is usually best: use a fast (but not the fastest) film-screen system, which will keep quantum mottle and screen unsharpness as favorable as possible and still allow reasonably short exposure times. Because

Table 15–5. Calculated MTF Caused by Object Motion

OBJECT MOTION (vt) (mm)	MOTION MTF (line pairs/mm)				
	2	3	5	8	10
0.1	0.94	0.85	0.64	0.24	0
0.25	0.64	0.30	0	0	0
0.5	0	0	0	0	0
1.0	0	0	0	0	0

magnification is useful when fast screen-film systems are used, the MTF of angiographic studies of moving vessels can usually be improved with magnification if the focal spot is of the correct size and shape. For example, consider an abdominal angiogram in which vessel motion is about 3 mm per second. Assume one uses Quanta II screens (Fig. 15–25), a 0.3-mm focal spot with uniform intensity distribution (Fig. 15–24A) and an exposure time of 0.033 seconds (vt = 3 × 0.033 = 0.1). At an information content of 4 line pairs per mm (i.e., blood vessels 0.125 mm in diameter), will system MTF be better at a magnification factor of 1.0, 1.2, 1.5, 2.0, or 3.0? The appropriate calculations are shown in Table 15–6, which shows system MTF to be best at a magnification factor of 2. Although calculation of MTF values does not tell the entire story of useful information content of the radiographic image, it does provide us with a means of beginning an objective analysis of a complex subjective problem (for example, this treatment neglects system noise, or quantum mottle).

HOW MUCH MAGNIFICATION IS BEST?

With a 0.3-mm focal spot there is a rather narrow range of magnification that will re-sult in improvement in resolution. No significant improvement greater than a magnification of about 2 is possible, so 2 × magnification is the upper limit with a 0.3-mm focal spot. This amount of magnification is calculated for structures inside the body, so magnification as calculated from the skin surface of the body nearest the tube will be about 1.6 to 1.8. Because the correct magnification factor will vary between tubes (i.e., focal spots are not the same), Milne has suggested that some experiments should be performed before clinical work is done.[8] For example, place a resolving power target in an appropriate phantom and then make a series of exposures at different degrees of magnification, using the same mA as will be used with patients. The degree of magnification that gives the best resolution is then determined. With small focal spots, information content will increase over much higher ranges of magnification (up to 8.0 × with a 0.1-mm focal spot).

QUANTUM MOTTLE

Quantum mottle is statistical fluctuation in the number of x-ray photons used by the imaging system to form the image. With magnification radiography, the num-

Table 15–6. Sample Calculations of MTF Values of Various Components of a Magnification Radiographic System*

MAGNIFICATION	SCREEN MTF	FOCAL SPOT MTF	MOTION MTF	TOTAL SYSTEM MTF
1.0	0.08	1.0	0.76	0.06
1.2	0.12	0.91	0.76	0.08
1.5	0.16	0.76	0.76	0.09
2.0	0.27	0.51	0.76	0.10
3.0	0.44	0.24	0.76	0.08

*Focal spot size: 0.3 × 0.3 mm; object motion: 3 mm/sec; exposure time: 0.033 sec; image frequency: 4 line pairs/mm; very fast screens: Du Pont Quanta II.

ber of x-ray photons per square millimeter required to produce the image is the same (if film density is the same) for any degree of magnification. That is, **quantum mottle does not change with radiographic magnification.** If a radiograph is photographically enlarged there is a change in quantum mottle. If 40,000 photons per mm² were used to form the radiographic image, photographic magnification of 2× will increase the area from 1 to 4 mm² and reduce the number of x-ray photons to 10,000 per mm². Thus, photographic enlargement increases quantum mottle in the magnified image by a factor of $\dfrac{N}{m^2}$, in which

N = number of photons used
m = magnification

How does quantum mottle (noise) affect the radiographic image? Quantum mottle influences the perception of low-contrast objects with poorly defined borders. By comparison, system MTF largely defines the ability to record small objects with sharp borders and high contrast. Therefore, radiographic magnification (as opposed to photographic or optical magnification) may improve visualization of low-contrast images because it does not increase noise.

PATIENT EXPOSURE

If 2× magnification radiography requires that the patient's body surface be twice as close to the x-ray tube as in non-magnification radiography, one would conclude that exposure to the skin would be increased by a factor of 2², or 4 (inverse square law). This is incorrect for the following reasons.

First, in routine radiography there is always some amount of magnification, usually by about 1.1 to 1.2 at the skin on the tube side of the body. The inverse square law calculated with these values shows skin exposure to increase by

$$\frac{2^2}{1.1^2} = 3.31, \text{ or } \frac{2^2}{1.2^2} = 2.78$$

Second, with magnification radiography a smaller portion of the body is exposed to x rays because a smaller body area now covers the film. With magnification only relatively small anatomic areas can be recorded. Because of the limited area that can be encompassed, careful collimation of the x-ray beam and accurate alignment of the part being examined with the central beam are mandatory. This improves image quality and decreases patient exposure.

Third, with magnification, high-speed or ultrahigh-speed screens are used, and a grid is not needed.

Because of these considerations, the increase in patient exposure with magnification is less than that anticipated by application of the inverse square law, and in some cases there might even be no increase or an actual decrease in skin exposure.

SUMMARY

Geometric factors that influence the quality of the radiographic image include magnification, distortion, penumbra, and motion. Absorption unsharpness produces a similar effect. Factors that will decrease unsharpness caused by

MAGNIFICATION
1. small object-film distance
2. large focal spot-film distance

PENUMBRA
1. small focal-spot size
2. small object-film distance
3. large focal spot-film distance

MOTION
1. short exposure time
2. maximum possible limitation of actual object motion

To minimize distortion, the object of interest should be kept parallel to the film and near the central portion of the x-ray beam, and magnification should be minimized.

The intensity of the x-ray beam varies inversely as the square of the distance from the x-ray tube.

Because x rays do not originate from a point source, calculations dealing with magnification of objects that are small compared to the size of the focal spot require an understanding of the relationship between geometric magnification (m) and true magnification (M). True magnification is a function of the ratio between focal spot size and object size $\left(\dfrac{f}{d}\right)$.

Specifications and measurements of focal spot size raise many issues. Industry standards define acceptable tolerance limits in focal spot size. Focal spot size varies with tube operating conditions, with the most significant variation being blooming with high mA/low-kVp techniques. The intensity distribution of radiation from the focal spot is important in determining the resolving power of the focal spot. The slit camera technique measures the physical size of the focal spot, and this measurement is used to calculate heat loading of the tube and magnification of small objects. Resolution chart (star pattern) measurements do not measure the physical size of a focal spot, but indicate the resolving power of the focal spot.

The resolution characteristics of magnification radiography may be studied in terms of the MTF of the various components of the imaging system. Film MTF is considered to be 1.0. Intensifying screen MTF improves with magnification, whereas focal spot MTF deteriorates rapidly with magnification. Magnification represents a compromise wherein deterioration of focal spot MTF and improvement in screen MTF combine to produce maximum MTF of the entire imaging system. Magnification offers advantages when high-speed screens are used and object motion is present. The amount of unsharpness caused by object motion is unrelated to magnification, and depends on the velocity of motion and the exposure time.

The optimum magnification for any system must be determined experimentally; with a 0.3-mm focal spot this will vary from about 1.6 to 2.0. Quantum mottle (noise) is not increased with radiographic magnification. Patient skin dose is usually increased with magnification, but the increase is less than the inverse square law would indicate.

REFERENCES

1. Bergeron, R.T.: Manufacturers' designation of diagnostic x-ray tube focal spot size: A time for candor. Radiology, *3*:487, 1974.
2. Bernstein, H., Bergeron, R.T., and Klein, D.J.: Routine evaluation of focal spots. Radiology, *3*:421, 1974.
3. Bernstein, F.: Specifications of focal spots and factors affecting their size. SPIE, *56*:159, 1975.
4. Bull, K.W.: The effects of the x-ray focal spot on primary beam magnification of small vessels. Master's thesis, the University of Texas Health Science Center at Dallas, May 1973.
5. Chaney, E.L., and Hendee, W.R.: Effects of x-ray tube current and voltage on effective focal-spot size. Med. Phys., *1*:141, 1974.
6. Dunisch, O., Pfeiler, M., and Kuhn, H.: Problems and aspects of the radiological magnification technique. Siemens Electro Medica, *3*:114, 1971.
7. Hendee, W.R., and Chaney, E.L.: X-ray focal spots: Practical considerations. Appl. Radiol., *3*:25, 1974.
8. Milne, E.N.C.: Magnification radiography. Appl. Radiol. Nucl. Med., *5*:12, 1976.
9. Milne, E.N.C.: Characterizing focal spot performance. Radiology, *3*:483, 1974.
10. Milne, E.N.C.: The role and performance of minute focal spots in roentgenology with special reference to magnification. CRC Crit. Rev. Radiol. Sci., *2*:269, 1971.
11. Rao, G.U.V., Clark, R.L., and Gayler, B.W.: Radiographic magnification: A critical, theoretical and practical analysis. Part I. Appl. Radiol., *1*:37, 1973.
12. Rao, G.U.V., Clark, R.L., and Gayler, B.W.: Radiographic magnification: A critical, theoretical and practical analysis. Part II. Appl. Radiol., *2*:25, 1973.
13. Spiegler, P., and Breckindidge, W.C.: Imaging of focal spots by means of the star test pattern. Radiology, *102*:679, 1972.
14. Weaver, K.E.: X-ray tube focal spots. Contained in the Syllabus of the AAPM 1975 Summer School, The Expanding Role of the Diagnostic Radiologic Physicist. Rice University, Houston, July 27–August 1, 1975.

16 *Body Section Radiography*

Body section radiography is a special x-ray technique that blurs out the shadows of superimposed structures to show more clearly the principal structures being examined. We must point out immediately that it is not a method of improving the sharpness of any part of a radiographic image. On the contrary, it is a process of controlled blurring that merely leaves some parts of the image less blurred than others. Various names have been used to describe body section radiography. Most were initially applied to a specifically designed unit. Over the years considerable confusion has developed over nomenclature. In 1962 the International Commission on Radiologic Units and Measurements adopted the term **tomography** to describe all types of body section techniques,[3] and we will use this term synonymously with body section radiography. Some commonly used names are

1. tomography (tomogram) preferred
2. planigraphy (planigram)
3. stratigraphy (stratigram)
4. laminography (laminogram)

BASIC METHOD OF TOMOGRAPHY

Many ingenious tomographic methods have been devised. We will begin by describing the simplest (Fig. 16–1A). The essential ingredients are an x-ray tube, an x-ray film, and a rigid connecting rod that rotates about a fixed fulcrum. When the tube moves in one direction, the film moves

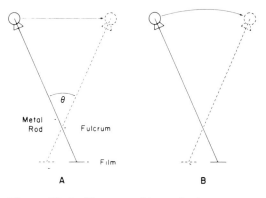

Figure 16–1 Tomographic method

in the opposite direction. The film is placed in a tray under the x-ray table so that it is free to move without disturbing the patient. The fulcrum is the only point in the system that remains stationary. The amplitude of tube travel is measured in degrees, and is called the tomographic angle (arc). The plane of interest within the patient is positioned at the level of the fulcrum, and it is the only plane that remains in sharp focus. All points above and below this plane are blurred.

A second type of tube motion is illustrated in Figure 16–1B. Both the x-ray tube and film move along an arc instead of in a straight line as they did in Figure 16–1A. Both methods give similar results. The primary advantage of a straight line motion is that it can be easily adapted to a standard x-ray table and requires no expensive equipment. It has more moving parts, however, including slip joints at both ends of

242

the connecting rod, which eventually wear and get out of adjustment. A tomographic system that moves the tube and film in an arc has fewer moving parts and is less likely to get out of adjustment, but it requires a special table and tube stand built specifically for tomography, so it is more expensive.

All points that are parallel to the x-ray film and on the same plane as the fulcrum are displayed in sharp focus on the tomogram. A whole plane is in focus, not just a point. In Figure 16–2, points A, B, and C are several centimeters apart on the same plane and their images all move exactly the same distance as the x-ray film; therefore, they are not blurred. When the tube moves to the left, the distance from point C to its image on the film is greater than the comparable distance of points B and A. The ratio of the object-tube and object-film distance for all three points is the same, and there is no difference in magnification of objects on the same plane.

Tomographic techniques blur all points that are outside (above or below) the focal plane. In Figure 16–3, point A is above and point C below the focal plane. As the x-ray tube moves, only the image of point B, which is on the focal plane, remains in sharp focus, because it is the only image that moves exactly the same distance as the film. The image of point A moves more than the film, and the image of point C less than the film, so both are blurred. The further an object is from the plane of the fulcrum, the more its image is blurred.

Types of Tube Motion

If we look down from the ceiling at the system we have just described, the x-ray tube and film move in a straight line. Appropriately, this is referred to as "linear tomography." Many other types of tube motion have been devised. Most of them circumscribe some sort of arc (not to be confused with the arc shown in Figure 16–1B, which is a side view). The six basic types of tube motion in common usage are

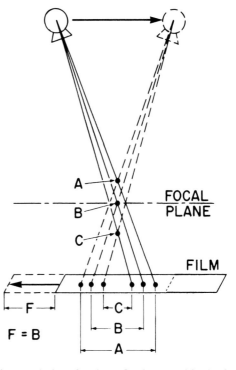

Figure 16–3 Blurring of points outside the focal plane

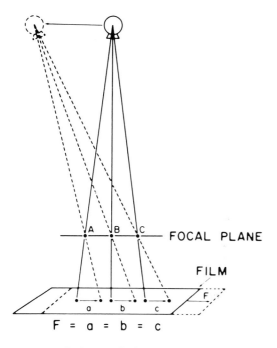

Figure 16–2 Focal plane

shown in Figure 16–4. Remember that these are patterns of tube and film motion as seen from above.

TERMINOLOGY

Before going further with our discussion of tomography, it will be helpful to define a few of the terms we have used. **Blurring** is the distortion of definition of objects outside the focal plane. The **fulcrum** is the pivot point about which the lever arm rotates. It determines the plane that will be in focus. Two mechanically different types of fulcrums are in common use. In the first, the relationship between the x-ray tube, fulcrum, and film is fixed. The patient is moved up and down on an adjustable table to bring the level of interest to the plane of the fulcrum. The second type has an adjustable fulcrum that is moved to the height of the desired plane, while the patient remains stationary on the table. The **focal plane** is the plane of maximal focus, and represents the axis (fulcrum) about which the x-ray tube and film rotate. The **focal plane level** is the height of the focal plane above the tabletop. The **tomographic angle** (arc) is the amplitude of tube travel expressed in degrees (Fig. 16–1*A*). The **exposure angle** is the angle through which the x-ray beam (or central ray) moves during the exposure. The tomographic angle and exposure angle are not always equal. Occasionally, x rays are not emitted during part of the tube travel, in which case the tomographic angle is greater than the exposure angle. Sometimes this is intentional, but usually it is the result of an equipment malfunction.

BLURRING

The whole purpose of tomography is to distort, or blur, the objects that might interfere with our perception of a particular radiographic image. To use our equipment to best advantage, we must understand the factors that control blurring. In tomography, the term "blurring" is used only with reference to objects outside the focal plane, and the same term should not be used to describe the image unsharpness inherent in all tomographic systems.

Width of the Blur

The width of the blur refers to the distance over which the image of an object is spread out on the film. It is determined by four factors:

1. amplitude of tube travel
2. distance from the focal plane
3. distance from the film
4. orientation of tube travel

Each of these will be discussed separately.

Amplitude of Tube Travel. The width of the blur is a direct linear function of the number of degrees of tube travel. As the amplitude of tube travel increases, the width of the blur increases. When the number of degrees of tube motion is doubled, the amount of blurring doubles.

Distance from Focal Plane. The farther an object is from the focal plane, the more it is blurred. Unfortunately, we have no control over this distance in diagnostic radiology. The relationships between anatomic parts and pathologic lesions are fixed in the patient, and we cannot change them.

Distance from Film. Objects far away from the film are blurred more than objects close to the film (assuming they are both the same distance from the focal plane). The patient should be positioned so that

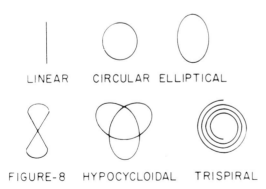

LINEAR   CIRCULAR ELLIPTICAL

FIGURE-8 HYPOCYCLOIDAL TRISPIRAL

Figure 16–4 Types of tomographic motions

the objects we want to blur are as far from the film as possible.

Orientation of Tube Travel. Many body parts are long and narrow and have a longitudinal axis. When the longitudinal axis of an object is oriented in the same direction that the x-ray tube travels, the image of the object is not blurred, even though it lies outside of the focal plane. Figure 16–5 shows a conventional radiograph (Fig. 16–5A) and a linear tomographic film (Fig. 16–5B) taken on a phantom consisting of multiple crossed and curved wires. The wires are located 1 cm below the focal plane on the tomogram. As you can see, the image of one of the wires is not blurred, and the unblurred wire is the one oriented in the direction of x-ray tube motion. Increasing the tomographic arc will not blur this wire but will merely elongate its image. Maximum blurring occurs when the long axis of the part to be blurred is perpendicular to the direction of tube travel.

Blur Margin

The edge of a blurred image is called the "blur margin." Figure 16–6 shows linear (Fig. 16–6A) and circular (Fig. 16–6B) tomograms of the same test phantom shown in Figure 16–5. As you can see, the blur

Figure 16–6 Character of blur margins for linear and circular tomography. (Courtesy of Dr. J.T. Littleton)

margins are different with these two types of tube motions. With linear tomography the entire image is uniformly blurred and fades off gradually at its edge. With a circular tube motion, however, the blurred image is not uniform. The margin appears whiter and more sharply defined on the film than the rest of the blur pattern. The reason for the sharply defined border is shown in Figure 16–7. The tube moves

Figure 16–5 Blur patterns with linear tomography. (Courtesy of Dr. J.T. Littleton)

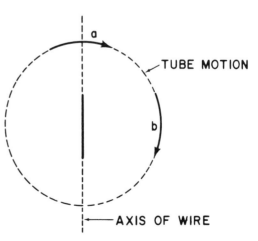

Figure 16–7 Circular tomographic motion superimposed on test wire (*top view*)

both across and parallel to the axis of the wire during different portions of its travel. Maximum blurring occurs as the tube moves across the axis of the wire (a), and this portion of the exposure produces the center of the blur pattern. Little blurring occurs while the tube is moving parallel to the wire's axis (b), and it is during this portion of the exposure that the incompletely blurred image is projected to the edge of the blur pattern. This sharply defined blur margin is important in phantom image formation, which we will discuss later in the chapter.

SECTION THICKNESS

There is no accurate way of defining section thickness. It means the thickness of the section that is in sharp focus on a tomogram. In theory, the focal plane is indeed a "plane" and has no thickness. The image that we see is actually made up of many thin planes superimposed on one another. The closer these planes are to the true focal plane, the sharper they are in focus. There is no abrupt cutoff in sharpness, just a gradual progressive deterioration of image quality as we move away from the focal plane. The point at which the image is no longer considered in focus is subjective. It varies from one observer to another.

Section thickness is inversely proportional to the amplitude of x-ray tube travel (in degrees), as shown in Figure 16–8. The larger the tomographic angle, the thinner the section. In Figure 16–8C, you can see the length of tube travel does not determine the number of degrees in the tomographic arc. The tube moves the same number of degrees going from point **m** to **n** as it does from point **o** to **p,** although it travels a greater distance between **m** and **n.** With greater target-film distances, the tube must move a greater distance to subscribe the same angle.

Although it is always desirable to have objects outside the focal plane maximally blurred, it is not always desirable to have the section as thin as possible. In fact, if we could cut an infinitely thin section, we would not be able to see it. Imagine a coronal section through the human body only one micron thick. If we could take this section out of the body and x ray it, we could not produce an x-ray image. There would be no contrast. Contrast depends on both the density and thickness of adjacent parts. Without some thickness, there is no contrast and, without contrast, there is no image.

Figure 16–9 shows section thicknesses for various tomographic angles and, as you can see, there is little change with angles larger than 10°. Even though the section thickness does not change with large tomographic arcs, the blurring of objects outside

Figure 16–8 Section thickness

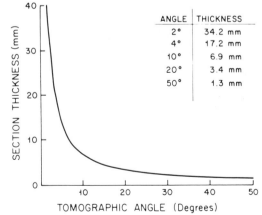

Figure 16–9 Section thickness for various tomographic angles

the focal plane does change. Blurring continues to increase as the amplitude of tube travel increases, which is why a film taken with a 10° angle looks a great deal different than one taken with a 50° angle.

NARROW- VERSUS WIDE-ANGLE TOMOGRAPHY

We can use tomography to approach a diagnostic problem in two different ways. One system uses a wide tomographic arc, and strives for maximal blurring of obscuring shadows. The other system, usually called zonography, uses a narrow tomographic arc, and attempts to present a view of the whole object, undistorted and sharply defined. The choice depends primarily on the type of tissue we are examining and the nature of the problem. At times the two systems are in conflict, but basically each is designed to do its own particular job.

Wide-Angle Tomography

The purpose of wide-angle tomography is to extend the limits of roentgen visibility to enable us to see objects that are completely obscured by overlying shadows on conventional roentgenograms. Figure 16–10 illustrates this principle. A series of lead letters are stacked on plastic shelves (*top*). On a standard roentgenogram all the letters are superimposed and obscure each other (*center*), but on the wide-angle tomogram (*bottom*) the letter C becomes clearly visible.

One disadvantage of wide-angle tomography is that it decreases contrast. Adjacent thick parts produce greater image contrast than thin parts of the same radiographic density, and because wide-angle tomography produces thin sections, it reduces image contrast. It is most effective in studying tissues that have a great deal of natural contrast, such as bone. It has been used extensively to examine the inner ear, in which there is still enough contrast to produce good images, even though the section thickness is very thin.

Figure 16–10 Extended visibility with wide-angle tomography. (The Fundamentals of Radiology. Rochester, NY, Eastman Kodak, Radiography Markets Division)

The sharpness of all images is decreased by wide-angle techniques, including those originating from the focal plane; the wider the tomographic arc, the more unsharp the images become. Theoretically, images from the focal plane should be in sharp focus, but in actual practice it is impossible to coordinate the motions of the x-ray tube and film perfectly. Minor vibrations cause unsharpness of the focal plane image, but the newer tomographic units are superbly engineered and unsharpness is minimal.

Narrow-Angle Tomography (Zonography)

Narrow-angle tomography refers to body section roentgenography employing an arc of less than 10°. Zonography is not efficient with linear tomography, and requires a multidirectional tube motion, which in practice is usually circular. Narrow-angle tomography produces undistorted, sharply defined images of the objects on the focal plane. An entire structure is displayed in sharp focus against a background of slight blurring. Our eyes tend to ignore the blurred images. The quality of the primary image is almost as good as it is with conventional roentgenograms, and interference from overlying shadows is diminished.

Zonography is especially useful when the tissues being examined have little natural contrast. Wide-angle techniques diminish contrast, while narrow-angle techniques retain all the natural contrast that is present. Contrast is usually minimal in soft tissue radiography, and zonography is the preferred tomographic method. The lung offers an ideal medium for this technique. Contrast is low, and the interfering ribs are usually several centimeters from our plane of interest. Rib blurring is sufficient to pre-vent them from interfering with visualization of the primary image.

One of the main objections to narrow-angle tomography is its tendency to produce phantom images. Both the narrow angle and circular motion contribute to phantom image formation. These images will be discussed in more detail later.

Table 16–1 summarizes the differences between wide- and narrow-angle tomography.

CIRCULAR TOMOGRAPHY

The more a tomographic motion differs from the shape of the object being examined, the less likely it is to produce phantom images, so tomographic units have been designed to operate with a wide variety of curvilinear tube motions, including circles, ellipses, hypocycloidals, sinusoids, spirals, and even a random motion. We will limit our discussion to circular tomography, although the same principles apply to all pluridirectional motions.

The movement of the x-ray tube, film, and grid for circular tomography is shown in Figure 16–11A. The x-ray tube and film are located at opposite ends of a rigid connecting rod. The tube moves in a circular motion, and the film follows at the opposite end of the rod. The film does not revolve as it moves. Point *a* in Figure 16–11A identifies one side of the film and, as you can see, it remains in the same relative position

Table 16–1. A Comparison of Wide- and Narrow-Angle Tomography

WIDE-ANGLE TOMOGRAPHY	NARROW-ANGLE TOMOGRAPHY
1. Tomographic arc of more than 10° (usually 30° to 50°)	1. Tomographic arc of less than 10°
2. Less section thickness	2. Greater section thickness
3. Considerable unsharpness of focal plane images	3. Very little unsharpness of focal plane images
4. Maximum blurring of objects outside focal plane	4. Minimum blurring of objects outside focal plane
5. Best for tissues with high contrast (bone)	5. Best for tissues with low contrast (lung)
6. Can be done with either linear or circular motion	6. Usually done with circular tomographic motion
7. Unlikely to cause phantom images	7. Frequently causes phantom images
8. Long exposure times	8. Short exposure times (with properly designed equipment)

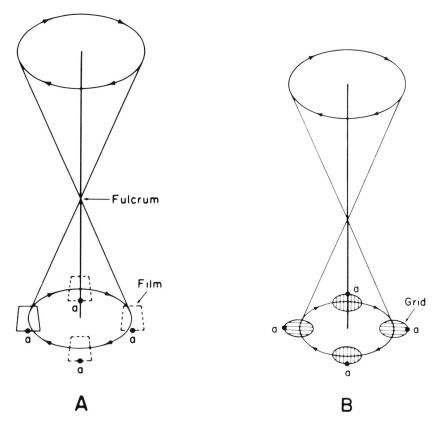

Figure 16–11 Position of film with circular tomography (*A*) and position of grid with circular tomography (*B*)

as the film moves through a 360° circle. The grid must revolve to avoid cutoff, however, because the entire exposure is made with the x-ray tube angled toward the grid. The only way cutoff can be avoided is to revolve the grid to keep the grid lines pointed toward the tube (Fig. 16–11*B*). Point *a* on the grid changes its position as the grid revolves, so that the lead strips of the grid maintain a constant orientation with the target of the x-ray tube. By examining Figure 16–11*A* and *B* together, you can see that the grid gradually rotates over the film throughout the 360° cycle. Grid lines are obscured by the relative motion of the x-ray tube and film, and no Bucky mechanism is necessary.

Advantages

The primary advantage of circular tomography is that it produces a uniform sec-tion thickness. Figure 16–6 shows the blur pattern of a test phantom obtained with both linear and circular tomographic motions. With a circular motion all portions of the phantom are uniformly blurred, no matter how they are oriented in space. Linear tomography does not produce a true section thickness. The amount of blurring is completely dependent on the orientation of the part with reference to tube motion. The only wire in the illustration that is maximally blurred is the one perpendicular to the direction of tube travel. Because linear tomography does not blur all parts uniformly, it frequently produces streaking or "parasite" lines that remain in sharp focus even though they are several centimeters from the focal plane. These lines represent the edges of linear objects oriented along the line of tube motion. They do not occur with circular tomography.

Disadvantages

To most radiologists the principal disadvantage of circular tomography is the high cost of the equipment. Circular tomographic units are much more expensive than linear units, which can usually be adapted to existing equipment. Another disadvantage is the length of time it takes to obtain an exposure. For a standard radiograph, the exposure time is determined primarily by the thickness and density of the part being examined. Tomographic exposure times, however, are determined by the length of time that it takes the tube to complete its arc, which is almost always considerably longer than the time that is needed to expose the film. One of the more popular tomographic units takes 3 seconds to complete a circular motion and 6 seconds for a hypocycloidal motion.* These long exposure times are a great disadvantage, especially for chest radiography, in which there is considerable involuntary motion.

Another disadvantage of circular tomography is the sharp cutoff of the blur patterns, which is conducive to phantom image formation.

Table 16–2 summarizes the differences between linear and circular tomography.

COMPLEX TOMOGRAPHIC MOTIONS

The tomographic objective is to blur images of objects outside of the focal plane

*Polytome, manufactured by Phillips.

as much as possible and as uniformly as possible. This can only by fully accomplished with a linear tube motion oriented at right angles to a linear structure. Figure 16–12B shows such an arrangement with three wires displaced 1 cm from the focal plane. The blur pattern of the wire oriented perpendicular to the tomographic motion is perfectly uniform. The blur pattern of the diagonal wire is also uniform, but not maximum. With a circular motion all the wires are blurred to the same degree, and all are maximally blurred, but the blurring is not uniform; that is, the blur margin is more sharply defined than the rest of the blur pattern (Fig. 16–12D). Because no anatomic part is shaped like a wire, the ideal can never be fully accomplished in a clinical setting. The more complex tomographic motions (e.g., ellipses, circles, trispirals, figure 8s, and hypocycloidals) are all designed to improve the uniformity of blurring.

Figure 16–13 demonstrates how the size of the tomographic arc is determined for complex motions. The number of degrees is measured from the extremes of tube motion. In the illustration, the arc is 35° from all four types of tube motion.

Table 16–3 compares the relative length of tube travel for four different tomographic motions. The numbers are only theoretic, because no manufacturer produces a unit that can perform all these motions with a 48° arc. As the type of motion becomes more complex, the length of tube travel increases. Using the 92-cm linear

Table 16–2. A Comparison of Linear and Circular Tomography

LINEAR TOMOGRAPHY	CIRCULAR TOMOGRAPHY
1. Equipment is inexpensive	1. Equipment is very expensive
2. Section thickness is dependent on orientation of body parts (no true section thickness)	2. Section thickness is independent of orientation of parts (produces a uniform section thickness)
3. Blur margins are tapered and indistinct	3. Blur margins are abrupt and sharply defined
4. Objects outside the focal plane may be incompletely blurred, producing "parasite" streaks	4. Objects outside the focal plane are uniformly blurred (no "parasite" streaks)
5. Does not produce phantom images	5. Likely to produce phantom images (with narrow-angle tomography)

Figure 16–12 Three wire phantoms (A) and blur patterns for linear (B), elliptic (C), circular (D), hypocycloidal (E), and figure 8 tomographic motions (F)

Table 16–3. Approximate Length of Tube Travel for Various Tomographic Motions

TYPE OF MOTION	TOMOGRAPHIC ARC (°)	LENGTH OF TUBE TRAVEL (cm)	SECTION THICKNESS (mm)	RELATIVE LENGTH OF TUBE TRAVEL
Linear	48°	92	1.3	1.0
Elliptic	48°	222	1.3	2.4
Circular	48°	292	1.3	3.9
Hypocycloidal*	48°	450	1.3	4.9

*Polytome, Medical Systems Division, North American Phillips Corporation, Shelton, CT; 45″ FFD.

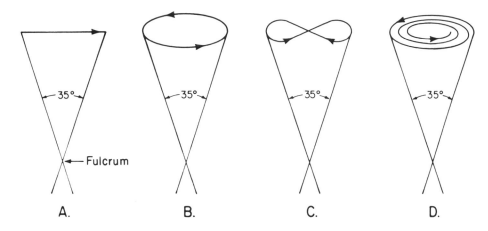

Figure 16–13 Method of determining the tomographic arc for complex motions

motion as the norm, the relative length of tube travel increases about five times for the hypocycloidal motion. The result is a considerable improvement in the uniformity of blurring. Figure 16–12 shows the blur patterns for several different tomographic motions. As you can see, blurring is more uniform for the more complex motions. Increasing the length of tube travel, however, does not necessarily improve blurring. The tomographic motion must be efficiently designed to be effective. For example, running the tube back and forth in a linear motion lengthens tube travel but does not improve the blur pattern. Section thickness is determined solely by the number of degrees in the tomographic arc, and is not affected by the complexity of the tube motion. Note in Table 16–3 that the section thickness is 1.3 mm for all four tomographic movements.

PHANTOM IMAGES

Phantom is defined by Webster as "something that appears to the sight but has no physical existence." Phantom images appear on tomograms, but they do not actually exist. These unreal images are always a little less dense and a little less sharp than real images, but they can still cause considerable difficulty in film interpretation.

Phantom images are produced by the blurred margins of structures outside of the focal plane, and they are most likely to occur with circular tomography and narrow-angle techniques. With a narrow-angle tube motion, objects outside the focal plane are only minimally blurred. The margins are still fairly distinct, and they tend to produce phantom images. Blurring is so complete with wide-angle tomography that phantom images are unlikely.

Phantom images are formed by two different mechanisms, which we will discuss separately. We should emphasize, however, that the parasite lines that occur in linear tomography are not phantom images. These lines represent the unblurred margins of structures oriented in the same di-

rection as the x-ray tube motion. The images are real and represent structures that do exist.

The first type of phantom image is produced by narrow-angle tomograms of regularly recurring objects, such as the wires shown in Figure 16–14. Three wires are equally spaced a short distance above the focal plane. Figure 16–14A represents a standard radiograph, and Figure 16–14B and C represent tomograms taken with two different arcs. In Figure 16–14A the images of the wires appear as dots. In Figure 16–14B the images are blurred but still separate. In Figure 16–14C the blur margins overlap slightly, and the overlapping edges produce the phantom images. These images are not real and, as you can see, it takes three wires to produce two phantom wires. Bony trabeculae, teeth, ribs, and dye-filled vessels are several of the anatomic parts that are apt to cause phantom image formation.

The second type of phantom image is formed by the displacement of the blurred image from an object outside the focal plane to simulate a less dense structure within the focal plane. Frequently, the blurred image of a bone will simulate a soft tissue structure. Figure 16–15 shows a narrow-angle tomogram of a dried skull. The apparent mucosal thickening along the floor of the nasal cavities represents the

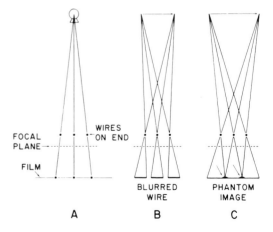

Figure 16–14 Phantom image formation

Figure 16–15 Phantom image formation. (Courtesy of Dr. J.T. Littleton)

blurred images of the bone in front of the focal plane. The films were taken with a circular tomographic motion, so the blur margins are fairly sharp. Because the images are from a dried skull, the apparent mucosal thickening must represent a phantom image. Bone is quite dense and, when it is minimally blurred by narrow-angle tomography, it retains enough density to simulate soft tissue. This type of phantom image formation is most likely to occur when the shape of the part being examined is similar to that of the x-ray tube motion, so it is common with circular tomography about the skull. The same mechanism, however, may produce phantom images in other anatomic areas. For example, a densely calcified granuloma in the chest, when incompletely blurred, may appear on a tomogram as a somewhat larger soft tissue nodule. The density of the calcification is spread out over a larger area so it becomes that of soft tissue, and the margins are sharply defined because of the circular tube motion.

Figure 16–16 shows a conventional ra-diograph of a nickel (Fig. 16–16A) and three circular tomograms taken with the same coin at slightly different distances from the image plane. One side of the coin is marked with a line that identifies the position of the same edge on all four films. The coin's image is blurred to exactly twice its original diameter in Figure 16–16C, a little less than twice its diameter in Figure 16–16B, and a little more in Figure 16–16D. If the original coin had represented a densely calcified pulmonary granuloma, then the exactly doubled image (Fig. 16–16C) would look like a larger, less dense soft tissue nodule, the less than doubled image (Fig. 16–16B) would look like a nodule with a calcific center, and the more than doubled image would exactly mimic a thick-walled cavitary lesion (Fig. 16–16D). Interpretive errors of this type can be avoided by carefully correlating the tomograms with the plain films.

In summary, phantom images are produced in two ways, by the superimposition of the blur margins of regularly recurring structures, and by displacement of the blur margins of dense objects to simulate less dense objects. They are most likely to occur with narrow-angle circular tomography, and they are never as dense or as sharply defined as real images.

DETERMINATION OF TOMOGRAPHIC ANGLE

Hundreds of different phantoms and multiple ingenious methods have been devised to study the characteristics of tomographic units. We will only discuss one, the pinhole camera technique described by Hodes and coworkers.[1] Figure 16–17 illustrates the principle. The only special equipment you need, in addition to the tomographic unit, is a sheet of lead with a small hole in its center. The lead is positioned at the level of the focal plane, and a film is placed on the x-ray table directly under the center of the pinhole. The film remains stationary throughout the test. It is exposed twice, the first time with the x-ray

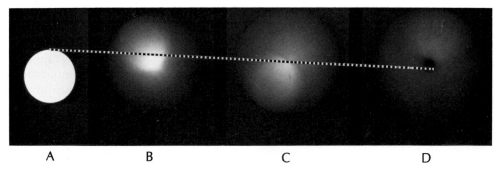

Figure 16–16   Plain film of a coin (*A*) and three circular tomograms taken with the coin at different distances from the focal plane (*B–D*)

tube perpendicular to the center of the film to mark the center of the tomographic arc, and the second time while the tube swings through its arc to record a series of superimposed dots that are a record of the tomographic motion. The line of dots produced on the film by the pinhole technique gives us the following information:

1. It is a geometric presentation of the type of tube motion (e.g., linear, circular, hypocycloidal, etc.).
2. It makes it possible for us to calculate

the length of the exposure angle, which is the number of degrees of tube motion during which x rays are emitted. We only need to know two sides of a triangle for the calculation. The first side is the distance between the pinhole and the film, and the second side is recorded on the film as shown in Figure 16–17 (*insert*). We can calculate the tomographic angle from the formula given in the illustration.

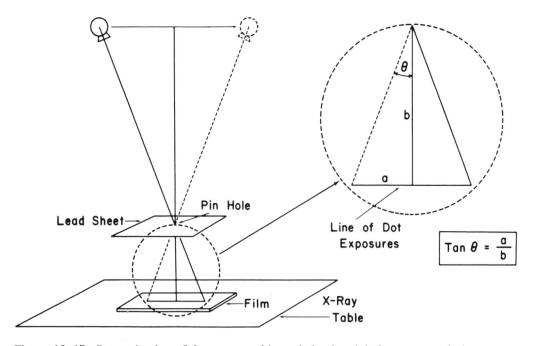

Figure 16–17   Determination of the tomographic angle by the pinhole camera technique

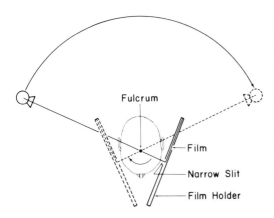

Figure 16–18 Pantomography

3. It shows us the symmetry of the exposure angle. With a properly functioning unit, the exposed dotted line will be equal in length on either side of the center of the tomographic arc. If the line is asymmetric, each side must be calculated separately, and then the two sides added to find the true exposure angle.

PANTOMOGRAPHY

Pantomography is a special radiographic technique that produces a panoramic roentgenogram of a curved surface. The patient sits in a chair and remains stationary through the examination (Fig. 16–18). The x-ray tube and film holder both rotate during the exposure. The film holder has a protective lead front, and is considerably longer than the film. The film is exposed through a narrow slit in its holder. The film moves across this slit as the x-ray tube rotates, and the radiographic image is "laid out" as the film passes by the slit, in much the same way that paint is applied to a wall with a roller. The resultant roentgenogram is a flattened out image of a curved surface. The rounded configuration of the mandible and teeth are especially well suited to pantomography, and it is widely used in dentistry. Pantomograms of the jaw show the temporomandibular joints on either side of the film with the teeth laid out between them (Fig. 16–19).

SUMMARY

Body section radiography is a special x-ray technique that blurs out the shadow of superimposed structures to show more clearly the principal structures being examined. The x-ray tube and film are connected by a rigid rod, which rotates about a fulcrum. When the tube moves in one

Figure 16–19 Pantomogram of the mandible

direction, the film moves in the opposite direction. The level of the fulcrum is called the "focal plane." Images originating at the focal plane level are in sharp focus on the film. The thickness of the section that is in focus depends on the amplitude of tube travel (in degrees). The larger the amplitude, the thinner the section.

If an object is located above or below the level of the focal plane, its image is blurred. The amount of blurring depends on the amplitude of tube travel, distance of the object from the focal plane and film and, in linear tomography, the orientation of the long axis of the part in relation to the direction of tube travel.

Pluridirectional tube motions (e.g., circles, ellipses, hypocycloidals, and spirals) are superior to linear motion because they produce a uniform section thickness—that is, one that is independent of the orientation of the long axis of the part to be blurred. Pluridirectional motions produce a sharply defined blur margin, however, and they are more likely to produce phantom images, especially with small tomographic angles. Pantomography is a special x-ray technique that produces a panoramic roentgenogram of a curved surface.

REFERENCES

1. Hodes, P.J., De Moor, J., and Ernst, R.: Body section radiography: Fundamentals. Radiol. Clin. North Am., 6:229, 1963.
2. Littleton, J.T.: A phantom method to evaluate the clinical effectiveness of tomographic devices. Am. J. Roentgenol., 108:847, 1970.
3. National Bureau of Standards: Methods of Evaluating Radiological Equipment and Materials. Washington, DC, National Bureau of Standards, 1963, Handbook 89.

CHAPTER

17 *Stereoscopy*

J. MacKenzie Davidson introduced stereoscopy to radiology in 1898, and it won immediate and widespread acceptance. Stereoscopy grew in popularity, and by 1930 most radiographs were taken stereoscopically. You can gain some insight into its popularity from a statement made by Jarre and Teschendorf in 1933:

A discussion of roentgen stereoscopy and some of its phases may seem rather unnecessary; no American roentgenologist doubts the advantages to be derived from the study of stereo-roentgenograms. To the well-informed observer it is even apparent that frequently overemphasis is placed upon the esthetic satisfaction of the tridimensional image, especially by many a young clinician using roentgenograms rather casually to the point of refusal of any non-stereo projection no matter how instructive it may be.[4]

Stereoscopy had reached the height of its popularity. Then, gradually, the pendulum began to swing.

The first step in the decline of stereoscopy was probably the result of its earlier overemphasis. When we expect too much we are frequently disappointed, and stereoscopy was no exception to this dictum. In addition, routine stereoscopy is expensive and time-consuming. The death blow came with the discovery that radiation causes mutations. The popularity of stereoscopy dropped precipitously, and the pendulum made its full swing. Unfortunately, stereoscopy is no longer used by many radiologists. Throughout the country stereoscopes are collecting dust, being placed in x-ray museums along with gas x-ray tubes as a remembrance of the past

or, even more humiliating, serving as stands for coffee pots.

Although we agree that stereoscopy was overemphasized in the past, this does not justify its present abandonment. Stereoscopic roentgenograms can give information that cannot be obtained in any other way, or at least not as easily in any other way. When properly used, it is still a valuable tool, and worthy of the attention of all radiologists.

PHYSIOLOGY OF DEPTH PERCEPTION

A basic knowledge of the physiology of depth perception is essential to an understanding of the principles behind stereoscopic filming and viewing systems. Depth perception is extremely complex and has some serious limitations. It depends on two completely independent mechanisms: the first, monocular or photographic depth perception, requires only one eye; the second, stereopsis, requires binocular vision. We will discuss each mechanism separately.

Monocular Depth Perception

Monocular depth perception is familiar to all accomplished artists. The artist depicts depth the same way we see depth with one eye. The mechanisms are as follows.

Size. Near objects are larger than distant objects.

Overlapping Contours. Near objects overlap distant objects.

Perspective. We see objects from a particular vantage point, or perspective. By following lines and contours we gain a sense of depth.

Shading. A sphere has the contour of a circle, but with proper shading we perceive its true shape.

Air Haze. Water vapor, dust, and smoke in the atmosphere absorb and reflect light, casting a veil over distant objects and causing them to appear farther away and less sharp.

These monocular mechanisms of depth perception are of little value in interpreting radiographs. Object size may occasionally give us some concept of depth, provided that two objects known to be the same size are both visible on one film. Perspective is of some value in determining depth, but only after we have become thoroughly familiar with anatomy. In a crude sort of way, unsharpness from penumbra is comparable to air haze; that is, objects close to the film are sharper than objects far from the film. Overlapping contours and shading contribute nothing to depth perception in radiography. In general, there is little that allows us to see depth on a single radiograph. In 3DCT, we will find that shading and perspective are used to give a three-dimensional appearance to a two-dimensional picture.

Stereopsis

Binocular depth perception, called "stereopsis," is a unique characteristic of man and other primates. It is dependent on the brain's ability to receive slightly different images from each eye, **discrepant images,** and then to fuse them into a single image that has depth. Discrepant images are the heart of stereopsis, and fusion occurs in the brain. The degree of discrepancy is of vital importance. If the images are too different, the brain cannot fuse them, and the stereoscopic effect is lost. If the difference is too small, the fused images appear flat.

Accommodation and Convergence. In the past, physiologists thought that accommodation and convergence were responsible for stereoscopic depth perception, but now it is known that they play only a passive role. Accommodation is the ability to

change the curvature of the lens with a change in visual distance. Convergence is a turning in of the optical axes so that both eyes can see the same object. The ciliary muscles, which regulate the curvature of the lens, and the internal rectus muscles, which converge the eyes, do not send the impulses that allow us to perceive depth.

Relative and Absolute Depth Perception. There are two types of depth perception: one relative, the other absolute. Relative depth perception is the ability to distinguish which of two objects is closer to the observer. Absolute depth perception is the ability to judge how far away an object is, or the distance between two objects. One is qualitative and the other quantitative. Stereopsis is relative. It only allows us to distinguish which of two objects is closer to us. To judge the distance between them accurately, we rely exclusively on monocular depth perception. Because monocular depth perception is of no value in interpreting radiographs, x-ray stereoscopy is only relative. It is a rank order type of depth perception. We can accurately rank objects in their order of closeness, but we cannot accurately judge the distance between them. A failure to appreciate this fact is one reason why some radiologists have been disappointed in stereoscopy.

Parallax. Parallax is the apparent displacement of an object when viewed from two different vantage points. In Figure 17–1, point A moves with respect to point B as the view shifts from one eye to the other eye. The convergent angle, α, is larger from A than from B (β), and the difference is called the angle of instanta-

PARALLAX = α - β

Figure 17–1   Parallax

neous parallax. As points A and B are moved closer together, eventually the angle of instantaneous parallax becomes so small that the brain can no longer recognize a difference between the images from the two eyes. The smallest recognizable angle has been found experimentally to be between 1.6 and 24 seconds of arc, depending on the investigator.[2] We can use this information to calculate the in-depth resolution of a stereoscopic filming system. If we use the largest reported angle of instantaneous parallax (24 sec), a 40-in. filming distance, and a 4-in. stereo tube shift, we should be able to recognize a difference in depth between two adjacent objects of slightly less than $\frac{1}{16}$ in., which is sufficiently accurate to meet most of our radiologic needs.

STEREOSCOPIC FILMING

Stereoscopic filming techniques are simple, and usually require no special equipment. Two films are exposed, one for each eye. Figure 17–2 shows the relationship between the x-ray tube, patient, and film. The film is changed between exposures. The second film should be placed in exactly the same position as the first film. The tube is shifted from the left to the right eye po-

sition between exposures, and it is the only part that moves. The patient must remain absolutely still. Usually the film is placed in a Bucky tray under the grid so that it can be changed without disturbing the patient. If the examination does not require a grid, the film is placed in a flat box with an open end (stereo tunnel), as shown in Figure 17–2.

Magnitude of Tube Shift

In the past, radiologists thought that the stereoscopic tube shift had to be equal to the interpupillary distance (2.6 in.), but now we know that this is neither necessary nor desirable. The optimal quantity of tube shift is empiric. We have learned by trial and error that a tube shift equal to 10% of the target-film distance produces satisfactory results. A 10% shift is simple to apply and produces discrepant images, which is the only prerequisite to stereoscopic image formation. For example, if the filming distance is 40 in., the tube shift will be 4 in.

In some radiographic units, especially head units, the x-ray tube and film are mounted on rigid connecting rods, so that the tube moves in an arc. With these units it is easier to shift the tube a certain number of degrees rather than a specific distance. Referring to Figure 17–3, and applying the 10% rule, you can see that a 10% tube shift is equal to an angle (θ) of approximately 6°. This angle will always be the same, regardless of the filming distance. The entire 4 in. tube shift in Figure 17–3 is in one direction, which is perfectly acceptable, al-

Figure 17–2 Stereoscopic filming

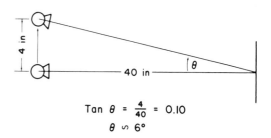

$$\text{Tan } \theta = \frac{4}{40} = 0.10$$

$$\theta \backsim 6°$$

Figure 17–3 Stereoscopic tube shift

though it is more customary to shift 2 in. on either side of center.

Direction of Tube Shift

The direction of tube shift is important for two reasons. First, many stereoscopic examinations are done with grid techniques, and it is undesirable to shift across the long axis of a grid because of grid cutoff from lateral decentering. In general, all grid-type techniques should be done with a longitudinal tube shift (i.e., along the long axis of the grid). If there is a compelling reason for using a cross shift, then you should use a low-ratio grid. Usually you can expect satisfactory films with a 10% cross shift on an 8:1 or lower ratio grid, but at the expense of increased patient exposure. Both exposures should be made with exactly the same tube shift to either side of grid center. If the shift is greater to one side, the films will not be equally exposed. Under no circumstances should you attempt a cross shift with a 12:1 or higher ratio grid. The chances of obtaining a satisfactory study are slight, and patient exposures are excessive because of grid cutoff from lateral decentering.

The direction of tube shift is important for a second reason. The objective in stereoscopic filming is to produce discrepant images. The tube shift should be in the direction that produces maximum discrepancy. In Figure 17–4, the tube was shifted

across the axes of the lines to produce maximum image discrepancy. If the tube had been shifted along the longitudinal axes of the lines, the difference between the two images would be less, and the stereoscopic effect would be correspondingly less. In this respect, stereoscopy is closely related to tomography. Both use a tube shift, and both yield best results when the tube is shifted across the long axis of the part being examined. You can think of the lines in Figure 17–4 as the tibia and fibula, the anterior and posterior ribs, or the front and back cortices of a joint. In each case the stereoscopic effect is greatest when the tube is shifted across the lines of interest.

STEREOSCOPIC VIEWING

The stereoscope is an optical instrument used to superimpose two pictures taken from slightly different vantage points. It was invented by Wheatstone in 1838, long before Roentgen discovered x rays. Since that time, many different designs have been described.

Preliminary Steps

Before we can view films stereoscopically, there are three preliminary steps we must follow to determine how the films should be oriented for stereoscopic viewing.

The first step is to **identify the tube side of the film,** that is, the side that is closer to

Figure 17–4 Stereoscopic images

the patient and thus facing the x-ray tube during the exposure. Usually we read x-ray films as if the patient were facing us. For example, frontal films of the skull are usually taken PA (i.e., with the patient facing the film). Most radiologists, however, read the films as if the patient were facing them. For stereoscopic viewing, we should think of our eyes as the tube, and view the patient as if he were standing between us and the film. If we do not do this, the left and right sides are likely to be reversed.

The next step is to **determine the direction of the x-ray tube shift.** In Figure 17–5, the films in the upper illustration were obtained with a cross shift, and those in the lower illustration with a longitudinal shift. The films must be viewed as shown to present the eyes with discrepant images. If the films are viewed in any other way, there will be no stereoscopic effect. Usually the direction of tube shift is determined by superimposing the images on the films (Fig. 17–6). The two edges of the film that superimpose (*upper* and *lower* in the illustration) represent the axis along which the x-ray tube shifted.

The last preliminary step is to **determine which film is to be viewed by the left eye, and which by the right eye.** Each eye must view its appropriate film. The whole concept of film placement is simplified if we merely think of ourselves as the x-ray tube. Our right eye represents the tube when it is on the right side, and our left eye represents the tube from the left side. Now, if we place the patient between us and the film, we are duplicating the manner in which the films were taken, and this is exactly the manner in which they must be viewed. Referring again to Figure 17–6, when the two films are superimposed, the right eye film will project out on the right side. If you just think of how they are taken, you can usually tell by inspection which is the right eye film. When the exposure is made from the right eye side, the image is projected over toward the left side

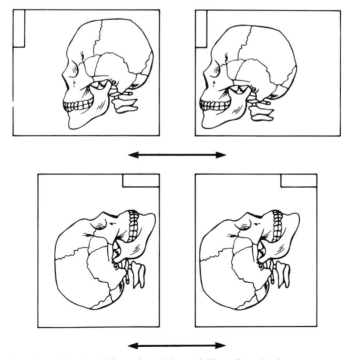

Figure 17–5 Direction of tube shift and position of films for viewing

L.E. FILM   R.E. FILM

TUBE SHIFT

Figure 17–6 Right and left eye films

of the film, and vice versa for the left eye exposure.

If you superimpose the images on a pair of stereo films, and the two edges of the films do not superimpose, then one (or more) of three things went wrong: (1) the patient moved, and the stereoscopic effect was lost; (2) the second film was put in a different position than the first film, in which case the study is still perfectly satisfactory, but the films must be viewed a little askew, with one film higher in the view box than the other (Fig. 17–7A); or (3) the tube moved in two directions during the stereo

A   B

Figure 17–7 Stereoscopic viewing of films taken improperly

shift. Again, the study is usually salvageable, but the films must be viewed diagonally so that our eyes converge along the true direction of tube shift (Fig. 17–7B). The only way of determining which of the three errors actually occurred is to put the films up in various positions and attempt to view them stereoscopically.

In summary, to keep the image of the patient properly oriented with regard to left and right, we must view stereoscopic films from the tube side, with our eyes converging along the direction of tube shift, and with each eye viewing its appropriate film.

Viewing Systems

Formerly, it was felt that the filming and viewing distances had to be the same or the distance between objects would be distorted. Before discussing individual viewing systems, we must clarify this point. Stereopsis, or binocular depth perception, is only qualitative. **With stereoscopic radiographs we are incapable of judging the absolute distance between objects.** All we can appreciate is which of two objects is closer to us (i.e., a rank order type of depth perception). All we need for stereopsis are discrepant images, and the degree of discrepancy must be sufficiently great to permit an appreciation of depth, and yet not so great that the brain cannot fuse the images. With this fact in mind, we can understand why the film reading distance is not important. Whatever distance is convenient and comfortable is perfectly adequate. The same stereoscope can be used to interpret all stereoscopic films, no matter what distance was used for the exposure.

Cross-Eyed Stereoscopy. In the routine interpretation of roentgenograms, both eyes are focused at a single area of interest, accommodation and convergence are coordinated, and both eyes see identical structures in sharp focus. With cross-eyed stereoscopy, two films are interpreted at the same time (Fig. 17–8). Accommodation and convergence must be dissociated. Our

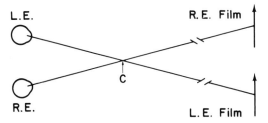

Figure 17–8 Cross-eyed stereoscopy

eyes cross so the right eye sees the film on the left side, and both eyes converge to point C in the illustration. If our eyes also accommodated for point C, the films would be out of focus because they are much farther away. Therefore we must converge on a point considerably in front of the films and still accommodate to the plane of the films. This dissociation requires a lot of practice, causes eye strain, and for many people, produces an image that is reduced in size or out of focus.

In spite of all these difficulties, many radiologists have become quite proficient at cross-eyed stereoscopy. You can test your own ability on Figure 17–4. Hold a finger between your eyes and the illustration, and focus both eyes on your finger. In the background you will see three images. The image in the center is formed by the fusion of the left and right eye images, and it has depth. Concentrate on it. If you are seeing stereoscopically, the right line will be suspended in space above the page. It takes a lot of practice to become proficient, but with enough effort you can master it.

Because no special equipment is needed, cross-eyed stereoscopy has two advantages over any other system. It costs nothing, and it is always available. It is certainly the most convenient system to use.

Wheatstone Stereoscope. The principal disadvantage of cross-eyed stereoscopy is that it requires a dissociation of accommodation and convergence. All other stereoscopic systems are designed to overcome this disadvantage. The Wheatstone stereoscope will be used to illustrate how they function. With a Wheatstone unit, conver-

gence is assisted by a pair of mirrors that are located halfway between the films (Fig. 17–9). We accommodate to the plane of the films and view reflected mirror images. The mirrors are adjusted to superimpose the right and left eye films without changing our convergent effort from what it would normally be for the viewing distance. We see a stereoscopic image hanging in space behind the mirrors and, because accommodation and convergence are coordinated to the same distance, our eyes feel no strain. All other stereoscopes operate on the same principle using either mirrors or prisms to assist the eye in convergence. In stereoscopes containing mirrors, the mirrors reverse the left and right sides of the patient's image; that is, they produce mirror images. To compensate for the reversal, the films must be turned over, so that they are viewed from the side away from the x-ray tube. This reverses the image again and brings it back into proper orientation.

Many other stereoscopes have been designed, but we will mention only a few of them. Figure 17–10 shows a stereoscope designed by Caldwell in 1906.[1] It consists of a pair of prisms mounted into binoculars. The unit is compact and convenient to use. Gass and Hatchett have described a similar system, in which they mounted a

Figure 17–9 Wheatstone stereoscope

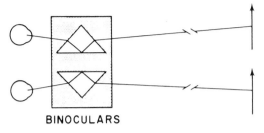

Figure 17–10   Binocular prism stereoscope

pair of thin prisms into eyeglasses.[3] The simplest stereoscope, described by Kerekes, requires only a small pocket mirror and a steady hand.[5] The mirror is held against the side of the nose and both eyes focus on the left eye film (Fig. 17–11). The mirror is adjusted to interrupt the view of the right eye, which then sees a mirror image of the right eye film. The mirror is carefully adjusted until the left and right eye images superimpose and are fused into a combined image having depth. Because the right eye sees a mirror image, the film must be reversed so that both images are seen in the same orientation. The mirror should be silvered on its front surface because of the high angle of reflection. The primary disadvantage of this system is that it is difficult to hold the mirror steady.

ADVANTAGES AND DISADVANTAGES

Advantages

The advantages (or perhaps **uses** is a better term) of stereoscopy depend on the skill of the stereoscopist. We will discuss only a few of the situations in which we have

Figure 17–11   Single-mirror stereoscope

found stereoscopy to be helpful. The list could be extended considerably.

Education. The teaching of normal anatomy is simplified with stereoscopic images. Lines that are superimposed into a confusing array for the novice migrate to their true position in depth, and they create a perspective that is not possible on a single film.

Foreign Body Localization. Stereoscopy cannot compete with a pair of right-angle radiographs for localization of a single foreign body. Stereoscopy is superior for the localization of many foreign bodies, such as multiple pellets from a shotgun wound. It allows us to localize each object from a single vantage point. With two right-angle films, it is not always possible to identify one particular foreign body on both films, because they all look alike.

Localization of Intracranial Calcifications. Some intracranial calcifications are so small that they can only be seen on the lateral view, and the only way they can be localized is with stereoscopic films. In fact, some calcifications can only be recognized stereoscopically.

Unimposing Confusing Shadows. The more confusing a radiograph is, the more likely stereoscopy is to be helpful. For example, a collection of gas in the colon may be impossible to differentiate from a destructive lesion in the pelvis on a single film. A good stereoscopist can recognize the true situation with ease. You can argue that a repeat film the next day would solve the problem, and you are correct. Almost all problems can be solved without resorting to stereoscopic films, but frequently stereoscopy offers the simplest solution.

Disadvantages

The disadvantages of stereoscopy are much better defined than the advantages.

Expense. Stereoscopy requires two films, which adds to the cost of an examination. It requires more technician time, is wearing on the equipment, and doubles the cost of films and processing.

Patient Exposure. The principal disadvantage of stereoscopy, the reason it should not be used routinely, is the increased patient exposure required to produce two films.

Need for Patient Cooperation. Because the patient must remain perfectly still between exposures, stereoscopy cannot be used on patients who are unable to cooperate.

Need for Practice. To become and remain a good stereoscopist, you must practice. The more stereoscopy you do, the better you will become. Most of us only dust off our stereoscopes when we have a problem and, in the long interval between examinations, we become rusty and lose our confidence. Stereoscopy should be practiced daily; routine lateral skull films are probably the most satisfactory study to use, because they frequently give information that cannot be obtained in any other way.

SUMMARY

Stereoscopic filming techniques are simple and require no special equipment. Two films are exposed, one for each eye. Between exposures, the x-ray tube is shifted 10% of the target-film distance (6°); the films are changed, taking care to position the second film in exactly the same position as the first film. The films of the stereoscopic pair present the eye with slightly different, or discrepant, images. Many viewing systems are available, but all accomplish the same purpose. They assist the eyes in coordinating accommodation and convergence. Stereoscopic depth perception is only relative, a rank order type of depth perception, which ranks objects in their order of closeness but does not disclose the distance between them. A failure to appreciate this fact is one reason why some radiologists have been disappointed in stereoscopy.

Stereoscopy has several serious disadvantages. The examination requires two films, so that it is costly and doubles the patient's radiation exposure. Because the patient must remain perfectly still between exposures, it cannot be used on patients who are unable to cooperate. In spite of these disadvantages, stereoscopy is still a valuable tool, and frequently offers the simplest solution to a difficult radiologic problem.

REFERENCES

1. Caldwell, E.W.: The stereoscope in roentgenology. Am. J. Roentgenol., 5:554, 1918.
2. Davson, H.: The Physiology of the Eye. 2nd Ed. Boston, Little, Brown and Company, 1963.
3. Gass, C.C., and Hatchett, C.S.: A simple inexpensive set of prisms for viewing stereoscopic roentgenograms. Am. J. Roentgenol., 61:715, 1949.
4. Jarre, H.A., and Teschendorf, O.E.W.: Roentgen stereoscopy: A review of its present status. Radiology, 21:139, 1933.
5. Kerekes, E.S.: A simple device for stereoscopic viewing of films. Am. J. Roentgenol., 75:140, 1956.

CHAPTER

18 *Xeroradiography*

Xeroradiography is the production of a visible image utilizing the charged surface of a photoconductor (amorphous selenium) as the detecting medium, partially dissipating the charge by exposure to x rays to form a latent image, and making the latent image visible by xerographic processing. Xerography was invented by a physicist, Chester F. Carlson, in 1937. In 1944 the Battelle Memorial Institute, and in 1947 the Haloid Company (now Xerox Corporation), began laboratory investigations of this process and its potential application to industrial and medical radiographic procedures. The Xerox Corporation has developed a highly automated xeroradiographic system that has allowed radiologists to make practical clinical use of this type of x-ray imaging. It is interesting to note that medical uses of xeroradiography were investigated as early as 1952 by Dr. John F. Roach of Albany Medical College, New York.

In August, 1989, Xerox Corporation and DuPont announced that they had signed a letter of intent for DuPont to acquire the Xerox Medical Systems Business.

GENERAL PRINCIPLES

Xeroradiography is a complex electrostatic process based on a special material called a photoconductor. A **photoconductor** will not conduct an electric current when shielded from radiation, but becomes conductive when exposed to radiation such as visible light or x rays. The photoconductor used in xeroradiography is **amorphous selenium**. The selenium is deposited as a thin layer onto a sheet of

aluminum to form the xeroradiographic plate, which is analogous to film used in conventional radiography. The plate is enclosed in a light-tight cassette.

The xeroradiographic imaging process consists of several steps:

1. A uniform charge is deposited onto the surface of the selenium. This sensitizes the plate before exposure to x rays.
2. The charged plate is placed in a light-tight cassette and exposed to x rays, just like a film-screen cassette. X rays reaching the plate cause the photoconductor layer to lose its charge in an amount corresponding to the intensity of the x-ray beam. The uniform charge is thus partly dissipated, and the remaining charge pattern forms the latent electrostatic image.
3. The latent electrostatic image is developed (made visible) by exposing the surface of the plate to fine-charged particles (called "toner") that are attracted to the plate surface in proportion to the intensity of the remaining charge.
4. The toner image is transferred to a receiver sheet by an electrostatic process.
5. The toner image is fixed to the sheet to make a permanent record.
6. The plate is cleaned of all remaining toner and prepared for reuse. The plate is not charged during storage.

PHOTOCONDUCTION

Solid materials may be classified as **conductors, semiconductors** (of which photoconductors are a special class), and **insulators**. This classification depends on whether or not the solid is capable of sustaining a current (moving electrons) if a voltage is applied. A brief review of the structure of an atom is necessary to understand why amorphous selenium, which is a photoconductor, is capable of forming the electrostatic latent image that is the basic physical phenomenon on which xeroradiography is based.

Let us again review solid crystalline structure. The atom is made up of a nucleus around which electrons are spinning in orbits. The forces existing within the atom are electrostatic forces (neglecting nuclear forces) that always exist between two electrical charges. Electron orbits represent precisely defined energy levels for the electrons, and no electron may exist at any level (or orbit) other than one of these permissible levels. Groups of permissible orbits are combined into electron shells. The number of electrons in the outer energy shells determines the chemical and electrical properties of the atom. The atomic number of selenium is 34, which means that selenium has 34 electrons: 2 in the K shell, 8 in the L shell, 18 in the M shell, and 6 in the N shell, which is the outermost occupied shell for selenium. The electrons in the outermost shell are called "valence electrons" (from the Latin *valere*, to have power) because they determine the action of the atom when it reacts with atoms of another element to form compounds (chemical reaction).

Electrons move in a curved orbit around the nucleus because of the electrostatic force of attraction provided by the nucleus. If the electron is provided with more energy, the orbit of the electron must change. The electron must obey structural laws, however, and move into a permissible higher energy (farther from the nucleus) orbit. **Electrons cannot exist between permissible orbits**. One way that the energy of an electron is increased is by the absorption of electromagnetic radiation.

Atoms are bound together to form solids by the interaction of valence electrons. The interactions not only bond the atoms together, but also slightly change the value of permissible energy that the valence electrons may have. The energy of the valence electrons in an isolated atom is defined by the discrete energy levels. **In solids the outer discrete energy levels are replaced by energy bands, and the electrons may have any energy within the energy band.** Inner shells may remain undisturbed by the bonding. In the isolated atom, the discrete energy levels are separated by nonpermissible energy values, and electrons may not exist with nonpermissible energy. The energy bands in solids may be separated by nonpermissible energy values or by forbidden energy bands.

In isolated atoms, the energy levels are filled to particular levels. Higher levels exist, but normally there are no electrons in these levels. Similarly, the energy bands in solids are filled to a particular level. The band with the highest energy that also has electrons is called the **valence band**. The next higher permissible band is called the **conduction band**. The two bands may be separated by the **forbidden gap**. Figure 18–1 shows the relationships of the conduction and valence bands for semiconductors.

The conduction band always has more energy states than electrons, and the electrons may move from one energy state to another. Therefore, the electrons are fairly

Figure 18–1 The valence, forbidden and conduction energy bands of a semiconductor

free to move when influenced by an external field in the form of a voltage (i.e., an electric current will flow). Solids that have many electrons in the conduction level are known as conductors, of which silver and copper are good examples.

The valence band is the highest energy band in which electrons normally exist at very low temperatures (at room temperature a few electrons will be thermally agitated into the conduction band). The electrons in the valence level are not free to move because nearly all the available energy states already are occupied by electrons, so an electron having no place to go must stay in the state it is in. With proper addition of energy, however, electrons in the valence band may be elevated to the conduction band. To do this, the electron must acquire sufficient energy to bridge the gap between the valence and conduction bands. This gap is known as the forbidden energy band. It is the energy difference across this forbidden energy band that determines whether a solid acts as a conductor, an insulator, or a semiconductor.

In a conductor there is no forbidden region between the valence band and the conduction band. Insulators are those solids in which the forbidden gap is so large that electrons seldom absorb enough energy to bridge the gap.

A semiconductor is a solid that contains a small forbidden gap. Addition of the appropriate quantity of energy will allow some electrons to bridge the forbidden gap and enter the conduction band. In a **photoconductor** the energy is provided by absorption of visible electromagnetic radiation (light). Energy added to a semiconductor will cause electrons in the valence band to enter the conduction band, and the semiconductor will then be able to conduct an electric current if an external force (voltage) is applied.

When an electron leaves the valence band, the area of the absent negative charge (electron) in the valence band is termed a "positive hole." Thus, the action of the energy of an absorbed light photon in selenium produces an electron and a positive hole, usually termed an "electron-hole pair." When an electron-hole pair is subjected to an electrical field, the two members of the pair migrate in opposite directions. The electron moves toward the positive electrode. The atom containing the positive hole does not actually move. Instead, the hole is transferred from one atom to another and the result is that the hole moves toward the negative electrode. Later in this chapter we will discuss the migration of the electron to the positively charged selenium surface of the xeroradiographic plate, and migration of the positive hole through the selenium toward the induced negative charge on the aluminum substrate of the plate.

XERORADIOGRAPHIC PLATE

The xeroradiographic plate is a sheet of aluminum approximately $9\frac{1}{2} \times 14$ inches in size on which a layer of amorphous (vitreous) selenium has been deposited. In addition, there is an interface layer between the selenium and aluminum, and an overcoating protecting the selenium surface (Fig. 18–2).

Aluminum Substrate. The aluminum plate on which the selenium is deposited is made of meticulously cleaned aluminum with an exceedingly smooth surface. Xeroradiographic sensitivity to any defect in the aluminum substrate is extremely high. Defects produce changes in the electrostatic charge in the selenium that may become visible during xerographic developing.

Interface Layer. Heat treatment of the

Figure 18–2 Cross section of a xeroradiographic plate

surface of the aluminum substrate serves to form a thin layer of aluminum oxide. Although aluminum is a conductor, aluminum oxide is an insulator. The thickness of the aluminum oxide layer is not critical. The purpose of this interface between the selenium and the aluminum substrate is to prevent negative charges induced in the aluminum from migrating into the selenium and dissipating the positive charge induced on the selenium surface. We will examine the nature of these induced charges shortly.

Selenium Coating. The photoconductive layer of the xeroradiographic plate is highly purified selenium in the amorphous, also called vitreous (i.e., not selenium crystals), form. It is deposited onto the aluminum substrate by condensation of vaporized liquid selenium in a high vacuum. The thickness of the selenium layer is 150 μm for powder toner development plates and 320 microns for liquid toner development plates.

Protective Overcoating. The selenium surface of xeroradiographic plates is protected by an overcoating. The material used for the overcoating is cellulose acetate, applied by dip-coating from solution to form a layer about 0.1 microns thick. Cellulose acetate bonds well to selenium. It has a resistance high enough to prevent lateral conduction of charges, which would degrade the electrostatic latent image. Overcoating extends the life of a xeroradiographic plate by a factor of about 10.

Photoconductive Layer

There are three properties required of the photoconductor used in xeroradiography. First, the electrical conductivity in the dark must be that of a good insulator so that a charge pattern present on the surface will be retained long enough to complete the steps of development. Second, the material must become electrically conducting during exposure to x rays so that an electrostatic image pattern can be formed on its surface by the exposure. Third, it

must have mechanical properties of durability and ease of fabrication. The photoconductor that presently fulfills these criteria for commercial use is selenium. Purification of selenium is very difficult, and any residual impurity may have a significant effect on its photoconductive properties.

The most stable form of selenium is its crystalline structure. This form is not used in xeroradiography because it has relatively high electrical conductivity. Crystalline selenium is used in selenium rectifiers. In addition to its crystalline structure, selenium also exists in an amorphous form, and it is this form that is used as the photoreceptor in xeroradiography. The amorphous form may be considered to be the super-cooled form of liquid selenium. It is formed by cooling the liquid suddenly so that crystals do not have time to form (the melting point of selenium is 216° C). In practice, amorphous selenium is deposited onto the aluminum plate by condensation of vaporized liquid selenium in a high vacuum. Pure amorphous selenium is mandatory as the presence of any impurity increases the dark decay rate. **Dark decay is the reduction of plate voltage while the plate remains in darkness**. For xeroradiography this rate should not exceed 5% per minute.

The selenium layer is 150 microns thick. **Sensitivity of the plate to x rays depends on selenium thickness and on the energy (kVp) of the x-ray beam.** For x rays in the energy range usually used in medical diagnostic xeroradiography, a selenium plate about 150 microns thick has been shown to exhibit high sensitivity. The recently introduced higher sensitivity liquid development xeroradiography system uses plates with a 320-micron thick selenium layer. This thicker photoreceptor results in an approximately 45% increase in x-ray absorption. We will discuss this new system in more detail at the end of the chapter.

Plate Charging. The first step in the xeroradiographic process is to sensitize the photoconductor by applying a uniform electrostatic charge to its surface in the dark. Because selenium is an insulator in the dark, during charging the xeroradiographic plate can be considered to be a parallel plate capacitor in which the outer (adjacent to protective coating) selenium surface and the aluminum backing (substrate) act as the parallel plates, and the selenium itself acts as the dielectric (see Fig. 18–4). The device used to produce a charge on the surface of the selenium operates on the principle of corona discharge in a gas. A brief review of capacitance and corona discharge is necessary.

Capacitance. A capacitor, or condenser, consists of two sheets of conducting material, with a sheet of insulating material between them. An electrical charge is placed on each plate (one plate is positive and the other negative); therefore, a potential difference, or voltage, exists between the two plates. The material between the plates has a strong influence on the amount of charge that can be placed on the plates. This material is an insulator, and is known as the "dielectric." When influenced by the electric field between the plates, the atoms of the dielectric become distorted into a configuration known as an "induced dipole." Consider Figure 18–3, in which a negatively charged rod is placed near an atom. The normal atom has its electron cloud centered on its nucleus (Fig. 18–3 A). The presence of the negative rod near the atom attracts the nucleus and repels the electrons so that the center of the electron cloud falls on the far side of the nucleus (Fig. 18–3 B). The atom now appears to have a positive side and a negative side; hence, it has become an induced dipole. Similar distortion exists in the atoms of the dielectric material between the charged plates of a capacitor.

Now consider the xeroradiographic plate. The outer surface of the selenium layer behaves like one plate of a capacitor, the aluminum backing (substrate) behaves like the other plate, and the photoconductor (selenium) acts as the dielectric (Fig. 18–4). If a positive charge is deposited onto the surface of the selenium, the remainder of the selenium atoms are distorted into the configuration of induced dipoles. The negative pole of each atom is attracted toward the positive charge, causing the atomic layer adjacent to the aluminum substrate to present a positive charge at the selenium-aluminum interface. Polarization of selenium atoms will attract negative charges (electrons) in the aluminum substrate toward the back of the selenium layer. In other words, a negative charge has been induced in the aluminum substrate by the presence of the positive charge on the free surface of the selenium. It is obvious that these induced negative charges cannot be allowed to enter the selenium if the positive charge on the selenium surface is to be retained. It is now easier to understand the function of the interface layer between the selenium and the aluminum. The interface layer (aluminum oxide) reduces negative charge leakage from the substrate into the selenium.

Corona. If a sufficiently high potential difference (called the corona threshold voltage) is applied between a fine wire and ground, the air near the wire becomes ionized. If the voltage is positive, free electrons in the gas near the wire will move toward the wire. These electrons will be of high

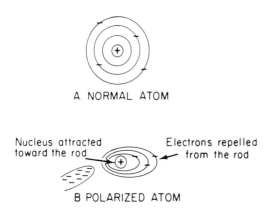

A. NORMAL ATOM

Nucleus attracted toward the rod   Electrons repelled from the rod

B POLARIZED ATOM

Figure 18–3 Polarization of an atom in an electric field

Figure 18–4   Charging of a parallel plate capacitor (*A*) and a xeroradiographic plate (*B*) is similar

energy and instead of going straight to the wire, they will interact with many molecules or atoms in the air and create many additional ions. The positive ions thus created will move outward from the wire. This movement of ions is called corona current. The corona around a wire with a positive voltage has the appearance of a uniform bluish-white sheath over the entire surface of the wire. When such a wire is placed close to the surface of the xeroradiographic plate (the distance is about $^{11}/_{16}$ in.) some positive ions repelled from the wire will be deposited onto the surface of the plate. The corona threshold voltage is quite high compared with the needed positive voltage on the surface of the plate.

Corona threshold voltage for such a wire is about 4400 V. By comparison, the positive voltage desired on the surface of the plate ranges from about 1000 to 1600 V. Plates used with the new liquid toner system are charged to about 2200 V. This creates two problems. First, overcharging the surface of the plate must be prevented, suggesting that the potential difference (voltage) on the charging wire should be kept as low as possible. Second, small variations in wire diameter or dirt on the wire will affect the threshold voltage at different points along the wire and cause nonuniformity of corona current. These variations can be minimized if the wire is operated considerably above the corona threshold voltage, at about 7500 V. Two devices have been developed to control the amount and uniformity of plate charging, the scorotron and the corotron.

Charging Devices. The **scorotron** in-

volves use of a control screen, or grid, that acts somewhat like the grid in a thyratron tube. This device consists of the corona-emitting wire (or wires) and a grounded backing plate. In addition, a grid of parallel wires about $^{3}/_{32}$ inch apart is placed between the corona wire and the surface of the xeroradiographic plate (Fig. 18–5). If the grid wires are operated at a positive potential, they will suppress the flow of positive ions from the corona wire to the surface of the plate (i.e., the positive charge on the grid will partially repel positive ions in the air attempting to reach the plate).

Assume that the grid is operated at + 1000 V. Initially, with no voltage on the plate surface, the entire 1000-V potential difference will repel positive air ions from the grid to the selenium surface. As a positive voltage begins to accumulate on the plate surface, the potential difference between the grid and plate will decrease. When the voltage on the plate surface reaches 1000 V, no potential difference will exist between the grid and plate, and the movement of positive air ions will stop. The grid allows more precise control of plate charging. Also, because it is now grid voltage rather than voltage on the corona wire

Figure 18–5   Cross-sectional schematic diagram of a grid-controlled corona-charging device (scorotron)

(wires) that controls plate charging, the corona wire may be operated at a voltage that produces a more uniform corona current (flow of ions). This corona voltage is usually about 7500 V DC, and is not under the control of the operator of the unit. The grid voltage can be regulated by local maintenance personnel to produce the contrast desired by the individual using the apparatus. The influence of initial plate voltage on the developed xeroradiographic image will be discussed later.

The **corotron** is a simpler device that has the same function as the scorotron. The corotron consists of a long U-shaped channel (called the shield) with inwardly bent lips and a single corona wire. A cross section of a corotron is illustrated in Figure 18–6. The shield is usually maintained at ground potential. The corona current to the plate is controlled by the corona wire voltage, the configuration of the shield, and the location of the wire within the shield.

The plate is charged by causing it to move at a uniform rate under the stationary charging device, which may be a scorotron or corotron. Because the charged photoconductor is sensitive to light as well as to x rays, plate charging and all subsequent operations leading to obtaining a developed xeroradiographic image must be carried out with the plate completely shielded from light.

EXPOSURE OF CHARGED PLATE

After the plate is sensitized by corona charging it must be enclosed in a cassette that is light-tight and rigid enough to provide mechanical protection for the fragile

plate. The plate-cassette combination is then used just as an x-ray film in its cassette would be used.

When the charged selenium plate is exposed to x rays (or light), **electron-hole pairs** are created (Fig. 18–7). These charged particles come under the influence of the corona-induced positive charge on the surface of the selenium, and the induced negative charge in the aluminum substrate. The electrons migrate to the plate surface and discharge the positive charge originally laid down. The positive holes "migrate" through the selenium toward the substrate, where they are neutralized by the induced negative charges. The amount of discharge of the positive charges on the surface of the plate is proportional to the intensity of x rays that penetrated the patient, so the variation of charge pattern remaining on the plate accurately reflects the pattern of attenuation of x rays caused by the patient. The remaining charge pattern on the plate is called the **electrostatic latent image**.

Conductivity Induced by X Rays

The energy gap between the valence band and conduction band (i.e., the forbidden energy band) in amorphous selenium is about 2.3 eV (electron volts). This corresponds to a wavelength of about

Figure 18–7 Exposure of the charged xeroradiographic plate to x rays creates an electrostatic latent image

Figure 18–6 Cross-sectional schematic diagram of a corotron

5400 Å, which is visible light in the green-yellow range:

$$E = \frac{12,400}{\lambda}$$

$$2.3 = \frac{12,400}{\lambda}$$

$$\lambda = \frac{12,400}{2.3} \text{ or } 5348 \text{ Å } (534.8 \text{ nm})$$

E = photon energy in eV
λ = wavelength in Angstroms (Å)

This calculation is a rough estimate used to illustrate the principle leading to creation of photoconductivity induced in selenium by light. Stated in another way, an electron in the valence band of amorphous selenium must absorb all the energy of a light photon of wavelength 5400 Å (540 nm) to be elevated into the conduction band, where it will be able to move when influenced by the positive voltage on the surface of the plate. Obviously, light is absorbed very near the surface of the selenium, with 63% of attenuation occurring within 0.125 μ of the incident surface.

Photoconductivity induced in amorphous selenium by x rays differs in two important ways from photoconductivity induced by light. First, the x-ray photons can penetrate further into the selenium, and their absorption may be almost uniform throughout the selenium layer. Second, the energy of an absorbed or scattered x-ray photon is transferred to a photoelectron or a recoil electron (Compton scattering), and each of these electrons will usually have enough kinetic energy to produce many more charge carrier (electron-hole) pairs along its track. The sensitivity of selenium plates of different thicknesses of selenium can be calculated by measuring the x-ray exposure required to reduce plate voltage to half its original value. This sensitivity will also vary with the quality (kVp) of the x rays. Figure 18–8 is a drawing taken from a series of curves in the literature, and shows the relative sensitivity of selenium plates of varying thickness to a 40-kVp x-ray beam.[2] The significantly greater sensitivity of plates in the 130- to 160-μ

Figure 18–8   Sensitivity of a selenium plate to 40-kVp x rays as a function of selenium thickness. (Modified from Boag[2])

range explains the choice of 150 μ as the thickness of standard commercially available xeroradiographic plates. Although **plate sensitivity is largely a function of the thickness of the selenium layer and the kVp** at which the exposure is made, it is also true that plate sensitivity can depend on the x-ray tube type, wave form of the x-ray generator, and amount of filtration.

Electrostatic Latent Image

After exposure by x rays there remains on the xeroradiographic plate surface a latent image composed of variations in the positive charge that represent the structure of the object examined. This is called the "electrostatic latent image," and it is accompanied by an electric field. The character of this electric field distribution above the latent image has a strong influence on the visible image formed when the image is developed. Because xeromammography is a well-established clinical application of xeroradiography, we will use this examination as a prototype to illustrate some basic principles. Typically, a xeroradiographic plate used for mammography will be charged to a positive potential of about 1625 V. After exposure, some areas of the plate will be almost completely discharged (e.g., areas outside the breast tissue), while other areas will retain almost all the 1625

V (e.g., under a large calcified fibroadenoma).

Electric Field Distribution Above Latent Image

Because the development of the electrostatic latent image depends on the attraction of charged toner particles to the surface of the plate, knowledge of local electric field strengths is necessary to understand the development process. This subject is highly complex, but for practical purposes we will confine our attention to two aspects of the electric fields existing above the latent image. First, the field has both a vertical and a horizontal component. Second, the field strength declines rapidly as one moves away from the charged surface.

Consider a plate that has been exposed so that a narrow strip retains its full initial charge (i.e., no x rays have reached the plate in that area), and the area on each side of the strip has been completely discharged. The lines of force existing above the plate will be similar to those shown in Figure 18–9, in which lines drawn close together represent stronger electrical fields. Note that the lines of force become further apart rapidly as distance from the plate surface increases by only a few microns. A negative charge at A, which is placed directly above the charged strip, will be attracted to the plate surface only by a nearly vertical force pulling it straight down to the surface of the plate. If the negative charge were located directly over

Figure 18–9 Electric field configuration above a narrow charged strip. (Modified from Boag[2])

the discharged portion of the plate, but near the charged area (B), both a vertical and a horizontal force act on the particle and cause it to pursue a curved path as it is attracted to the edge of the charged area. Because of this horizontal force component, negatively charged particles will be "stolen" from the area adjacent to a charged zone on the plate. We will use this concept to explain the phenomena of edge enhancement and deletion that are encountered in the developed xeroradiographic image.

Sensitometry

Xeroradiography is unique in that the response of the plate to x-ray exposure can be measured independently of the development process. To do this, the plate is usually exposed using an aluminum step wedge, just as film sensitometry is done. For measurements in the mammographic range, a nine-step aluminum test object with thicknesses ranging from 0 to 0.4 in. is used. Then an electrometer is positioned over the plate and the voltage remaining on the plate under the center of each step of the wedge is measured (this must be done in the dark). The results are plotted as a discharge curve, giving the voltage remaining on a plate after exposure through a given thickness of the aluminum step wedge. Such a curve is illustrated in Figure 18–10, in which response for variation in x-ray tube kVp is plotted. In this illustration plate voltage may be considered to be the equivalent of film density in the more familiar film characteristic curve. Note that these curves have a toe, straight line portion, and shoulder, similar to x-ray film characteristic curves. Also note that **the effect of increasing kVp is to decrease the slope of the straight-line portion of the curve (decrease contrast)**. This is an important difference compared to an x-ray film characteristic curve. The characteristic curve of a film is established by the manufacturer; inherent film contrast cannot be changed by the radiologist.

Figure 18–10 Effect of kVp on the electrostatic latent image. (Modified from Thourson[7])

The effect of changing mAs (kVp constant) is illustrated in Figure 18–11. **Increasing exposure shifts the curve to the right** (i.e., greater exposure more completely discharges the plate under each step of the wedge) without making any significant change in the slope of the straight-line portion of the curve. This result should be easily understood based on knowledge of the effect of mAs and x-ray film exposure.

Xeroradiographic Undercutting

Xeroradiographic undercutting is caused by ionization of the air in the space between the selenium surface of the xero-

Figure 18–11 Effect of mAs on the electrostatic latent image. (Modified from Thourson[7])

radiographic plate and the lid of the cassette. This ionization can be caused by interaction of x rays directly with air molecules, or it may be caused by high-speed electrons being able to escape from the selenium and enter the air space. This results in the presence of positive and negative air ions in the dark space between the selenium surface and the cassette lid. At the same time these air ions are being created, the x-ray exposure has caused some areas of the selenium plate to be discharged more than others (i.e., the electrostatic latent image has been formed).

Assume that a test exposure has been made in which part of the cassette has been covered by a lead bar that prevents any x rays from reaching the selenium plate (Fig. 18–12A). This will cause an abrupt step in charge density on the plate surface, with charge varying from virtually zero to almost the initial voltage on the plate. Across this step strong electrostatic fields will exist in the air space immediately above the plate. Because the initial charge on the plate surface is positive, the electrostatic forces will cause negative air ions to be deposited on the edge of the high plate charge and tend to neutralize the charge. This **deposition of negative ions would tend to "move" the edge of the electrostatic image toward the shielded side of the plate** (Fig. 18–12B) and, in extreme cases, could actually **cause the image to become considerably smaller** than the object being imaged. To eliminate this problem, a DC voltage is applied between the cassette lid and the aluminum backing of the plate. This will cause any air ions formed to move in a direction perpendicular to the plate so that they cannot be pulled from any area into the charge field at the edge of an image. If the cassette lid is made positive, negative air ions can be attracted away from the plate surface. The problem of xeroradiographic undercutting is rarely serious in medical xeroradiography, but can occur frequently in industrial radiography at the border of totally absorbing metal parts.

Figure 18–12   Xeroradiographic undercutting

Because of the highly localized nature of the electrostatic fields at the edge of a sharp charge difference, the results of xeroradiographic undercutting tend to move the charge pattern toward the center of the more highly charged area. Note that this differs from the more familiar concept of edge unsharpness on film radiographs, which causes a sharp edge to become less sharp but does not move the position of the edge.

POWDER DEVELOPMENT

Development of the xeroradiographic image may be defined as the selective deposition of imaging material onto a surface in response to electrostatic forces. Development consists of attracting small charged dust particles, called **toner**, to the electrostatic latent image on the selenium surface of the plate. The most commonly used toner in xerographic copy machines is charcoal, with a particle size of about 1 micron. Xeroradiography, however, requires use of a pigmented thermoplastic material. Average diameter of the particles is 4 μ.

Powder Cloud Development

The terms "powder cloud development" and "aerosol development" are synonyms. This is one form of development used in xeroradiography. It is fast, relatively simple, and **provides the edge enhancement** that is so characteristic and desirable in the developed image.

The exposed xeroradiographic plate is placed on top of a dark box into which an aerosol of charged toner particles is sprayed through a nozzle (Fig. 18–13).

Aerosol Generation and Toner Charging. If pressurized gas (commonly nitrogen gas) is used to force toner through a small bore tube, an aerosol of toner particles is created. An aerosol is a suspension of small liquid or solid particles in a gaseous medium. Aerosol particles have random movement. It has been found that a conventional paint spray gun will produce satisfactory aerosols from dry powders. Agglomeration of toner into unacceptably large particles is prevented because of the turbulent flow produced when the aerosol passes through the small bore nozzle.

The electric charge on the toner particles

Figure 18–13   Powder cloud development chamber

is produced by friction between the toner and the wall of the nozzle. This process is called "triboelectrification" (from the Greek *tribein* meaning "to rub"), or contact electrification. Charging particles by contact electrification involves complex processes, and a discussion of the physics involved is beyond the scope of this text. Toner particles with both a positive and a negative charge are produced in roughly equal numbers, and it is possible to attract either the positive or negative particles to the surface of the selenium. "Positive" developing involves attracting negatively charged toner particles to the remaining positive charge on the surface of the selenium.

Development Process

Xeroradiographic development consists of attracting the charged toner particles to the configuration of residual positive electrostatic charges on the selenium surface. The plate containing the electrostatic latent image is clamped onto the top of a powder cloud chamber, and toner is introduced into the chamber as an aerosol (Fig. 18–13). Diffusion air is also introduced into the chamber to create air turbulence. The toner cloud contains both positive and negative particles of pigmented thermoplastic, but particles of only one polarity

are used to form the image. To get a "positive" image a positive voltage is applied to the aluminum backing of the plate to attract only negatively charged toner. It is necessary to use this positive voltage applied to the plate back (termed the "back-bias" voltage) to attract negatively charged toner particles close enough to the plate to allow the electrostatic forces of the latent image to act on the toner. There are now two electrostatic forces influencing the motion of the particles: the uniform electric field of the back-bias voltage, and the nonuniform field caused by the latent image. For typical positive development the back-bias potential in the range of 2000 V DC. Conversely, a "negative" image can be produced by applying a negative bias voltage to the back (about −3350 V DC is a typical value) and attracting positive toner to the plate. This is done by moving one switch in the development processor. In the positive mode, positive toner particles are repelled by the positive potential on the plate and are directed to the grounded bottom of the powder cloud chamber.

With positive development, unexposed or minimally exposed areas of the plate will be dark blue. With negative development, these areas will be white to light blue. An example is the image of a breast containing a large calcification that absorbs almost all x rays. Positive development will show the calcification as a blue area; negative development will show calcification as a white area. The negative mode requires less radiation for a properly exposed image of the breast, with a decrease of about 20 to 25% being typical. A change from the positive mode to the negative mode involves reducing mAs by about one third and reducing kVp by about 1 to 2 kVp. The new Xerox 175 system allows an even greater reduction in radiation. We will examine this new system at the end of this chapter.

We must now examine what happens to the negatively charged toner particles (all examples will be for positive development) as they approach the surface of the selenium in the region of an image representing a high-contrast edge. For example, we might consider a step wedge image in which an abrupt change in charge on the selenium surface of 100 V is produced (e.g., +900 versus +1000 V) by the abrupt change in x-ray exposure at one step. Examination of this high-contrast edge will help in understanding the concepts of edge enhancement and deletion.

Edge enhancement arises from the electric field pattern associated with any abrupt change in charge density on the surface of the plate. The negatively charged toner particle in the powder cloud moves toward the plate under the influence of both the back-bias voltage and the latent image electric field. Although a uniform flow of toner approaches the plate, the electrostatic latent image electric field will cause significant change in "flow" as toner gets very near (e.g., 100 microns) the plate surface. Near an abrupt step in charge the electrostatic lines of force actually form closed loops, and charged toner particles moving along these lines of force are thrown toward the side of highest charge and excluded from the other side. The increase in toner deposited on the more highly charged side of the edge will be at the expense of toner deposition on the lower charge side. At some distance from the

edge, in either direction, the influence of the edge gradient is greatly diminished, and the uniform back-bias field dominates to cause even more deposition of toner.

Deletions can also be explained in terms of the electric field distribution. In Figure 18–14 it can be seen that if toner particles strictly followed the lines of force, no toner would be deposited in the region marked "X". Air turbulence in the development chamber, however, causes some toner to break through the "shield" formed by the lines of force, but toner that does penetrate will be attracted only to the highly charged side of the edge. This causes development to occur completely to the edge of the area of higher charge (A, Fig 18–14), but still leaves the region immediately adjacent to the edge (B, Fig. 18–14) undeveloped. This undeveloped region is called a "deletion." Although small deletions may sometimes be desirable, a large deletion may result in loss of information in the deletion zone.

There is a relationship between edge enhancement (or edge contrast), initial xeroradiographic plate voltage, the back-bias voltage, and the size of a deletion. The size of a deletion depends on the voltage contrast (voltage difference) at an edge and on the magnitude of the back-bias voltage. Large contrasts lead to large deletions,

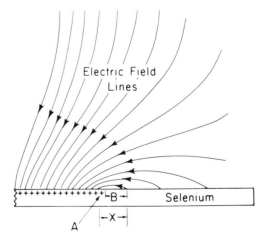

Figure 18–14 Deletions are caused by electric field lines of force

while increasing the bias voltage reduces deletion width. If the back-bias voltage is too high, low contrast detail in other parts of the image may be obscured. A lower initial plate voltage will reduce overall image contrast, and this will also reduce deletion width. For the low contrast encountered in mammography, however, higher initial plate voltage is usually used.

To review,

	CONTRAST	DELETION WIDTH
High back-bias	Low	Small
High plate voltage	High	Large
High contrast image	High	Large
Low contrast image	Low	Small

Development Electrode. The development electrode is an electrode placed in front of the plate during powder cloud development, and is given a voltage of appropriate sign (+ voltage for "positive" development) to superimpose a uniform helping field in the direction of the plate for the toner particles of desired charge (Fig. 18–13). **One major effect of the development electrode is to cause a visible image to be developed in uniformly exposed regions of the electrostatic latent image.** Otherwise these areas would go undeveloped. For example, use of a development electrode with xeromammography will make possible imaging of skin and large soft tissue areas of the breast. Additionally, the development electrode can be used to influence edge enhancement and the width of deletions, such as those that surround dense breast calcifications. The developing electrode is actually a grid (series of wires) placed close (1.5 to 2.5 mm) to the surface of the plate. The potential applied to the grid is usually +500 V DC.

We will use a specific example to explain the way in which a development electrode influences the electrostatic field of the latent image. Assume a selenium plate with an initial surface charge of +1625 V has been exposed so that a large area (e.g., a 2-cm^2 area of normal dense breast tissue) retains a uniform charge of +1200 V.

Close to this large area there is a small area (e.g., a 50-μm^2 area under a breast calcification) in which the plate receives little x-ray exposure and retains a +1500-V charge. Figure 18–15A diagrams the electric field that exists above both these areas (it is assumed that the space between these two areas has been completely discharged). Above the small area there is a strong electric field, but the electric field strength and potential have decreased significantly at a distance of 1.5 mm from the surface of the plate (we will assume that +600 V remain). Above the broad area the electric field is weak, and the potential drop is minimal, so that at 1.5 mm most of the original potential persists. The voltage above each area must fall to zero volts at the opposite side of the development chamber (this side of the chamber is grounded to keep it at zero volts potential; see Fig. 18–13), but the potential drop over the small charged area is very rapid near the plate while the potential over the large area drops rather evenly from the plate to the grounded development chamber bottom.

To summarize, (1) the electric field strength above the small area is strong and drops rapidly with distance from the plate, and (2) the electric field strength above the large area is weak, and drops slowly. Charged toner particles approaching the surface of the plate in Figure 18–15A would be strongly attracted to the narrow area, and to the edge of the broad area, but would have little attraction to the central part of the broad area. Thus, edge enhancement and deletions would be maximal, but there would be little visualization of structures in broad areas of relatively uniform exposure (e.g., normal breast tissue or skin).

Now, let us place a development electrode 1.5 mm from the surface of the plate, and place a potential of +500 V on the development electrode. What effect does this electrode have on the electric field above the 50-μm^2 and the 2-cm^2 areas of the plate? Above the small area (50 μm^2),

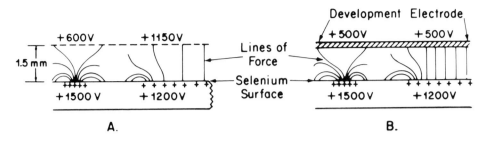

Figure 18–15 Effect of the development electrode

almost no effect. Above the large area (2 cm²) there will be a marked increase in strength of the electric field, shown by the increased number of lines of force drawn in Figure 18–14B. We must explain why this happens.

The electric field (E) between two parallel plates is equal to the voltage (V) divided by the distance (d) between the plates, provided d is small compared to the area of the plates:

$$E = \frac{V}{d}$$

If the distance (d) can be made smaller, the electric field (E) will increase if voltages are the same. Without the development electrode in place, the potential above the 2-cm² field falls to zero across the entire distance from the surface of the plate to the grounded bottom of the development chamber (i.e., d is large, so $\frac{V}{d}$ is small). The addition of a development electrode with a +500-V potential, 1.5 mm from the surface of the plate, will force the voltage above the 2-cm² field to drop from +1200 to +500 V over a small (1.5-mm) distance. This causes a large potential difference (V) to occur in a short distance (d), so the expression $\frac{V}{d}$ is now large, and the electric field (E) between the plate and development electrode has become much stronger. Conversely, the strength of the electric field above the small (50-μ²) area is minimally affected because a strong electric field (E) associated with a rapid potential

drop (V) existed without the development electrode being present.

The important concept is the change the development electrode has caused in the electric field above each area. The development electrode has little effect on the field near fine detail, but greatly increases the strength of the electric field over more uniformly charged areas. Properly used, **the development electrode allows satisfactory detail to be developed in broad exposure areas without sacrificing information in areas of fine detail.**

SENSITOMETRY OF DEVELOPED IMAGE

We have previously explored the way in which kVp affects the contrast present in the electrostatic latent image. It is now necessary to consider the characteristics of the developed optical density of the xeroradiographic print. Figure 18–16 shows developed optical density as a function of plate voltage, using positive development and a plate initially charged to +1625 V. Note that there is little change in developed optical density, or contrast, across the entire range of voltage in the electrostatic latent image. This provides a system with **great latitude**, in that all variations in plate voltage can be developed, but the resulting image would have so little contrast that it would be of almost no diagnostic value. More important than this total density range is the **contrast** (change in optical density) **across an image edge**. Because of the edge enhancement inherent in xeroradiography, the developed optical density

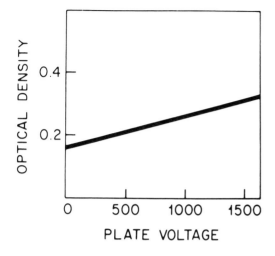

Figure 18–16 Developed optical density as a function of plate voltage (positive development)

on the high-voltage side of the edge falls above the general density level of the plate (positive development), while the density on the low-voltage side of the edge falls below the general density level. A density peak and valley exist at the edge. The perceptibility of an edge depends on the difference in optical density (contrast between the high-density peak and low-density valley) that exists at an edge. This density difference is a function of the voltage contrast that exists at the edge of the electrostatic latent image with more voltage contrast resulting in greater density difference.

Figure 18–17 shows examples of densi-

Figure 18–17 Densitometer scans across step edges of different voltage contrast

tometer scans across step edges of various voltage contrasts. You will recall that it is possible to measure voltages on the selenium plate before the electrostatic latent image is developed. In Figure 18–17 the average optical density is about 0.5, and at edge gradients developed optical density falls above and below the average density. Because of edge enhancement, a voltage difference of only 1 V across an edge can be detected in the developed image.

QUALITY OF XERORADIOGRAPHIC IMAGE

The quality of the developed xeroradiograph may be evaluated by its resolving power (line pairs per mm) and by its modulation transfer function (MTF).

The inherent resolution of the latent image on the surface of a selenium plate is high, with resolution as high as 2000 line pairs per millimeter being reported in laboratory experiments using liquid developer. When powder cloud development is used, the size of the toner particles sets a limit on resolving power. For toner with a mean particle diameter of 5 microns, this limit is thought to be about 50 line pairs per mm. Other factors, such as the charge on the toner particles and the thickness of the selenium layer, have some influence on resolution. The inherent resolving power of both the selenium plate and the powder cloud development process are not limiting factors in resolution in the xeroradiographic image as it is used for medical diagnosis. Limitations imposed by the focal spot of the x-ray tube and by patient motion are the two major factors in limiting resolving power.

The modulation transfer function of xeroradiography is quite different from that of film. Curves comparing the MTF of xeroradiography and film have been published, and such a diagram is presented in Figure 18–18.[4] Notice that for xeroradiography, the low spatial frequencies are poorly reproduced, whereas frequencies near 1 line pair per mm are greatly accen-

Figure 18–18 Comparison of the modulation transfer function of film and xeroradiography. (Modified from Kilgore et al.[4])

tuated. Film has its best response at lower spatial frequencies (i.e., the less information to be recorded, the better job film can do). The upper limit of both film and xeroradiography MTF curves is about the same because this represents a limit imposed by factors other than the film or xeroradiographic plate (e.g., x-ray tube focal spot and patient motion). The unusual shape of the MTF curve of a xeroradiograph is compatible with clinical observations that large homogeneous structures, such as areas of normal dense breast tissue, are difficult to image. Stated another way, **xeroradiography may be said to exhibit enhanced fine structure contrast and subdued broad area contrast**.

Exposure Latitude

Xeroradiography exhibits broad exposure latitude compared to x-ray film exposure. Experimental data show that xeroradiography will produce satisfactory image resolution over a wider range of kVp selections than will film. In other words, it may be said that with xeroradiography the resolution capability is less sensitive to exposure, and a single exposure will produce good image resolution in all portions of a breast (thick and thin areas). Using film, obtaining good resolving power of the

image under thin breast areas often requires a significantly different kVp than that required to produce a similar image under thick breast areas. With xeroradiography an appropriate kVp that produces satisfactory resolution in all portions of the image is more easily found. Another illustration of this concept of broad exposure latitude of xeroradiography is that objects such as blood vessels will exhibit equal contrast over wide variations in breast thickness.

IMAGE TRANSFER AND FIXING

It is necessary for the powder image on the surface of the xeroradiographic plate to be transferred to paper and fixed there to form a permanent image. An electrostatic transfer process is used. The paper is coated with a slightly deformable layer of plastic, such as a low-molecular weight polyethylene material. When this paper is pushed against the powder image under relatively high pressure, the toner particles become slightly embedded in the plastic.

After development, the plate is removed from the development chamber and prepared for this transfer process by being passed over a pretransfer corotron that has a negative charge. This negative corona loosens the attraction between toner particles and the selenium surface of the plate, and gives the toner a negative charge to prepare it for the transfer process. The plate then comes in contact with the paper over a transfer corotron, and the image is transferred to the paper. The transfer corotron has a positive charge that attracts the negatively charged toner to the paper. The paper is also mechanically pressed against the powder image. After the image is transferred, the paper is peeled off the plate, and the loosely held powder image is made into a permanent bonded image by heating the paper to about 475° F. The heat softens the plastic coating on the paper and allows toner particles to sink into and become bonded to the plastic. The toner particles do not melt or flow.

After fixing, also called "fusing," the

imaging portion of the xeroradiographic process is complete, and the completed image is delivered from the processor ready for viewing. With positive development, areas that received little x-ray exposure (such as dense breast calcification) will appear dark blue on the print, and areas receiving heavy x-ray exposure will appear light blue. If a charged plate is inadvertently exposed to room light and then developed (positive), the paper will be almost devoid of toner. Conversely, a charged but unexposed plate will produce a uniformly deep blue print if it is subjected to positive development.

PLATE CLEANING AND STORAGE

After transfer of the toner to paper, some toner remains on the plate surface. All toner must be removed before the plate can be used again. After the transfer process is completed, the plate is exposed to a light source (electroluminescent strip) that reduces the bond holding residual toner to the plate. Next, a preclean corotron exposes the plate to an alternating current that serves to neutralize the electrostatic forces holding toner to the plate. A cleaning brush then mechanically brushes the residual toner from the plate.

Relaxation (Plate Fatigue)

Relaxation is done to prevent faint "ghost" images from appearing (this phenomenon is sometimes called "plate fatigue"). Absorption of x rays in the selenium produces an alteration in the physical state of the selenium atoms that causes some photoconductivity to persist for as long as several hours after exposure. If the plate were charged for a new exposure without allowing it to rest for several hours, this residual photoconductivity would cause some discharge in the dark and create a faint "ghost" image of the previous exposure to appear when the plate was developed. This rest period can be reduced to only 2 or 3 minutes if the plate is relaxed by heating it to 140° F for 150 sec. The cleaned and relaxed plate is then held in the storage compartment of the conditioner module of the xeroradiographic system at 89° F until needed for another exposure.

The life of a xeroradiographic plate is of the order of several thousand exposures. Exposure to x rays or to light does not shorten the life span. The main cause of plate failure is physical damage caused by handling and the cleaning process.

AUTOMATIC XERORADIOGRAPHIC SYSTEM

Processing of a xeroradiographic plate takes place in two units that have been termed the "conditioner" (prepares the plates for exposure) and the "processor." (Fig. 18–19).[5] Following processing, cleaned plates are stored in a box (1) in the processor unit. The box can hold as many as six plates. When this storage box is inserted into the input station of the conditioner, the plates are extracted one at a time and transported to the relaxing oven (2). The relaxed plates are stored in the storage unit (3) for an indefinite period of time. When a sensitized plate is needed, an empty cassette is inserted into the cassette station of the conditioner (5). This causes a plate to be removed from the storage area and passed under the charging device (4). Immediately after charging, the plate is moved into the cassette (5), and is ready for use. The conditioner requires about 15 sec to charge a stored plate and place the plate in a cassette.

After exposure, the cassette (5) is placed in the processor where development transfer and cleaning take place. The exposed plate is extracted from the cassette and transported (6) to the back of the processor unit, where it is sealed to the top of the development chamber (7). During development, a sheet of paper is transported from the paper storage tray (9) to the transfer station (10). The developed plate passes the pretransfer station (8) and then proceeds to the transfer station (10), where the

CONDITIONER

PROCESSOR

1. Plate storage box
2. Relaxation oven
3. Plate storage compartment
4. Plate charging
5. Cassette
6. Plate transport mechanism
7. Development chamber
8. Pre-transfer station
9. Paper storage and feeder
10. Transfer station
11. Fusing oven
12. Paper print tray
13. Pre-cleaning station
14. Plate cleaning station

Figure 18–19 Diagram of the automatic xero-radiographic processing system. (Modified from McMaster and Hoyt[5])

image is transferred from the plate to the paper. The paper is then pulled away from the plate and into the fusing oven (*11*), where the image is fixed to form a permanent image. The paper then proceeds to the output tray (*12*). At the same time the paper is being processed, the plate passes through the precleaning (*13*) and cleaning (*14*) stations. The clean plates may be stored in the storage box (*1*) until six plates have accumulated, or transferred

back to the conditioner before the box is full. The processor is able to produce a completed print in about 2 minutes. In many processors it is possible to begin transport of a plate to the developing chamber while another plate is in the transfer and cleaning areas, thus speeding the rate of processing of multiple plates.

The front of the conditioner of the Xerox 125 conditioner has a control knob labeled "B", "C", and "D". This control changes the initial plate voltage, and corresponds to approximately 975 V (B), 1300 V (C), and 1625 V (D). The D setting is generally used in xeromammography because high contrast is desirable.

The front of the Xerox 125 processor has two control knobs, labeled "Mode" and "Density." The mode knob determines whether a positive or negative print is obtained. The density knob is used only with the negative mode, and determines the number of powder bursts that will be introduced into the development chamber during plate development. The stations on the density knob are labeled "B", "C", and "D", and correspond to 10 (B), 18 (C) and 26 (D) powder bursts. In the positive mode, development is accomplished with 10 powder bursts.

LIQUID TONER XERORADIOGRAPHY

The Xerox Corporation introduced powder cloud xeroradiography in 1971 with the 125 System. Efforts to reduce patient dose resulted in the introduction of a liquid development system, called the Xerox 175 System, in 1985. Actually, the first liquid development system was a unit used for intraoral radiography. This dental unit, called the Xerox 110 dental x-ray imaging system, was made commercially available in 1981.

The Xerox 175 System is sold as a single unit that incorporates plate preparation and processing in a single unit, similar to the older 125 System. The 175 System has no external operator controls.

Patient exposure with the 175 System is reduced by about half when compared to the 125 System (all comparisons between these two systems refer to xeromammographic examinations). Three factors contribute to this dose reduction:

1. A different photoreceptor manufacturing process
2. A thicker photoreceptor
3. A more sensitive developer

We will discuss the photoreceptor and liquid developer of this higher sensitivity xeromammography system.

Photoreceptor

The photoreceptor in the higher sensitivity xeromammography system remains amorphous selenium. Two factors contribute to the increased sensitivity of the new photoreceptor:

1. A thicker photoreceptor layer increases x-ray absorption
2. A higher conversion of absorbed x-ray energy to charge signals

Absorptions of the x-ray beam by the 175 System were increased by increasing the thickness of the photoreceptor layer from 150 microns (as in the 125 System) to 320 microns. This thickness increase resulted in an approximately 45% increase in x-ray absorption.

In addition to a thicker photoreceptor layer the 175 System photoreceptor layer has an improved conversion efficiency. This concept is analogous to the x ray to light conversion efficiency in intensifying screen phosphors. For Xerox plates, conversion efficiency is a measure of the amount of discharge of the positive charges on the surface of the plate. Photoreceptors for the 125 and 175 Systems were prepared in equal thicknesses and subjected to identical x-ray exposures. It was found that the newer (175 System) photoreceptor layer had a 15 to 20% greater discharge in plate voltage. The higher sensitivity is the result of higher efficiency in converting absorbed

energy to charge signals. A change in the manufacturing process of the amorphous selenium layer is responsible for this increased conversion efficiency; details of the process are proprietary. Since 1986 the higher conversion efficiency photoreceptor has been used in Xerox 125 plates, making them about 20% more sensitive than the pre-1986 plates.

The combination of higher absorption and discharge efficiency of the 175 photoreceptor results in a photoreceptor that requires about one-half the exposure (mAs) needed for the 125 photoreceptor. Discharge curves for the two systems demonstrate that the 175 photoreceptor yields an electrostatic latent image that retains the characteristics needed to maintain the object latitude and edge enhancement that are important in xeromammography.

Liquid Development

The search for a more sensitive toner led to a liquid toner development system. Liquid toner particles are black (compared to blue powder toner). Two characteristics of liquid toner that contribute to an improved image are toner particle size and the charge per particle.

Since the new xeroradiography system requires only half the radiation exposure of the old system, quantum mottle (photon noise) will be greater. Toner granularity is also a source of noise that will reduce the signal-to-noise ratio. Since the particles on the liquid toner are smaller, signal-to-noise ratio should improve. Use of smaller toner particles will decrease toner granularity and offset some of the expected increase in quantum mottle. Average particle size of standard blue powder toner is about 4 microns. Average size of black liquid toner particles is about 1.7 microns.

Liquid toner particles are smaller in size, and they also have a smaller charge per particle. The charge on toner particles is expressed as elementary charges per particle, with an elementary charge being the charge of an electron. Powder cloud toner has about 1000 elementary charges per particle, whereas the smaller liquid toner particles have about 150 elementary charges per particle. Smaller particles plus less charge per particle results in more toner particles being deposited per image on the imaging plate. Cancelling all the charge on the plate may mean that toner particles have to be stacked several layers deep on the plate. Toner particles stacked on top of each other will increase optical density in the final image recorded on paper. Liquid toner particles also allow visible development of much smaller charge signal differences than powder toner. What does this mean? Suppose identical areas of charge on a plate are developed with both powder toner and liquid toner. The deposited toners are than transferred to paper and the net optical density is determined for both toners. Toner covering power is defined as the net optical density per deposited charge density. Liquid toner has about 2.5 times the covering power of powder toner. This means that, for the two images we have just developed, the one with liquid toner will have a toner covering about 2.5 times the one with powder toner. The higher covering power of liquid toner means that liquid toner development will allow a visible image of charge signals that are too small to be imaged with powder toner.

The actual process of liquid toner development, like powder toner development, is fully automated. Liquid toner is pumped through multiple small ports called "fountain heads." The photoreceptor plate moves across the fountain heads (as opposed to the stationary plate in powder cloud development). The liquid toner image is then transferred to a receiver sheet by an electrostatic process, similar to powder cloud development.

Readers interested in more details of the Xerox 175 System are referred to the paper by Jeromin and Speiser.[3]

PATIENT EXPOSURE FROM FILM-SCREEN AND XERORADIOGRAPHIC MAMMOGRAPHY

Several years ago the radiation dose received during mammography was measured as the entrance dose to the skin of the breast. It is presumed that it is the breast glandular tissue that is at risk for developing cancer in the future, and estimates of radiation dose to the glandular tissue is now the measurement considered most important. In particular, measurement of the average glandular dose (given the symbol $\overline{D}g$) is now recommended. The National Council on Radiation Protection and Measurements (NCRP) has published a report dealing with the entire subject of mammography. The report is NCRP Report No. 85: Mammography—A User's Guide (NCRP, 7910 Woodmont Avenue, Bethesda, MD 20814), This report reviews the subject of mean glandular dose in detail.

Mean glandular dose calculations are made easy by tables contained in NCRP Report No. 85. These tables require measurement of the x-ray exposure in air required to produce a good mammographic examination (film-screen or xeromammography). Also taken into account is breast size and the type of x-ray beam (kVp, molybdenum or tungsten target, and molybdenum or aluminum filter). Remember that the unit of exposure is the **roentgen (R).** In the SI system, the unit of exposure is **coulombs per kilogram (CKg⁻¹),** with one R equal to 2.58×10^{-4} CKg⁻¹. The unit of absorbed dose is the **rad,** which is the absorption of 10^{-2} joules of energy per kilogram of tissue, or 100 ergs per gram. A joule is a unit of energy equivalent to 10^7 ergs, which explains why 10^{-2} joules per kilogram is the same as 10^2 ergs per gram. The SI unit for absorbed dose is the **gray (Gy),** which is one joule per kilogram. **One Gy is the equivalent of 100 rads. One cen-**

tigray (cGY), or 10^{-2}Gy, **is the equivalent of one rad.**

Comparing mean glandular dose for film versus xerox mammography is now a fairly standardized procedure. Two aspects should be emphasized. First, exposure techniques for film and xerox are usually different. Film exposures usually use a molybdenum target x-ray tube with a molybdenum filter of 0.03 mm thickness, and kVp of about 28 with a half value layer (HVL) of about 0.31 mm Al. Xeroradiography usually uses a tungsten target x-ray tube with an aluminum filter of 1.5 mm thickness at a kVp of about 44 to 48 with a HVL of about 1.21 mm Al. The second point to emphasize is that data regarding mean glandular dose are only available in newer publications. NCRP Report No. 85 was published in March, 1986. The Xerox System 175 became available in 1985, and higher sensitivity System 125 plates appeared in 1986. Older publications may give doses calculated as skin dose, midplane dose to the glandular tissue, or average whole breast absorbed dose. Table 18−1 lists recently published skin doses and mean glandular doses for a breast phantom made of BR12 material.[7] The film-screen system uses a Kodak Min-R screen. Kodak Min-R film is a medium-speed film, and Kodak Ortho M is a high-speed film. A grid (5:1 ratio) is often used, so grid and no-grid techniques were evaluated. Xeroradiography was evaluated using the standard 125 System in the negative mode, and using the newer 175 System. We present only measurements made with the BR12 phantom at 5 cm thickness.

SUMMARY

The summary is contained in the beginning of this chapter under the heading "General Principles."

Xeroradiography is a radiographic method that has imaging characteristics different from those of film, which include:

1. Edge enhancement
2. Subdued broad area response
3. Deletions
4. Broad exposure latitude

This system is useful for imaging low-contrast objects defined by sharp edges. Because of subdued broad area response and edge enhancement, object latitude is large, and a single image can contain useful information over a wide range of object thicknesses.

In 1985, a higher sensitivity Xerox system, the 175 System, was introduced. Exposure factors for xeromammography are reduced to about half those previously required. The higher sensitivity of the new system is achieved by two improvements:

1. A more sensitive photoreceptor (thicker layer and greater conversion efficiency)
2. Higher sensitivity development (liquid toner with smaller particles)

Table 18–1. Mean Glandular Dose Estimates for a Single Cranio-Caudal Mammogram Using a BR12 Phantom, 5 cm Thickness

	SKIN EXPOSURE (R)	MEAN GLANDULAR DOSE (cGy)
Min-R screen:		
Ortho M film/grid	1.41	0.19
Ortho M film/no grid	0.57	0.078
Min-R film/grid	2.7	0.38
Min-R film/no grid	1.07	0.15
Xeroradiography		
125 System, negative	0.595	0.255
175 System	0.31	0.13

REFERENCES

1. Boag, J.W.: Electrostatic imaging. Contained in the syllabus of the AAPM, 1975 Summer School, The Expanding Role of the Diagnostic Radiologic Physicist, Rice University, Houston, July–August 1, 1975, p. 159.
2. Boag, J.W.: Xeroradiography. Phys. Med. Biol., *18*:3, 1973.
3. Jeromin, L.S., and Speiser, R.C.: Process studies on higher sensitivity xeromammography. SPIE Vol 555: Medical Imaging and Instrumentation '85, 1985, 127–136.
4. Kilgore, R.A., Gregg, E.C., and Rao, P.S.: Transfer functions for xeroradiographs and electronic image enhancement systems. Opt. Eng., *13*:130, 1974.
5. McMaster, R.C., and Hoyt, H.L.: Xeroradiography in the 1970's. Mater. Eval., *29*:265, 1971.

6. NCRP Report No. 85. Mammography—A User's Guide. National Council on Radiation Protection and Measurements. 7910 Woodmont Avenue, Bethesda, MD. 20814.

7. Speiser, R.C., Zanrosso, E.M., and Jeromin, L.S.: Dose comparisons for mammographic systems. Med. Phys. 13(5), Sept/Oct 1986, 667–673.

8. Technical Application Bulletin 7. Negative De-velopment in Xeroradiography of the Breast. Jan 1977. Xerox Corporation. Xerox Medical Systems, 125 North Venedo Avenue, Pasadena, CA. 91107.

9. Thourson, T.L.: Xeroradiography. In Encyclopedia of Medical Devices and Instrumentation. Vol. 2, 1146–1168. John Wiley & Sons. 1988.

19 *Computed Tomography*

At the Annual Congress of the British Institute of Radiology, in April of 1972, G.N. Hounsfield, a senior research scientist at EMI Limited in Middlesex, England, announced the invention of a revolutionary new imaging technique, which he called "computerized axial transverse scanning." The basic concept was quite simple: a thin cross section of the head, a tomographic slice, was examined from multiple angles with a pencil-like x-ray beam. The transmitted radiation was counted by a scintillation detector, fed into a computer for analysis by a mathematical algorithm, and reconstructed as a tomographic image. The image had a remarkable characteristic, one never before seen in an x-ray image: it demonstrated a radiographic difference in the various soft tissues; blood clots, gray matter, white matter, cerebrospinal fluid, tumors, and cerebral edema all appeared as separate entities. The soft tissues could no longer be assigned the physical characteristics of water. The computer had changed that concept.

Computed tomography has had many names, each referring to at least one aspect of the technique. Two of the more popular names are computerized axial tomography (CAT) and computed (computerized) tomography (CT). Computed (computerized) tomography (CT) is currently the preferred name and the one we will use in this text.

Like most great discoveries, CT was the end product of years of work by numerous investigators. An Austrian mathematician, J. Radon, working with gravitational theory, proved in 1917 that a two- or three-dimensional object could be reproduced from an infinite set of all its projections. Thus, the mathematical concept was established 55 years before the production of a commercial CT scanner. Workers in several unrelated fields (i.e., electron microscopy, astronomy, optics) were all struggling with a similar problem. In 1956, Bracewell, working in radioastronomy, constructed a solar map from ray projections. Oldendorf in 1961 and Cormack in 1963 understood the concept of computed tomography and built laboratory models. Kuhl and Edwards in 1968 built a successful mechanical scanner for nuclear imaging, but did not extend their work into diagnostic radiology. It remained for Hounsfield to put a CT system together and demonstrate its remarkable ability.

As with all fields in radiology, CT units are being continuously changed and upgraded by manufacturers. The mathematics of image reconstruction are beyond the scope of this text. The physical principles are probably most easily explained in terms of rotation and translation motion because radiation attenuation information may be collected by a pencil x-ray beam and a single detector. Since this is how the original EMI scanner was constructed, that scanner may be used to describe the basic principles. By necessity the discussion of the software, or mathematics, will be superficial.

BASIC PRINCIPLE

The basic principle behind CT is that **the internal structure of an object can be reconstructed from multiple projections of the object.** The principle is illustrated in

Figure 19–1. The object is made up of multiple square blocks, five of which have been removed to form a central cross (Fig. 19–1A). Projections could be obtained by passing an x-ray beam through the blocks and measuring the transmitted radiation. For the sake of simplicity, we will represent the ray projections that represent attenuated radiation, by the number of blocks in each row. The horizontal sums (called "ray projections") are shown on the right; the vertical ray sums are shown below the object. All the horizontal and vertical ray sums are added, like the two shown in Figure 19–1B, to produce a numerical reconstruction of the object (Fig. 19–1C). The numbers included in the reconstruction are 4, 6, 7, 8, 9, and 10. A gray scale value is then assigned to the numbers to produce an image like the one shown in Figure 19–1D. The image can be manipulated to highlight certain areas; that is, contrast can be adjusted. For example, the gray scale can be narrowed to include only black and white, and applied at any point along the numerical sequence. In Figure 19–1E, the scale is centered at the 9–10 level. Blocks with the number 10 are white and all other blocks are black. A perfect reproduction is achieved in Figure 19–1F by centering the black-white scale at the 6–7 level. This simple method of reconstructing an object may illustrate the basic idea, but unfortunately will not work in practice.

In x-ray CT the method of forming the ray projections is different than in our illustration, and the number of projections and picture elements is much greater, but the principle is exactly the same. The ray projections are formed by scanning a thin cross section of the body with a narrow x-ray beam and measuring the transmitted radiation with a sensitive radiation detector. The detector does not form the image. It merely adds up the energy of all the transmitted photons. The numerical data from multiple ray sums are then computer-processed to reconstruct an image.

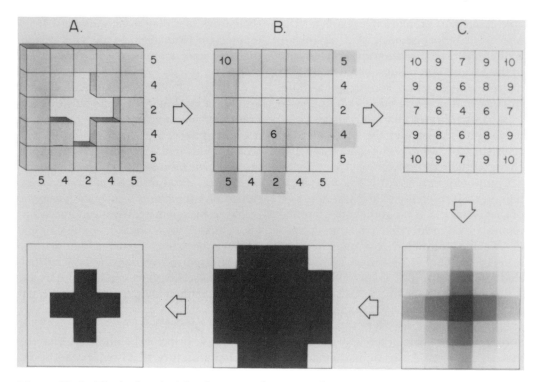

Figure 19–1   The basic principle of computed tomography

DATA ACCUMULATION

Data-gathering techniques have developed by stages. These stages have been called "generations." We would like to get away from this terminology and, except for first and second generation units that are no longer used, describe technologies in terms of their x-ray and detector configuration. Such descriptions will divide currently used CT units into categories but will not imply that one category is superior to another. Improvements being made in each category are as important as the introduction of a different category. As an example, improvements in computer technology fall in the range of improvements that do not define a new type (or "generation") of CT unit. Before going through the various configurations, the original EMI scanner will be used as the prototype to show how data are accumulated. We hope you will be impressed with the fact that the number of ray projections increases from 28,800 in the original scanner to more than one million in newer scanners. Image quality is related to the number of ray projections used to reconstruct each CT scan image. This statement assumes that each ray contains new information (described as non-redundant information). Notice in Figure 19–3, the original EMI scanner, that the non-redundant ray projections were collected by translation motion and rotational motion. Each ray represented in the figure is completely different from any other ray. Therefore, each ray contains new information and is not redundant.

Original EMI Scanner

The original EMI scanner was designed specifically for evaluation of the brain. In this unit, the head was enclosed in a water bath between the x-ray tube above and a pair of detectors below (Fig. 19–2). A third, a reference detector, intercepted a portion of the beam before it reached the patient. A rigid scanner gantry maintained the relative position of the x-ray tube and detec-

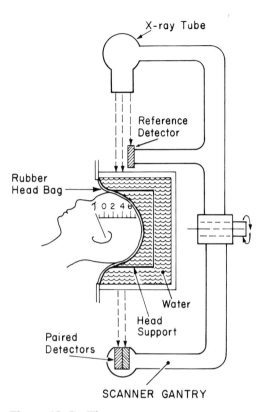

Figure 19–2 The scanner gantry

tors and ensured their proper alignment. The x-ray beam was collimated to the exact size of the two side-by-side detectors.

The patient remained in one position throughout the scan. The gantry moved through two different types of motion, one linear and the other rotary (Fig. 19–3). The linear motion was repeated over and over 180 times. Between each of these 180 linear movements, the gantry rotated 1°. Thus, the total rotary motion encompassed a 180° semicircle. The axis of rotation passed through the center of the patient's head. In Figure 19–3 the linear motions are called "scans." Only 3 of the 180 linear motions are shown (i.e., numbers 45, 90, and 135). The x-ray beam was "on" throughout the linear movement and "off" during the rotary movements. The transmitted radiation was measured 160 times during each linear movement. The total number of transmission measurements was

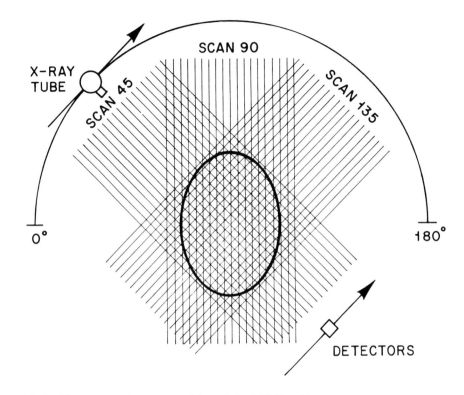

Figure 19–3 First-generation scanner (the original EMI unit)

the product of the number of linear measurements (160) and rotary steps (180), which was 28,800 in the original EMI scanner. The total scan time was between 4.5 and 5 minutes. Each scan simultaneously examined two tomographic sections, one for each of the paired detectors. Multiple tomographic sections were required for most patients, frequently as many as ten. Each pair of tomographic sections took 5 minutes, so the total scan time for a clinical study was approximately 25 minutes.

The x-ray tube and paired detectors moved continuously and in unison during the linear scanning movement. They did not stop for the 160 transmission readings. The transmission readings represented a composite of the absorption characteristics of all the elements in the path of the beam. In the original EMI scanner, the CT image was reconstructed and then displayed on an 80 × 80 matrix in two different formats: a paper printout of CT numbers and

a visual image on a cathode ray tube. The CT numbers were proportional to the linear attenuation coefficient. (They will be discussed in more detail later.) Each square in the image matrix was called a **pixel,** and it represented a tiny elongated block of tissue called a **voxel.** Figure 19–4 shows the sizes of the x-ray field (Fig. 19–4*A*), distance between transmission readings (Fig. 19–4*B)*, and sizes of the pixel and voxel (Fig. 19–4*C* and *D)* for the original EMI scanner. The x-ray field was collimated to 3 × 13 mm (the actual length was 26 mm, which produced two parallel slices per scan, one for each of the paired detectors). This field moved across the 17-cm wide water bath making 160 transmission measurements, one every 1.7 mm (270 mm ÷ 160). The data from these measurements were computer-processed and presented in multiple little squares (pixels), each representing 3 × 3 mm of patient cross section. The CT number for each pixel rep-

Figure 19–4 Comparison of the width of the x-ray beam (*A*), distance between detectors (*B*), pixel size (*C*), and voxel size (*D*) of the original EMI scanner

resented the average attenuation coefficient for all the elements in a block of tissue (voxel) $3 \times 3 \times 13$ mm in size. The size of the pixel was determined by the computer program and not by the dimensions of the x-ray beam. The same transmission data could be computer-processed for any pixel size. With a modified program, the original EMI data could be displayed with either 1.5- or 3-mm pixels. The length of the voxel, 13 mm in Figure 19–4, was determined by the width of the x-ray beam. This dimension could not be changed once the transmission data had been collected. It could only be changed by recollimating the x-ray beam and repeating the scan.

An oil-cooled stationary anode tube was used in the original EMI scanner. Its nominal focal spot size was 2.25×12 mm. The tube was operated at 120 kVp and 33 mA. The x-ray beam was heavily filtered with a half-value layer of 6 mm of aluminum (0.22 mm of copper). The mean, or effective, energy of the 120-kVp beam when it reached the detectors was 70 keV. Beam size was restricted by a pair of slitlike collimators, one near the tube and the other near the detectors. The detectors were so-

dium iodide scintillation crystals coupled to photomultiplier tubes. The reference detector furnished an exposure factor to compensate for moment-to-moment variations in x-ray output.

A large difference in attenuation between adjacent areas, such as air surrounding the head, makes computations more difficult. The patient's head was incorporated into a water bath in the original EMI unit to facilitate data analysis within the computer. A slip ring between the rubber head cap and water bath allowed the bath to rotate independently of the head.

Scanning Motions

CT scanners have gone through a number of design changes since the technology was first introduced in 1971. We will discuss geometry of design in five categories:

First generation (translate-rotate, one detector)

Second generation (translate-rotate, multiple detectors)

Rotate-rotate (third generation)

Rotate-fixed (fourth generation)

Other geometries

Time reduction is the predominant reason for introducing new configurations. Scan time has been reduced in newer configurations by the reduction or simplification of mechanical motion. For example, the stop-start motion in the first two generations has been replaced by continuous rotation. We will discuss a device that has no moving parts and an extremely short scan time.

First Generation. The original EMI unit was a first-generation scanner. It employed a pencil-like x-ray beam and a single detector; that is, one detector per tomographic section. The x-ray tube-detector movements were both linear and rotary (usually termed "translate-rotate motion"). A five-view study of the head took about 25 to 30 minutes.

Second Generation. One major objective of second-generation scanners, and of all later configurations, was to shorten the scanning time for each tomographic section. The increased speed was accomplished by abandoning the single detector and pencil beam of the original EMI scanner and adopting a fan-shaped beam and multiple detectors.

Figure 19–5 shows the physical makeup and movements of a typical second-generation scanner. The number of detectors in the fan beam array varied from one manufacturer to another. Only a few detectors are shown in the illustration, but there may be as many as 30. The movements of the x-ray tube-detector array are both linear and rotary, just like a first-generation scanner, but the rotary steps are larger. The 30 detectors gather more data per linear scan, so fewer linear movements are needed to gather an adequate data base. Instead of moving 1° at the end of each linear scan, the gantry rotates through a greater arc, up to 30°. The number of repetitions is determined by the number of detectors in the detector array. With 30 detectors, the linear movements only have to be repeated six times rather than the 180 linear movements of the original EMI unit.

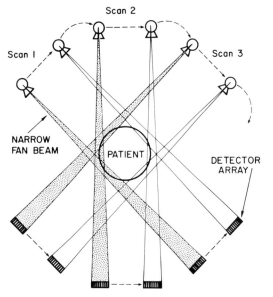

Figure 19–5 Second-generation scanner

Second-generation scanners produced a tomographic section in between 10 and 90 sec, depending on the manufacturer.

Rotate-Rotate (Third Generation). In 1975, the General Electric Company introduced a CT scanner in which the translation motion was completely eliminated. Only rotation motion was required, with both the x-ray tube and detectors rotating around the patient. This scanning geometry came to be known as "fan beam" geometry, or "third-generation" geometry, and the original unit could produce a scan in 4.9 sec. Multiple detectors are aligned along the arc of a circle whose center is the x-ray tube focal spot (the detectors are always perfectly aligned with the x-ray tube). The x-ray beam is collimated into a fan beam. Both the x-ray tube and detectors rotate about the patient (rotate-rotate geometry) in concentric circles whose centers approximately coincide with the center of the patient as illustrated in Figure 19–6. The original rotate-rotate scanner used 288 detectors, but newer versions of some units use over 700 detectors. The fan beam must completely cover the object to be imaged. Both xenon and scintillation crystal detectors can be used with this configuration because the detectors and x-ray tube are in precise alignment throughout the entire scan motion (more about this concept when we discuss detectors). In the original rotate-rotate scanners the x-ray tube was pulsed. Each pulse of the tube produced one projection, and the number of scan lines in each projection was equal to the number of detectors. A single image is computed from many projections, often more than 1000 projections. In some rotate-rotate scanners the x-ray tube is continuously on, and individual projections are obtained by reading the output of the detectors at rapid intervals (more about this later). More than 1000 projections may be obtained in a time as short as 1 sec (or slightly less). The topic of the number of projections and the number of individual lines in each projection will require more

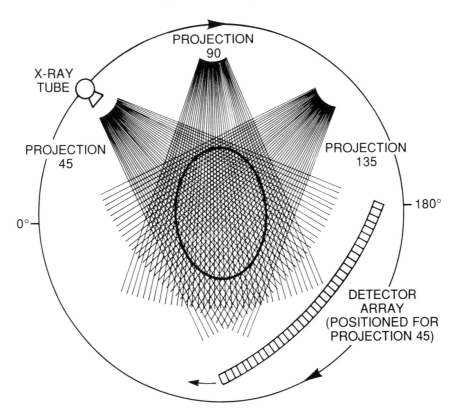

Figure 19–6   Rotate-rotate scanner (third generation)

attention when we discuss image quality. Rotate-rotate, or so-called third-generation, scanners continue to produce excellent images with short scan times. This emphasizes the point that "third-generation" units are not better or worse than "fourth generation" units.

We wish to be certain that our use of the terms "line," "projection," and "CT image" do not cause confusion. The CT image is the image of one CT slice that is viewed on the TV monitor or on film. The image is computed from many projections. A projection is produced each time the detectors are read. Therefore, the data contained in a projection is a set of readings composed of one signal from each detector that has been exposed to the x-ray beam. We describe the data (signal) collected from one exposed detector as a line, or scan line. This means that one projection contains many scan lines. The number of scan lines

is equal to the number of detectors exposed. Unfortunately, terms are sometimes used somewhat ambiguously. For example, the final image of one CT section may be called a scan or a slice or an image or a projection. We wish to be sure our readers know exactly what we mean when we use the terms image, projection, and line.

Rotate-Fixed (Fourth Generation). Figure 19–7 shows the configuration of a rotate-fixed scanner. The detectors form a ring that completely surrounds the patient. The detectors do not move. The x-ray tube rotates in a circle inside the detector ring, and the x-ray beam is collimated to form a fan beam. A fan of detectors is always in the x-ray beam. Some designs have used more than 2000 detectors. When the x-ray tube is at predescribed angles, the exposed detectors are read. For example, an angular sampling rate of one projection each $\frac{1}{3}°$ will produce 1080 projections in one

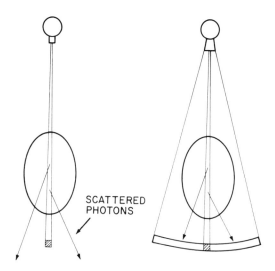

Figure 19–7 Rotate-fixed scanner (fourth generation)

360° rotation. Projections are taken at many angles during the rotation of the x-ray tube, with numbers of projections greater than 1000 being common. Thus, one CT scan will be made up of many projections, each projection taken at a slightly different angle. This is why continuous-on x-ray tubes are generally used today. It requires a less complex unit to read the detectors 1000 or more times in 1 sec. than to pulse an x-ray tube on and off 1000 times in 1 sec.

Both rotate-rotate and rotate-fixed CT units continue to give excellent results, with no clear advantage of one over the other.

The advantage of a fan-beam/multiple-detector array is speed. Obviously, multiple detectors can gather data faster than a single detector. One principal disadvantage of the fan beam is an increased amount of scattered radiation. At the high energies used for CT, usually 120 kVp, Compton scattering is a common basic interaction. The total number of Compton reactions is nearly the same for pencil beam and fan beam scanners, but the scattered photons are more likely to be recorded by a fan beam unit. Figure 19–8 shows the comparison diagrammatically. Two scattered photons are generated by a narrow pencil beam but both miss the detector and go unrecognized. In the fan beam scanner the same two scattered photons, generated

Figure 19–8 Pencil beam scanner (A) is less likely to record scattered radiation than fan beam scanner (B)

from the same volume of tissue, strike a detector and are recorded as noise. The problem of scatter radiation is exaggerated by the illustration for two reasons. First, the likelihood of a photon striking the detectors depends on the solid angle between the point of origin of the scatter radiation and the detectors. The scattered photons shown in Figure 19–8 may have been scattered into or out of the page, and thus they would go undetected. Secondly, the detectors in a fan beam array have their own individual collimators. Most scattered photons are absorbed by these collimators.

Other Scan Configurations. Rotate-rotate and rotate-fixed CT scanners cannot achieve scan times much shorter than 1 sec because of mechanical constraints. Rotating a heavy x-ray tube takes time. Interest in faster scan times evolves from a desire to image moving structures, such as the wall of the heart or contrast material in blood vessels and heart chambers.

One proposed solution to the problem of producing an image in a very short time is to use multiple x-ray tubes. An example of this concept is the Mayo Clinic's dynamic spatial reconstructor, which uses 28 x-ray tubes positioned around a semicircular gantry. The x-ray tubes are aligned with 28 light amplifiers and TV cameras that are placed behind a single curved fluorescent screen that surrounds the patient. The gantry of x-ray tubes and imaging systems rotates about the patient at a rate of 15 revolutions per minute. This system can acquire the data for an image in about 16 ms. Disadvantages include high cost and the fact that mechanical motion is not eliminated.

Another approach to very fast CT scans eliminates all motion of the x-ray tube or detectors. Magnetic focusing and deflection of an electronic beam replaces x-ray tube motion. In effect, this system positions the patient within the curvature of a giant x-ray tube. The system was developed by Imatron, Inc.* We will describe the basic concept, more details are available in Reference 5. The device is commonly referred to as a cardiovascular computed tomography scanner, or CVCT scanner.

The three basic components of the CVCT scanner are an electron gun with its focusing and deflecting coils, a tungsten target ring 180 cm in diameter, and a ring of detectors. The electron gun has a thermionic cathode and an elaborate set of coils that allow magnetic control of the electron beam. The electron gun is 320 cm long (about 10.5 ft). Electrons are accelerated to about 130 keV and focused onto one of four 180-cm diameter tungsten target rings. When the focused electron beam scans this large target, x-rays are produced and collimated into a 2-cm-wide fan beam by a set of circular collimators. The x-ray beam passes through the patient and is detected by an array of luminescent crystals. Both the tungsten targets and the detector array cover an arc of 210°. The current commercial model contains two rows of 432 detectors each. One scan can be obtained in 50 ms (.05 sec), or a high-resolution mode with a scan time of 100 ms can be used. Because there are four anode targets and two rings of detectors, this scanner can produce eight contiguous tomographic images, each 1 cm thick, without moving the patient. With a 47-cm-diameter scan aperture, this device looks similar to a conventional CT scanner except for the long extension to the rear that is the electron gun and its controls.

X-Ray Tubes

Ideally, the radiation source for CT would supply a monochromatic x-ray beam (i.e., one made up of photons all having the same wavelength). With a monochromatic beam, image reconstruction is simpler and more accurate. Early experimental models used radionuclides to supply such a beam, but radiation intensities were too low to be clinically useful. X-ray tubes are currently being used in all commercial scanners. Earlier models used oil-cooled, fixed-anode, relatively large (2 × 16 mm) focal spot tubes at energies of about 120 kV (constant potential) and 30 mA. The beam was heavily filtered to remove low-energy photons and to increase the mean energy of the radiation.

New fan beam units have a diagnostic-type x-ray tube with a rotating anode and a much smaller focal spot, in some units down to 0.6 mm. These tubes have large heat loading and heat dissipation capabilities to withstand the very high heat loads generated when multiple slices are acquired in rapid sequence. Anode heat capacities as high as 3,500,000 heat units are available, with tube currents of over 600 mA possible.

Collimators

The x-ray beam is collimated at two points, one close to the x-ray tube and the other at the detector(s). Perfect alignment between the two is essential. The collimator at the detector is the sole means of controlling scatter radiation. Each detector has its own collimator. The collimators also regulate the thickness of the tomographic slice (i.e., the voxel length). Most scanners have

---

*Imatron, Inc., San Francisco, CA 94080.

collimators that can be varied to produce different slice thicknesses, typically from 1 to 10 or 15 mm. Choice of slice thickness is usually limited to one of several predetermined values, with choices of 1, 2, 5, or 10 mm being typical examples. Pixel size is determined by the computer program and not by the collimator. The computer can use the input data to print out an image on any size matrix, assuming that there is sufficient data.

Detectors

There are two types of detectors used in CT scanners. These are:

Scintillation crystals

Xenon gas ionization chambers

Xenon gas ionization detectors are limited in use to rotate-rotate (i.e., "third-generation") type scanners, although these scanners may also use scintillation crystal detectors. Rotate-fixed scanners ("fourth generation") must use scintillation crystal detectors. The reasons for these limitations should become clear as we discuss each type of detector.

Scintillation Crystals. Scintillation crystals are any of an extremely large number of materials that produce light as a result of some external influence. More specifically, these materials are those that will produce light (scintillate) when ionizing radiation reacts with them. This is just what an x-ray intensifying screen does. The difference is that an intensifying screen consists of many tiny crystals imbedded in a matrix. Scintillation crystals are normally single crystals of the material. Aside from their larger size, the crystals look different because their surfaces are polished to facilitate extraction of the light. In this polished state they look somewhat like a piece of clear glass or plexiglass.

On a single interaction of a photon with a crystal the energy of the x-ray photon will be converted to light photons, with the number of light photons proportional to the energy of the incident x-ray photon.

Some of these light photons will be emitted promptly and produce the desired signal. Some light photons will be delayed and produce what we will call "afterglow." As in rare earth screens, the color of light emitted is determined by the type crystal and which dopant (activator) it contains. This is pertinent only to those that must match the output light to a light detector. All crystals must be matched to a light detector to convert the light output to an electrical signal.

The combination of a **scintillation crystal** and the **light detector** is called a **scintillation detector.** Scintillation detectors are used by physicists to study radionuclide decay. This is because the electrical signal output of the detector is proportional to the energy of the decay photon. The first two generations of CT scanners used thallium-activated sodium iodide scintillation crystals optically attached to photomultiplier tubes.

Unfortunately, photomultiplier tubes are fairly big (the smallest commercially available being about $\frac{1}{2}$ in. in diameter), and would not easily fit into the large array of detectors used in current CT geometry. In addition, NaI has problems. First, it is hygroscopic and requires an air-tight container. Second, it has a very long afterglow. Most of the light is emitted within 230 nanoseconds (.23 ms), but 9% of the light will be emitted over a time of 0.15 sec (150 ms). It is the buildup of this 9% fraction that causes the afterglow problem with NaI. These problems prompted a search for a different scintillation detector that could be used with newer CT geometry. Large numbers of detectors (over 1000) negate the use of photomultiplier tubes. Fast scan times (over 1000 exposures in 1 sec) negate the use of NaI with its long afterglow.

Photomultiplier tubes have been replaced with silicon photodiodes (sometimes called solid-state photodiodes). A photodiode can convert a light signal into an electron flow (electric current) output that is proportional to the intensity of the light signal. Photodiodes offer the advantage of smaller size, greater stability, and lower cost.

There are several possibilities for replacing NaI. These include cesium iodide (CsI), bismuth germinate (BGO) and cadmium tungstate (CdWO$_4$). Note that some of these chemical formulas are not correct, but this is the form of abbreviation for these crystals that is in common use. All these have short enough decay times that afterglow is not a problem. Their stopping power for x-rays used with CT is almost 100%. A quick survey of manufacturers' specifications (25 units from 6 manufacturers, Jan. 1989) shows that CdWO$_4$ is the scintillator most commonly used in CT units that use scintillation detectors. For example, the Picker International 1200 Expert unit uses 1200 CdWO$_4$ crystals in a rotate-fixed geometry configuration.

All rotate-fixed, and some rotate-rotate, units use scintillation crystal detectors. With rotate-fixed geometry, alignment between rotating x-ray tube and the fixed detectors is constantly changing because the geometry dictates that the detectors must be aligned with (point at) the center of rotation and not the x-ray tube. Thus, as the x-ray tube rotates, the angle from the x-ray tube to the crystal face is constantly changing. Since the angle of incidence can change, detectors with high stopping power must be used to prevent detector crosstalk. Detector crosstalk occurs when a photon strikes a detector, is partially absorbed, and then enters the adjacent detector and is detected again. Crosstalk produces two weak signals coming from two different detectors. Crosstalk is bad because it decreases resolution. Crosstalk is minimized by using a crystal that is highly efficient in absorbing x rays.

Xenon Gas Ionization Chambers

Those rotate-rotate CT units that do not use scintillating crystals use xenon gas ionization chambers. Our review of 25 CT units in January 1989 revealed that 22 are

rotate-rotate units and 3 are rotate-fixed units. Of the 22 rotate-rotate units, 18 use xenon gas detectors (remember that rotate-fixed units may not use xenon gas detectors).

Figure 19–9 illustrates a single gas filled detector. In all detectors there must be:

1. An anode and a cathode
2. A counting gas (inert gas)
3. A voltage between the anode and cathode
4. Walls that separate the detector from the rest of the world
5. A window for the radiation photon to enter the detector

Gas-filled detectors come in a variety of sizes and shapes. Usually a size and shape is selected for a particular application; the gas-filled detectors used with phototimers, therefore, are thin and flat. The one illustrated in Figure 19–9 is more than likely a cyclindrical one. But regardless of the shape or size, all gas-filled detectors use ionization of the gas by the incoming radiation to produce a signal.

Suppose a photon enters a detector. The photon interacts with a gas atom by ionizing the atom into an electron-ion pair. The voltage between the anode and cathode will cause the electron (negative ion) to move toward the anode, and the positive ion (atom minus an electron) to move toward the cathode. When the electrons reach the anode, they produce a small current in the anode. This small current is the output signal from the detector.

Gas-filled detectors may operate in one of three modes. *Which* mode is determined by the voltage. For low voltage, only the negative ions produced by the photon are collected by the anode. A gas-filled detector operating in this mode is called an **ionization chamber. The important characteristic is that the current is directly proportional to the intensity of the incoming radiation.** As the voltage increases, the ions moving under the influence of the voltage acquire sufficient energy to produce sec-

Fig. 19-9 A xenon gas ionization detector

ondary ionization of the gas atoms. For a small range of voltage, the number of secondary ionizations is proportional to the energy of the photons. In this mode of operation the gas-filled detector is called a "proportional counter." Its main characteristic is that the output signal is proportional to the energy of the photon (just like a scintillation detector). With higher voltage, the secondary ionization is so large that the energy proportionality is lost, and all incoming photons register the same-size pulse. In this mode, the gas-filled detector is called a "Geiger counter." Its main characteristic is large signals that are easily recorded. Hand carried survey meters are this type of detector. In CT scanners, we are interested in the x-ray beam intensity, not in the energy of the individual photons. So, the xenon gas-filled detectors are operated in the ionization chamber mode. Thus, the term **xenon gas ionization chamber.**

The principal disadvantage of ionization chambers is their inefficiency. Because of the relatively low density of gases as compared to solids, many x-ray photons pass through the chamber undetected. This problem is at least partially overcome in three ways: (1) by using xenon, the heaviest of the inert gases (atomic number 54); (2) by compressing the xenon 8 to 10 atmospheres to increase its density; and (3) by using a long chamber to increase the number of atoms along the path of the beam. Typical size of a chamber is 1 to 2 mm wide, 10 mm high, and 8 to 10 cm deep. In one scanner, the anode is made of copper and

the cathode side plates are made of tantalum. These 10-cm-long side plates are the reason xenon detectors cannot be used in rotate-fixed type scanners in which the angle at which x rays hit the detector changes constantly. The long plates act as collimators. Obliquely entering x rays would pass through only a short distance of gas before they hit the wall of the detector. In such a case, the x rays are absorbed in the detector walls, and the information they carry is lost for all time. In rotate-rotate type scanners the x-ray tube and detectors maintain a fixed relationship, so the beam is always aligned with the long axis of each detector.

The disadvantage of the xenon gas detector is reduced efficiency. The efficiency of these detectors is in the 50% to 60% range. This low efficiency is caused by two factors: the low density of the absorbing material, and absorption of x rays by the front window, which is needed to contain the high pressure gas.

The selection of detector type is a choice of the manufacturers. Since one cannot tell by looking at the image which type of detector was used, the type of detector becomes relatively unimportant when one is evaluating CT scanners for clinical use today.

IMAGE RECONSTRUCTION

In computed tomography a cross-sectional layer of the body is divided into many tiny blocks such as the ones shown in Figure 19-10, and then each block is assigned a number proportional to the degree that the block attenuated the x-ray

TISSUE SECTION
REPRESENTED IN
COMPUTER MATRIX

Figure 19–10   The tissue section represented in the computer matrix

beam. The individual blocks are called "voxels." Their composition and thickness, along with the quality of the beam, determine the degree of attenuation. The linear attenuation coefficient (μ) is used to quantitate attenuation. The mathematics are really quite simple. We will start by describing the simplest case, a single block of homogeneous tissue (an isolated voxel) and a monochromatic beam of x rays:

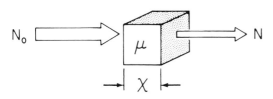

The value of μ, the linear attenuation coefficient, can be calculated with the equation for exponential attenuation described earlier in Chapter 5:

$$N = N_0 e^{-\mu x}$$

In this equation, e is the base of the natural logarithm (2.718). The number of initial photons (N_0), transmitted photons (N), and thickness (x) can all be measured. The linear attenuation coefficient (μ) is the only unknown in the equation.

If two blocks of tissue with different linear attenuation coefficients are placed in the path of the beam, the problem immediately becomes more complex:

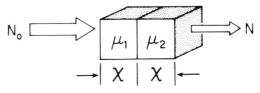

Now the equation has two unknowns, μ_1 and μ_2, and is written as

$$N = N_0 e^{-(\mu_1 + \mu_2)x}$$

The values of μ_1 and μ_2 cannot be determined without additional information. At least one additional equation is required. The additional equation must contain different information than the first, otherwise it is a redundant equation. We must have an independent equation for each unknown in our sample. If we have such independent equations, we can find a unique value for each of the unknowns. If one of the equations is a redundant equation, the very best we can do is determine rations of the unknowns and sometimes we cannot even do that. For example, consider the equations:

$$x + y = 5$$
$$x + 2y = 7$$

These equations can be solved to yield:

$$x = 3$$
$$y = 2$$

and there are no other values that satisfy these equations. This is called a "unique solution." Now consider the equations:

$$x + y = 5$$
$$2x \times 2y = 10$$

These equations cannot be solved for unique values of x and y, and are redundant (obviously, the second equation is nothing more than 2 times the first one). Though the redundancy in this pair of equations is obvious, redundant equations hidden among a few thousand might not be so easy to spot. Additional equations can be obtained by examining the blocks from different directions (i.e., different lines). In this case we will also increase the number of blocks in our example to four, so that each reading represents the composite of two blocks:

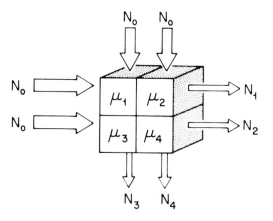

We have gone from two to four unknowns, but we can now construct four different equations:

$$N_1 = N_0 e^{-(\mu_1 + \mu_2)x}$$
$$N_2 = N_0 e^{-(\mu_3 + \mu_4)x}$$
$$N_3 = N_0 e^{-(\mu_1 + \mu_3)x}$$
$$N_4 = N_0 e^{-(\mu_2 + \mu_4)x}$$

This array looks formidable, but the equations can all be simultaneously solved for the value of the linear attenuation coefficient with the aid of a computer. Exactly the same principle applies to computed tomography, but the number of unknowns is much larger. For example, in the original EMI scanner, the matrix in the computer contained 80×80, or 6400, separate picture elements. Each transmission measurement records the composite of 80 separate linear attenuation coefficients:

The equation is longer and looks more awesome, but it has exactly the same format:

$$N = N_0 e^{-(\mu_1 + \mu_2 + \mu_3 + \cdots \mu_{80})x}$$

To solve this equation, we must have transmission readings taken from at least two different directions, just as we did for the simple example above. The number of separate equations and unknowns now becomes at least 6400. The original EMI unit took 28,800 readings (160 linear readings $\times$ 180°). A fan beam scanner may take between 1,000,000 and 2,000,000. The more projections and lines that are collected, the more equations that may be constructed. Therefore, the little voxels may be smaller. An equation like the one shown above can be reconstructed for each of these readings. Even though Radon understood the mathematical principles in 1917, he could not put his knowledge to practical use. The mathematics were so tediously long that before computers it would have taken years to construct a single image.

Two correction factors are incorporated into the CT program. The first is a correction for the heterochromatic (polychromatic) nature of the beam. As heterochromatic radiation passes through an absorber, filtration increases its mean energy. The linear attenuation coefficient changes with energy, as shown in Figure 19–11. The illustration compares the linear attenuation coefficients of water for 70-keV monochromatic and 120-kVp heterochromatic beams. The initial mean energy of the heterochromatic beam is 70 keV. The monochromatic linear attenuation coefficient (μ) is constant, but the heterochromatic μ strays down on the graph as filtration increases its mean energy from 70 to 75 keV. The CT program must be written to compensate for this stray and bring the calculated μ back to a straight line.

The second program correction is a weighting factor to compensate the differences between the size and shape of the scanning beam and the picture matrix. Figure 19–12A shows the problem geometrically. In Figure 19–12A, the parallel rays of a linear-type scanning motion exactly coincide with the size and square shape of the picture elements. In Figure 19–12B, the

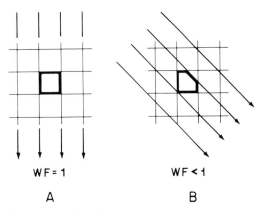

WF = 1   WF < 1

A   B

Figure 19–12 When only a portion of a pixel is included in the scanning beam, a weighting factor (WF) is used in the mathematical reconstruction

scanning rays cross the picture elements obliquely. A weighting factor (WF) is used to compensate for the difference in size between the actual elements and that seen by the beam. In these examples, the weighting factor would be 1 in Figure 19–12A and less than 1 in Figure 19–12B.

Algorithms for Image Reconstruction

An algorithm is a mathematical method for solving a problem. Thousands of equations must be solved to determine the linear attenuation coefficients of all the pixels in the image matrix. Several different methods, or algorithms, are in current use. They all attempt to solve the equations as rapidly as possible without compromising accuracy. The original EMI scanner took 4 to 5 minutes to process the data for a single CT section. This long processing time seriously limited the number of patients that could be handled in a working day. More recent algorithms are much faster and can display a picture immediately after the tomographic slice is completed. We have tried to make the discussion more pictorial than mathematical, because the actual mathematics go beyond the intended scope of this text. The following three mathematical methods of image reconstruction will be described:

Figure 19–11 The linear attenuation coefficient of a heterochromatic beam decreases as filtration increases its mean energy

1. Back-projection
2. Iterative methods
3. Analytical methods

The object of all the methods is to produce an accurate cross-sectional display of the linear attenuation coefficients of each element in the image matrix.

Back-Projection. Back-projection, sometimes called the "summation method," is the oldest means of image reconstruction. None of the commercial CT scanners uses simple back-projection, but it is the easiest method to describe so we will use it as a prototype. The principle is shown schematically in Figure 19–13, which demonstrates a two-dimensional reconstruction of a cross cut from the center of a solid block. The block is scanned (Fig. 19–13A) from both the top and left sides by a moving x-ray beam to produce the image profile shown in Figure 19–13B. The image pro-

files look like steps. The height of the steps is proportional to the amount of radiation that passed through the block. The center transmitted the most radiation, so it is the highest step in the image profile. The steps are then assigned to a gray scale density that is proportional to their height. These densities are arranged in rows, called "rays" (Fig. 19–13C). The width of the rays is the same as the width of the steps in the profile. In the illustration the ray length is equal to the height of the original object, but in an actual clinical situation, in which the image is displayed on a television monitor, these heights and widths could be any convenient size. When the rays from the two projections are superimposed, or back-projected, they produce a crude reproduction of the original object (Fig. 19–13D). In practice many more projections would be added to improve image quality, but the principle is the same.

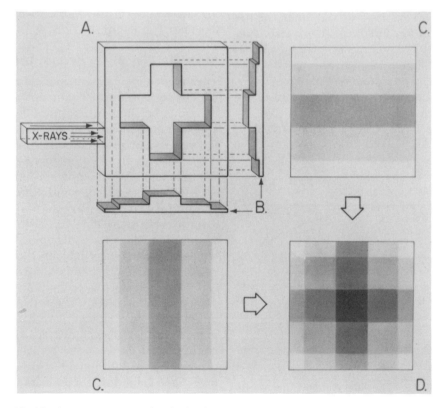

Figure 19–13 Image reconstruction by back-projection

All points in the back-projected image receive density contributions from neighboring structures. The result of these contributions is dramatized in Figure 19–14. The black dot in Figure 19–14A represents a radiodense material, such as a surgical clip. The radiodense material severely attenuates the beam and produces localized spikes in the image profiles. Back-projection of the rays from these spikes produces a star pattern like the one shown in Figure 19–14B. A great number of projections will obscure the star pattern, but the background density remains as noise to deteriorate the quality of the CT image.

Iterative Methods. An iterative reconstruction starts with an assumption (for example, that all points in the matrix have the same value) and compares this assumption with measured values, makes corrections to bring the two into agreement, and then repeats the process over and over until the assumed and measured values are the same or within acceptable limits. There are three variations of itera-

tive reconstructions, depending on whether the correction sequence involves the whole matrix, one ray, or a single point.

Simultaneous Reconstruction. All projections for the entire matrix are calculated at the beginning of the iteration, and all corrections are made simultaneously for each iteration.

Ray-by-Ray Correction. One ray sum is calculated and corrected, and these corrections are incorporated into future ray sums, with the process being repeated for every ray in each iteration.

Point-by-Point Correction. The calculations and corrections are made for all rays passing through one point, and these corrections are used in ensuing calculations, again with the process being repeated for every point.

Figure 19–15 illustrates a ray-by-ray iterative reconstruction for a four-element square. Horizontal, vertical, and diagonal ray sums are shown in the adjacent blocks. In the first step, the two horizontal ray sums (16 and 6 in the hatched blocks) are

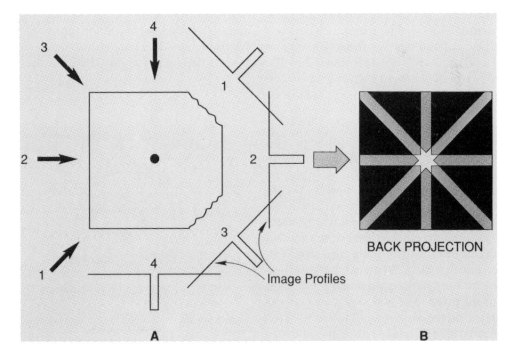

Figure 19–14 Star pattern from back-projection of a dense object

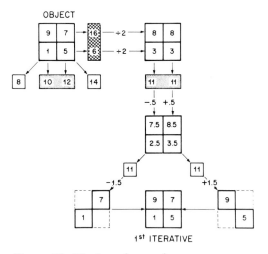

Figure 19–15 Iterative ray-by-ray reconstruction of a four-element object

divided equally among the two elements in the ray. If the ray sums had represented 10 elements, the sum would have been divided equally among all 10 elements. Next, the new numbers in the vertical row are added to produce the new ray sums (11 and 11 in the shaded blocks) and compared with the original measured ray sums (also in shaded blocks). The difference between the original and new ray sums $(10 - 11 = -1$ and $12 - 11 = +1)$ is divided by the number of elements in the ray $(-1 \div 2 = -0.5$ and $+1 \div 2 = +0.5)$. These differences are algebraically added to each element $(8 - 0.5 = 7.5, 3 - 0.5 = 2.5, 8 + 0.5 = 8.5,$ and $3 + 0.5 = 3.5)$. The process is repeated for diagonal ray sums to complete the first iteration. In this example, the first iteration produces a perfect reconstruction. With more complex data, iterations may have to be repeated 6 to 12 times to reach an acceptable level of agreement between the calculated and measured values. The first 80×80 matrix EMI scanner used an iterative reconstruction, but most manufacturers are now using one of the analytic methods.

Analytic Methods. Analytic methods are used in almost all x-ray CT today. These algorithms differ from iterative methods in

that exact formulas are utilized for the analytical reconstructions. These formulas are frighteningly complex to most radiologists, although mathematicians say they are really quite simple. We will only attempt a pictorial explanation of the two popular analytic methods, two-dimensional Fourier analysis and filtered backprojection.

Two-Dimensional Fourier Analysis. The basis of Fourier analysis is that any function of time or space can be represented by the sum of various frequencies and amplitudes of sine and cosine waves. Figure 19–16 shows three functions: projections of a phantom skull containing bone, air, and calcium. The ray projections are shown with squared edges, which is the most difficult wave form to reproduce. The actual projected images would be more rounded than those shown, which would simplify a Fourier reconstruction.

Figure 19–17 shows progressively improving Fourier reconstructions. A single cosine wave of the appropriate height (amplitude) and length (frequency) makes a first approximation of the square wave, and each subsequent addition improves the reproduction. The last reconstruction represents the sum of eight cosine waves, but

Figure 19–16 Projections of a skull phantom

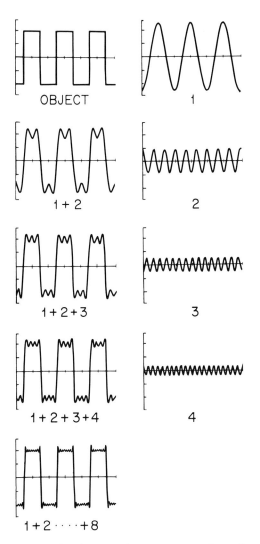

OBJECT

1 + 2

1 + 2 + 3

1 + 2 + 3 + 4

1 + 2 · · · · + 8

1

2

3

4

Figure 19–17 Fourier reconstruction of a square wave form

only the first four steps are shown. This type of mathematical manipulation is easily and quickly processed in a computer. The construction is a little more complex for a two-dimensional image such as a CT section, but the basic principle is the same.

Filtered Back-Projection. Filtered back-projection is similar to back-projection except that the image is filtered, or modified, to exactly counterbalance the effect of sudden density changes, which causes blurring (the star pattern) in simple back-projection. The projected information is filtered much like light is filtered by a polarizing lens. Those frequencies responsible for blurring are eliminated to enhance more desirable frequencies. Figure 19–18 is a two-dimensional filtered back-projection of a square object. The density of the projected rays is adjusted to compensate for the star effect; that is, the inside margins of dense areas are enhanced while the centers and immediately adjacent areas are repressed. The net effect is an image more closely resembling the original object than could have been achieved with back-projection alone. Image quality is further improved with each additional projection. Most CT units use a Fourier reconstruction or filtered back-projection.

Comparison of Mathematical Methods

No general agreement exists as to which mathematical method is superior and, indeed, a system's superiority under one set of circumstances may disappear under new circumstances. In terms of speed, analytical reconstructions are clearly faster than iterative methods. A projection can be processed immediately after recording, so the entire reconstruction can be displayed seconds after completion of the last projection. Iterative reconstructions may take several minutes to process after scan completion. Both methods are equally accurate if the projection data are complete. With incomplete data (i.e., insufficient to determine the image fully), iterative methods are superior. Analytic methods must do time-consuming interpolations to fill in missing data, whereas iterative methods simply average adjacent points. Thus, with incomplete data, analytical methods are slowed while iterative methods are actually made faster than they would be with complete data.

CT Numbers

The CT scanner calculates, from the collected data, the linear attenuation coefficient (μ) of each pixel. After the CT computer calculates a value for the linear

FILTRATION

Figure 19–18 Filtered back-projection of a square object

attenuation coefficient of each pixel, the value is converted to a new number called a "CT" number. Why do this calculation? The calculation allows the computer to present the information as a picture with a large gray scale.

How is a CT number determined? The computer calculates a relationship between the linear absorption coefficient of a pixel and μ for water. The calculation follows the equation:

$$CT\ number = \frac{K\ (\mu_p - \mu_w)}{\mu_w}$$

K = Magnification constant
μ_p = Pixel linear attenuation coefficient
μ_w = Water linear attenuation coefficient

It is rather easy to see that the CT number for air (we will assume air stops little or no x rays) will be equal to $-K$, and that the CT number for water will be 0. If dense

bone has a linear attenuation coefficient of about 0.38 cm^{-1} and water has a linear attenuation coefficient of about 0.19 cm^{-1}, then the CT number for this bone will be $+K$ because:

$$CT\ number\ bone = K\left(\frac{.38 - .19}{.19}\right) = K\left(\frac{.19}{.19}\right) = K$$

In currently available CT units, K has a value of 1000. With this value of K, the CT number for air becomes -1000, for water the CT number is still 0, and for dense bone becomes 1000. To image materials with a higher linear attenuation coefficient than dense bone, such as a metallic surgical clip, CT numbers larger than 1000 should be available. In fact, the 1989 survey shows that most units have CT numbers from about -1000 to $+4000$. To honor Hounsfield, CT numbers based on a magnification constant of 1000 are also called Hounsfield units (H). Since new CT scanners use a magnification constant of 1000, CT numbers and H units are equivalent for these scanners.

The original EMI scanner used a magnification constant of 500, and its CT numbers ranged from -500 (air) to $+500$ (dense bone).

An interesting exercise will help us appreciate the accuracy with which a CT scanner must calculate linear absorption coefficients for each pixel. Water has a linear absorption coefficient of about 0.191 cm^{-1}.

CT Number	μ_p(cm^{-1})
868	.35679
869	.35698
870	.35717
871	.35736
872	.35755

Notice that the change in μ_p takes place in the fourth decimal place. We include five of these calculations because manufacturers indicate that the noise error is about ± 2 CT numbers, and the calculated μ_p gives a feel for the extreme accuracy of these new scanners. Note also that our use of 0.191 cm^{-1} for μ_w is inadequate for calculations requiring this degree of accuracy.

Image Display

A CT image is usually displayed on a television monitor for immediate viewing, and recorded on film for interpretation and permanent storage. Our 1989 survey shows that the display matrix was on the average 512×512, with some units having 1024×1024 (this is really rather variable among manufacturers). All but one display had 256 shades of gray. We find ourselves in an interesting situation from two points of view. The first interesting thing is that we are going to image CT numbers ranging from -1000 to about $+1000$ with 256 shades of gray. The second interesting thing deals with pixel size. Pixel size is, on the average, about 0.1 mm (this again varies from one manufacturer to another). If we displayed the full image, we would have several pixels per TV matrix point. For ex-

ample, a typical scan field of view is as large as 40 cm. With a pixel size of 0.1 mm, a 40-cm scan field will contain 4000 pixels per line. These 4000 pixels, displayed on a 512×512 TV monitor, will result in about 8 pixels per matrix element in the monitor. In normal display of the full field of view of a scan, the CT scanner system does not take advantage of the full range of information. On the other hand, if we use only 512×512 pixels (of the 4000×4000 available) for the display, we will have unique information for each matrix point in the display image (and we will have magnified the image displayed by a factor of 8).

Now let us return to the first interesting thing, which is how to display CT numbers from -1000 to $+1000$ with only 256 shades of gray. Obviously, one could simply assign about 8 CT numbers to the same shade of gray, and display the entire range of information in a compressed scale. This is rarely done. Instead, one usually selects a CT number that will be about the average CT number of the body tissue being examined. Such a CT number might be -200 for air (lung), $+20$ to $+40$ for retroperitoneal soft tissues, or $+200$ for bone. The computer may then be instructed to assign one shade of gray to each of the 128 CT numbers below and each of the 128 CT numbers above the baseline CT number. For example, a general view of the abdomen will center at CT number 20, and display CT numbers -108 to $+148$ as 256 gray levels. The center CT number is called the "window level," and the range of CT numbers above and below the window level is called the "window width." It is possible to set the window level at any desired CT number. Window width is also variable to any width desired by the operator. Generally one does not pick a window width of exactly 256, and window width will vary widely depending on the type of examination or pathology. Windowing obviously limits viewing to a narrow portion of the total information available. In practice, multiple window levels and multiple window widths may be examined in an effort to extract maximum diagnostic information from each examination.

Recording the image produced by the CT scanner is usually done with a multi-format camera. The manner in which the CT scan information is presented to the camera is variable and often complex, and we will not discuss the topic. The resulting image is recorded on film designed especially for such purposes. A more recently introduced recording system uses a laser to directly record images on film. The digital information from the CT scanner is used to modulate a laser beam that scans and exposes the film. Direct use of digital information to produce a photographic image is useful in many imaging modalities, including ultrasound, nuclear medicine, magnetic resonance imaging, CT scanning, and digital radiography.

IMAGE QUALITY

Image quality is not accurately defined for computed tomography. We will attempt to use the same terms and definitions described for the radiographic image. Image quality (clarity) is the visibility of diagnostically important structures in the CT image. The factors that affect quality are all interrelated, so when we discuss one we will frequently refer to the others. The more important factors are defined below under three separate headings:

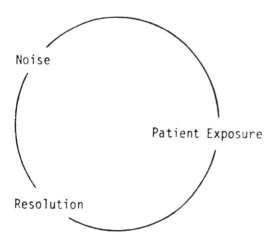

These three factors are intimately tied together, but we will discuss them separately. All other factors affecting image quality will be included under these three headings.

Quantum Mottle (Noise)

Precision in computed tomography is a measure of background, or matrix uniformity. If a perfectly homogeneous object such as a water bath is examined with a CT scanner, all elements in the picture matrix should have exactly the same CT number. Deviations from uniformity represent statistical fluctuations, called "quantum mottle." We will use the terms "quantum mottle" and "noise" interchangeably. **A lack of precision, or the presence of mottle, is the limiting factor in CT performance at the present time.** Contemporary scanners have noise values in the range of 0.2 to 0.4%. Expressed in H units, this means that pixels must vary by more than 2 to 4 H units for the variation to be statistically significant. The quantum mottle is due to the statistical emission of photons from the x-ray tube. The statistical fluctuation is a function of the number of photons emitted. The standard deviation is a measure of noise, and is:

$$\sigma = \frac{\sqrt{N}}{N}$$

σ = Standard deviation
N = Number of x-ray photons

Figure 19–19 shows anticipated statistical fluctuations as a function of the number of counts in a ray projection. Counts of 100, 1000, 10,000, and 100,000 are shown as paired bar graphs, with each bar in the pair representing 1 standard deviation (SD) above and below the anticipated value. The counts are normalized to demonstrate the decrease in percentage fluctuation. At 100 counts, the statistical fluctuation is $\pm 10\%$, or from 90 to 110 counts. As the number of counts increases, the percent fluctuation decreases. At 10,000 counts, 1 SD is 100 counts ($10,000^{1/2} = 100$), which

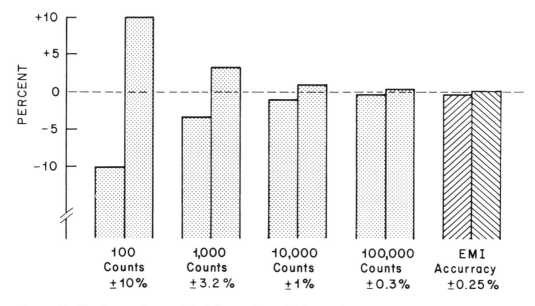

Figure 19–19 Decreasing statistical fluctuations with increasing count rates

is a percentage fluctuation of ±1% (100 ÷ 10,000 = 1%).

The statistical nature of the x-ray beam is generated in the x-ray tube, carried through the patient, and recorded by the detectors. Remember this important fact. **Quantum mottle, or noise, is variation in the number of x-ray photons absorbed by the detector.** At the detector, noise is still determined by the number of photons absorbed (detected). The only way to decrease noise is to increase the number of photons absorbed by the detector. The way to increase the number of photons absorbed is to increase x-ray dose to the patient.

Precision cannot be improved by a more accurate mathematical reconstruction. In fact, mottle becomes more visible as the accuracy of the reconstruction improves. This principle is shown diagrammatically in Figure 19–20, a bar graph similar to the one shown earlier in Figure 19–19. The heights of the shaded bars depict the actual number of counts in two adjacent ray projections of a water phantom. Because the phantom is homogeneous, the difference in the counts between the two bars repre-

sents noise (statistical fluctuations). Employing an iterative algorithm after the first iteration, the two bars are almost the same height and, if the image were displayed at this time, the noise would be smoothed out and the image would appear quite homogeneous. Each iteration more closely approximates the reconstructed image to the original data until finally, after many iterations, the two are nearly identical. The image will then show the noise more accurately than the earlier reconstruction. **Most of the noise in current CT images is a result of statistical fluctuations and is not related to the mathematical reconstruction.**

The number of counts per picture element is determined by numerous factors, including the quantity and quality of the x-ray beam, the number and efficiency of the detectors, the amount of absorber in the path of the beam, the number and volume of the picture element, and the scan time. Short scan times are generally desirable because they minimize the effect of patient motion. For any given scanner and voxel size, however, scan times can only be shortened at the expense of precision.

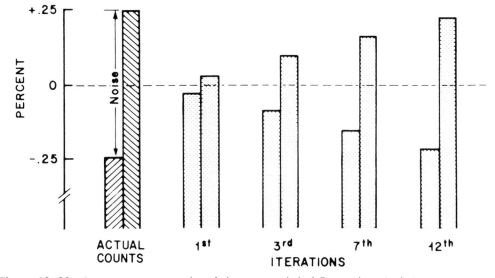

Figure 19–20   Accurate reconstructions bring out statistical fluctuations (noise)

When high-quality images are essential, scan times may have to be lengthened to produce a statistically more accurate reconstruction. Contemporary scanners offer scan times as fast as 1 sec, or a little less. The same units, in a high resolution mode, have scan times of about 8 to 10 sec.

Counting statistics are intimately related to voxel size. **A voxel is a volume element, as opposed to a pixel, which is a picture element.** A pixel is a flat surface without thickness. The image is displayed on a television monitor as thousands of tiny pixels, each representing a specific tiny cross-sectional area in the patient. The stated size of a pixel, such as 3 × 3 mm, refers to the size of the patient. Their actual size in a video image is determined by the size of the television monitor. A given size of pixel will appear larger on a large TV monitor than it would on a smaller monitor, but in both cases it would represent the same area in the patient. A voxel adds the third dimension to the area represented by the pixel, so the voxel is a volume element. A 1-mm square pixel might represent a 5- or 10-mm thick section; the first would be a 5-mm³ and the second a 10-mm³ voxel. Diminishing voxel size decreases the number of counts per each element, assuming that

other factors remain constant. In the next two paragraphs we will use pixel size of the original EMI scanner. We recognize that this is larger than current pixel sizes, and that the display matrix is considerably smaller than in newer units. Contemporary CT scanners have pixel sizes of about 0.1 to 1.0 mm, and display matrices ranging from 256 × 256 to 1024 × 1024. The figures used aptly illustrate the points to be discussed. Table 19–1 shows the size of some EMI voxels with volume factors and patient exposure factors normalized to the original 3- × 3-mm pixel (80 × 80 matrix) and the 13-mm thick section of the original EMI scanner. Assuming that the counting statistics (precision) are kept constant, the superior resolution of the smallest sized (18-mm³) voxel can only be realized with a 6.5-fold increase in patient exposure. An important point to keep in mind when selecting techniques is that noise is less with an 80 × 80 matrix than with a 160 × 160 matrix for any given patient exposure.

Matrix size, field size, and pixel size are all interrelated as shown in Figure 19–21. Matrix size is the number of points in a picture matrix, 6400 (80 × 80) in Figure 19–21A and 25,600 (160 × 160) in both Figure 19–21B and C. The name **matrix**

Table 19–1. Relationship Between Voxel Size and Patient Exposure

VOXEL SIZE (mm)	VOLUME (mm³)	VOLUME FACTOR	PATIENT EXPOSURE FACTOR*
3 × 3 × 13	117	1.0	1.0
3 × 3 × 8	72	0.62	1.6
1.5 × 1.5 × 13	29.3	0.25	4.0
1.5 × 1.5 × 8	18	0.15	6.5

*For comparable counting statistics.

size is firmly entrenched in the CT literature, but it is a confusing name, because the "size" refers to the size of a unitless number and not to a physical size. **Field size** (x and 2x in Figure 19–21) refers to the outside dimensions of the CT slice (e.g., 27 × 27 cm in the original EMI scanner). Field size dictates the maximum size of anatomic part that can be examined. The smaller field size shown in Figure 19–21A and B might be used for head scans, while the larger size in Figure 19–21C could accommodate a larger part and might be used for body scans. Note that the matrix size is the same in Figure 19–21A and B and the pixel size is the same in Figure 19–21A and C. In current rotate-rotate and rotate-fixed CT units the scan field of view generally ranges from about 40 cm to 50 cm. The entire field is scanned for any CT image, but one may choose to display only a small segment of this area. Small areas of display may be used in high resolution modes which we will discuss shortly.

Continuing with Figure 19–21, if exactly the same precision (counting statistics) were required for the pixel in all three blocks, the patient exposure would have to be increased four times in going from the 80 × 80 to either of the 160 × 160 matrices, because there are four times as many pixels in the larger matrix. As we shall discuss next, resolution is a function of pixel size. With equal exposures per voxel (equal noise), resolution would be better in Figure 19–21B than in Figure 19–21A because the pixels are smaller in Figure 19–21B. Resolution would be equal in both Figure 19–21A and C, because both have the same-sized pixels. Remember that a voxel (volume element) is a small volume of the patient in the scan beam. This three-di-

Figure 19–21 Comparison of field size (×, 2×), matrix size (80 × 80, 160 × 160), and pixel size (1.5 mm, 3 mm)

mensional voxel attenuates the incident x-ray beam. The image resulting from the x-ray beam attenuation in one voxel is displayed on the TV monitor as a pixel (picture element). A pixel lives on the TV monitor and is derived from a voxel that lives inside the patient. If you look at the voxel on end you will see the size of a pixel. Suppose you look at the end of a voxel in a patient and see a square 1 mm on each side. Without magnification, the pixel size to be displayed for this voxel would be 1 mm^3. With magnification at the detectors, the displayed pixel would be slightly larger than 1 mm^2. This is why we said a few paragraphs back that pixel size refers to size of the patient.

Resolution

Resolution has two components, **spatial resolution** and **contrast resolution.** Spatial resolution of a CT unit is its ability to display, as separate images, two objects that are very close to each other. Contrast resolution of a CT unit is the ability to display, as distinct images, areas that differ in density by a small amount. Contrast and spatial resolution are intimately related to each other and to the radiation dose absorbed by the detector (i.e., noise or quantum mottle). Attempts to improve spatial resolution may cause increased noise levels that decrease contrast resolution. Attempts to improve contrast resolution by increasing scan times (larger dose) may decrease spatial resolution by increasing the effects of patient motion.

Spatial Resolution. Spatial resolution is the ability of the CT scanner to display separate images of two objects placed close together. Spatial resolution measurements are determined by using test objects of high contrast. High contrast test objects make it possible to ignore the effect of noise on spatial resolution measurements. The usual test object consists of small holes drilled at varying distances from each other in a piece of plexiglass (for CT units air versus plexiglass is very high contrast).

High contrast spatial resolution is determined by the **scanner design, computer reconstruction,** and the **display** (this list excludes patient motion over which design engineers have no control).

Scanner design includes x-ray tube focal spot size, detector size, and magnification. X-ray tubes have been designed for CT scanners to have fairly small focal spots and high anode heat storage capabilities. Typical focal spot sizes range from slightly under to slightly over 1 mm (dual focal spots are available in some units), with anode heat storage capacities ranging from roughly 1,000,000 to over 2,500,000 heat units.

Detector size influences spatial resolution of a CT scanner. Detector size places a limit on maximum spatial resolution. To increase resolution, it is possible to put an aperture in front of a detector and effectively reduce detector size. The detectors in some contemporary CT units are apertured by sliding metal pins in front of the detector when a high resolution mode is required. Note that there is one pin for each detector. In rotate-rotate and rotate-fixed scanners there is built-in magnification because the patient is near the center of axis of rotation. It is not possible to place a patient close to the detectors and far from the x-ray tube as we do in routine film-screen radiography. The magnification factor will vary from about 1.6 or 1.7 to 2.0. Resolution is measured at the detectors, but is referred back into the patient. We would expect magnification to increase resolution of the unit (since we assure the focal spot is small enough that it does not limit resolution in the rather gross ranges we will be considering). To record a line pair, we must have one detector for the opaque line and one detector for the space adjacent to the opaque object. If the line pair is smaller, the detector will average the opaque and adjacent line in some fashion and the line pair will not be resolved. Some manufacturers list resolution in mm; others list resolution as line pairs per cm. We will interpret a resolution of 0.5 mm as 10 line pairs per centimeter (i.e., 10 lines 0.5 mm wide separated by 10 spaces 0.5 mm wide). Resolution of 10 line pairs per cm means the same as resolution of 0.5 mm. Remember, this is resolution in the patient. Detector size recording the image of the 0.5 mm object may be larger than 0.5 mm (multiply object size by magnification to arrive at minimum detector size). Contemporary CT units have advertised resolution capabilities of up to 15 line pairs per cm. Note that resolution is expressed in line pairs per centimeter, not line pairs per mm as in film-screen radiography.

Although we have listed **computer reconstruction** as a determining factor for resolution, in reality the resolution capability is determined by the scanner design discussed above. What is required of the reconstruction matrix is that it be large enough to distinguish the high contrast resolution. If we are going to have a 10 lp/cm resolution in a 40-cm CT field, we can determine the minimum size of the reconstruction matrix that will reconstruct such a resolution. First, it is again necessary to have a minimum of one pixel for an opaque line and one pixel for the adjacent space. To meet this criterion of a minimum of one pixel per line, 10 lp/cm information would require 20 pixels per cm. A 40-cm line would require 40 × 20, or 800 pixels minimum. Obviously, for equal resolution throughout the image, we will require 800 × 800 pixels. Thus, we require a minimum reconstruction matrix of 800 × 800, or 640,000 matrix point (pixels) for our example (in this example we would be required to collect a minimum of 640,000 non-redundant scan lines). The reconstruction matrix must be large enough to reconstruct all available information, or information will be lost. But, the reconstruction matrix can never add information.

The **display** is what you look at. Really, the display is the unit that shows you the picture. This unit looks like a TV monitor, but it is not a TV monitor. What is the difference? A TV monitor, such as your home TV or routine fluoroscopic TVs, uses interlaced scanning. The number of scan lines available for displaying an image is significantly less than the total scan lines. Interlaced scanning is used when motion must be displayed without flicker. Interlacing makes the display of a moving object pleasing to the eye. In all computed tomography, motion in a single displayed image is not a consideration (in fact it is not available). Therefore, for CT, a non-interlaced full matrix monitor can be used. This means that a 512 × 512 monitor will display a full 512-pixel resolution in both horizontal and vertical dimensions. Most contemporary CT units have a display matrix of 512 × 512, a few units have less and a few have as high as 1024 × 1024. If we assume a 512 × 512 matrix, we could not display the example given in the last paragraph where an 800 × 800 matrix would be required. We can overcome this problem by selecting an area of interest that is smaller than the full field, in which case the display monitor will be able to show sufficient resolution. Contemporary CT units allow some choice of field of view and resolving power. For example, a unit with a 50-cm field of view may be used with a resolving power of 5 lp/cm to produce lines with 500 pixels of information per line. A 512 × 512 monitor will display this information. The same unit using a 50-cm field of view with a resolving power of 10 lp/cm would require a 1000 × 1000 matrix monitor to display the full field and show 10 lp/cm any place in the image. Actually, a 512 × 512 matrix monitor could display a pleasing image of this high resolution matrix by adding four adjacent pixels (two in each direction) together and displaying them as one pixel. Obviously, such pixel averaging will reduce resolution in the displayed image by a factor of two. The effect of pixel size, either in the image data or in the display, is illustrated in Figure 19–22. The letters EMI are first displayed on a 32 × 32 matrix (1024 pixels). There is a

Figure 19–22   Resolution improves with a large matrix (smaller pixels)

marked improvement in image quality when the letters are displayed in an 80 × 80 matrix (6400 pixels). The unobtainable goal is a matrix with an infinite number of points, which would resolve anything. A display with a 1024 × 1024 matrix (1,048,576 pixels) would come close to the ideal. We can at least appreciate how increasing the matrix size (decreasing pixel size) will improve high contrast spatial resolution.

Perhaps high contrast should be more accurately defined. In computed tomography the difference between Plexiglas and water is considered to be high contrast, and their linear attenuation coefficients differ by approximately 12% at an effective energy of 70 keV. With this sort of contrast, resolution is pixel-size limited. The differences between air and water, or between water and bone, are enormous by CT standards. For example, a tiny fleck of calcium in a pineal gland, a fleck too small to be seen on a radiograph, may be easily seen on a CT scan. **The calculated linear attenuation coefficient for a pixel is a weighted average of all materials in the pixel.** Photoelectric attenuation is so much greater for calcium than for water that a small amount of calcium weights the average toward the higher linear attenuation coefficient of calcium. With even a small amount of calcium, a whole picture element appears white. This effect is called **partial volume averaging.** The predominance of calcium over water has a deleterious effect on

imaging in some circumstances. Figure 19–23 shows how the skull can obscure large areas of brain, especially in the more superficial cuts in which the tomographic slice traverses the calvarium obliquely. In slice A, five picture elements contain bone (shaded pixels), whereas only two contain bone in slice B. In the shaded area the brain is hidden from view by the calvarium.

Contrast Resolution. Contrast resolution may be defined as the ability of an imaging system to display an image of a relatively large (2- or 3-mm) object that is only slightly different in density from its surroundings. For the image to be visible, the object must produce enough change in the number of transmitted photons to overcome statistical fluctuations in transmitted photons caused by noise. Low contrast visibility is determined by noise. The more homogeneous the background, the better the visibility of low contrast images. And, of course, homogeneity of the background is a function of noise. The only way that resolution can be improved for low contrast objects is with better counting statistics, which produces a more homogeneous background. Low contrast resolution may be studied quantitatively by comparing two plastics whose linear attenuation coefficients differ by approximately 1%. With a 1-cm object, a subject contrast of 1%, and a fixed patient exposure, visibility may be better with 3-mm pixels than it is with 0.5 mm pixels because the counting statistics are better with the large pixels

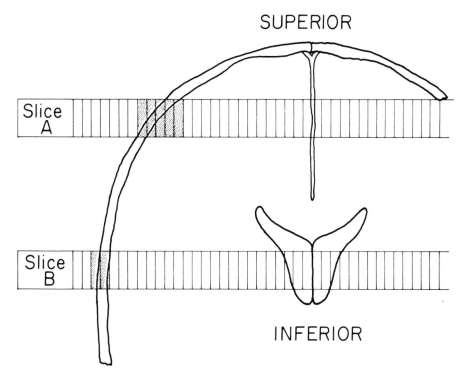

SUPERIOR

Slice A

Slice B

INFERIOR

Figure 19–23 Apparent increase in skull thickness when the bone is cut obliquely, such as by slice A.

(Fig. 19–24). The illustration represents a portion of a CT matrix, uniformly radiated to 10,000 counts per unit element (i.e., small squares). The number of counts in the smaller squares will vary statistically by 1%. This is the same percentage as the subject contrast, and the object will be obscured in this noisy background. With the larger pixels, the statistical fluctuation is only 0.5%, and the 1% subject contrast should be visible against this more uniform background.

With film-screen radiography, a density difference of about 10% is required for contrast resolution (the density of fat is about 0.92, and muscle about 1.06). Contemporary CT scanners can display objects about 3 mm in diameter with density differences of 0.5% or less. These data indicate there has been an almost overwhelming improvement in low contrast visibility with CT scanning (let us remind you that high contrast resolution is not as great in

CT scanning as in film-screen radiography). Even with improved low contrast resolution some pathologic processes remain undetected. Use of iodinated contrast materials to enhance subject contrast is an accepted practice in most head and body CT scanning protocols.

PATIENT EXPOSURE

Theoretically, each small increment of tissue in a CT scan is exposed only during the time that the slice containing the increment is being tomogrammed. At other times the increment is exposed only to scatter radiation, which is minimal because of the narrow beam. Because the scan fields do not overlap, the absorbed doses are not compounded. The theory is only partially true. Dose measurements are usually determined with an appropriate phantom. A single measurement made at the slice level is not sufficient because a slice receives a small dose of scatter radiation when adja-

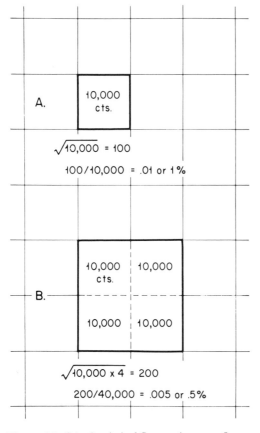

Figure 19–24 Statistical fluctuations are fewer with large pixels

cent slices are scanned. A dosimeter is placed in a phantom at the center of a slice, then scans are made through the center slice and for several slices on each side (perhaps three on each side). Typical doses range from about 2 cGy (rads) to about 4.0 cGy. It is interesting that dose rates have remained about the same in all types of CT scanners.

Dose is intimately related to contrast resolution and spatial resolution. Contrast resolution improves only if counting statistics improve, and the only way to improve counting statistics (i.e., decrease noise) is with more x-ray photons. Improved spatial resolution requires smaller pixel size, which requires smaller voxel size. If one decreases the volume of tissue from which a signal is generated and leaves dose the same, the dose per volume will decrease. Thus, improved spatial resolution will be at the expense of increased noise unless dose is increased. Improvement of both contrast resolution and spatial resolution always requires increased patient dose.

ARTIFACTS

With contemporary CT units, artifacts due to equipment defects are rare. Short scan times have diminished but not eliminated motion artifacts. Artifacts at the edge of high contrast objects may also be seen (we will call these "streak artifacts"). Beam-hardening effects are minimized by reconstruction programs, but we need to understand the concept. The one equipment defect that may be seen is a ring artifact caused by failure of a detector.

Motion Artifacts

Patient motion has a devastating effect on image quality. This is the primary reason for developing faster scan units, including the 50-μsec unit used to image cardiovascular structures. When the patient moves during scan acquisition, the reconstruction program has no ability to make appropriate corrections because motion is random and unpredictable. The reconstructed image will display an object in motion as a streak in the direction of motion. On reconstruction the scanner will average the density of the pixels covering the motion area. In some fashion, the intensity of the streak artifact will depend on the density of the object in motion. Motion of objects that have densities much different from their surroundings produces more intense artifacts. Thus, motion of metallic or gas-containing structures produce striking artifacts. Figure 19–25 illustrates motion artifacts produced when a patient sneezed during the examination. Notice how the artifact produced by motion of gas in the stomach produces large streaks in the image.

Figure 19–25 Motion artifacts produced by a sneeze (A) compared to the normal appearance of stomach gas (B).

Streak Artifacts

One of the basic assumptions in CT scanning is that each detector, at every position, will observe some transmitted radiation. If a high density material severely reduces the transmission, the detector may record no transmission. This violates the basic assumption, and the reconstruction program will not account for such a violation. Streaks will appear in the image. Even for high density materials that do transmit some x rays, the filter in the reconstruction program is not designed to perfectly reproduce the high density to average density interface. Some CT units expand the CT numbers well above those numbers associated with dense bone in order to assign a linear absorption coefficient to materials that are denser than bone. A 1989 survey indicates that almost all units now have CT numbers that range from at least -1000 to $+3000$, and some have a greater range. In these cases the CT numbers $+1000$ to $+3000$ are for materials whose densities are greater than dense bone, whose density is about 2 gm cm^{-3}. Figure 19–26 illustrates an artifact caused by a shotgun pellet in the soft tissues of the flank. This is the same patient who sneezed to give us Figure 19–25.

Beam-Hardening Artifacts

Unfortunately, the x-ray beam producing the CT image is not a monochromatic beam. The beam contains x rays with many energies, although we speak of the average energy of a CT x-ray beam as being about 70 keV. As a heterogeneous x-ray beam passes through the patient, the low energy protons are rapidly absorbed. This means the x-ray beam exiting the patient contains a lower percentage of energy photons than the beam had when it entered the patient. This effect is called "beam hardening." The linear attenuation coefficient of a tissue is directly related to the average energy of the x-ray beam. The measured linear attenuation coefficient (μ) of a tissue near the beam entry site will be higher than the measured μ of the same tissue after the beam has been hardened by passage through a volume of tissue. Reconstruction programs anticipate and correct for variation in linear attenuation coefficients caused by beam hardening, but such corrections are not precise. Generally, beam hardening artifacts are not a problem. In the head, a so-called "cup artifact" may be produced. This results from reconstructing an image from a 360° tube rotation. All points in the periphery of the brain will

Figure 19–26 Streak artifact produced by a shotgun pellet (B). Scout film (A) shows location of pellet (arrow)

"see" both a hardened and a non-hardened beam, but the central area of the brain will always "see" a beam that has been partially hardened. Linear attenuation coefficients from the center of the brain will be decreased compared to the periphery and the reconstructed image will be less dark centrally than peripherally.

Ring Artifact

Ring artifacts are the result of miscalibration of one detector in a rotate-rotate geometry scanner. (Of course, detector failure would also produce a ring artifact.) If a detector is miscalibrated, it will record incorrect data in every projection. This misinformation is reconstructed as a ring in the image, with the radius of the ring determined by the position of the faulty detector in the detector array. Faulty detectors in rotate-fixed units also record false information. However, this information is not visible in the reconstructed image because the faulty detector collects data from many angles (rings may appear in rotate-fixed geometry if the x-ray tube is not aligned correctly). Ring artifacts have virtually disappeared in contemporary CT units.

3-D IMAGING

Three-dimensional reconstruction of CT scan data is an option now available on many contemporary units. Whether the technology will prove to be of significant clinical usefulness is still being evaluated. There are two modes of 3-D reconstruction:

1. Surface reconstruction shows only the surface of the object.
2. Volumetric reconstruction shows the surface of the object in relation to its surroundings.

Three-dimensional reconstruction is simply the result of computer manipulation of CT scan data obtained in a routine manner. That is, there is no additional information obtained for the specific purpose of obtaining a 3-D image. It is true that a high resolution set of CT scans is obtained for good 3-D reconstruction; a typical scan might consist of 4-mm-thick slices with no gap between slices.

Surface Reconstruction

Display of the 3-D surface of an object can be accomplished if the object is displayed with shading, and by making surfaces appear opaque (e.g., one cannot see the petrous pyramids through the maxilla when looking at the front of a facial image). We assume the computer graphics program used to reproduce 3-D surfaces is complicated, and we have no intention of delving into the depths of computer programming. Essentially, the computer is told to scan the data bank of CT numbers and find all the CT numbers corresponding to the CT number of the object to be displayed. For example, we may be interested in a bone, and the CT numbers searched for would be of high value. Similarly, the computer may be told to search for soft tissue CT numbers. The computer has the task of locating the required CT numbers, then must keep tract of the pixel and slice location at which those CT numbers occur. Once the pixels have been selected and located, 3-D reconstruction of the surface may begin. There is sufficient information to present the object from any orientation, and the selection of which orientation must be made by the operator. In the skull, for example, one may choose anterior, posterior, or either lateral view. In fact, some programs allow rotation of the object, which is simply the selection of different views in rapid sequence. Once a view is selected, shading of pixels is used to enhance the perception of depth in the image. Pixels that are perceived as being closer to the viewer may be shaded light, while those that are perceived as farther away are shaded darker. And, of course, pixels that are perceived to be behind an opaque structure will be disregarded. An image formed in this fashion will appear as an object illuminated with light coming from directly behind the observer. Of course, we could select shading that would make the light appear to come from the left or right. If light is assigned a position other than directly behind the observer, one might have to use shadows as well as shading. The computer must at times interpolate to form a continuous image from matrix data points. Such things as artifacts, gaps between slices, and volume averaging will degrade the image.

Volumetric Reconstruction

Volumetric reconstruction requires two additional things. The first is to give the computer a window of CT numbers to look for. This window represents the material surrounding the area of interest in the volumetric reconstruction. For example, one may wish to display the muscles surrounding the bony pelvis. Therefore, at least two windows of CT numbers would be set (one for bone and one for muscle in our example). Second, the computer must display the pixels as translucent. This means that objects behind a displayed pixel will also be displayed. In our example, transparency will allow us to see bone surfaces through overlying muscle.

Surface reconstruction allows us to see objects as if they were anatomic specimens (i.e., their surfaces are opaque). Volumetric reconstruction presents objects more like they would appear during fluoroscopy.

In reality, one can show volumetric reconstruction with only one window of CT numbers by requiring the computer to assign a transparency to an object perceived to be closer to the viewer. For example, one may choose to view the bony pelvis isolated from surrounding soft tissues but still displayed with volumetric reconstruction. Such a display would allow visualization of the acetabulum through the femoral head.

SUMMARY

The basic principle behind CT is that the internal structure of an object can be reconstructed from multiple projections of an object. Today, CT units use either rotate-rotate or rotate-fixed geometry. Scan times of slightly less than 1 sec are possible. One ultra-fast design using magnetic focusing and deflection of an electron beam allows scan times to be as short as .05 sec.

High capacity rotating anode x-ray tubes

allow short scan times and have small focal spots that improve spatial resolution.

Two types of detectors are used. Scintillation crystals must be coupled with photodiodes, and may be used with rotate-rotate or rotate-fixed geometry. Xenon gas ionization detectors are the most common detector in contemporary units, and must be used in rotate-rotate geometry only.

Image reconstruction requires adequate non-redundant data. Analytic methods use 2-D Fourier transform or filtered back-projection to reconstruct the image.

CT numbers are also called Hounsfield units (H). CT numbers are derived by comparing the liner attenuation coefficient of a pixel with the linear attenuation coefficient of water. Most CT units cover a range of at least 4000 CT numbers.

Resolving power of CT units may be as high as 14 line pairs per cm when used in a high resolution mode. Spatial resolution is the ability of the CT scanner to display separate images of high contrast objects placed close together. Spatial resolution is determined by scanner design, computer reconstruction, and the display. Contrast resolution is the ability of the system to display an image of a relatively large object only slightly different in density from its surroundings. Contrast resolution is limited by noise.

Patient dose from a CT scan is intimately related to contrast resolution and spatial resolution. Typical doses range from about 2 cGy to 4 cGy.

Computer programs can produce 3-D reconstruction of CT images.

REFERENCES

1. Brooks, R.A.: Comparative Evaluation of CT Scanner Technology. In: Medical Physics Monograph No. 6. Medical Physics of CT and Ultrasound: Tissue Imaging and Characterization. Published by the American Institute of Physics, 335 East 45 Street, New York, NY 10017, 1980. p. 53–69.
2. Hendee, W.R.: The Physical Principles of Computed Tomography. Little, Brown and Co., Boston, 1983.
3. Hounsfield, G.N.: Computerized transverse axial scanning (tomography). Br. J. Radiol., *46*:1016, 1973.
4. Kak, A.C., Slaney, M.: Principles of Computerized Tomographic Imaging. IEEE Press. 345 East 47th Street, New York, NY 10017, 1988.
5. Peschmann, K.R., Napel, S., Boyd, D.P., et al.: High-speed computed tomography: systems and performance. Applied Optics, 24:4052–4060, 1985.
6. Trefler, M.: Computed Tomography. In: A Practical Approach to Modern Imaging Equipment. Thompson, T. Ed. Little, Brown and Co., Boston, 1985.

CHAPTER

20 *Ultrasound*

X rays were put to practical use the moment they were discovered, and improvements in equipment and techniques progressed rapidly during the first few years. In contrast, ultrasound has been notoriously slow in its medical evolution. The technology for producing ultrasound and the characteristics of sonic waves have been known for many years. The first major attempt at a practical application was made in the unsuccessful search for the sunken Titanic in the North Atlantic in 1912. Other early attempts at applying ultrasound to medical diagnosis met with the same fate. Techniques were not sufficiently developed, especially imaging techniques, until the massive military research effort that accompanied World War II. Sonar (**SO**und **N**avigation **A**nd **R**anging) was the first important successful application. Successful medical applications began shortly after the war, in the late 1940s and early 1950s. Since then progress has been rapid.

CHARACTERISTICS OF SOUND

A sound beam is similar to an x-ray beam in that both are waves transmitting energy. A more important difference is that x rays pass readily through a vacuum whereas sound requires a medium for its transmission. The velocity of sound depends on the nature of the medium. A useful way to picture matter (the medium) is as a series of spherical particles, representing either atoms or molecules, separated by tiny springs (Fig. 20–1A). When the first particle is pushed, it moves and compresses the attached spring, thus exerting a force on the adjacent particle (Fig. 20–1B). This sets up

Figure 20–1 Propagation of a sound wave

a chain reaction, but each subsequent particle moves a little less than its neighbor. The tension or pressure applied to the spring is greatest between the first two particles and less between any two down the line. If the driving force reverses its direction, the particles also reverse their direction. If the force vibrates to and fro like a cymbal that has been struck, the particles respond by oscillating back and forth. The particles in a sound beam behave in the same manner; that is, they oscillate back and forth, but over a short distance of only a few microns in liquids and even less in solids.

Although the individual particles move only a few microns, you can see from Figure 20–1 that the effect of their motion is transmitted through their neighbors over a much longer distance. During the same time, or almost the same time, that the first particle moves through a distance **a,** the effect of the motion is transmitted over a distance **b.** The velocity of sound is determined by the rate at which the force is transmitted from one molecule to another.

Longitudinal Waves

Ultrasonic pulses are transmitted through liquids as longitudinal waves. The term "longitudinal wave" means that the

323

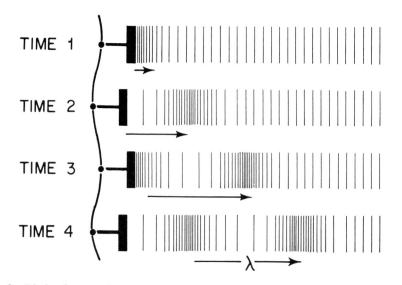

Figure 20-2   Birth of a sound wave

motion of the particles in the medium is parallel to the direction of wave propagation. The molecules of the conducting liquid move back and forth, producing bands of compression and rarefaction (Fig. 20–2). The wave front starts at time 1 in Figure 20–2 when a vibrating drum compresses the adjacent material. A band of rarefaction is produced at time 2, when the drum reverses it direction. Each repetition of this back-and-forth motion is called a cycle, and each cycle produces a new wave. **The length of the wave is the distance between two bands of compression, or rarefaction,** and is represented by the symbol λ. Once the sound wave has been generated, it continues in its original direction until it is either reflected, refracted, or absorbed. The motion of the vibrating drum, plotted against time, forms the sinusoidal curve shown along the left side of Figure 20–2. Ultrasound, by definition, has a frequency of greater than 20,000 cycles per second. Audible sound has a frequency between 15 and 20,000 cycles per second (the frequency of the average man's voice is about 100 cycles per second, and that of the average woman is about 200). The sonic beams used in diagnostic imaging have frequencies from 1,000,000 to 20,000,000 cy-

cles per second. One cycle per second is called a Hertz; a million cycles per second is a megahertz (abbreviated MHz). The term "Hertz" honors the famous German physicist Heinrich R. Hertz, who died in 1894.

Velocity of Sound

For body tissues in the medical ultrasound range, **the velocity of transmission of sound is independent of frequency, and depends primarily on the physical makeup of the material through which the sound is being transmitted.** The important characteristics of the transmitting medium are (1) its compressibility and (2) density. Table 20–1 shows the velocity of sound in some common materials, including several types of body tissue. The materials are listed in order of increasing speed of transmission, and you can see that sound travels slowest in gases, at intermediate velocity in liquids, and most rapidly in solids. Note that all body tissues, except bone, behave like liquids, and therefore they all transmit sound at about the same velocity. A velocity of 1540 m per second is used as an average for body tissue.

Compressibility. The velocity of sound is inversely related to the compressibility of

Table 20–1. Velocity of Sound in Various Materials

MATERIAL	VELOCITY (m/sec)
Air	331
Fat	1450
Mercury	1450
Castor oil	1500
Water (50° C)	1540
"HUMAN SOFT TISSUE"	1540
Brain	1541
Liver	1549
Kidney	1561
Blood	1570
Muscle	1585
Lens of eye	1620
PZT-5A	3780
PZT-4	4000
Skull (bone)	4080
Brass	4490
Quartz	5740
Aluminum	6400

the conducting material; that is, the less compressible a material, the more rapidly it transmits sound. Sound waves move slowly in gases because the molecules are far apart and are easily compressed. They behave as though they are held together by loose springs. A particle must move a relatively long distance before it can affect a neighbor. Liquids and solids are less compressible because their molecules are closer together. They only need to move a short distance to affect a neighbor, so liquids and solids propagate sound more rapidly than gases.

Density. Dense materials tend to be composed of massive molecules, and these molecules have a great deal of inertia. They are difficult to move or to stop once they are moving. Because the propagation of sound involves the rhythmic starting and stopping of particulate motion, we would not expect a material made up of large molecules (i.e., large in mass) such as mercury to transmit sound at as great a velocity as a material composed of smaller molecules, such as water. Mercury is 13.9 times denser than water, so we would expect water to conduct sound much more rapidly. Nevertheless, you can see from Table 20–1 that

water and mercury transmit sound at fairly similar velocities. The apparent discrepancy is explained by the greater compressibility of water, which is 13.4 times as compressible as mercury.[5] The loss in mercury's ability to transmit sound rapidly because of its greater mass is almost exactly balanced by a gain because of its lesser compressibility. As a general rule, this same principle applies to all liquids, that is, density and compressibility are inversely proportional. Consequently, all liquids transmit sound within a narrow range of velocities.

The relationship between wavelength and wave velocity is as follows:

$$v = \nu\lambda$$

v = Velocity of sound in conducting media (m/sec)
ν = Frequency (Hz)
λ = Wavelength (m)

In the ultrasonic frequency range, the velocity of sound is constant in any particular medium. When the frequency is increased, the wavelength must decrease. This is shown in Figure 20–3. In Figure 20–3A, the vibrator has a frequency of 1.5 MHz. Assuming the medium to be water, which propagates sound at a velocity of 1540 m/sec, the wavelength will be

$$1540 \text{ m/sec} = 1,500,000 \ (1/\text{sec})\lambda$$

and

$$\lambda = 0.001 \text{ m}$$

Therefore, 0.001 m (1.0 mm) is as far as the wave can propagate in the time available before a new wave starts. In Figure 20–3B, frequency is doubled to 3.0 MHz, but the waves move away at the same velocity, so their length is halved to 0.0005 m (0.5 mm).

Intensity

The intensity of sound, or loudness in the audible range, is determined by the length of oscillation of the particles conducting the waves. The greater the amplitude of oscillation, the more intense the sound. Figure 20–4 shows high- and low-intensity longitudinal waves of the same

Figure 20–3   The wavelength of sound decreases as its frequency (MHz) increases

frequency, wavelength, and velocity. The compression bands are more compacted in the high-intensity beam. The harder the vibrator is struck, the more energy it receives and the wider its vibrations. These wider excursions are transmitted to the adjacent conducting media and produce a more intense beam. In time, the vibrations diminish in intensity, although not in frequency, and the sound intensity decreases, producing a lower intensity beam. Ultrasonic intensities are expressed in watts (power) per square centimeter (note that these units are a mixture of SI and cgs units, but that's the way we do it). The mathematical expression that relates intensity to particle velocity, wave velocity, and medium density is rather complex and of no practical importance to radiologists, so we will not attempt to explain it here.

Relative Sound Intensity. Sound intensity is measured in **decibels.** A decibel is a relative unit, not an absolute one. Simply defined, a decibel (dB) is one tenth of a bel (B). A **bel** is a comparison of the relative

power of two sound beams expressed logarithmically using the base 10. For those who may have forgotten, we will briefly review logarithms. Starting with the number 10 and raising it to various positive and negative powers, we get a series of numbers, as follows:

10 Raised to a Power	Corresponding Number	Log (base 10)
10^4	10,000	4
10^3	1,000	3
10^2	100	2
10^1	10	1
10^0	1	0
10^{-1}	0.1	-1
10^{-2}	0.01	-2
10^{-3}	0.001	-3

For example, 10 raised to the fourth power (10^4) is 10,000. The log of 10,000 is 4. Note that there is no zero in the center column. The log of zero is undefined. The number 10 raised to the 0 power is 1, and not 0 as might be expected at first glance.

Returning to our definition of a bel, it is a logarithmic comparison of the relative in-

Figure 20–4   A larger amplitude of vibration produces denser compression bands and a higher intensity of sound

tensity of two sound beams. Table 20–2 summarizes the relationships between the bel, decibel, and intensity (or power) of an ultrasonic beam. Note that increasing intensity from 1 to 2 B increases relative intensity by a factor of 10. The number of decibels is obtained by multiplying the number of bels by 10. If an ultrasonic beam has an original intensity of 10 watts/cm², and the returning echo is 0.001 watts/cm², their relative intensity will be

$$\log \frac{0.001}{10} = \log 0.0001 = -4 \text{ B, or } -40 \text{ dB}$$

Decibels may have either a positive or negative sign. Positive decibels indicate a gain in power, whereas negative decibels express a power loss. Ultrasound loses power as it passes through tissue, so in the above example, the intensity of the returning echo relative to the original beam is −40 dB. Table 20–2 shows a column of negative decibels and the percentage of sound remaining in the beam at the new decibel level. In our example, the intensity of the returning echo (−40 dB) is only 0.01% that of the original intensity.

TRANSDUCERS

A transducer is a device that can convert one form of energy into another. Ultra-sonic transducers are used to convert an electric signal into ultrasonic energy that can be transmitted into tissues, and to convert ultrasonic energy reflected back from the tissues into an electric signal.

The general composition of an ultra-sonic transducer is shown in Figure 20–5. The most important component is a thin (approximately 0.5-mm) **piezoelectric crystal** element located near the face of the transducer. The front and back faces of the crystal are coated with a thin conducting film to ensure good contact with the two electrodes that will supply the electric field used to strain the crystal. The term "strain" refers to deformity of the crystal caused when a voltage is applied to the crystal. The surfaces of the crystal are plated with gold or silver electrodes. The outside electrode is grounded to protect the patient from electrical shock, and its outside surface is coated with a watertight electrical insulator. The inside electrode abuts against a thick backing block that absorbs sound waves transmitted back into the transducer. The housing is usually a strong plastic. An acoustic insulator of rubber or cork prevents the sound from passing into the housing. A large variety of sizes and shapes of transducers are available to perform spe-

Table 20–2. Comparison of Relative Intensity, Bels, Positive and Negative Decibels, and Percentage of Sound Remaining in Ultrasonic Beam

BELS (B)	POSITIVE DECIBELS (dB)	INTENSITY (Watts/cm²)	NEGATIVE DECIBELS (−dB)	SOUND REMAINING IN BEAM (%)
0	0	1	0	100
1/10	1	1.26	−1	79
2/10	2	1.59	−2	63
3/10	3	2.00	−3	50
4/10	4	2.51	−4	40
5/10	5	3.16	−5	32
6/10	6	3.98	−6	25
7/10	7	5.01	−7	19
8/10	8	6.31	−8	16
9/10	9	7.94	−9	13
1	10	10	−10	10
2	20	100	−20	1
3	30	1,000	−30	0.1
4	40	10,000	−40	0.01
5	50	100,000	−50	0.001
6	60	1,000,000	−60	0.0001

Figure 20–5 Ultrasound transducer

Figure 20–6 An electric field realigns the dipoles in a piezoelectric crystal

cific functions, but they all have this general design.

The Characteristics of Piezoelectric Crystals

Certain materials are such that the application of an electric field causes a change in their physical dimensions, and vice versa. This is called the "piezoelectric effect," first described by Pierre and Jacques Curie in 1880. Piezoelectric materials are made up of innumerable **dipoles** arranged in a geometric pattern (Fig. 20–6). An electric dipole is a distorted molecule that appears to have a positive charge on one end and a negative charge on the other (Fig. 20–6A). The positive and negative ends are arranged so that an electric field will cause them to realign, thus changing the dimensions of the crystal (Fig. 20–6B). The illustration shows a considerable change in thickness, but actually the change is only a few microns. Note that no current flows through the crystal. The plating electrodes behave as capacitors, and it is the voltage between them that produces the electric field, which in turn causes the crystal to change shape. If the voltage is applied in

a sudden burst, or pulse, the crystal vibrates like a cymbal that has been struck a sharp blow and generates sound waves. The backing block quickly dampens the vibrations to prime the transducer for its second function, which is to detect returning echoes.

As the sound pulse passes through the body, echoes reflect back toward the transducer from each tissue interface. These echoes carry energy and they transmit their energy to the transducer, causing a physical compression of the crystal element. This compression forces the tiny dipoles to change their orientation, which induces a voltage between the electrodes. The voltage is amplified and serves as the ultrasonic signal for display on an oscilloscope or television monitor. Incidentally, the compression force and associated voltage are responsible for the name piezoelectricity, which means "pressure" electricity.

Some naturally occurring materials possess piezoelectric properties (e.g., quartz), but most crystals used in medical ultrasound are man-made. This group of artificial piezoelectric materials is known as

ferroelectrics, of which a great variety exist. Barium titanate was the first of the ceramic ferroelectrics to be discovered. This has been largely replaced by lead zirconate titanate, commonly known as **PZT.*** Several types of PZT are available, with slight variations in chemical additions and thermal treatment producing different properties.

A great advantage of piezoelectric ceramics is that they can be formed into different shapes, depending on the application for which they are intended. Piezoelectric crystals can be designed to vibrate in either the thickness or radial mode (Fig. 20–7). Medical crystals are designed to vibrate in the thickness mode. They still vibrate to a lesser extent in the radial mode, however, so the receiving amplifier is gated to tune out all frequencies except those from the thickness mode.

Curie Temperature. Ceramic crystals are made up of innumerable tiny dipoles but,

to possess piezoelectric characteristics, the dipoles must be arranged in a specific geometric configuration. To produce this polarization, the ceramic is heated to a high temperature in a strong electric field. At a high temperature the dipoles are free to move, and the electric field brings them into the desired alignment. The crystal is then gradually cooled while subjected to a constant high voltage. As room temperature is reached, the dipoles become fixed, and the crystal then possesses piezoelectric properties. The Curie temperature is the temperature at which this polarization is lost. Heating a piezoelectric crystal above the Curie temperature reduces it to a useless piece of ceramic, so obviously transducers should never be autoclaved. The approximate Curie temperatures for several crystals are as follows:

Quartz	573° C
Barium titanate	100° C
PZT-4	328° C
PZT-5A	365° C

THICKNESS MODE

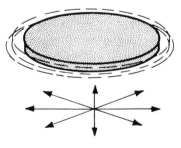

RADIAL MODE

Figure 20–7 Modes of vibration of a piezoelectric crystal

*PZT is a registered trade name of PZT materials from the Clevite Corporation.

Resonant Frequency. An ultrasound transducer is designed to be maximally sensitive to a certain natural frequency. The thickness of a piezoelectric crystal determines its natural frequency, called its "resonant frequency." Crystal thickness is analogous to the length of a pipe in a pipe organ. Just as a long pipe produces a low-pitched audible sound, a thick crystal produces a low-frequency ultrasound. The surfaces of a piezoelectric crystal behave like two identical cymbals, facing each other but separated in an open space. When one cymbal is struck, its vibrations set up sound waves that cause the other cymbal to vibrate. Vibrations are maximum in the second cymbal when the space separating the two is equal to one half of the wavelength of the sound. At this distance the sound waves from and vibrations of the two cymbals are exactly synchronized. The sound from one reinforces the vibrations of the other. A vibrating piezoelectric crystal transmits sound in both directions from each surface. The internally transmitted waves cross the transducer to synchronize with vibrations from the other side, just like the two cymbals in our example. When a crystal is struck with a single sharp voltage spike, it vibrates at its natural frequency, which is determined by its thickness. The natural frequency is the one that produces internal wavelengths that are twice the thickness of the crystal.

The crystal is designed so that its thickness is equal to exactly half the wavelength of the ultrasound to be produced by the transducer. The crystal is said to **resonate** (i.e., oscillate most efficiently) at the frequency determined by its thickness. The frequency that corresponds to half of the wavelength thickness is called the "fundamental resonance frequency" of the transducer. As an example, let us calculate the fundamental resonance frequency of a PZT-4 crystal that is 0.001 m (1 mm) thick. The velocity (v) of sound in PZT-4 is 4000 m/sec (Table 20–1), and we are told that the crystal will resonate at a frequency (v) equal to twice the crystal thickness (i.e., λ = $2v$ = 0.002 m). Substituting these values in the equation relating frequency, wavelength, and velocity of sound, we obtain

$$v = v\lambda$$
$$v = \frac{v}{\lambda}$$
$$v = \frac{4000 \text{ m/sec}}{0.002 \text{ m}}$$
$$v = 2{,}000{,}000/\text{sec} = 2 \text{ MHz}$$

Thus, a 2-MHz piezoelectric crystal made of PZT-4 will have a thickness of 0.001 m (1 mm). Similarly, a 1-MHz crystal will be 0.002 m thick. Note how crystals designed to resonate at high megahertz frequencies will be extremely thin.

A crystal can be forced to vibrate at the frequency of any alternating voltage, but the intensity of this sound is much less than it would be for a comparable voltage at the crystal's natural frequency. In medical ultrasound equipment the transducer is driven at its resonant frequency. A special circuit is used to generate an oscillating voltage waveform that is applied to the electrodes of the piezoelectric crystal. The output ultrasound frequency will reproduce the voltage waveform. The voltage frequency and the resonant frequency of the crystal are carefully matched. The fact that piezoelectric crystals have a natural frequency has considerable practical importance. With an x-ray machine the wavelength, or kilovoltage, can be adjusted by simply turning a few dials on a control panel. We do not have this freedom with ultrasound imaging. A frequency change requires another transducer, one designed for the desired frequency. Only a few different sizes and frequencies are needed to handle most clinical situations, which is fortunate because transducers are rather expensive.

Transducer Q Factor. The Q factor refers to two characteristics of piezoelectric crystals: the purity of their sound and the length of time that the sound persists. A high-Q transducer produces a nearly pure sound made up of a narrow range of frequencies, whereas a low-Q transducer produces a whole spectrum of sound covering a much wider range of frequencies. Almost all the internal sound waves of a high-Q transducer are of the appropriate wavelength to reinforce vibrations within the crystal. When an unsupported high-Q crystal (i.e., a crystal without a backing block) is struck by a short voltage pulse, it vibrates for a long time and produces a long continuous sound. The interval between initiation of the wave and complete cessation of vibrations is called the "ring down-time." Figure 20–8 shows the ring down-time for high-Q and low-Q crystals.

The Q factor can also be defined mathematically in terms of the purity of the sound. As the result of the sudden application of an electrical pulse, a transducer will ring at its resonance frequency, but will also produce sound waves at frequencies above and below the resonance frequency. The Q factor of a transducer system de-

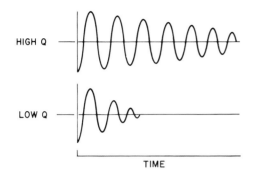

HIGH Q

LOW Q

TIME

Figure 20–8 Ring down-time of a high Q and low Q transducer

scribes this frequency response. If the frequency response of a crystal is plotted, curves similar to those in Figure 20–9 are obtained. The points f_2 and f_1 represent the frequencies above and below the resonance frequency where the sound intensity has been reduced to half. The Q factor of a transducer system describes the shape of the frequency response curve, and is defined as

$$Q = \frac{f_0}{f_2 - f_1}$$

Q = Q factor
f_0 = resonance frequency
f_2 = frequency above resonance at which intensity is reduced by half
f_1 = frequency below resonance at which intensity is reduced by half

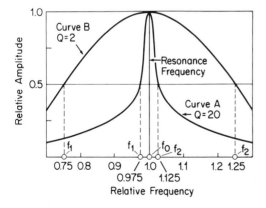

Figure 20–9 The Q factor related to frequency response for a high Q (curve A) and a low Q (curve B) transducer

In Figure 20–9, curve A illustrates a Q factor of 20. The transducer system generating curve A produces a narrow range of sound frequencies and has a long ring down-time. Such a system is useful for Doppler ultrasound transducers (we will discuss this in detail later). The transducer system producing curve B in Figure 20–9 has a Q factor of 2. This type of system will produce sound with a broad frequency range and will have a short ring down-time. Such a transducer (i.e., low Q) is needed for organ imaging (pulse-echo operation) because it can furnish short ultrasound pulses and will respond to a broad range of returning frequencies.

A long continuous sound is unsatisfactory for sonic imaging. **The transducer is both a transmitter and a receiver,** but it cannot send and receive at the same time. When continuous sound is being transmitted, the associated vibrations in the crystal produce continuously fluctuating voltages between the electrodes. If the internally generated sound waves are stronger than the returning echoes, as they may be, the returning signal is lost in the noise of the system. Another reason why continuous sound is undesirable for imaging is that depth resolution is generally determined by the length of the sonic pulse. (Depth resolution will be defined later in this chapter.) The length of the sonic pulse, called the **spatial pulse length,** is the number of waves multiplied by their wavelength. The sonic pulse from an unsupported high-Q crystal is long because the sound persists for a long time.

The approximate Q factor of several piezoelectric materials is as follows:

Quartz	>25,000
PZT-4	>500
PZT-5A	75
Piezoelectric polymers	3

The Q factor of piezoelectric materials can be controlled by altering the characteristics of the backing block of the transducer. **A backing block is incorporated to quench**

the vibrations and to shorten the sonic pulse. If the wavelength of sound from a transducer is 0.5 mm (0.0005 m), and the pulse is quenched after two wavelengths, the spatial pulse length is 1 mm (0.001 m). Ideally, the ultrasonic pulse should be a single wavelength. Transducers used in ultrasound imaging are pulsed for 2 or 3 cycles, with between 500 and 3000 pulses per second (1000 pulses per second is about average). We will discuss pulse rate in some detail later. The ideal backing material should accept all sound waves that reach it (i.e., not reflect any back into the crystal) and should then completely absorb the energy from these waves. This means that the backing material must have a characteristic impedance similar to that of the transducer crystal (don't worry about characteristic impedance right now; we will discuss it shortly). Backing blocks are generally made of a combination of tungsten and rubber powder in an epoxy resin. The ratio of tungsten to resin is chosen to satisfy the impedance requirements, and the rubber powder is added to increase the attenuation of sound in the backing block. For example, addition of 5% by volume of rubber powder to a 10% by volume mixture of tungsten powder in epoxy increases the attenuation from 5.6 to 8.0 dB cm^{-1} at 1 MHz. As a general rule, high-Q crystals are more efficient transmitters and low-Q crystals are more efficient receivers.

Three other important topics concerning transducers are focused transducers, impedance matching, and quarter-wavelength matching. These will be dealt with later in the chapter after the appropriate background material has been introduced.

CHARACTERISTICS OF AN ULTRASONIC BEAM

A single vibrating point sends out waves in all directions, much like those produced by a pebble thrown into a quiet pond; the waves move away from their point of origin as concentric circles. If two pebbles simultaneously land side by side, they each cause ringlike waves, and these waves may either reinforce or cancel each other, depending on their phase when they meet (Fig. 20–10). At time A, two waves are approaching each other from opposite directions. At time B, they are touching but not overlapping. One half-cycle later, at time C, the valley of one has reached the crest of the other and they cancel each other. Another half-cycle later, at time D, the crest and valleys are exactly superimposed, reinforcing themselves and doubling the height and depth of the peaks and valleys. Another half-cycle later, at time E, the waves have separated, and finally go their own way, at time F, as two separate waves moving in the opposite direction.

Piezoelectric crystals behave as a series of vibrating points and not as the pistonlike surface that we have implied previously.

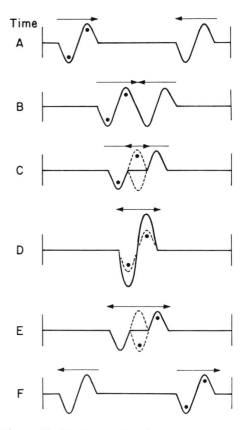

Figure 20–10 Interactions between two sound waves traveling in opposite directions

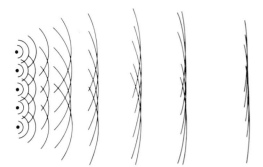

Figure 20–11 Superimposition of waves to form a wavefront

The wave fronts are not uniform, at least not close to the crystal. In Figure 20–11 the crystal is depicted as five vibrating points, with each point producing multiple concentric rings or waves that eventually form a continuous front as they reinforce each other along a line parallel to the face of the crystal. The distance at which the waves become synchronous depends on their wavelengths. The shorter the wavelength, the closer the front forms to the surface of the transducer.

The intensity of ultrasound varies longitudinally along the length of the beam. The simplest way of depicting a beam is that shown in Figure 20–12, in which the beam is drawn as a parallel bundle for a certain distance, beyond which it disperses. The parallel component is called the near or **Fresnel** (pronounced Fre-nel) **zone.** The diverging portion of the beam, that beyond **x′** is called the far or **Fraunhofer zone.** The notation **x′** is used to identify the transition point between the Fresnel and Fraunhofer zones.

The length of the Fresnel zone is determined by the diameter of the transducer and the wavelength of the ultrasound:

$$x' = \frac{r^2}{\lambda}$$

x′ = length of the Fresnel zone (cm)
r = radius of the transducer (cm)
λ = wavelength (cm)

Note that we have left this illustration in cgs units (cm), rather than switching to SI units (m). Table 20–3 shows the length of the Fresnel zone for various wavelengths and transducer diameters. The zone is longest with a large transducer and high-frequency sound, and shortest with a small transducer and low-frequency sound. For those who have difficulty interpreting tables, the same type of data are visually displayed in Figures 20–13 and 20–14. In Figure 20–13, the size of the transducer is constant at 1.5 cm, and the frequency of the sound is increased in stages from 1 to 3 MHz. The near zone increases in length with increasing frequency. In Figure 20–14, the frequency is fixed at 1 MHz and the size of the transducer is increased in stages from 1 to 2.5 cm. Again, the near zone increases in length with larger transducers.

High-frequency beams have two advantages over low-frequency beams: depth resolution is superior, and the Fresnel zone is longer. It would seem logical to use high frequencies for all imaging. High frequencies, however, have a major drawback re-

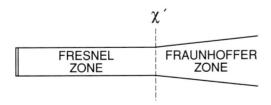

Figure 20–12 The Fresnel and Fraunhofer zones of an ultrasound beam

Table 20–3. The Length of the Fresnel Zone for Various Sized Transducers and Frequencies*

FREQUENCY (MHz)	LENGTH OF FRESNEL ZONE (cm)				
	DIAMETER OF TRANSDUCER (cm)				
	0.5	1.0	1.5	2.0	2.5
1.0	0.37	1.6	3.4	6.5	10
1.5	0.58	2.4	5.1	9.7	15
2.0	0.79	3.2	6.8	13.0	20
2.5	1.01	4.0	8.5	16.0	25
5.0	2.01	8.1	17.0	32.0	50
7.5	2.97	11.9	25.0	48.0	75

*Based on a sound velocity of 1540 m/sec.

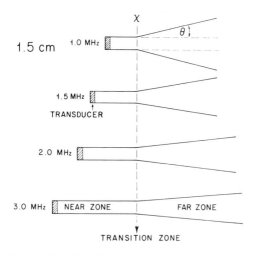

Figure 20–13 Elongation of the near zone with increasing frequencies

lated to penetration. **Tissue absorption increases with increasing frequency,** so a relatively low-frequency beam is required to penetrate thick parts. It would also seem logical to increase the size of the transducer to keep the beam coherent for sufficient depth to reach the point of interest. Although larger transducers improve coherence, they deteriorate side-to-side resolution. This dilemma is at least partially resolved with the use of focused transducers (to be discussed later). The amount of dispersion in the far zone is shown in the

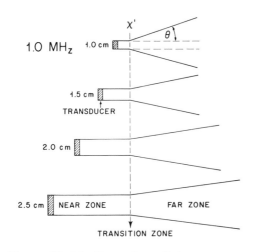

Figure 20–14 Elongation of the near zone with increasing transducer size

uppermost illustration in Figure 20–14. The size of the angle is determined as follows:

$$\sin \theta = 1.22 \frac{\lambda}{D}$$

θ = dispersion angle of far zone
λ = wavelength (mm)
D = diameter of transducer (mm)

The equation is rather simple to use with mathematical tables or a calculator with trigonometric functions. For example, the dispersion angle for a 10-mm transducer and a wavelength of 1 mm (a frequency of 1.5 MHz) may be determined as follows:

$$\sin \theta = 1.22 \frac{1.0}{10} = 0.122$$
$$\theta = 7°$$

If the wavelength is shortened to 0.5 mm (a frequency of 3 MHz), and the transducer size is kept at 10 mm, the dispersion angle is 3.5°.

INTERACTIONS BETWEEN ULTRASOUND AND MATTER

The types of interactions between sound and matter are similar to those of light, and include the following: (1) reflection, (2) refraction, and (3) absorption.

Reflection

In x-ray imaging, the transmitted radiation blackens the film and creates the actual image. Attenuated radiation creates defects or holes in the transmitted beam, contributing to image formation in a passive way. Scattered radiation fogs the film and is detrimental to image quality. With ultrasound, however, the image is produced by the reflected portion of the beam. Transmitted sound contributes nothing to image formation, but transmission must be strong enough to produce echoes at deeper levels. The percentage of the beam reflected at tissue interfaces depends on (1) the tissue's acoustic impedance, and (2) the beam's angle of incidence.

Acoustic Impedance. Acoustic impedance is a fundamental property of matter.

The impedance of a material is the product of its density and the velocity of sound in the material.

$$Z = \rho v$$
Z = acoustic impedance (Rayls)
ρ = density (g/cm³)
v = velocity of sound (cm/sec)

For example, the acoustic impedance of water is the velocity of sound in water (154,000 cm/sec) times the density of water (1 g/cm³), or

cm/sec × g/cm³ = g/cm² sec
154,000 × 1 = 154,000 g/cm² sec

This is an inconveniently large number, so it is divided by 100,000 (the same as multiplying by 10^{-5}) to reduce it to a more convenient size. Thus, the unit for acoustic impedance in the cgs system, the Rayl, is defined as g/cm² sec × 10^{-5}. The Rayl is named in honor of the English physicist Lord Rayleigh, who received the Nobel prize in 1904 for isolating the inert gas argon. **The velocity of sound in tissue is fairly constant over a wide range of frequencies, so a substance's acoustic impedance is a constant.** Table 20–4 lists the acoustic impedance, in Rayls, of various materials, including several body tissues

Table 20–4. Approximate Acoustic Impedance of Various Materials

MATERIAL	ACOUSTIC IMPEDANCE (Rayls—g/cm² sec × 10⁻⁵)
Air	0.0004
Fat	1.38
Castor oil	1.4
Water (50° C)	1.54
Brain	1.58
Blood	1.61
Kidney	1.62
Liver	1.65
Muscle	1.70
Lens of eye	1.84
Piezoelectric polymers	4.0
Skull (bone)	7.8
Quartz	15.2
Mercury	19.7
PZT-5A	29.3
PZT-4	30.0
Brass	38.0

and some piezoelectric materials used in ultrasound transducers. As sound waves pass from one tissue plane to another, the amount of reflection is determined by the difference in the impedances of the two tissues. The greater the difference, the greater the percentage reflected. Note that the difference between most body structures is fairly small, the two exceptions being air and bone. A soft tissue-air interface reflects almost the entire beam, and a soft tissue-bone interface reflects a major portion of it. The sum of the reflected and transmitted portions is 100%. For example, if 90% of a beam is reflected, 10% will be transmitted. At a tissue-air interface, more than 99.9% of the beam is reflected, so none is available for further imaging. Transducers, therefore, must be directly coupled to the patient's skin without an air gap. Coupling is accomplished by use of a slippery material such as mineral oil for contact scanning or by a water bath when the transducer cannot be placed directly on the patient.

Let us pause a moment and consider the unpleasant subject of the units used to express various quantities. In discussing acoustic impedance we have used the unit of the Rayl, which is a member of the cgs (centimeter-gram-second) system. In Chapter 1 we pointed out that it is now becoming more common to encounter units based on the SI system. In the SI system we must express the velocity of sound (v) in units of meters per second (m/s) and density (ρ) in units of kilograms per cubic meter (kg/m³), so acoustic impedance becomes

$$Z = \rho v = \frac{kg \cdot m}{m^3 s} = \frac{kg}{m^2 s} = kg \; m^{-2}s^{-1}$$

Table 20–5 lists acoustic impedance (Z) expressed in the cgs and SI systems for several materials.

Angle of Incidence. The amount of reflection is determined by the angle of incidence between the sound beam and the reflecting surface. The higher the angle of

Table 20–5. Acoustic Impedance as Written in the cgs and SI Systems

| MATERIAL | ACOUSTIC IMPEDANCE | |
	cgs System ($g\ cm^{-2}\ s^{-1}$)	SI System ($kg\ m^{-2}\ s^{-1}$)
Air	0.0004×10^5	0.0004×10^6
Water	1.54×10^5	1.54×10^6
Quartz	1.52×10^6	1.52×10^7
PZT-4	3.0×10^6	3.0×10^7

incidence (i.e., the closer it is to a right angle), the less the amount of reflected sound. The angles of incidence and reflection are equal, just as they are for visible light. In medical ultrasound, in which the same transducer both transmits and receives ultrasound, almost no reflected sound will be detected if the ultrasound strikes the patient's surface at an angle of more than 3° from perpendicular. When a sound beam strikes a smooth interface that is perpendicular to the beam, the amount of reflection is given by

$$R = \left(\frac{Z_2 - Z_1}{Z_2 + Z_1}\right)^2 \times 100$$

R = percentage of beam reflected
Z_1 = acoustic impedance of medium 1
Z_2 = acoustic impedance of medium 2

For example, to determine the percentage of a sonic beam reflected in going from the chest wall to the lung, substitute the acoustic impedance of lung and chest wall (muscle) from Table 20–4:

$$R = \left(\frac{1.70 - 0.0004}{1.70 + 0.0004}\right)^2 \times 100 = 99.9\%$$

As you can see, the number 0.0004 is so small that for practical purposes it can be ignored, and the beam is almost totally reflected, giving an intense echo but leaving no beam for further imaging. At a kidney-fat interface, the amount of reflection is

$$R = \left(\frac{1.62 - 1.38}{1.62 + 1.38}\right)^2 \times 100$$
$$R = \left(\frac{0.24}{3}\right)^2 \times 100 = 0.64\%$$

Approximately 0.64% of the beam is reflected at a kidney-fat interface. The brain

is intermediate between the soft tissues and air. At a skull-brain interface, approximately 44% of the beam is reflected. The preceding equation applies only to perpendicular reflections.

It is also possible to calculate the amount of transmission of a sound beam that strikes a smooth interface perpendicular to the beam. The equation is

$$T = \frac{4Z_1 Z_2}{(Z_1 + Z_2)^2} \times 100$$

T = percentage of beam transmitted
Z_1 = acoustic impedance of medium 1
Z_2 = acoustic impedance of medium 2

Remembering that the sum of the reflected and transmitted portions of the sound beam must be 100%, let us calculate the percentage transmission at a kidney-fat interface and see if it balances the 0.64% reflection calculated in the preceding paragraph:

$$T = \frac{4\ (1.62)\ (1.38)}{(1.62 + 1.38)^2} \times 100$$
$$T = 99.36\%$$

Refraction

When sound passes from one medium to another its frequency remains constant but its wavelength changes to accommodate a new velocity in the second medium (Fig. 20–15). In the illustration, the velocity of sound is twice as fast in the first medium as in the second. Each wave is shown as a single horizontal line and reflection is ignored. When the waves reach the surface of the second medium they are slowed to half-speed, but they keep coming at the same frequency. Their spacing, or wavelength, must be reduced by half to accommodate the decrease in velocity ($\lambda' = \frac{1}{2}$).

Exactly the same thing happens when the sound beam strikes the second medium at an angle, but the change in wavelength necessitates a change in direction. The reason for the direction change is shown in Figure 20–16. At time 1, a wave front approaching from a 45° angle just barely

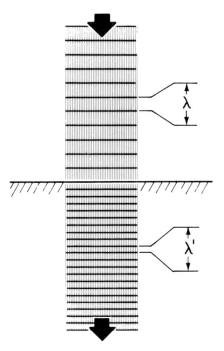

Figure 20–15 The wavelength of sound shortens when its velocity decreases

makes contact with the second medium. As it progresses, straddling the two media, one edge is traveling at a different velocity than the other. The wave front remains continuous, but one edge lags behind the other until the beam finally emerges in the second medium with a different wavelength and a different direction. This bending of waves as they pass from one medium to another is called **refraction.** Exactly the same process occurs in optics. Because the beam could be traveling in either direction, the arrows can be reversed in the illustrations to demonstrate the change that occurs when velocity increases in the second medium.

The angles of reflection (θ_x) and refraction (θ_t) are shown in Figure 20–17. The angle of refraction is governed by **Snell's law,** which is

$$\frac{\sin \theta_i}{\sin \theta_t} = \frac{V_1}{V_2}$$

θ_i = incidence angle (see Fig. 20–17)

θ_t = transmitted angle

V_1 = velocity of sound for incident medium

V_2 = velocity of sound for transmitting medium

Refraction can cause artifacts. Refraction artifacts cause spatial distortion (real structures are imaged in the wrong location) and loss of resolution in the image.

Absorption

Absorption of ultrasound in fluids is a result of frictional forces that oppose the motion of the particles in the medium. The energy removed from the ultrasound beam is converted into heat. To be precise, the term "absorption" refers to the conversion of ultrasonic to thermal energy, and "attenuation" refers to total propagation loss, including absorption, scattering, and reflection.

The mechanisms involved in absorption are rather complex, and our explanation will be greatly simplified. Three factors determine the amount of absorption: (1) the frequency of the sound, (2) the viscosity of the conducting medium, and (3) the "relaxation time" of the medium. We will discuss frequency last because it is affected by the other two factors.

If we picture sound as being composed of vibrating particles, the importance of viscosity is obvious. Particle freedom decreases and internal friction increases with increasing viscosity. This internal friction absorbs the beam, or decreases its intensity, by converting sound into heat. In liquids, which have low viscosity, very little absorption takes place. In soft tissues viscosity is higher and a medium amount of absorption occurs, whereas bone shows high absorption of ultrasound.

The relaxation time is the time that it takes for a molecule to return to its original position after it has been displaced. It refers to the resilience of a material. Two substances with the same viscosity may have different relaxation times. The relaxation time is a constant for any particular material. When a molecule with a short relaxation time is pushed by a longitudinal compression wave, the molecule has time to return to its resting state before the next compression wave arrives. A molecule with a longer relaxation time may not be able to

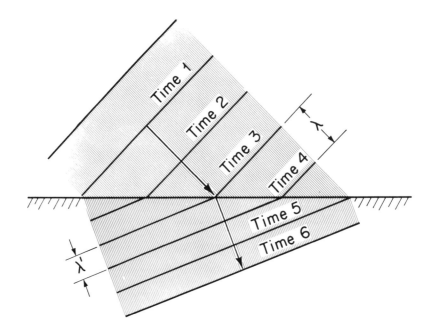

Figure 20–16 Refraction of sound waves

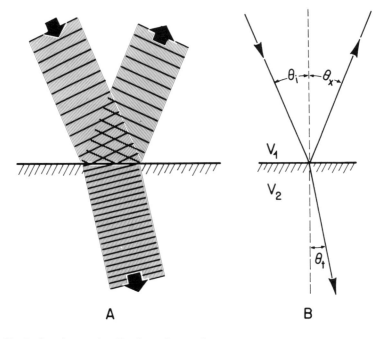

Figure 20–17 Refraction and reflection of sound waves

return completely before a second compression wave arrives. When this happens, the compression wave is moving in one direction and the molecule in the opposite direction. More energy is required to reverse the direction of the molecule than was needed to move it originally. The additional energy is converted to heat.

In soft tissues there is a linear relationship between absorption of ultrasound and frequency. Doubling the frequency approximately doubles absorption and approximately halves the intensity of the transmitted beam. Knowledge of the absorption allows the correct transducer for a particular job to be selected. The common transducer frequencies available are 1, 2.25, 3.5, 5, 7, and 10 MHz. The proper frequency is a compromise between the best resolution (higher frequency) and the ability to propagate the energy into the tissues (lower frequency).

The attenuation of ultrasound also varies with the temperature of the tissues, but the relationship varies with different tissues. For example, at a temperature range of 7° to 35° C and a frequency range of 0.4 to 10 MHz, physiologic hemoglobin solutions show a decreasing attenuation with increasing temperature. By contrast, central nervous system tissues have been shown to exhibit increasing attenuation with increasing temperature.

The frequency of sound effects the amount of absorption produced by the viscosity of a material. The higher the frequency (i.e., the more often a particle moves back and forth in a given time), the more its motion is affected by the drag of a viscous material. Frequency also affects the amount of absorption produced by the relaxation time. At low frequencies, molecules have sufficient time to relax between cycles but, as frequencies increase, the relaxation time consumes a greater and greater proportion of the total cycle. These effects are already appreciable in the lower range of diagnostic frequencies (1 MHz),

and they continue to increase at higher frequencies.

Only rather fragmentary data are available to quantitate the absorption of ultrasound. An absorption coefficient is usually employed. This coefficient is identical in concept to the linear attenuation coefficient described for x-rays. The unit for the absorption coefficient is decibels/cm of thickness at a frequency of 1 MHz. The stipulation of 1 MHz is essential because absorption is frequency-dependent. At 2 MHz, the absorption coefficient is about twice as large. Table 20–6 lists absorption coefficients for various materials. A 1-cm thick slice of kidney, with an absorption coefficient of 1 dB/cm, reduces the sound intensity by 1 dB. Table 20–2 shows that −1 dB represents an absorption of 21% of the beam, and that 79% of the beam remains. A 1-cm thick slice of lung absorbs 41 dB, which reduces intensity by a factor of more than 10,000, leaving less than 0.01% of the beam remaining.

QUARTER-WAVE MATCHING

Now that we have developed a better understanding of absorption, reflection, and acoustic impedance, let us reconsider the ultrasound transducer. When a short electrical shock is applied to the piezoelectric

Table 20–6. Absorption Coefficients for Various Materials at a Frequency of 1 MHz

MATERIAL	ABSORPTION COEFFICIENT (dB/cm)
Lung	41
Skull (bone)	20
Air	12
Muscle (across fiber)	3.3
Lens of eye	2.0
Kidney	1.0
Castor oil	0.95
Liver	0.94
Brain	0.85
Fat	0.63
Blood	0.18
Aluminum	0.018
Water	0.0022
Mercury	0.00048

crystal, four ultrasonic pulses are generated, two at each face of the crystal. Two pulses travel back into the transducer; one pulse from the back travels into the backing block, and one pulse from the front travels into the patient's tissues. We have discussed how the acoustic impedance (Z) of the backing block is matched to that of the crystal so that the sound directed away from the patient will be transmitted into, and absorbed by, the backing block. Another important consideration is the transmission of the ultrasound wave into the patient with a minimum loss of energy. The use of mineral oil between the transducer and the patient's skin is an effective means of transmitting energy from the transducer to the patient. Another method of improving energy transfer is that of mechanical impedance matching. If a layer of material (called the "matching layer") of suitable thickness and characteristic impedance is placed on the front surface of the transducer, the energy is transmitted into the patient more efficiently (Fig. 20–18). The thickness of the matching layer must be equal to one fourth the wavelength of sound in the matching layer: hence the name "quarter-wave matching." In addition, the impedance of the matching layer must be about the mean of the impedances on each side of the layer (this is probably not exactly true, but is close enough for our purposes).

$$Z_{matching\ layer} \cong \sqrt{Z_{transducer} \times Z_{soft\ tissue}}$$

For example, impedance of about 6.8×10^6 kg m^{-2}s^{-1} is required for the matching layer between PZT-4 ($Z = 3.0 \times 10^7$ kg m^{-2}s^{-1}) and water ($Z = 1.54 \times 10^6$ kg m^{-2}s^{-1}). Such a layer could be manufactured using a mixture of aluminum powder and epoxy resin.

Use of quarter-wave matching will also improve the transmission of ultrasound pulses returning from tissues back into the transducer. The equations explaining the theory of quarter-wave matching have been described by Wells, and will not be discussed here.[18]

ULTRASONIC DISPLAY

The ultrasonic image is an electronic representation of data generated from returning echoes and displayed on a TV monitor. The image is assembled, one bit at a time, much like a television image. Each returning echo generates one bit of data, and many bits together form the electronic image. The evolution of sonic imaging began slowly from a static one-dimensional base (A mode), improved somewhat when a component of motion was added

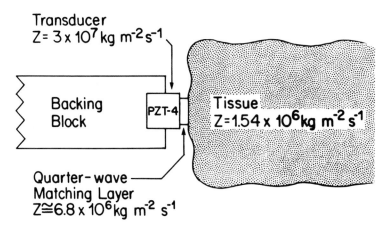

Figure 20–18 Quarter-wave matching

(TM mode), and made giant leaps forward with two-dimensional imaging (B mode) and with gray-scale imaging. These advancements can all be attributed to refinements in electronic instrumentation. In this edition we will continue to describe A mode, TM mode, and B mode scanning. Almost all ultrasound examinations today involve real-time imaging. The old articulating scanning arm, gray-scale B mode scanners, may be encountered on rare occasion, but they are museum pieces in most institutions. Reading about bistable images and analog scan converters may provide some appreciation of the phenomenal speed with which technology has changed the field of ultrasound imaging. We suggest you read and enjoy the next five pages, realizing that they describe technology that was current only a decade ago. We will discuss real-time imaging in following sections.

A Mode

In the A mode, echoes are displayed as spikes projecting from a baseline (Fig. 20–19A). The baseline identifies the central axis of the beam. Spike height is proportional to echo intensity, with strong echoes producing large spikes. A series of sonic pulses is used for A-mode imaging but, for simplicity, we will begin with a single pulse. When a voltage pulse strikes a transducer, an echo spike is generated on the monitor to mark the beginning of the sonic pulse. As the pulse passes through the patient, sound is reflected to the transducer from each tissue interface. The depth of the interface recorded on the display is proportional to the time that it takes for the echo to return. Using a sound velocity of 1540 m/sec in average soft tissue, it is a simple mathematical task to convert time into distance. At a velocity of 154,000 cm/sec, sound travels 1 cm in 6.5 microseconds (μsec). An echo must make a round trip, however, so when the echo takes 13 μsec to return, it is displayed at a depth of 1 cm.

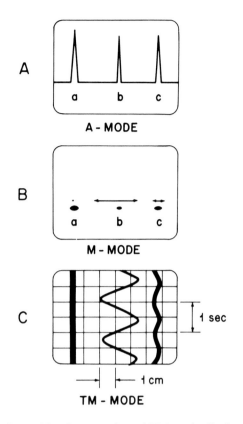

Figure 20–19 A mode and TM mode displays

If the tissue planes are in a fixed position, and the transducer is held stationary between pulses, as is customary, then the echo spikes from subsequent pulses will fall in the same positions as those from the initial pulse. No memory is built into the display mechanism, so it discards previous pulses as it receives new ones. A permanent record is made by photographing the electronic display. In the A mode, or amplitude mode, the display on the cathode ray tube contains information about the depth of structures and the amplitude of the returning echo. Generally, little use is made of the amplitude of the echo spike. A mode is used in ophthalmology, echoencephalography, echocardiology, and as an adjunct to B-mode displays when accurate depth measurements are required. The A-mode cathode ray tube will display about 40 dB of amplitude information, corre-

TM Mode

In the A mode, if the echoes are produced by moving structures, then the echo spikes will also move. If the echoes shown in Figure 20–19A had originated from the anterior chest wall (a), the posterior leaflet of the mitral valve (b), and the posterior heart wall (c), the echoes from the moving structures would move back and forth along the baseline. At any moment they might appear as shown in the illustration. A moment later, however, the mitral valve and heart wall would be in a different position, with the mitral valve moving more than the heart wall. For the TM mode, the spikes are converted into "dots" as shown in Figure 20–19B (M mode). The dots move back and forth, as indicated by the arrows. The M mode is an intermediate mode that cannot be meaningfully recorded. To make a permanent record, the motion must be recorded over a period of time. This is accomplished by moving the line of dots to the top of the scope and then gradually dropping them to the bottom. A record of the sweep is made with a camera using an exposure time longer than the sweep time. Such a record is shown in Figure 20–19C. Because this is a time-motion study, it is referred to as the TM mode. The sweep time in the illustration is 3 sec. If a longer sweep time is used, more beats are recorded and they are compacted from top to bottom, but their back-and-forth excursions remain unchanged. The obvious disadvantage of this method is the short time that can be recorded. A longer record can be made with an electronic strip chart recorder that can also simultaneously display several other parameters, such as the electrocardiogram. A strip chart record can be as long as the operator desires, and this method is increasing in popularity for echocardiography, in which the TM mode is most useful.

B Mode

Sonography came of age as an imaging technique with development of the B mode. The other modes produced valuable information, but they were only useful in limited areas. The B mode greatly expanded the role of ultrasound as a diagnostic tool, especially in abdominal diseases. **The B mode produces a picture of a slice of tissue.** Echoes are displayed as dots, similar to that in the TM mode but, in contrast to the TM mode, the transducer is moved so that the sound beam traverses a plane of the body. The transducer is like the handle of a saber, with the ultrasonic beam as the blade. The blade images a sagittal section when it cuts through the length of the body, and images a transverse or cross section when drawn from side to side. The images are similar to what we would see if the section could be exposed and viewed face-on.

In most B-mode scanning techniques the transducer is placed on the patient's skin, with mineral oil on the skin acting to exclude air and to ensure good acoustic coupling between transducer and skin. This is called contact scanning. The transducer may be left in one spot and rocked back and forth, producing a simple sector scan (Fig. 20–20A). More often, the transducer is moved across the body while it is being rotated, producing a compound contact scan (Fig. 20–20B). This compound motion is required because anatomic structures in the body present various angles from which the ultrasound waves are reflected. If the angle between the perpendicular from the transducer surface and

Figure 20–20 Simple sector B scan (A) and compound contact B scan (B)

the interface to be imaged is greater than about 5°, the amount of reflected ultrasound returning to the transducer will be too little to produce an image. Thus, the compound scanning motion is required to present the surface of the transducer to the wide variety of interface angles requiring imaging. Assembling the echoes generated by compound scanning into a meaningful scan picture requires precise synchronization between the transducer motions and the cathode ray tube display.

In assembling the image, the localization of one echo relative to another is accomplished with a small computer that is fed information by an arm containing three joints (Fig. 20–21). The computer calculates the alignment of the baseline by the number of degrees in the three joints. Echo depth is determined by the time delay, as in the A mode. When the transducer moves from one position to another, from A to B in the illustration, the computer recalculates the angles and time delays to position returning signals in the display properly. Even though the echoes arise from two completely different transducer positions (A and B), the computer correctly interprets them as originating from one point (P). Many thousands of these calculations and echoes produce an image that appears on the scope as a cut section. Various manufacturers employ different methods for measuring the three angles. The angles of

the joints of the arm may be measured by potentiometers or by optical digital encoders that generate signals that change with transducer position and orientation.

To review, the scanning arm serves two functions: (1) it determines the spatial orientation of the sound beam; and (2) it constrains the motion of the transducer so that all components of a single image slice through the same plane in the patient.

The method used to display the image obtained by B-mode scanning must be different from the ordinary cathode ray tube used to display A-mode images. Two requirements must be met. First, the image must persist on the viewing screen long enough to allow it to be studied (the image on a routine cathode ray tube is only visible for a fraction of a second). Second, persistence of the image is required to allow a picture to be "built up" as a result of the compound scanning motion of the transducer. These requirements were initially met by displaying the B-mode scan on a modification of the cathode ray tube called a "storage" (or "variable persistence") cathode ray tube. These tubes allowed the operator to view the B-mode scan as it was produced (an image could be viewed continuously for about 10 minutes). The design and function of a variable persistence cathode ray tube are not considered pertinent, so we will spare you (and ourselves) the agony of exploring the technical details. Also, this type of display is not used on current B-mode scanners. The overwhelming disadvantage of these direct viewing storage tubes is their limited ability to display shades of gray. In fact, some of them show no shades of gray, with the image being composed of only light or dark areas on the screen. This is termed a "bistable image."

Gray-Scale Imaging

B-mode scanning took a major step forward with the advent of gray-scale imaging in 1972. The purpose of gray-scale imaging is to display the great variation of the am-

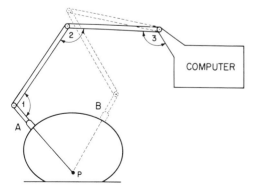

Figure 20–21 Computer localization of transducer alignment

plitudes of the echoes arising from tissues as varying shades of gray on a television monitor. This contrasts with the bistable or limited gray-scale image possible with direct viewing storage cathode ray tubes. Gray-scale imaging was made possible by the development of the scan conversion memory tube (usually called a "scan converter"). Unlike storage cathode ray tubes, the scan converter tube does not produce a visible image. Instead, the scan converter stores the information received from a transducer and then uses the stored information to generate a signal that is used to produce a visible image on a television monitor. A scan converter tube is similar to a cathode ray tube in that an electron beam is caused to scan a target capable of storing the information it receives. The electron beam is used alternately to "write" the information on the target, "read" the information to generate the signal sent to a television monitor, and "erase" the target in preparation for receiving a new set of information. The target of the scan converter tube is a complex affair made up of a silicon backplate about 25 mm in diameter on which more than a million tiny (about 10 μm) squares of silicon "wafers" are placed. It is reasonable to assume that, as a transducer is used to scan a patient in a compound contact scanning maneuver, several returning echoes from the same point will be received by the transducer. When the target of the scan converter receives multiple signals to the same area, it records only the strongest signal and discards all others. In this way the final "picture" is composed only of the strongest echo detected from each point of the scan, rather than of a random addition of numerous signals (called "overwriting"). This is why the operator is able to build up a more diagnostic picture by repeated movements of the transducer through the plane of each image. Once the image has been stored on the target of a scan converter tube, the electron beam can be made to scan the target and generate a signal suit-

able for display on an ordinary television monitor.

Two types of scan conversion memory tubes are in use. The analog scan converter was developed in 1972. More recently, the digital scan converter has replaced the analog unit. The terms "analog" and "digital" are rather vague to most physicians. Because of the explosion of "digital" components being introduced to diagnostic imaging procedures, we are making this topic the subject of an entire chapter. Briefly stated, a digital scan converter converts variations in amplitude of the echo signal received by the transducer into binary numbers. The information is sorted into 16 (4-bit) or 32 (5-bit) or more levels of gray that can be displayed on a television monitor.

The analog scan converters present some difficulty in clinical use because the gray-scale levels assigned to the echo amplitude tend to drift, causing deterioration of images and making comparison of scans obtained at different dates difficult. There is also an objectionable flicker of the image viewed on the television monitor. This flicker is related to the fact that a scan converter tube must simultaneously store (write) the image and transmit (read) the image to the television monitor. The tube must switch between writing and reading modes during the time an image is being received. An analog converter tube is able to do this switching at a rate of about ten times per television frame, producing visible on-off flicker. Once stored by an analog converter, an image can be viewed for about 10 min before image deterioration begins.

Digital scan converter tubes are free of gray-scale drift. They have a much faster writing speed than the analog unit, thereby eliminating the flicker on the television monitor. Once stored, the image on a digital storage tube can be viewed indefinitely. Digital scan converters are suitable for advanced computer processing and are adaptable to real-time imaging developments. Thus, the digital scan conversion memory tube promises to replace the analog systems.

Being able to read the information stored by a scan converter tube on a regular TV monitor offers several advantages. Such monitors are inexpensive, and accessories such as character generators (i.e., letters) can be easily employed to identify scans. The controls of the TV monitor can be used to adjust contrast and brightness. Other television accessories such as color, video tape, and video disc options can be adapted. A "zoom" display can also be employed by using only a portion of the stored image to generate the TV image. It is also possible to store several complete images on different parts of the scan converter target.

Let us briefly review the advantages of a digital scan conversion memory tube over direct view cathode ray storage tubes:

1. Reading the image on a routine TV monitor allows use of numerous accessories and additional image control.
2. Computer data processing options are available.
3. Gray-scale display is available.
4. Zoom display is available.
5. More than one image can be stored.
6. Resolution is better.
7. Prolonged viewing does not degrade the image.
8. There is negligible overwriting (only the strongest signal from each point in the scan is recorded).

Controls

The number and intensity of echoes from any particular area are extremely variable, and setting the scanner to demonstrate one area optimally frequently detracts from image quality in another area. Multiple controls are built into ultrasonic units, and all are designed to regulate the intensity of echoes from various depths. Usually several controls are manipulated

simultaneously, so there is no logical sequence for discussion. The following controls may be available, although they may not all be provided by a single manufacturer:

1. Time gain compensator
2. Delay
3. Intensity
4. Coarse gain
5. Reject
6. Near gain
7. Far gain
8. Enhancement

The echoes from deep structures are much weaker than those from closer structures. The two may differ by a factor of one million. If an echo from an object close to the surface produces a 10-cm spike, as displayed in the A mode, the echoes from deeper structures may be a mere 0.001 mm, less than the thickness of a hair. Obviously, something must be done to remedy this, and most controls are designed for just that purpose. The **time gain compensator (TGC)** is the most important control. Its function is shown in Figure 20–22. The echoes from deep structures are severely attenuated and produce small spikes (Fig. 20–22B). The TGC is depicted in Figure 20–22C as a sloping line, and the height of the slope is added to that of the pulses. The result, shown in Figure 20–22D, is a series of pulses of similar amplitude. The slope of the TGC adjusts the degree of amplification. The slope is shown as a straight line but it is actually exponential, because the deeper echoes require more of a boost than it would appear from the illustration. They may actually be amplified more than a thousand times. The delay control regulates the depth at which the TGC begins to augment weaker signals.

Three controls govern amplitude across the entire display without discrimination for or against a particular depth. The first is the **intensity control,** which determines the potential difference across the transducer (i.e., the strength of the voltage pulse). Increasing intensity produces a more energetic ultrasonic beam and thus stronger echoes at all levels. The second amplitude control is the **coarse gain,** which

Figure 20–22   Time gain compensation

Figure 20–23   Coarse gain and reject controls

regulates the height of echoes from all depths. Increasing the coarse gain control enhances all echoes proportionately (Fig. 20–23). The initial echoes (Fig. 20–23A) are all enhanced to nearly twice their amplitude by increasing coarse gain (Fig. 20–23B). The third amplitude regulator is the **reject control,** and it is slightly different from the other two. Although it does not discriminate against echoes from a particular depth, it does discriminate against those below a minimum amplitude (Fig. 20–23C and D). Reject cleans up the image by removing small useless signals. Selective rejection of weaker signals enhances the clarity of the stronger ones.

A **delay control** regulates the depth at which the TGC begins to augment the weaker signals (Fig. 20–24). Obviously the strong superficial echoes do not require amplification by the TGC; in fact, they may have to be dampened. This is accomplished with the **near gain control,** which is used primarily to diminish and not to enhance near echoes. The distance over which near gain operates is controlled by the delay.

Two additional methods may be used to supplement distant echoes (i.e., those originating deep in the tissues): the **far gain** and the **enhancement controls.** Far gain is similar to near gain only at the opposite end of the TGC curve and is used to enhance all distant echoes. The enhancement controls augment a localized portion of the TGC curve (Fig. 20–24). It gates a specific depth and enhances echoes within the gate to any desired level. For example, the gate can be set to "frame" the near and far extremes of mitral valve motion; echoes from this specific region will then be amplified to delineate the valve more clearly.

The interplay between all these controls is extremely complex, and it is impossible to learn their effect on imaging from a book.

Pulse Rate

Pulse rate and frequency are different and unrelated. Frequency refers to a characteristic of the sound; that is, the number of times that conduction particles vibrate back and forth per second, usually between 1 and 20 MHz in medical sonography. **Pulse rate refers to the number of separate little packets of sound that are sent out each second** (Fig. 20–25). Each sonic pulse is short (typically two or three wavelengths), and its duration varies with the Q factor of the transducer. Between pulses, the transducer serves as a receiver. A commonly used rate is 1000 pulses/sec (with a range of 500 to 3000). At this rate, the total time available for each pulse is 0.001 sec. Approximately one millionth of a second is devoted to transmission, so the transducer is a receiver almost 1000 times longer than it is a transmitter.

The pulse rate determines the total number of echoes returning to the transducer in a unit of time. Doubling the rate from 1000 to 2000 pulses/sec will double the number of echoes returning to the transducer each second.

Obviously, a high pulse rate is desirable, but too high a rate creates another problem. The transducer cannot send and receive at the same time. As the pulse rate increases, the receiving time decreases. If the receiving time is too short, echoes from distant parts may still be out, or on their way in, when the next pulse starts. The time between pulses, or the pulse rate, must be set to accommodate the thickest part that might be examined. This thickness is half the distance between pulses. Remember, the sound is making a round trip, so the maximum thickness that can be examined is only half of the distance that the sound can travel. Table 20–7 shows the maximum part thickness that can be imaged at various pulse rates. At the commonly used rate of 1000 pulses/sec, a 75-cm thick part can be examined. At a rate of 10,000, the thickest part is 7.5 cm, which is satisfactory for ophthalmology but not for abdominal imaging.

IMAGING PRINCIPLES

The sonographic image is influenced by the size and shape of both the object and the transducer. The same principle applies to x-ray imaging. The effect of the x-ray focal spot size is made readily apparent if

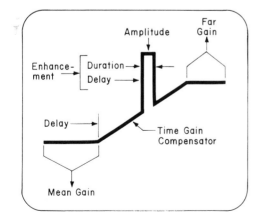

Figure 20–24 Various controls for the sonic display

Figure 20–25 Multiple sonic pulses

a pinhole is placed halfway between the target and film, with the resultant image being a picture of the focal spot, not the pinhole. At shorter object-film distances, or with larger objects, the effect is much less dramatic, and we call it "penumbra" or "edge gradient," but the effect is there just the same. Transducers are much larger than focal spots, so transducer images are more evident. Figure 20–26 shows a B-mode scan of five equally spaced wire rods imaged with a focused transducer. (Focused transducers will be described later in this section.) The wires are small in diameter relative to the sound beam. As the beam moves from left to right, echoes begin when the leading edge of the beam reaches a wire and continue until the beam has passed beyond all the wires. The resulting images are pictures of the sound beam, not of the wire. Because beam width varies with depth, image width also varies with depth, being closest to the shape of the wire when the beam is narrowest. The wire is the sonographer's pinhole.

Resolution

When we talk about resolution with the A mode, we are only concerned with the ability of the beam to separate two objects

Table 20–7. Maximum Part Thicknesses that can be Imaged at Various Pulse Rates

PULSE RATE (per second)	MAXIMUM PART THICKNESS (cm)*
1,000	75
3,000	25
6,000	12.5
10,000	7.5

*Based on a velocity of sound of 150,000 cm/sec; the sound must travel twice as far as the thickness to complete a round trip.

at different depths. In the B mode, however, we must also be concerned with horizontal, or lateral, resolution: that is, the ability to separate two adjacent objects. We will refer to these as depth and lateral resolution. Neither is accurately defined, at least not by x-ray imaging standards, so our discussion will be in terms of general principles, and not of line pairs per mm.

Depth (Axial) Resolution. Depth resolution is the ability of the beam to separate two objects lying in tandem along the axis of the beam. Figure 20–27 shows a time sequence of an ultrasonic pulse resolving two surfaces, a and b, separated by x distance. At times 2 and 3, portions of the beam are reflected from surfaces a and b respectively. The reflected pulses are completely separated, and each produces its own signal. The separation of their leading edges is 2x, or twice the original separation, because the second echo had to travel back and forth across the distance x. The length of the sonic pulse, called the "spatial pulse length," equals the wavelength of the sound multiplied by the number of wavelengths in the pulse. The number of wavelengths will depend on the Q factor of the transducer. For example, at a frequency of 1.5 MHz, the wavelength of the sound in water is 1 mm (λ = 1,500,000 cycles/sec ÷ 1,500,000 mm/sec). If each sonic pulse consists of three wavelengths, the spatial pulse length will be 3 mm. Two objects will be resolved (recognized as being separate) if the spatial pulse length is less than twice the separation. Figure 20–28 shows two objects separated by exactly half a spatial pulse length. At time 2 the pulse splits, but the first reflected pulse does not clear surface a before the second reflected pulse re-

Figure 20–26 "Imaging" the sonic beam

turns from surface b. The transducer only sees one pulse, so the two surfaces are not resolved.

Reverberation Echoes. When we discussed tomography we described phantom images as images that appear to the eye but have no physical existence. A similar image, called a **reverberation image,** occurs in sonography. Figure 20–29 shows how these spurious images are produced. The critical event occurs at time 4 when the returning echoes from b reflect off the back surface of a and initiate a third echo (time 5), which the transducer interprets as another object. Thus three surfaces are displayed, with the third being a reverberation image. Time 6 shows the beginning of a fourth image and, with a geometric configuration such as the one shown in the illustration, the number of reverberation images is limited only by the penetrating power of the beam and the sensitivity of the detector.

The transducer itself may act as a reflecting surface and produce a reverberation artifact, especially in ophthalmologic sonography. The artifact is recognized by manually changing the distance between the transducer and the globe of the eye. The factitious image moves in synchrony with the transducer.

Lateral (Horizontal) Resolution. Lateral resolution is the ability to separate two adjacent objects. Figure 20–30 shows two objects separated by a narrow space. To recognize the objects as discrete entities, the beam must be narrower than the space separating the objects. In Figure 20–30*A* the

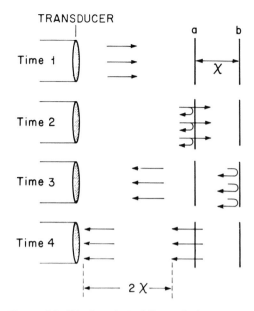

Figure 20–27 Depth (axial) resolution

beam is too wide, so that even when it strad-
dles the space, echoes return from both
objects, the display interprets an edge, and
the space goes unrecognized. An obvious
way to narrow the beam and to improve
resolution is to use a smaller transducer.

Figure 20–29 Reverberation images

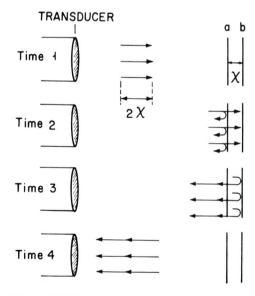

Figure 20–28 Unsatisfactory or unsuccessful
depth resolution

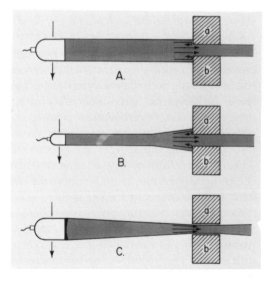

Figure 20–30 Lateral (horizontal) resolution

This works well in some clinical situations, for example in ophthalmology in which small diameter high-frequency transducers are used to produce superb resolution. The advantages of small transducers, however, are lost in the much thicker abdomen. The Fresnel zone is too short, even at high frequencies, to reach deep structures. Figure 20–30B illustrates the problem. The beam is well into the Fraunhofer zone at the object plane, and may actually be wider than the beam from a larger transducer.

Focused Transducers. The solution to the above imaging problem is use of a focused transducer, such as the one shown in Figure 20–30C. Focused transducers restrict beam width and improve lateral resolution but they are designed to focus at a specific depth or depth range, so they must be selected for optimal display of the depth of interest. In Figure 20–30C the beam is focused at the proper depth so that it can pass through the space between objects a and b, thus permitting them to appear as separate entities.

Sonic beams can be focused with either a curved piezoelectric crystal or with an acoustic lens. The lens material, usually polystyrene or an epoxy resin, propagates sound at a greater velocity than body tissues, so the sound is refracted, or bent, toward a point in space. Knowing the radius of curvature of the lens and the velocities of sound in the lens material and body tissues, the exact focal point can be calculated. **A close approximation of the focal length is the diameter of curvature of the lens** (Fig. 20–31). Focusing moves the transition point between the near and far zones from its anticipated position at x′ back toward the transducer to a new position at x′$_f$. The beam is maximally restricted and of greatest intensity at the focal point, but the point is not sharply defined. Like an optical lens, an acoustic lens has a focal zone, a distance over which the focal properties are fairly well maintained. The focal zone is shortest with a large diameter, short focal length lens. Focused transduc-

ers are classified as short, medium, or long, depending on the depth at which they focus, as follows:

Short	4–6 cm
Medium	6–8 cm
Long	8–11 cm

Tomographic Thickness. The expression "tomographic thickness" is only meaningful with B-mode scanning. It refers to the thickness of the slice in sharp focus or to the thickness that the sonic beam "sees." It is closely related to lateral resolution. We described a B-mode scanner as a saber cutting a gash through the body. Two sabers would be more accurate: two sabers side by side separated by the width of the beam and cutting out a slice of tissue. The thinner the slice, the more accurately the images will depict a plane. The final image is a composite of all objects in the slice. The thickness and shape of the tomographic slice are the same as those of the sonic beam. A cylindrical beam (unfocused) produces a pancakelike slice with parallel sides in the Fresnel zone and a flared-out bottom in the Fraunhofer zone. Slices from focused transducers flare out at both the top and bottom, and are narrowest in the center. The top flare is limited by the width of the transducer but the bottom flare increases with increasing depth.

DOPPLER TECHNIQUES

The Doppler effect is a change in the perceived frequency of sound emitted by a moving source. The effect was first described by Christian Doppler in 1843. The cause of the frequency change is shown in Figure 20–32. In Figure 20–32A a vibrating source (p) produces a series of concentric waves, all moving out from the center, with the oldest in the most peripheral location (time 1) and the newest at the center (time 6). The velocity of sound in the particular medium and the frequency of the oscillator determine the wavelength (λ), or distance between crests. In Figure 20–32B the sound source is moving to the right as

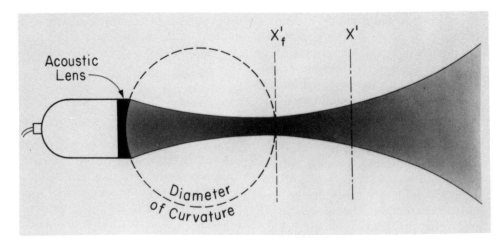

Figure 20–31   Focused transducer

it vibrates. It sends out a wave crest and then runs after the crest in one direction and away in the opposite direction. The sound usually moves faster than the source, so the source never catches the crest. Source motion does change the gap between crests, increasing the frequency and decreasing the wavelength to the right and decreasing the frequency and increasing the wavelength to the left. Sound velocity is not affected by source motion, so the sound moves at the same velocity in all directions. The wavelength change is caused by the source motion changing the spacing between crests.

The magnitude of the Doppler shift is shown in Figure 20–33. An ambulance moving 27 m/sec (60 miles/hr) is blowing its siren at a frequency of 1000 Hz. The frequency ahead of the siren is 1086 Hz, while the frequency behind it is 926 Hz. A pedestrian would hear a frequency shift of 160 Hz as the ambulance passed. The only persons hearing the true frequency of 1000 Hz would be the passengers in the vehicle. Doppler techniques are used to study motion, primarily that of the circulatory system. Two transducers are used in the audio mode, one as a transmitter and the other as a receiver. Both operate continuously.

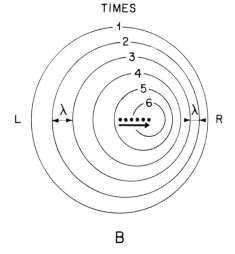

Figure 20–32   The Doppler shift

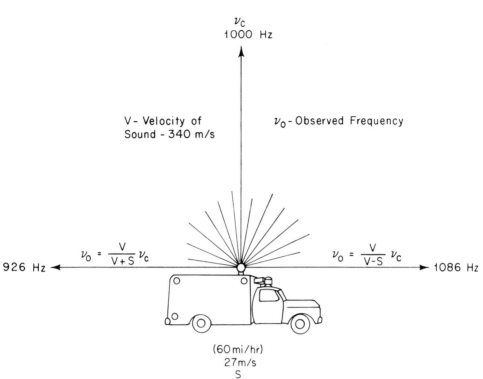

Figure 20–33   Magnitude of the Doppler shift

Pulsed Doppler devices that allow discrimination of Doppler signals from different tissue depths are much different from continuous wave Doppler, and will be described separately.

Continuous Wave Doppler

The continuous wave Doppler mode employs two piezoelectric elements, both contained in a single head (Fig. 20–34). One crystal transmits a continuous sonic signal at a known frequency, usually between 3 and 8 MHz. The other crystal receives the returning echoes and records their frequency. The frequency of the initial signal is algebraically subtracted from that of the returning echoes. The difference, the **Doppler shift,** usually falls within the frequency range detectable by the human ear and, after amplification, this Doppler shift is the audio signal. Returning echoes originate from the cellular elements of the blood, particularly the red blood cell. The

Doppler beam is used to detect the motion of the blood within the vessel rather than the motion of the vessel wall.

In contrast to pulsed sonography, in which the intensity of returning echoes is greatest when the beam is perpendicular to a reflecting surface, the Doppler shift is

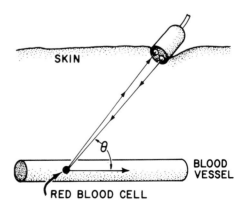

Figure 20–34   Audio mode Doppler transducer

greatest when the beam strikes a vessel at a small angle. Figure 20–34 shows a vector of red blood cell motion toward the transducer even though the transducer is not in the direct path of flow. The smaller the angle between the sonic beam and the flow direction (θ), the greater the vector of motion toward the transducer, and the greater the Doppler shift. Theoretically, motion cannot be detected when the transducer is perpendicular to the direction of blood flow, but this situation does not actually occur because of divergence of the beam (i.e., some part of the beam is always off of the perpendicular). The frequency change of back-scattered echoes can be calculated with the Doppler shift equation:

$$\Delta v = \frac{2\ vs}{v} \cos\theta$$

Δv = frequency change (Doppler shift-Hz)
v = frequency of initial beam (Hz)
s = velocity of blood (m/s)
v = velocity of sound (1540 m/s)
θ = angle between sound beam and direction of blood flow (Fig. 20–34)

The vector of blood cell motion toward the transducer is represented by cos θ in the equation. If the angle is increased, there is a smaller vector of motion toward the transducer and consequently cos θ is smaller. If the number of degrees in the angle is decreased, the cos θ is larger, and it approaches 1 as the transducer looks directly into the blood stream.

Why does the number 2 appear in the Doppler shift equation? When a Doppler shift is caused by moving red blood cells, two successive Doppler shifts are involved. First, the sound from a stationary transducer is received by moving red blood cells. Second, the moving red cells act as a moving source when they reradiate the sound back toward the transducer. A Doppler shift is generated when the moving red cells receive the ultrasound wave, and a second Doppler shift is generated when the moving cells reflect the ultrasound back to the stationary transducer. These two Dop-

pler shifts are nearly equal and add to each other. This double Doppler shift accounts for the factor of 2 appearing in the Doppler shift equation.

At frequencies between 2 and 10 MHz, the Doppler shift falls in the audible range for most physiologic motions. An experienced listener can learn a great deal about the status of the circulatory system with a Doppler device. It can be used to detect blood flow or its absence in both arteries and veins, to identify vascular constrictions with their associated eddy currents and venturi jets, and to detect fetal heart motion earlier than with any other method. It should be understood that the Doppler shift signal may be electronically processed to give the power spectrum of the signal (i.e., the range of frequencies and relative strength of each frequency). This processed signal may be observed and recorded to provide objective analysis of the Doppler shift signal.

Let us calculate the Doppler shift that might be encountered in a typical examination of arterial blood flow. Assume blood flow to be at an average velocity of 20 cm/sec (s = 0.2 m/s), the operating frequency of the transducer to be 5 MHz (v = 5,000,000 Hz), and the angle θ that the sound beam makes with respect to the vessel lumen to be 60° (cos 60° = 0.5):

$$\Delta v = \frac{2(5,000,000)\ (0.2)}{1540}\ (0.5)$$
$$\Delta v \cong 650\ \text{Hz}$$

Thus, for relatively slow-moving structures, the Doppler shift signal falls within the audible range. Note that the Doppler shift equation tells us that the change in frequency of the ultrasound signal received by the transducer will be 650 Hz, but does not designate whether the change will be positive or negative (i.e., we may receive 5,000,650 Hz or 4,999,350 Hz). If the flow of blood is toward the transducer, the higher frequency is received; if blood flow is away from the transducer, the Doppler shift will be negative. Thus, the sign of the frequency change carries information about the direction of blood flow. Some Doppler systems are able to use this information to measure flow direction. Most simple Doppler systems only indicate that flow is present and do not indicate direction.

A review of the Doppler shift equation reveals that the magnitude of the shift (Δv) will vary with the velocity of blood flow and the frequency of the transmitted ultrasound beam. For ultrasound frequencies in the range of 2 to 10 MHz, Δv will range from 0 to about 10 KHz for velocities ranging from 0 to 100 cm/sec.

Scattering of Ultrasound by Blood. The composition of blood causes important differences between the Doppler signal generated by blood and that generated by solid moving structures. Sound reflection from solid structures is usually referred to as **specular reflection.** Specular reflection implies a nice smooth surface. As an example, consider light reflected from a smooth mirror and a very rough surface. The light from the mirror is reflected in an orderly fashion, and as a result produces a nice sharp image. On the other hand, light from the rough surface is reflected in many different directions causing the light to be diffused or scattered. Similarly, the wall of a blood vessel is relatively smooth, whereas the red cells are not continuous and act as a rough surface. Ultrasound encountering blood is not reflected; it is scattered in all directions. This scattering is referred to as **Rayleigh-Tyndall scattering,** and is caused by the red blood cells (erythrocytes) in the blood. Red cells are the particulate components of blood that interact with ultrasound (platelets are too small and white blood cells too few in number). If the primary ultrasound wavelength is much larger than the size of the object encountered, the primary ultrasound wave will be scattered in all directions. The average diameter of a red blood cell is 7 μm (7 μm = 7/1,000,000 m = .000007 m = .007 mm). The wavelength of ultrasound is about .44 mm at 3.5 mHz and .154 mm at 10 mHz. Therefore, erythrocytes act as scatterers. The size of the echo from blood is small compared to that produced by specular reflection from solid tissue interfaces. A typical sonogram displays blood vessels as echo-free structures because of the scattering produced by erythrocytes.

The intensity of the scattered ultrasound wave in Rayleigh-Tyndall scattering increases with the fourth power of the frequency. Doubling the ultrasonic frequency causes the echo from blood to become 16 times as strong ($2^4 = 16$). Images of blood vessel lumens will be significantly different when Doppler instruments of different frequencies are compared.

Transducers for Continuous Wave Doppler. The typical transducer used in continuous wave Doppler instruments contains two separate piezoelectric elements, one for transmitting and the other for receiving ultrasonic waves. The transmitted sound beam and the receiving pattern of the receiver are very directional. To obtain maximum sensitivity for detecting returning echo signals, the beam regions of the transmitter and receiver are caused to overlap. This overlap is achieved by inclining the transducer elements (Fig. 20–35) or by using focused elements. The region of beam overlap defines the most sensitive region of the transducer.

Several technical considerations apply to the design of a transducer for continuous Doppler operation. Because one is concerned with the Doppler frequency shift, it is important to produce a transmitted signal that has a minimum of frequencies outside the resonant frequency of the transmitting transducer. This is done by using a high-Q transducer material, which means that the transducer will produce a narrow range of sound frequencies. With continuous Doppler operation as much of the generated power must be transmitted into the patient as possible. There are two requirements for this: all the energy transmitted to the back face of the transducer

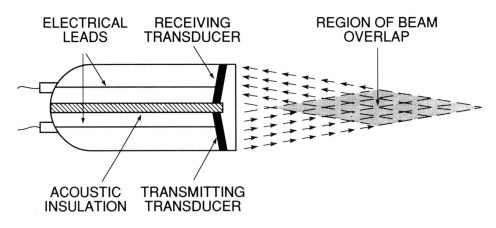

Figure 20–35 A typical Doppler ultrasound transducer with inclined transducer elements

must be reflected back to the front face; and all the power from the front face of the transducer must be transmitted to the patient. Reflection of energy from the back face of the transducer is accomplished by mismatching the acoustic impedance of the transducer material and the material behind it. This may be done by backing the transducer with air, which has an impedance much lower than that of the piezoelectric transducer (usually PZT). Acoustic transmission from the transducer face into the patient is now often accomplished with quarter-wave matching (previously discussed).

Doppler units designed to detect movement of the fetal heart must have as broad a beam as possible, so that small changes in the position of the fetus do not cause loss of the signal. Transducers for this purpose have several wide-angle transmitters surrounded by an array of similar receivers.

Figure 20–36 is a block diagram of the basic elements of a continuous wave Doppler instrument. The oscillator produces an electrical voltage varying at the resonant frequency of the transducer. Ultrasound is continuously transmitted by the transmitting transducer and continuously received by the receiving transducer. After amplification, the received echoes are fed to the demodulator, which also receives a signal

from the oscillator. The function of the demodulator is to compare the frequency of the received echoes to that of the oscillator, and to produce a signal equal to the difference in frequencies. The frequency difference in transmitted versus received signals is, obviously, the Doppler shift signal. Stationary interfaces produce a signal whose frequency is identical to that of the oscillator, and these signals are rejected by the demodulator. Most demodulators are also able to distinguish between signals whose frequency is higher and those whose frequency is lower than that of the transmitted signal (how this is done involves a lot of mathematics that we will not discuss). This is the way Doppler instruments provide information about the direction of the blood flow (i.e., toward or away from the transducer).

One addition problem must be considered. The receiving transducer and de-

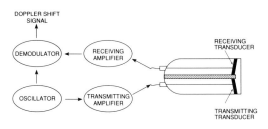

Figure 20–36. Block diagram of a continuous wave Doppler instrument

modulator will detect any moving structures within the sensitive volume of the beam. Slow moving solid structures within the sensitive volume, such as the wall of the aorta, will produce low frequency Doppler shift signals much stronger than the signal produced by scattering in blood. This very strong signal from the solid reflector may overload the demodulator, resulting in loss of part of the blood flow signal. For this reason, most instruments contain circuits that filter out and eliminate Doppler signals below a specified limit (typically 100 to 250 Hz in a 10-mHz system).

Choice of Operating Frequency. Remember that the transmitted Doppler frequency actually has a frequency spectrum rather than a single frequency spike, but we will continue to assume a single transmitted frequency signal to simplify our analysis.

The choice of the transmitted Doppler frequency is generally controlled by the need to obtain an adequate signal strength at the receiving transducer. As a general rule, the reduction in signal strength of a sound beam traveling through soft tissue is about 1 dB per cm per MHz. Thus, a 4-MHz wave traveling through 5 cm will have a loss of about 20 dB. Now, what does 20 dB mean? The answer is complicated, and we must be satisfied with only a partial answer. The definition of decibel given earlier in this chapter described a ratio between sound intensities:

$$\text{Intensity ratio in dB} = 10 \log_{10} \frac{\text{intensity}_1}{\text{intensity}_2}$$

A difference in the intensity ratio of 20 dB corresponds to a 100-fold difference in relative intensity between two sound beams:

$$20 \text{ dB} = 10 \log_{10} \frac{100}{1} = 10 \ (2) = 20$$

Here is the complication. The decibel system is also frequently used to express the relative amplitude of sound reflections. You may think of amplitude as the amount of displacement the sound beam causes on a certain area (such as the face of a piezoelectric crystal). Intensity and amplitude are related as

$$I = A^2 \ (\log I = 2 \log A)$$
$$I = \text{intensity}$$
$$A = \text{amplitude}$$

Therefore, the equation expressing amplitude ratio in the decibel system becomes

$$\text{Amplitude ratio in dB} = 20 \log_{10} \frac{\text{Amplitude}_1}{\text{Amplitude}_2}$$

When discussing attenuation of a sound beam in soft tissue, we are using the amplitude ratio. Therefore, a 20-dB loss in amplitude ratio represents a loss by a factor of 10:

$$20 \text{ dB} = 20 \log_{10} \frac{10}{1} = 20 \ (1) = 20$$

Similarly, a 40-dB loss in amplitude corresponds to a factor of 100, and a 60-dB loss represents a factor of 1000. When discussing attenuation of sound traveling through body tissues, we are using the decibel system to relate a change in relative amplitude. The answer to the original question of what a 20-dB loss in relative amplitude means is this: loss in relative amplitude by a factor of 10:1.

Because higher frequency sound is more rapidly attenuated by soft tissue, why not use lower frequencies for Doppler examinations? Use of a higher frequency offers several advantages. A higher frequency transducer will produce a stronger scattered signal because the intensity of the scattered wave increases with the fourth power of the frequency. Higher frequency beams produce two other desirable effects: higher frequency sound beams can be more sharply defined, and higher frequency input also causes a larger Doppler shift, which increases the sensitivity of the unit.

Continuous wave Doppler is very sensitive to weak signals. When there are several blood vessels within the sensitive region of beam overlap, a confusing superimposition of several Doppler signals can result. In the abdomen there are usually too many vessels present to allow continuous wave systems to be very useful. Continuous wave techniques are usually confined to examination of more superficial structures, such as the carotid arteries and vessels in the limbs. This may be done by using 7- to 10-mHz transducers. The high frequency limits penetration of the beam, thus limiting the sensitive region of beam overlap to superficial structures. Because of its extreme sensitivity, continuous wave Doppler is useful for examination of arteries within the eye and the female breast. One exception to use of high frequency is found in obstetrics. Continuous wave Doppler with a 3-mHz frequency is used to monitor the fetal heart sounds.

To review, choice of operating frequency of a continuous wave Doppler unit is a compromise between (1) high frequency, which gives a stronger returning signal, a larger Doppler shift, and a better defined beam, and (2) low frequency, which decreases amplitude attenuation of the beam in the body soft tissues.

Pulsed Doppler

With continuous wave Doppler instruments, reflectors and scatterers anywhere within the beam of the transducer contribute to the Doppler signal. Continuous wave Doppler lacks any form of depth resolution, and is thus not useful in the heart, in which everything is in constant motion. **Pulsed Doppler has provided the means of detecting the depth at which a returning signal has originated.** The depth can be positioned at any point along the axis of the pulsed Doppler ultrasound beam.

Pulsed Doppler is similar to a conventional pulse echo instrument in that bursts of ultrasound are emitted repetitively at a precisely controlled rate into the tissues. A new pulse is not transmitted until the echoes from the previous pulse have been detected. The depth at which a returning signal originated can be determined by knowing the time of transmission of the

signal and the time of its return (i.e., the "time of flight" to an interface and the subsequent return). Short bursts of ultrasound, about 0.5 to 1.0 μsec, can yield good axial resolution with separation of interfaces to within about 1 mm.

To summarize, continuous wave Doppler instruments provide velocity information and pulsed Doppler instruments provide both velocity and position information simultaneously.

To determine the Doppler shift of an echo at a specific depth requires that the ultrasonic transducer produce very short duration (such as 1 μsec) bursts at a precise rate of repetition. After transmission of this short burst of ultrasound, the receiving transducer may be turned on (termed "gating on") for a short period at a specific time. Therefore, only signals arriving from a specific tissue depth are available for detection. The "gate" position may be adjusted by the operator to select Doppler signals from any depth along the axis of the transducer. The same transducer is usually used for transmitting and receiving.

The operator controls the depth from which the Doppler shift signal will be received by changing the length of time the system waits after sending a pulse before opening the gate that allows the transducer to receive the signal. Also under operator control is the axial length along the beam from which the signal will be read. Axial length is determined by the length of time that the gate is open. The length of beam over which signals are detected typically varies from about 1.5 mm to 15 mm. The width of the beam is a function of the transducer and is often not under the control of the operator. Some scanners do allow some lateral beam focusing.

A brief review will emphasize the last two points, that is, the way a pulsed Doppler transducer is used to control the depth and axial length of the received Doppler shift signal. The depth (often called "range") from which the signal originates is controlled by the length of time after pulse transmission before the transducer is allowed to receive returning signals (the time at which the gate is turned on). The axial length over which the signal originates is determined by the length of time the gate is turned on. Some units allow further control of the volume of tissue in the sensitive region by allowing lateral focusing of the transducer.

The basic facts of pulsed Doppler have now been presented. A very short burst of ultrasound traveling through soft tissues generates a Doppler shift signal from all moving structures along the beam's path. By gating on the receiving transducer for a short period at a specified time following transmission of the burst, only Doppler signals originating from a specified depth are recorded. As you have come to expect, certain technical considerations turn the simple into the complex.

Let us first calculate how much time "time of flight" is talking about. Remember the speed of sound in soft tissues is 154,000 cm per second. A simple calculation (e.g., 1 ÷ 154,000) reveals that sound travels 1 cm in soft tissue in about 0.0000065 sec, usually expressed as 6.5 μsec. So, a round trip of 1 cm requires 13 μsec. This sets a time limit on the repetition rate of the pulses: the required time between successive pulses is at least 13 μsec per cm of range in the sample volume. For example, a time of 80 μsec between ultrasound bursts would allow detection of flow from vessels as deep as 6 cm, because 6 cm × 13 μsec/cm = 78 μsec. A new pulse cannot be transmitted until the desired echoes from the previous pulse have been recorded.

To determine the Doppler shift originating at a particular depth requires that the transmitted bursts of sound be repeated at a precise rate. As an example, let us consider how a 1-μsec burst might be generated every 80 μsec. The "clock" used to time the events is a master oscillator, which operates in a continuous mode. The rate at which this master oscillator clock fires the repetitive bursts is expressed in terms of kilohertz, which can be confusing. As an example, suppose we have a 2 MHz master oscillator that must generate a 1 μsec pulse every 80 μsec (this means a 1 μsec pulse with 79 μsec between pulses). To have the electronics respond in this fashion requires a counting circuit to count the cycles in the master oscillator. Since the master oscillator is 2 MHz, two oscillations will occur in 1 μsec. In 80 μsec, 160 oscillations (cycles) will occur. All that is necessary is to have the counter tell the transmitting amplifier to drive the transducer for two cycles and to be off for 158 cycles (these counting circuits are very easy for engineers to design, and even physicists can build them with only moderate effort). Therefore, the transducer will be driven for 1 μsec and will be off (able to detect returning signals) for 79 μsec. Since we get a pulse every 80 μsec, we can have a total of 12,500 pulses per second (1,000,000 μsec/sec ÷ 80 μsec = 12,500/sec). This example places two important limitations on the pulsed Doppler examination. First, the maximum depth from which a Doppler shift signal can be detected is 6 cm. Second, the maximum number of signals that can be detected in one second is 12,500. This pulse sequence will usually be described as a 12.5 kHz pulse repetition frequency, and each pulse will be exactly in step with the master oscillator so that precise depth measurements are possible. It may be that a higher frequency master oscillator is used, such as 5 MHz, in which case a burst of 1-μsec duration would require the counter to count 5-cycles for the 1 μsec pulse, and 400 cycles for the 12.5 kHz rate (on for 5-cycles, off for 395). Because the time between pulses must be at least 13 μsec per cm of tissue being examined, the maximum allowable pulse repetition frequency of pulsed Doppler ultrasound is in the 8 to 15-KHz range. As a review, consider a pulsed Doppler using a pulse repetition frequency of 5 kHz, 8 kHz, and 15 kHz. A repetition frequency of 5 kHz means there will be 5000 pulses per second (or per 1,000,000 μsec), with 200 μsec between pulses. Similarly, an 8 kHz pulse has 8000 pulses per second spaced at 125 μsec intervals. A 5 kHz pulse can detect a Doppler shift that originates from a maximum depth of about 15 cm, an 8 kHz about 9.5 cm, and a 15 kHz about 5 cm.

There is a reason that the pulse repetition frequency of a pulsed Doppler ultrasound system must be variable. It can be shown mathematically (but not by one of us) that the maximum Doppler shift frequency that can be detected by a pulsed Doppler system is equal to half the pulse repetition frequency. With the 12.5-KHz pulse repetition frequency used in the previous example, the maximum Doppler shift frequency that could be detected would be 6.25 KHz. For practice you should now calculate the velocity corresponding to a 6.25-KHz Doppler shift assuming a 5-MHz transducer and an angle θ of 0° (the answer is about 96 cm per second). The maximum depth at which this velocity could be detected is about 6 cm, as explained earlier. The maximum depth for a 5-kHz pulse repetition frequency is about 15 cm (200 μsec divided by 13 μsec per cm), and that of a 15-kHz pulse is about 5 cm (66 divided by 13). In these calculations we choose to ignore the approximately 0.5 to 1 μsec used to generate each pulse of transmitted ultrasound. Remember that a new ultrasound pulse cannot be emitted before the echo caused by the preceding pulse has been received. Thus, a high pulse repetition frequency limits the depth at which a pulsed Doppler transducer can receive echoes. Pulse-repetition frequency also determines the maximum Doppler shift frequency that can be detected. A 5-kHz pulse repetition frequency will allow samples to be obtained from a depth of 15 cm, but can detect Doppler shift signals of no greater than 2.5 kHz. Occasions arise when the Doppler shift frequency of moving blood is greater than the detectable fre-

quency when deep vessels are being examined. This results in the system producing an incorrect Doppler shift frequency, a phenomenon known as "aliasing." Attempts to correct aliasing by increasing the pulse repetition frequency may be successful (remember the detectable Doppler shift is equal to half the pulse repetition frequency). However, the higher pulse repetition frequency may not allow detection of signals from a sufficient depth of tissue. A second approach to deal with aliasing is to lower the ultrasound frequency, because this will also lower the Doppler shift frequency that must be detected. One may also lower the Doppler frequency by approaching the vessel being examined from a steeper angle, which will lower the value of cos θ in the Doppler shift equation. It is obvious that clinical use of pulsed Doppler ultrasound requires that the operator understand the equipment in considerable detail. By way of review of pulsed Doppler ultrasound techniques, we submit the following statements.

Pulse repetition frequency determines the depth at which a Doppler shift signal can be detected and the maximum Doppler shift that can be detected without encountering aliasing.

The Doppler shift frequency is directly related to the frequency of the initially transmitted ultrasound beam.

The Doppler shift frequency is directly related to the cosine of the angle between the transducer and the blood vessel being examined.

When a sound beam passes through a blood vessel, the back-scattered signal will consist of all the Doppler shifts produced by all the red cells moving through the sound beam. Because velocities of the red cells range from almost zero at the vessel wall to a peak velocity near the center of the vessel, a spectrum of Doppler shift frequencies will also be present. This spectrum may be quite complex with pulsating blood flow, especially when areas of vessel stenosis produce rapid and turbulent flow patterns. An experienced observer can hear the typical Doppler frequency shifts encountered with vessel stenosis. Frequency information is usually displayed on a pulsed Doppler image as a spectral display that depicts the Doppler shift frequencies in a blood vessel as they vary with time. The spectrum is determined by analyzing the returning Doppler shift spectrum. Mathematical spectral analysis (usually using a technique called "fast Fourier transform") of the complex signal can reduce the signal to a graph that shows the relative amplitude of each of the frequency components in the signal. The analysis can be performed at a very high speed. Three variables (time, frequency, and amplitude) are then available to make up the spectral display. The spectral display is displayed on the TV monitor in real time during the clinical examination.

The Duplex Scanner. We have reviewed the way in which the location and volume of a pulsed Doppler beam can be controlled. For such control to be useful, it is necessary for the operator to know where this sensitive volume is located within the patient. This is done by coupling the Doppler system with real-time ultrasound imaging. Most systems combine pulsed Doppler with real-time sector imaging (real-time imaging is our next topic). In general, a real-time image of the anatomy of interest is obtained and the image is frozen on the viewing screen. Then the Doppler mode is switched on, and the operator positions the location and axial length from which the Doppler signal will be obtained by locating appropriate cursors on the frozen real-time image. In this way, one can accurately define the area of interest by direct visualization. Usually, different transducers, often operating at different frequencies, perform the imaging and Doppler parts of the examination (examples might be 7-MHz imaging and 5-MHz Doppler in the carotid, or 5-MHz imaging and 3-MHz Doppler in the abdomen).

Many duplex systems can be used to estimate the velocity of flow in a blood vessel. First, the Doppler shift frequency of blood moving in the sensitive area of the beam is calculated. This calculation is a complex mathematical analysis performed by the system's computer, and we will not discuss these details. Second, the angle between the Doppler beam and long axis of the blood vessel must be measured from the ultrasound image. With these two determinations, plus knowledge of the frequency of the original beam and the velocity of sound in soft tissue, a simple algebraic calculation will solve the Doppler shift equation for the velocity of blood flow in the sensitive region of the pulsed Doppler beam. Clinical applications of this concept may be difficult, because arteries are not always nice and straight, and blood flow may not be exactly parallel to the wall of the vessel.

Doppler Color Flow Imaging

One limit of duplex ultrasonic imaging is that flow information is obtained only from the small area for which the Doppler signals are determined, and flow is not evaluated in the rest of the image. This requires that the examiner sample the proper sites throughout the lumen of a vessel. Doppler color flow imaging has been developed to produce imaging of flow throughout an entire real-time image, allowing visualization of blood vessels and their flow characteristics plus images of tissues surrounding the vessels. Clinical applications include carotid, cardiac, and peripheral arterial and venous imaging, evaluation of deep vessels in the abdomen, pelvis and fetus, and investigation of organ and tumor perfusion.

We will present the principles of Doppler color flow imaging and leave technical details to the engineers. First, consider duplex Doppler for a moment. Doppler shift information was obtained along a single ultrasound beam, or line, by gating on the receiving transducer to receive Doppler shift signal from one point (tissue depth) along the line. Such a system is called a "single range-gate" system. It is also possible to obtain a large number of Doppler signals simultaneously from selected points along the ultrasound beam. This is done by having multiple gates in the receiving transducer circuit, each gate controlled by a different time delay. The gates can be arranged to be close to each other so they can simultaneously sample Doppler shift information (amplitude, velocity, and direction) across the entire lumen of a large vessel. An arrangement of this type is called a "multigate" system. A typical multigate system will contain 16 to 32 gates, each with an axial length of about 1 mm.

A multigate system allows us to obtain Doppler shift information from many points along a single line, or ultrasound beam. As we will discuss in the next section, a real-time ultrasound image is made up of many lines of information obtained at a rapid rate. Typical numbers of lines for a single ultrasound frame range from about 100 to over 200 per frame (with about 15 to 30 frames per second). It is easy to visualize how a multigate system could be combined with a real-time system to obtain Doppler signals across an entire ultrasound image. Such an approach would require an enormous amount of circuitry, and would be too expensive. But this approach illustrates the principle of Doppler color flow imaging. In practice, the required Doppler information is obtained at each point along a single line by comparing the change in Doppler shift information (actually phase shift, which we will not discuss) that occurs during four to eight rapidly repeated pulses along the line. Color flow mapping requires that the beam remain stationary at one line for a brief time, then move to the next line, and so on. An electronic steered-array (or phased-array) transducer is used to obtain this type of scan. We will discuss steered-array transducers in the section on real-time ultrasound.

Color Doppler presents flow information by superimposing a color image on the gray-scale real-time image. This presents a real-time image of both anatomy and blood flow. Detected motion is assigned a color, usually red or blue. Color choice is arbitrary and usually under the control of the operator. Usually red is assigned to arteries and blue to veins. The hue and intensity of color change with changes on Doppler shift frequency. Usually a dim color is used to designate high velocity.

Color Doppler systems have two technical disadvantages. First, they compute mean, rather than maximum, velocity at each point in the sample. Second, the pulse repetition frequency is limited, limiting the Doppler shift frequency that can be detected. Color Doppler can be useful to rapidly identify areas of abnormal flow in blood vessels, but more detailed study of these abnormalities using standard range gated Doppler techniques is usually required. The real usefulness of color Doppler techniques has not been fully evaluated at this time (1989).

REAL-TIME ULTRASOUND

Real-time imaging systems are those that have frame rates fast enough to allow movement to be followed. With a conventional B-mode system the operator produces a single image frame with the transducer. This single frame is viewed until it is erased and a new image is generated. A real-time ultrasound transducer can produce multiple frames in a very short time, typically at least 10 frames per second. This fast frame rate allows movement to be viewed in "real-time" as the images are generated. Because of the short persistence of vision, a flicker-free display requires at least 16 frames per second.

Line Density and Frame Rate

Line density refers to the number of vertical lines per field of view. The lines can be parallel to each other, as in a linear array, or can radiate from a point, as in sector scanners. The greater the number of lines per frame, the higher the resolution of the image (Fig. 20–37). Obviously, we assume that each line contains new information. In some early units the number of lines per frame was increased by duplicating lines, a maneuver that will produce a pleasant image but does not add any information.

The maximum pulse repetition rate, or frame rate, is limited by the speed of ultrasound in tissue. Consider a structure 20 cm deep in a patient. The time required for an ultrasound pulse originating at the skin to reach the structure and then return to the transducer (a round trip of 40 cm) will be about 260/1,000,000 of a second, usually expressed as 260 μsec. Because a new pulse cannot be generated until all echoes from the first pulse have returned, the maximum number of individual lines that can be generated in our example is 3846 per second (1,000,000 ÷ 260). If there were 113 lines per frame (this is a common situation), the circumstances in

our example would allow a maximum of 34 frames per second. With 225 lines per frame, however, we are limited to 17 frames per second.

The purpose of the previous example is to illustrate the possible tradeoffs that must be considered with real-time imaging. Visualizing deep structures will require a slower frame rate (pulse repetition rate). High frame rates are desirable, however, when imaging fast-moving structures such as the heart. High line density is desirable to improve image quality, but more lines per frame requires a lower number of frames per second. As in film-screen radiography, some compromise is required.

Types of Real-Time Instruments

There are two basic techniques for producing real-time ultrasonic images. In one type a conventional single-element transducer, or group of single-element transducers, is mechanically moved to form images in real time. This is the group of **mechanical scanners.** The other technique uses an array of transducers. The transducers do not move, but are activated electronically so as to cause the ultrasonic beam to sweep across the patient. This is called **electronic array** real-time scanning.

Mechanical Scanning. Essentially there are three types of mechanical real-time scanning instruments. Two of these use a single transducer that is caused to oscillate, whereas the third uses two, three, or four transducers mounted on a rotating wheel. All produce an image with a sector format, usually encompassing an arc between 45° and 90°. This design produces a relatively rugged transducer that has a minimum of electronics and is of comparatively less complex design. The frame rate and sector angle can be varied in some instruments. Decreasing the sector angle will produce higher resolution, because the same number of vertical lines are compressed into a smaller area. Wide-angle sectors give lower resolution but allow a larger field of view. One disadvantage of sector scanners is that

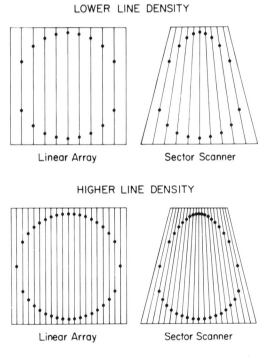

LOWER LINE DENSITY

Linear Array   Sector Scanner

HIGHER LINE DENSITY

Linear Array   Sector Scanner

Figure 20–37 Image resolution improves in both linear array and sector real time images as the number of lines per frame increases the scan format is relatively fixed for any transducer, requiring a change of transducers if any special imaging is required (such as an M-mode recording of the heart). Let us look briefly at the three types of mechanical real-time transducers.

Oscillating Transducer: Unenclosed Crystal. A single transducer crystal is caused to oscillate through an angle. The frame rate depends on the rate of oscillation, and can be varied. The motor driving the transducer is connected to the transducer by gears or a lever (Fig. 20–38). Because the oscillating transducer touches the patient's skin (i.e., there is no interposed water bath), both the operator and patient can feel vibrations caused by the moving crystal. A sector-shaped image is produced. This oscillating transducer is often called a wobbler sector scanner. The angle of wobble can be varied from about 15° to 60°, and frame rates are generally about 15 to 30 per second.

With mechanical scanners the ultrasound beam may be reflected from a reflecting mirror, making it possible to move the mirror rather than the transducer crystal. We will not describe mirror systems in any more detail.

Oscillating Transducer: Enclosed Crystal. In this type of sector scanner the transducer is enclosed in an oil- or water-filled container. Castor oil is commonly used as the fluid. The transducer may be driven by mechanical linkage to a motor. Another design attaches a permanent magnet to the

back of the transducer and mounts the combination between the poles of an electromagnet. Changing the direction of current flow through the coils of the electromagnet causes the magnet and transducer to oscillate. The type of image produced by this system depends on the distance between the transducer and the front surface of the casing that is in contact with the patient's skin. If the transducer is near the surface, a sector image (similar to that in Fig. 20–38*B*) is produced. When the transducer is mounted several centimeters behind the front surface, a trapezoidal image is produced (Fig. 20–39). With this type of system the patient does not feel any vibration because the moving transducer does not touch the skin. The ultrasonic, or acoustic, window through which the ultrasound beam emerges is made of a flexible membrane, and it is this window that contacts the patient's skin.

Rotating Wheel Transducer. This type usually employs three or four transducers that are mounted 120° or 90° apart on a wheel (Fig. 20–40). The wheel diameter is usually between 2 and 5 cm. Several different methods are used to connect the wheel to a motor, which rotates the wheel at a constant rate in one direction only. The ultrasound beam emerges through an acoustically transparent window. Only the transducer that is behind the acoustic window is allowed to transmit and receive ul-

Figure 20–38 An oscillating transducer with an unenclosed crystal (*A*) produces a sector image (*B*)

Figure 20–39 An oscillating transducer with an enclosed crystal (*A*) may produce a trapezoidal image (*B*)

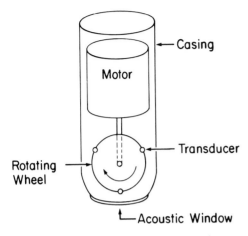

Figure 20–40 A rotating wheel transducer

trasound waves. Depending on design, either a sector- or trapezoid-shaped image may be produced.

Rotating transducer systems can also be designed to use a reflecting mirror. The sector or trapezoid field may be operated at an opening angle up to 90°. If only two transducers are used, it is possible to use a sector angle as large as 180°.

Electronic Array Scanning. There are basically two types of electronic real-time scanners. Both use arrays of transducers composed of many small rectangular transducer elements (about 2 × 10 mm) arranged adjacent to each other. The two types are **linear array** (which produces a rectangular scan format) and **phased** or **steered array** (which produces sector scans). Unlike mechanical systems, the transducers in an electronic array real-time system do not move. The ultrasound beam is caused to move by electronic controls. We will attempt to describe the design of these transducers and to explain how electronics causes the ultrasound beam to move and become focused.

Linear Array. This consists of a number of small rectangular transducer elements (about 2 mm × 10 mm) arranged in a line, with their narrow dimensions touching. There could be 64 to 200 transducers forming an assembly from 4 to 10 cm long.

In our examples we will assume an assembly of 64 transducers. From our earlier discussion you will recall that a good ultrasound image requires a satisfactory number of vertical lines per image. Early linear array instruments had 20 transducer elements, with each transducer being larger than those in more recent units. The resulting image had only 20 lines per frame, which did not produce a very satisfactory picture.

Increasing the number of lines per frame without increasing the total length of the transducer assembly would seem to have a simple solution: use more but smaller transducers. This is exactly how the problem has been solved, but a new problem is created. Please refer back to Figures 20–13 and 20–14 to remind yourself that the length of the Fresnel (near, or nondivergent) zone of an ultrasound beam is determined by the diameter of the transducer and the wavelength of the ultrasound:

$$x' = \frac{r^2}{\lambda}$$

x' = length of Fresnel zone
r = radius of the transducer
λ = wavelength

Thus, for a constant wavelength, decreasing transducer size will shorten the Fresnel zone and increase the angle of dispersion. If each transducer in a 64-unit assembly were fired separately, the resulting beam pattern would disperse rapidly and be of no diagnostic usefulness (Fig. 20–41A).

The problem of a sufficient number of lines per frame versus the need for satisfactory beam focusing (i.e., a long Fresnel zone) has been solved in two ways: first, by using an array with many narrow transducer elements to produce high line density; and second, by firing the transducers in groups, causing the group to act as a single larger transducer and thus provide better resolution (Fig. 20–41B).

The pulsed sequence of firing of groups of transducers in a linear array is illustrated

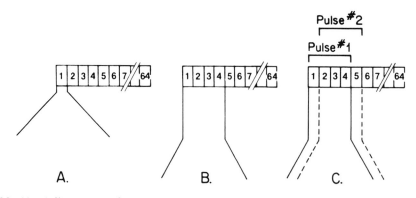

Figure 20–41   A linear transducer array

in Figure 20–41*C*. We will assume that four transducer elements are operated as a group. In the illustration, pulse 1 is generated by simultaneously pulsing elements 1, 2, 3, and 4. After the echoes return to this first group, the next line in the frame is generated (pulse 2) by pulsing elements 2, 3, 4, and 5. This sequence continues until elements 61, 62, 63, and 64 form the final line in the frame. By this mechanism a linear array of 64 elements (individual transducers) pulsed in groups of four and stepped one element between lines will produce a frame with 61 lines. This is the origin of the 61-line frame we mentioned in the introduction to this section. The entire array will be pulsed in approximately 1/20 to 1/50 sec, producing 20 to 50 frames per second. The number of lines per frame will depend on the number of transducers in the array, the number of transducers pulsed at one time, and the sequence of pulsing.

We must now turn to the question of how the ultrasound beam originating from a linear array is focused. This is done electronically in one dimension, and with a plastic lens in another dimension.

You will recall that an ultrasound beam can be focused in a manner similar to the effect of lenses and mirrors on visible light. Focusing can increase the intensity of an ultrasound beam by factors greater than 100. Plastics are used as the lens material. Because the speed of sound in plastic is greater than that in water and soft tissue, a concave lens is necessary for focusing an ultrasonic beam (note that this is the opposite of the effect of optical lenses on visible light). For our example, we will consider that the linear array is made up of a series of 2-mm × 10-mm transducers (elements). Focusing along the 10-mm dimension is accomplished by placing a long concave lens in front of the elements (Fig. 20–42). Remember, the concave lens will not bring the beam to a focus at a single point, but will create a focal zone (i.e., a distance over which the focal properties are

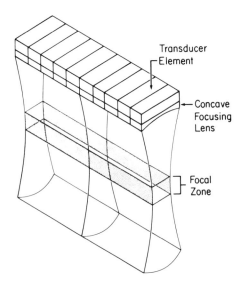

Figure 20–42   A concave lens used to focus a linear array

fairly well maintained). This focusing lens determines the width of the ultrasound beam in the plane perpendicular to the image plane, and determines the thickness of the image slice.

A fixed lens cannot be used to focus the beam in the plane parallel to the image because the location of the beam is constantly moving along the array as the elements are switched on and off. Focusing to improve resolution in this plane is termed "improved azimuthal resolution," and is accomplished electronically (Fig. 20–43). How can an ultrasonic beam generated by a group of transducers be focused electronically? We will discuss this in some detail because the same principle applies to steered array real-time scanners. The student interested in details about electronic focusing should consult the elegant article and illustrations of Wells.[17]

To improve azimuthal resolution, the method of pulsing each individual transducer element within each group is changed. Figure 20–44 shows how a group of four transducer elements can be focused electronically. First, refer back to Figure 20–11, which shows that the concentric rings of sound originating from different points within a single piezoelectric crystal reinforce each other to form a wave front in front of the crystal. Similarly, each element in a group can be considered to emit a circular wavelet when stimulated. When each transducer element in the group is stimulated at the same time, the wavelets will reinforce each other to form a wave front that travels normal to the surface of the array (Fig. 20–44A). When all elements in a group are pulsed at the same time, the resultant wave front behaves like a non-focused single-element transducer equal in diameter to the width of all the elements in the group.

Producing a focused beam using a group of transducer elements can be accomplished by stimulating the individual elements at slightly different times (Fig. 20–44B). If the two central elements are pulsed several nanoseconds (1 nanosecond = 10^{-9} sec) after the outer two elements, the wavelets from the individual elements combine to form a focused beam. When speaking of ultrasound propagation in tissue, a nanosecond is a very short time. You will recall that ultrasound travels one centimeter in soft tissue in about 6.5 μseconds (microsecond = 10^{-6} second), and the timing between pulses is usually slower than one pulse every 80 μsec (the time required for a round trip of 6 cm). It is possible to vary the sharpness of the focus (length of the focal zone) and the depth of focus by varying the time delay between the pulsing of the central and outer elements of the group. In some systems the operator has some control of sharpness of focus and depth of focus. As the operating group of elements is switched along the entire array, the associated delay (i.e., focusing) signals must be appropriately switched along the array to maintain the focusing action.

The typical linear array real-time scanning transducer used in adult abdominal examinations employs a transducer array about 120 mm long by 10 mm wide, and a frequency of between 2 and 3 MHz. The basic principles of the instrumentation are said to be relatively simple, allowing portable battery-operated units to be designed. ***Steered or Phased Array.*** The term

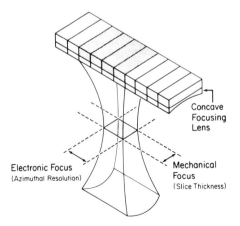

Figure 20–43 Focusing a linear array transducer

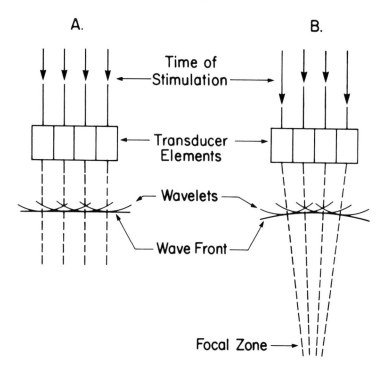

Figure 20–44   Electronic focusing of the ultrasonic beam produced by a transducer array

"steered array" or "phased array" may be used for this type of real-time scanning.

With a steered array transducer a sector scan is obtained, but the transducer is not moved while the scan is being generated. Rather, the ultrasound beam is caused to sweep back and forth across the patient by using electronically controlled steering and focusing.

For linear array scanning we discussed how an ultrasound beam produced by a group of transducers could be focused by the appropriate choice of time delays. Similarly, the beam may be directed, or steered, to a desired angle by a similar mechanism of time delays. By choosing the appropriate delay between stimulation of the individual elements of the transducer, it is possible to steer the beam, or to steer and focus the beam simultaneously. This concept is illustrated with simple block diagrams in Figure 20–45. Note that it is necessary to change the pulsing sequence constantly for each element in the array.

A steered array transducer is similar in size to a single-element transducer used for conventional B-mode scanning. A typical transducer contains 32 elements and operates at a frequency of 2 to 3 MHz. With a steered array transducer all the elements are pulsed to form each line of the image, as opposed to the linear array in which only a few (typically four) elements produce each line in the image. The scan format is a sector with its apex at the center of the array. The ultrasound beam is caused to sweep through the sector angle at a rate fast enough to form a real-time image. A similar delay pattern is introduced into the received signals, which causes the transducer to be sensitive only to echoes returning along the same path as the transmitted beam.

The steered array system can be used to produce a time-motion tracing from a single line, while simultaneously displaying the entire sector image. It has found its major application in cardiac imaging and in evaluation of vessel pulsation in abdominal imaging. Two problems presently limit

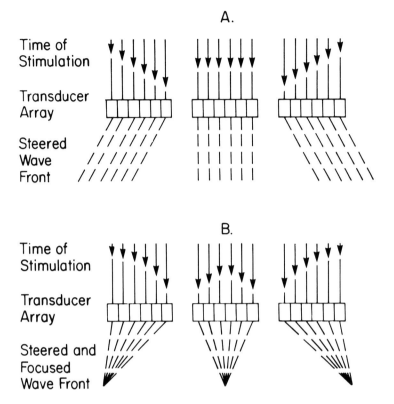

Figure 20–45   A steered array transducer system showing a nonfocused (*A*) and an electronically focused (*B*) beam

more general use of this technique. First, image quality is not uniform across the entire beam pattern, and resolution may not be as good at the edges of the sector as in the center. Second, this instrument is very expensive because of the complex computer-controlled electronics necessary to steer and focus the beam.

SUMMARY

Ultrasound is sound with a frequency greater than 20,000 cycles/sec (Hertz, Hz). Medical sonography employs frequencies between 1 megahertz (MHz) and 20 MHz. These high frequencies are produced by subjecting a special ceramic material, a piezoelectric crystal, to a short-voltage spike. A group of synthetic piezoelectric materials called "ceramic ferroelectrics" have replaced the piezoelectric crystal materials that were used earlier. Although PZT is currently the most widely used material, research suggests that certain plastic polymers may soon replace these synthetic ceramics in the construction of ultrasound transducers. The electric field created by the voltage spike realigns crystalline elements (dipoles) in the ceramic, thereby suddenly changing the crystal's thickness. This sudden change in thickness starts a series of vibrations that produces sound waves.

The piezoelectric crystal is housed in the front of a transducer, a plastic box that protects the crystal from mechanical trauma and provides sonic and electrical insulation. Electrodes are plated onto the surface of the crystal, and the outside electrode is grounded to protect the patient from electrical shock. A backing block dampens vibrations between voltage spikes, so the transducer can be used to generate multiple short pulses of sound. If a clinical situation dictates a different frequency, another transducer must be selected, one designed with the appropriate frequency. Piezoelectric crystals can be damaged by heat. Above a critical temperature, called the "Curie temperature," a crystal loses its piezoelectric properties and becomes a worthless piece of ceramic. The Q factor is a measure of the purity of tone (narrowness of frequency range). The ring down-time is the time that it takes a transducer to stop vibrating.

An ultrasonic beam is a series of longitudinal waves that transmit energy. These waves travel through average body tissue at a velocity of 1540 m/sec. Their velocity is independent of frequency. The velocity of sound depends on the density and compressibility of the conducting medium, and is equal to the frequency multiplied by the wavelength. As a sound beam passes through the body, the beam is attenuated, or reduced in intensity, by a combination of diffusion, reflection, refraction, and absorption. The sonic beam is fairly coherent with parallel sides in the near, or Fresnel, zone. Beyond a certain critical distance, the transition point, the beam reaches the far, or Fraunhofer, zone and begins to flare out and disperse. The length of the near zone is proportional to the square of the diameter of the transducer and inversely proportional to the wavelength of the sound. The beam is rapidly attenuated by dispersion in the far zone. Reflection occurs at tissue interfaces. The incident and reflected angles are equal. The amount of reflection depends on the difference in the acoustic impedance of the two surfaces and on the angle of incidence of the beam. Acoustic impedance is the product of the density and velocity of sound in the conducting medium. Reflection is greatest with a large difference between the acoustic impedance of the two media and with a small incident angle. Reflection is least, and transmission greatest, at an incident angle of 90°.

When the velocity of sound changes as it passes from one medium to another, the frequency remains constant but the wavelength changes. If the wave front strikes the second medium at an angle, the sound is refracted, or bent. The degree of refraction depends on the angle of incidence and on the difference in the velocity of sound in the two media. Absorption, which is the conversion of sound into heat, depends on the frequency of the sound and on both the viscosity and relaxation time of the conducting medium. Absorption in tissue is proportional to frequency; that is, increasing from 1 to 2 MHz doubles absorption and halves the penetrating power of the beam. Therefore, high-frequency sound cannot be used to examine thick body parts.

A longitudinal wave is propagated by multiple particles (molecules) oscillating in the direction of propagation to produce bands of compression and rarefaction in the conducting medium. When these bands are back-scattered to the piezoelectric crystal as echoes they change the crystal's thickness, which produces an electrical signal. This signal forms the basis of the ultrasonic image. The sound is transmitted in short bursts, or pulses, usually 1000/sec. The pulses are short, about 0.000001 sec in duration. Between pulses the transducer acts as a receiver, recording returning echoes. The time delay between the initiation of a pulse and the return of an echo is converted into depth in all imaging modes. The images can be displayed in several modes. Multiple controls are provided to augment weaker echoes. The most important control is the time gain compensator, which logarithmically enhances echoes from selected depths after an adjustable delay.

Depth resolution, the ability to separate two objects in tandem, depends on the spatial pulse length, which is the number of waves in a pulse multiplied by the wavelength. Depth resolution is best with transducers that have a short spatial pulse length. Lateral resolution, the ability to separate two adjacent objects, depends on the width of the sonic beam. The beam can be narrowed with an acoustic lens, which bends the sound toward a focal point.

The Doppler effect is a change in the perceived frequency of a sound emitted by a moving source. Doppler devices are used to detect motion. They accomplish this by transmitting a sound beam and recording and demodulating returning echoes. The difference between the two frequencies usually falls in the audible range for most physiologic motions. After amplification the difference becomes an audio signal. Continuous wave Doppler instruments can provide velocity information, but lack any form of depth resolution. Pulsed Doppler instruments provide both depth and velocity information simultaneously. A pulsed Doppler instrument is usually combined with some other form of ultrasound imaging system in a "piggybacked" system. Spectral analysis of a Doppler signal, by allowing evaluation of the spectrum of frequencies making up a Doppler signal, allow evaluation of the nature of blood flow in normal and stenotic blood vessels.

Real-time imaging systems produce image frames fast enough to allow motion to be followed. A compromise between line density per frame and frame rate is required. Frame rates are usually at least 16 frames per second. The real-time image may be generated by a mechanical scanner or by an electronic array arrangement. Mechanical scanners generate a sector format image with either an oscillating transducer or a rotating wheel transducer. Electronic array real-time scanners may use a linear array transducer, which produces a rectangular scan format, or a steered array transducer, which produces a sector format image. Focusing the electronic array ultrasound beam requires both a concave plastic lens and electronic focusing. Satisfactory beam geometry requires that the individual elements in a linear array transducer be pulsed in groups, commonly four elements

at a time, with each group producing one line in the resulting image. With a steered array transducer, all elements of the transducer are pulsed to form each line of the image.

REFERENCES

1. Baker, D.W.: Applications of pulsed Doppler techniques. Radiol. Clin. North Am., *18*:79, 1980.
2. Barnes, R.W.: Ultrasound techniques for evaluation of lower extremity venous disease. Semin. Ultrasound, *11*:276, 1981.
3. Burns, P.N.: The physical principles of Doppler and spectral analysis. J. Clin. Ultrasound, *15*:567, 1987.
4. Burns, P.N., Jaffe, C.C.: Quantitative flow measurements with Doppler Ultrasound: techniques, accuracy, and limitations. Radiologic Clinics of N.A., *23*:641, 1985.
5. Carpenter, D.A.: Ultrasonic transducers. Clin. Diagn. Ultrasound, *5*:31, 1980.
6. Cooperberg, P.L., David, K.B., Sauerbrei, E.C.: Abdominal and peripheral applications of real-time ultrasound. Radiol. Clin. North Am., *18*:59, 1980.
7. Hendee, W.R.: Medical Radiation Physics. Chicago, Year Book Medical Publishers, 1979.
8. James, A.E., Fleischer, A.C., et al.: Ultrasound: Certain considerations of equipment usage. *In* The Physical Basis of Medical Imaging. Edited by G.M. Coulam, et al. New York, Appleton-Century-Crofts, 1981, p. 169.
9. James, A.E., Goddard, J., et al.: Advances in instrument design and image recording. Radiol. Clin. North Am., *18*:3, 1980.
10. Merritt, C.R.B.: Doppler color flow imaging. J. Clin. Ultrasound, *15*:591, 1987.
11. Price, R.R., Jones, T., Fleischer, A.C., and James, A.E.: Ultrasound: Basic principles. *In* The Physical Basis of Medical Imaging. Edited by G.M. Coulam, et al. New York, Appleton-Century-Crofts, 1981, p. 155.
12. Rose, J.L., and Goldberg, B.B.: Basic Physics in Diagnostic Ultrasound. New York, John Wiley and Sons, 1979.
13. Sanders, R.C., and James, A.E.: The Principles and Practice of Ultrasonography in Obstetrics and Gynecology. New York, Appleton-Century-Crofts, 1980.
14. Sarti, D.A.: Diagnostic Ultrasound Text and Cases. Year Book Medical Publishers, Inc. Chicago, London. 1987.
15. Skolnick, M.L.: Real-Time Ultrasound Imaging in the Abdomen. New York, Springer-Verlag, 1981.
16. Souquet, J., Defranould, P., and Desbois, J.: Design of low-loss wide-band ultrasonic transducers for noninvasive medical application. IEEE Trans. Sonics Ultrasonics, *Su-26*:75, 1979.
17. Wells, P.N.T.: Real-time scanning systems. Clin. Diagn. Ultrasound, *5*:69, 1980.
18. Wells, P.N.T.: Biomedical Ultrasonics. London, Academic Press, 1977.

CHAPTER

21 *Protection*

HISTORICAL REVIEW

Many somatic dangers of radiation became evident a few months after x rays were discovered. Roentgen announced his discovery in December of 1895. In 1896, 23 cases of radiodermatitis were reported in the world literature.[1] Between 1911 and 1914, three review articles identified 54 cancer deaths and 198 cases of radiation-induced malignancy. The first American radiation fatality occurred in 1904 when Thomas Edison's assistant, Clarence M. Dally, died of cancer. A few farsighted individuals cried out for radiation controls, but their pleas were largely ignored. Catastrophes continued until the whole medical community became alarmed. Finally, in 1921, the first official action was taken when the British X-Ray and Radium Protection Committee was founded to investigate methods for reducing exposures. Their efforts were severely hampered, however, because they did not have a satisfactory unit of radiation measurement. The crude units of the time, the erythema dose and "slight film fogging," proved completely inadequate. In 1928, the Second International Congress of Radiology (ICR) appointed a committee to define the Roentgen (R) as a unit of exposure. The committee did not finish its assignment until 1937, but the Roentgen became the accepted unit of measurement even though it was not accurately defined.

The first dose-limiting recommendation was made by a group of American scientists, the Advisory Committee on X-Ray and Radium Protection, in 1931, 46 years after Roentgen's discovery. The recommendation was 0.2 R per day. The name of the committee has been changed several times, and it is now called the National Council on Radiation Protection and Measurements (NCRP). It is a private organization of scientists, experts in various aspects of radiation, who operate under a congressional charter but without legal status. The NCRP publishes its recommendations periodically in handbooks. These are purely advisory, but most state and federal laws are based on NCRP recommendations. Since the first recommendation of 50 R per year (0.2 R per workday), made in 1931, the maximum permissible dose (MPD) has been lowered on three separate occasions (Table 21–1). The MPD is now only one tenth of its initial level. Recommended exposures have been lowered because of growing concern over the increasing use of diagnostic radiation, and apprehension about the mounting evidence that small doses can cause leukemia and carcinoma.

BIOLOGICAL EFFECTS OF RADIATION

All ionizing radiation is harmful! This is the premise that mandates a radiation

Table 21–1. Historical Review of Maximum Permissible Dose (MPD) Recommendations of the National Council on Radiation Protection and Measurements

DATE	ANNUAL MPD (rem)
1931	50
1936	30
1948	15
1958	5

protection policy. The harmful effects fall into two broad categories: somatic, those effects harmful to the person being irradiated; and genetic, those effects harmful to future generations. We are not qualified to discuss the biologic effects of radiation in any detail, so our description will be quite superficial. The interested reader should read one of the texts listed at the end of this chapter.[2,3,6] **One important point must be emphasized: the data are not available to indicate if there is a threshold below which no harmful effect will occur.** Without this knowledge, we cannot say that there is a safe dose. Therefore, a recommendation that 5 rem per year is the maximum permissible dose really means "that, in light of present knowledge, this dose is not expected to cause appreciable bodily injury to a person at any time during his lifetime."[5] **In actual practice, radiation levels should be kept at the lowest practicable level, and we should not think of permissible doses as being perfectly safe.**

The most important somatic effect of radiation is carcinogenesis, and leukemia is the most common neoplasia. The exact risk is unknown. Hall made the statement that "the 20-year risk from leukemia plus all other radiation-induced neoplastic diseases is 6 cases per 100,000 individuals exposed per rem."[2] He admitted that this estimate was made on limited data and involved many tenuous assumptions. Nevertheless, most experts agree that low doses of radiation can cause neoplasms. Usually there is a long latent period, ranging from 5 to 20 years for leukemia and from 10 to 30 years for other tumors.

The genetic effects of radiation are more frightening than the somatic ones, because they may not manifest themselves for several generations. Each new mutant constitutes a potential burden to society, and the burden must be kept at the lowest level consistent with good medical practice. Because of the fear of these genetic effects, dose limits are placed on exposures to large segments of the population, as opposed to maximum permissible doses. This emphasizes the need to restrict exposures. The **genetically significant dose (GSD)** is defined as the dose that, if received by every member of the population, would be expected to produce the same total genetic injury as the actual doses received by the various individuals. For example, if the world population consisted of 1000 individuals and each received a radiation dose of 0.1 rem, the genetic effect would be the same as if 10 individuals received 10 rem and the other 990 received nothing:

$$1000 \times 0.1 = (10 \times 10) + (990 \times 0)$$

The concept implies that the effect of large exposures to a few individuals is greatly diluted by the total population and thus has little overall genetic impact. Radiation workers may receive relatively large exposures without significantly changing the population's genetically significant dose.

RADIATION UNITS

Before discussing maximum permissible dose (MPD) recommendations, we are going to digress and define three units of radiation measurement: the roentgen, the rad, and the rem.

The roentgen (R) is defined as a unit of **radiation exposure** that will liberate a charge of 2.58×10^{-4} coulombs per kilogram of air.[4] Please recall from Chapter 1, and Table 1–3, that no special SI unit corresponds to the familiar radiation exposure unit of the roentgen. In the SI system, exposure is expressed in terms of coulombs per kilogram. This definition is relatively meaningless to most radiologists, because the coulomb is not part of our daily vocabulary. In more familiar terms, a roentgen is the approximate exposure to the body surface for an AP film of the abdomen for a patient of average thickness. As a measure of exposure, the roentgen is independent of area, or field size (Fig. 21–1). When a large square (A) is exposed to 1 R, each increment of the square receives 1 R. If the square is divided into multiple

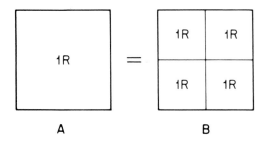

Figure 21–1 The exposures in A and B are identical

smaller squares (B), each of these squares receives 1 R of exposure. It would be improper to add the exposures of the smaller squares and say the total was 4 R, because no area has received that much exposure. This is a familiar concept in other areas of our daily lives. For example, rainfall is measured in inches without regard to area. A 1-in. rain produces a 1-in. deep layer of water in a drinking glass or a washtub, provided they both have flat bottoms and perpendicular sides. Roentgen exposures are exactly the same.

The **rad** is the unit of **absorbed dose.** One rad is equal to the radiation necessary to deposit energy of 100 ergs in 1 gram of irradiated material (100 erg/g). The **gray (Gy)** is the SI unit for absorbed dose. Louis Harold Gray (1905–1965) made one of the most fundamental contributions to radiation dosimetry, the principle now known as the Bragg-Gray Theory (this theory deals with radiation therapy, so we do not discuss it). One Gy is defined to be the radiation necessary to deposit energy of one joule in one kilogram of tissue (Gy = J/kg). The relationship between the Gy and the rad is:

$$1 \text{ Gy} = 100 \text{ rads}$$
$$1 \text{ rad} = 1 \text{ cGy (centigray)}$$

One gray is equivalent to 100 rads. **One centigray (cGy) is the same as one rad.** Values of absorbed dose are being increasingly reported in the literature in terms of the cGy, which is really just our old friend the rad with a new name.

The absorbed dose is independent of the composition of the radiated material and energy of the beam. The number of rads (cGy) deposited per roentgen of exposure, however, varies both with energy of the beam and with the composition of the absorber (Table 21–2). The energy deposited in soft tissue per roentgen is approximately 95 erg/g in the diagnostic energy range. It may be five times as much in bone at low energies and actually a little less than 95 erg/g at 1 MeV. As a general rule, the absorbed dose is proportional to the degree of attenuation.

The **rem** is a unit of **absorbed dose equivalent.** The rem is a unit used only in radiation protection. The rem is a measure of the biological effectiveness of radiation. The SI unit of absorbed dose equivalent is the **sievert** (in honor of the Swedish scientist who was active in the ICRP for many years). The relationship between the sievert (Sv) and the rem is:

$$1 \text{ sievert (Sv)} = 100 \text{ rems}$$

In this chapter we will continue to use rems.

The absorbed dose equivalent is equal to the absorbed dose multiplied by a **quality factor (QF):**

$$\text{Rem} = \text{rads} \times \text{quality factor}$$

The rem is a measure of the biologic effectiveness of irradiation. Some practical quality factors are shown in Table 21–3.[8] These are only approximations; the actual numbers depend on the energy of the beam. Because the quality factor for x rays is 1, the rad and rem are equal. In fact, at diagnostic energy levels the rad, rem, and roentgen may all be considered to be equal,

Table 21–2. Approximate Absorbed Dose (Rad) per Roentgen of Exposure

TYPE OF TISSUE	RAD PER ROENTGEN OF EXPOSURE	
	50 kVp	1 MeV
Soft tissue	0.95	0.95
Bone	5.0	0.90

Table 21–3. Recommended Quality Factor Values for Various Types of Radiation

TYPE OF RADIATION	APPROXIMATE VALUE OF QUALITY FACTOR
X rays	1
Gamma rays	1
Beta particles	1
Electrons	1
Thermal neutrons	5
Other neutrons*	20
Protons*	20
Alpha particles	20

*These are the worst case (maximum) values. Since Q is a function of particle type and energy, Q values for a particular particle may be significantly lower.[8]

because the energy deposited in soft tissues by 1 R of exposure is only 5% more than a rad:

$$1 \ R \simeq 1 \ rad = 1 \ rem$$

X rays and beta particles have the same quality factor. This is logical, because the beta particle is a moving electron and the end product of x-ray attenuation is also a moving electron. They are used as the standard, and assigned a quality factor of 1. Larger particles deposit more energy per unit length of travel. The amount of energy deposited per unit length of travel, expressed in keV per micron, is called the **linear energy transfer (LET)**. If an electron and proton start with the same energy, the proton will be attenuated more quickly. Because of the proton's large size, it encounters more "friction" as it passes between atoms. Having started with the same amount of energy as the electron, the proton deposits more energy per unit length of travel, so it is a higher LET radiation. The amount of biologic damage is determined by the linear energy transfer of the radiation. A tissue absorbing 100 rads of thermal neutron radiation sustains five times as much biologic damage as a tissue absorbing the same quantity of x rays. Thus, thermal neutrons have a quality factor of 5. For radiation protection purposes the quality factor is multiplied by the ab-

sorbed dose in rads to determine the dose equivalent in rems.

The **relative biologic effectiveness (RBE)** is another expression used to compare the effectiveness of several types of radiation. It must be determined for each type of radiation and biologic system and, by convention, is reserved for laboratory investigation.

POPULATION EXPOSURES

All individuals are exposed to radiation in low doses. Of concern is the risk involved in this low dose radiation, especially the induction of cancer or genetic defects.

Risk assessment is in some way related to the absorbed dose. This risk cannot be a simple linear function of just the absorbed dose because irradiation from the external environment affects the entire body, whereas medical diagnostic procedures generally affect only selected areas of the body. In an attempt to make some comparison in the risk assessment for all types of exposures, the concept of **effective dose equivalent (H_E)** has been developed.[5] **The purpose of the effective dose equivalent is to relate exposure to risk.**

It is difficult to evaluate risk of radiation absorbed in local regions of the body (e.g., skull, chest, or ankle radiographs) compared to radiation to the entire body (e.g., cosmic radiation). What one must do is assign a weighting factor to each type of radiation exposure in an attempt to express the risk involved in that exposure compared to the risk involved from total body radiation. This weighting is accomplished by the effective dose equivalent (H_E). Consider an example. The H_E resulting from a chest radiographic examination is .06 mSv (6 mrem). An H_E of .06 mSv means that the risk involved from a chest examination is the same as the risk involved in exposing the entire body to an x-ray exposure of .06 mSv. Notice that H_E does not measure exposure to the chest; H_E does assign a risk value resulting from an exposure to the chest. This concept of effective dose equivalent is described in detail in NCRP Report No. 93, (Reference 5), and you are advised to review this short document.

Annual exposures (expressed as H_E) in the United States from the various types of radiation are summarized in Table 21–4.[5] Note that radiation sources are divided into natural sources and medical sources. We will discuss each category.

Natural Radiation

Natural radiation exposure arises from **external** and **internal** sources. The external sources are **cosmic radiation** from outer space and **terrestrial gamma radiation** from radionuclides in the environment. Internal exposure comes from **radionuclides within the body.**

External Sources. The average cosmic-ray annual dose equivalent is about 0.26 mSv (26 mrem) at sea level. This exposure varies with latitude and altitude. Denver (a mile high) has an annual exposure of about 0.5 mSv (50 mrem) from cosmic radiation. Cosmic radiation exposure approximately doubles for each 2000-m increase in altitude (a mile is about 1600 m).

The average annual gamma-ray effective dose equivalent is about 0.28 mSv (28 mrem), but varies geographically from about 0.16 mSv to 0.63 mSv. The exposure comes primarily from radionuclides in rock and building materials. The three major components of terrestrial gamma radiation are ^{40}K and the members of the thorium and uranium series.

Internal Sources. Internal exposure comes from radionuclides within the body. There are two groups of these radionuclides; those that are **ingested** in food and water and those that are **inhaled.**

Ingested radionuclides include ^{40}K, ^{87}Rb, ^{14}C, and members of the thorium and uranium series. Annual effective dose equivalent from these radionuclides is 0.39 mSv (39 mrem).

Among natural sources, inhaled radon (with radon decay products) is the largest contributor to the average annual effective dose equivalent. The estimated annual effective dose equivalent from radon sources is 2 mSv (200 mrem).

Medical Radiation

The concept of effective dose equivalent is particularly useful when describing medical x-ray exposures. In fact, this is a major reason for this concept. There are two categories of medical radiation: **diagnostic medical x rays** and **nuclear medicine** (dental x rays and therapy radiation are excluded because of minimal general population exposure). The estimated annual effective dose equivalent from nuclear medicine studies is 0.14 mSv (14 mrem).

The estimated annual effective dose equivalent from diagnostic x-ray examinations is 0.39 mSv (39 mrem). It is emphasized that three procedures provide more than half this total dose: lumbar spine, upper gastrointestinal, and barium enema examinations. Table 21–5 lists the annual effective dose equivalents for several medical x-ray examinations.[5]

Summary of Population Exposure

The average annual effective dose equivalent to people in the United States is estimated to be 3.6 mSv (360 mrem). Most of this exposure is from natural background radiation (3.0 mSv), and the largest segment of natural background radiation is 2 mSv from radon and its decay prod-

Table 21–4. Annual Effective Dose Equivalent in the U.S. Population

SOURCE OF RADIATION	ANNUAL DOSE (mSv)
Natural Radiation	
External	
Cosmic	.26
Gamma	.28
Internal	
In the body	.39
Inhaled	2.00
Medical Procedures	.53
1 mSv = 100 mrem	

Table 21–5. Effective Dose Equivalent for Diagnostic Medical X-Ray Examinations[5]

EXAMINATION	EFFECTIVE DOSE EQUIVALENT (mSv) PER EXAMINATION
Chest	.06
Skull	.2
Lumbar Spine	1.3
Upper GI	2.45
Abdomen	.55
Barium enema	4.05
Pelvis	.65
Intravenous urogram	1.6
Extremities	.01

ucts. Medical diagnostic use of radiation contributes about .5 mSv per year.

DOSE-LIMITING RECOMMENDATIONS

The National Council on Radiation Protection and Measurements (NCRP) works under a charter from Congress that includes making recommendations on limits of exposure to ionizing radiation. These limits are certainly not easy to define, and from time to time must be updated as new information becomes available. As a result, the new report on radiation limits was published in 1987 in the form of NCRP Report No. 91. The information in this report supersedes NCRP Report No. 39, published in 1971. We recommend that you get a copy of NCRP Report No. 91 and read it. (Available from the National Council on Radiation Protection and Measurements, 7910 Woodmont Avenue, Bethesda, MD 20814.) However, we would like to summarize the recommendations.

Table 21–6 is a summary of pertinent recommendations on limits. Note that there are four classes of individuals:

1. Occupationally exposed individuals
2. The general public
3. Trainees under 18 years of age
4. Embryo-fetus

Occupational Exposure

The occupationally exposed individual accepts some risk. He takes this slight risk for some tangible benefit, usually gainful employment. As a general rule, he is somewhat knowledgeable of the risks involved and his numbers are relatively small, so his exposure does not contribute appreciably to the genetically significant dose. For this reason, his maximal permissible dose is larger than that of the other groups.

We would like to give our interpretation of what the terms in Table 21–6 mean. Since we have already discussed effective dose equivalent, we can go directly to "stochastic" and "nonstochastic" effects.

The **stochastic effect** of radiation exposure is defined as an effect in which the probability of occurrence increases with increasing absorbed dose, but the severity of the effect does not depend on the magnitude of the absorbed dose. A stochastic effect is an all-or-none phenomenon, and is assumed to have no dose threshold. Examples of stochastic effects that may be caused by radiation exposure are cancers and genetic effects.

A **nonstochastic effect** of radiation exposure is defined as a somatic effect that increases in severity with increasing absorbed dose. Nonstochastic effects are usually degenerative effects severe enough to be clinically significant, such as organ atrophy and fibrosis. Examples of radiation exposure are lens opacification, blood changes, and decreased sperm production.

For occupational exposures, the NCRP recommends an annual effective dose equivalent limit of 5 rem (50 mSv).

For avoidance of nonstochastic effects, the recommended annual dose equivalent limits are: 15 rem (150 mSv) for the lens of the eye and 50 rem (500 mSv) for all other tissues or organs, including the skin and extremities.

There is a new recommendation for accumulation of lifetime exposure. The NCRP recommends that the limit calculated by (age − 18) × 5 rem by replaced by

Age in years × 1 rem

Table 21–6. Summary of NCRP Recommendations for Radiation Dose Limits*

CLASS OF EXPOSED INDIVIDUAL	REMS	mSv
Occupational exposures (annual)		
Stochastic effects	5	50
Nonstochastic effects		
Lens of eye	15	150
All other areas (e.g., red bone marrow, breast, lung, gonads, skin, and extremities)	50	500
Lifetime cumulative exposure	1 ($\times$ age in years)	10 ($\times$ age in years)
Public exposure (annual)		
Effective dose equivalent limit	0.5	5
Dose equivalent limits for lens of eye, skin, and extremities	5	50
Trainees under 18 years of age		
Effective dose equivalent limit	0.1	1
Dose equivalent limit for lens of eye, skin, and extremities	5	50
Embryo-fetus exposures		
Total dose equivalent limit	0.5	5
Dose equivalent limit in a month	0.05	0.5

*Excluding background and medical exposures, but including both internal and external exposures

An individual's lifetime effective dose equivalent in rems should not exceed the value of his or her age in years.

Public (Nonoccupational) Exposure

The nonoccupationally exposed individual is in a different situation than the radiation worker. Usually the occasionally exposed individual has no knowledge of the risk involved, receives no compensation for taking a risk and, most important, has no freedom to decide if he will accept the risk. When a member of the general population—for example, a visitor—enters a radiation area, he becomes an occasionally exposed individual. The radiation is thrust on him, frequently without his knowledge. Also, the population size of the occasionally exposed is not controlled, so large numbers of individuals could be involved, which would have a greater impact on the genetically significant dose. **For all these reasons, the dose limits for the occasionally exposed is 0.5 rem/year, or one tenth of the MPD for the occupationally exposed.**

The 0.5-rem (5 mSv) annual effective dose equivalent limit for members of the public will keep the annual dose equivalent to those organs and tissues that are considered in the effective dose equivalent system to be below levels of concern for nonstochastic effects. However, because some organs and tissues are not routinely included in the calculation of effective dose equivalent (such as extremities, skin, and lens of the eye), an annual dose equivalent of 5 rem (50 mSv) is recommended for these organs or tissues.

Trainees Under 18 Years of Age

It is recognized that some individuals beginning training in industrial or medical use of radiation will be under the age of 18 years. The NCRP recommends that exposure to these trainees should result in an annual effective dose equivalent of less than 0.1 rem (1 mSv), and that intentional exposure of trainees should be avoided.

Embryo-Fetus Exposures

This recommendation is intended to limit exposure to a fetus of an occupationally exposed mother. However, the special sensitivity of the fetus should be considered in all situations, including those involving medical exposures of the expectant mother.

The NCRP recommends a total dose equivalent limit (excluding medical exposure) of 0.5 rem (50 mSv) for the embryo-fetus. Once a pregnancy becomes known, exposure of the embryo-fetus should be no greater than 0.05 rem (0.5 mSv) in any month (excluding medical exposure).

PROTECTIVE BARRIERS

Three methods can be used to control radiation exposure levels: distance, time, and barriers. Distance is obviously an effective method, because beam intensity is governed by the inverse square law. Exposures can be controlled with time in various ways: by limiting the time that the generator is turned on; by limiting the time that the beam is directed at a certain area; or by limiting the time that the area is occupied. All these factors are taken into consideration in planning a new installation. When they prove inadequate, however, the only alternative is a protective barrier, usually lead or concrete. Barriers are designated as either primary or secondary depending on whether they protect from primary radiation (the useful beam) or stray radiation (a combination of leakage and scatter radiation).

Primary Barriers

Figure 21–2 summarizes the factors that must be considered in determining primary barrier requirements for a radiographic installation. The number of factors seems imposing, but the total concept is quite simple.

Our first task is to evaluate the exposure to the area in question. Once we know the exposure, we can use either half-value layers or tables to determine barrier requirements. Five factors must be evaluated in exposure calculations. These are shown

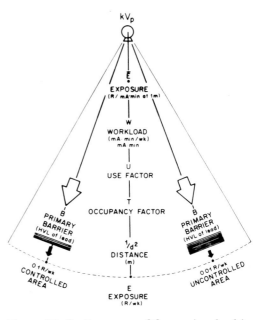

Figure 21–2 Summary of factors involved in primary barrier determinations

along the central axis of the illustration and include the following:

1. Workload (W) in mA · min/wk
2. R per mA · min at 1 m ($\overline{E}$)
3. Use factor (U)
4. Occupancy factor (T)
5. Distance (d) in meters

We will go through the list one step at a time, but first note that no mention is made of attenuation by the patient. Even though patient attenuation may be 90%, it is completely ignored in calculating barrier requirements. The x-ray energy used for protection calculations is the maximum voltage (kVp) of the generator, even though the machine will frequently be operated at lower potentials. No distinction is made between single- and three-phase generators.

Step 1. The **workload (W)** is the quantity of x rays generated per week. It is the product of tube current in mA and time in minutes of exposure per week (mA · min/wk). For example, if a 125-kVp chest room is being designed to handle 12 patients/

hour, the workload is calculated by multiplying the mAs per exposure times the number of exposures per week and then dividing by 60 to convert seconds into minutes. At 125 kVp, we will estimate 2 mAs for a PA and 8 mAs for a lateral film (i.e., 10 mAs/patient):

$$\frac{mAs}{pt} \times \frac{pts}{hr} \times \frac{hr}{wk} = mAs/wk$$
$$10 \times 12 \times 40 = 4800 \ mAs/wk$$

To convert mAs to mA · min, we simply divide by 60:

$$4800 \div 60 = 80 \ mA \cdot min/wk$$

The workload recommended by the NCRP can be used when more specific information is not available. Their recommendations are given in Table 21–7. The recommendations for our 125-kVp chest room is 400 mA · min/wk, which is five times the 80 mA · min/wk that we calculated. The NCRP recommendations provide a generous margin for error, which is the goal of radiation protection policies. Note in the table that the workload diminishes as energy increases. The workload for a radiographic room is 1000 mA · min/wk at 100 kVp and only 200 mA · min/wk at 150 kVp. The recommended workload is diminished because fewer mAs are required to expose a film at the higher kVp. Patient handling limits the number of procedures that can be accomplished in a day. Therefore, the recommended workloads in Table 21–7 are all considered equal. This may not seem logical, but it makes good sense. A room can only handle a certain number of patients a day. It takes approximately the same number of milliroentgens to expose a film at 100 kVp as

it does at 150 kVp. When the kVp is raised, the mAs can be lowered and the net mR output stays about the same.

Step 2. Because the recommendations regarding maximal permissible dose are all given in roentgens, we must have a way of converting workload into roentgens. The customary way of expressing exposures is in terms of **roentgens/mA · min at a distance of 1 m** from the x-ray source. Table 21–8 shows the x-ray output for various x-ray energies.[7] This exposure is multiplied by the workload to determine the total roentgen output per week. For example, at a maximum energy of 100 kVp with a workload of 1000 mA · min/wk, Table 21–8 shows an exposure of 0.9 R/mA · min at 1 m. This is a weekly exposure of (1000 mA · min/wk × 0.9 R/mA · min) 900 R/wk at 1 m. The inverse square law is used to determine the exposure at other distances. Note that the exposure per mA · min increases with increasing kVp, and this compensates for the lower workload recommendation described in the previous section.

Step 3. The **use factor (U),** which should really be called the **beam direction factor,** is the fraction of time that the beam is directed at a particular barrier. If it is anticipated that the beam will only be directed at a wall 10% of the time, then U is 0.1. If a wall holds a fixed film changer for chest radiography, where the direction of the beam cannot be changed, then U for that particular wall is 1.0; all other walls are secondary barriers. When specific information is not available, recommended use factors can be obtained from Table 21–9.[4]

Table 21–7. Recommended Workloads for Radiographic and Fluoroscopic Installations

MAXIMUM ENERGY (kVp)	WORKLOAD (mA · min/wk)	
	RADIOGRAPHIC ROOM	FLUOROSCOPIC ROOM
100	1000	1500
125	400	600
150	200	300

Table 21–8. X-Ray Output in R per mA·min at 1 m ($\overline{E}$) for Various Energies

PEAK KILOVOLTAGE (kVp)	$\overline{E}$ (R/mA · min at 1 m)
50	0.15
70	0.40
100	0.90
125	1.4
150	2.0

Table 21–9. Use Factors for Diagnostic
Exposure Rooms

	USEFUL BEAM (Primary Barrier)	STRAY RADIATION* (Secondary Barrier)
Floor	1	1
Walls	1/16	1
Ceiling	0	1

*Stray radiation is the sum of leakage and scatter
radiation

U for ceilings is always zero, because the beam is rarely directed at the ceiling. **U for secondary barriers is always 1,** because the entire room is exposed to stray radiation whenever the x-ray beam is turned on.

Step 4. The **occupancy factor (T)** is the fraction that the workload should be decreased to correct for the degree of occupancy of the area in question. It has the same basis as U, and is expressed as a fraction that represents the amount of time that the area will be occupied. If the floor of an exposure room is in the basement of a hospital, and no subbasement will ever be constructed, then the floor's T is 0, and it is neither a primary nor a secondary barrier. The following list shows recommended occupancy factors for various areas for nonoccupationally exposed persons when more specific information is not available:

Full occupancy (T = 1): Areas that will be occupied by the same individuals for their full work day, such as offices, laboratories, and nurses' stations.

Partial occupancy (T = 1/4): includes corridors, restrooms, and elevators using operators.

Occasional occupancy (T = 1/16): includes waiting rooms, stairways, unattended elevators, janitor closets, and outside areas used for pedestrian and vehicular traffic.

If the area in question is **a controlled area** (i.e., within the x-ray department), it **is assigned an occupancy factor of one.** A radiation worker may spend only a small amount of time in any particular area, but

wherever he goes in the department, he will be in a position of potential exposure, so all areas are assumed to be continuously occupied. Therefore, the occupancy factors listed above are only for areas occupied by nonoccupationally exposed individuals.

Step 5. Distance (d) is one of the most effective means of radiation protection, because exposures change inversely with the square of the distance (the inverse square law). Distances are measured in meters to be consistent with the units used in Table 21–8. If an exposure is 2 R at 1 m, then at 4 m it will be

$$2R \times \frac{1}{4^2} = 0.13R$$

It is usually assumed that an individual will be at least 1 ft from a barrier for distance measurements. Some radiation is absorbed in air, but with energies over 50 kVp and distances less than 100 ft, the amount is negligible, and it is ignored.

The product of the factors described in steps 1 through 5 gives the "effective" weekly exposure to any particular point. The term "effective" is used here to emphasize that the actual exposure may be different, depending on the occupancy factor:

$$E = \bar{E}WUT \times \frac{1}{d^2}$$

E = weekly exposure reaching the point in
 question (R/wk)
$\bar{E}$ = R/mA · min at 1 m
W = workload (mA · min/wk)
U = use factor (no units)
T = occupancy factor (no units)
d = distance in meters from the x-ray tube to
 the point in question

The categories of protected areas were discussed earlier ("Dose-Limiting Recommendations"). Two types of areas require protection, those occupied by occupationally exposed individuals and those occupied by persons only occasionally exposed. The recommendations are 5 rem/year for the occupationally exposed and 0.5 rem/

year for the occasionally exposed. Dividing by a 50-wk work year, the weekly maximum permissible exposures are 0.1 R for occupationally occupied and only 0.01 R for occasionally occupied areas. After an area has been assigned to a category, its weekly exposure must be kept below recommended levels. If the total exposure (E) at the point in question is less than 0.1 R/wk for a controlled area, or 0.01 R/wk for an uncontrolled area, no barrier is required. If E is greater than these maximal permissible exposures, then a protective barrier is required. Calculation of its thickness is discussed next.

Methods for Calculating Primary Barrier Thickness

Having determined the amount of radiation reaching the area in question, we must reduce this exposure to an acceptable level that depends on the category of the area. This is accomplished by interposing a barrier of either lead or concrete. Two methods are commonly used to calculate barrier requirements for diagnostic installations: (1) half-value layers (HVL), and (2) precalculated shielding requirement tables. A third method, employing attenuation curves, is commonly used for therapy installations. The attenuation curves are difficult to read at diagnostic exposure levels and are rarely used by physicists, so we will not bother describing the method.

Half-Value Layers (HVL). The first method for calculating barrier requirements, and the simplest to understand, is with half-value layers (HVL). The concept of HVL was first used in radiation therapy to express the quality of an x-ray beam. **The half-value layer is the thickness of a specific substance that, when introduced into the path of a beam of radiation, reduces the exposure rate by one half.** A beam with a HVL of 0.2 mm of lead is more penetrating than a beam with a HVL of 0.1 mm of lead. HVLs in millimeters of lead and inches of concrete are given in Table 21–10.[4] Barrier thickness is calculated by

Table 21–10. Half-Value Layer (HVL) Thicknesses of Lead and Concrete for Various X-Ray Energies[4]

PEAK KILOVOLTAGE (kVp)	LEAD (mm)	CONCRETE (in.)
50	0.05	0.17
70	0.15	0.33
100	0.24	0.6
125	0.27	0.8
150	0.29	0.88

repetitively halving the exposure until it reaches a permissible level, and then multiplying the number of halves times the HVL of the beam. For example, if the actual exposure at some point is 3.2 R/wk, and the permissible exposure 0.1 R/wk, the required number of HVLs is determined as follows:

$$3.2 \div 2 = 1.6$$
$$1.6 \div 2 = 0.8$$
$$0.8 \div 2 = 0.4$$
$$0.4 \div 2 = 0.2$$
$$0.2 \div 2 = 0.1$$

Five HVLs reduces 3.2 R/wk down to 0.1 R/wk. If the HVL of the beam were 0.25 mm of lead, the barrier would be

$$0.25 \times 5 = 1.25 \text{ mm of lead}$$

A problem arises in using half value layers with heterochromatic radiation. Remember, filtration changes the quality of a diagnostic beam as it passes through a barrier. The beam increases in mean energy, or is hardened, so if we use its initial HVL we could underestimate barrier requirements.

Table 21–11 explains how this problem arises. We start with a 150-kVp heterochromatic beam with a mean energy of 50 keV, a HVL of 0.29 mm of lead, and a hypothetical 100 R/wk from the beam. These are the characteristics of the beam as it emerges from the x-ray tube. It has already been filtered by both inherent and added filtration. To reduce the intensity to 50 R, we place 0.29 mm (1 HVL) of lead at point A. The 0.29 mm of lead further filters the radiation, increases its mean energy from 50 to 57 keV, and therefore in-

Table 21–11. Filtration Changes the Quality of a Diagnostic X-Ray Beam

		0.29 mm Pb	+	0.32 mm Pb	+	0.34 mm Pb	=	0.95 mm Pb
		A		B		C		P
Peak Energy (kVp)	150	150		150				150
Mean Energy (keV)	50	57		63				66
HVL (mm lead)	0.29	0.32		0.34				0.35
R in beam*	100	50		25				12.5

*Assumes no reduction in intensity from the inverse square law; that is, the distance between points A, B, and C is zero.

creases its HVL. Now we must place 0.32 mm of lead at point B to reduce intensity by one half. In the example given, it is assumed that there is no intensity loss from inverse square. As we continue adding newly determined HVLs to reduce intensity to 12.5 R at point P in the table, we change the mean energy from 50 to 66 keV and the HVL of the beam from 0.29 to 0.35 mm of lead, 0.06 mm more than its initial thickness. Summing the three HVLs placed at points A, B, and C shows that 0.95 mm of lead is required to reduce the intensity at point P to 12.5 R. If we had assumed that three of the original HVLs would have accomplished this objective, we would have underestimated the barrier, because 0.29 × 3 is only 0.87, which is 0.08 mm less than that actually required. The error is not significant, however, if the original HVL is for an already hardened beam. The numbers given in Table 21–11 are for such a beam. In other words, the radiation has been passed through numerous HVLs, and the last one is used to express beam quality.

Precalculated Shielding Requirement Tables. Most physicists use precalculated tables such as Table 21–12 to determine barrier requirements for diagnostic installations.[4] The tables are easy to use because the inverse square effect and barrier thicknesses are precalculated. All that needs to be done is to determine the effective workload by multiplying the actual workload (W) by the use factor (U) and occupancy factor (T). The effective workload is still in mA · min/wk, because the use and occupancy factors have no units. Knowing the kVp and distance, the table indicates primary and secondary barrier requirements in both lead and concrete. For example, to determine the barrier requirements at 10 feet for a busy 100-kVp radiographic room with a workload of 1000 mA · min/wk with the use and occupancy factors both 0.25, we would multiply the workload by the use and occupancy factors:

$$W \cdot U \cdot T = mA \cdot min/wk$$
$$1000 \cdot 0.25 \cdot 0.25 = 62.5$$

We then go to Table 21–12 and find 62.5 mA · min/wk in the 100-kVp column. Moving to the right to a distance of 10 ft, we find primary barrier requirements of 0.5 mm of lead for a controlled and 1.25 mm for an uncontrolled area. In the same column we can find barrier requirements in concrete and also secondary barrier thicknesses. All this is accomplished with little mathematical manipulation, which explains the popularity of the tables.

Secondary Barriers

Secondary barriers provide protection from scatter and leakage radiation, which we will lump together and call stray radiation. As a general rule, **no secondary barrier is required for areas protected by a primary barrier;** that is, the primary serves

Table 21–12. Shielding Requirements for Radiographic Installations[4]

WUT* in mA·min/week 100 kVp	125 kVp	150 kVp	DISTANCE IN FEET FROM SOURCE (X-RAY TUBE TARGET) TO OCCUPIED AREA									
1000	400	200	5	7	10	14	20	28	40			
500	200	100		5	7	10	14	20	28	40		
250	100	50			5	7	10	14	20	28	40	
125	50	25				5	7	10	14	20	28	40
62.5	25	12.5					5	7	10	14	20	28
TYPE OF AREA	**MATERIAL**		**PRIMARY PROTECTIVE BARRIER THICKNESS**									
Controlled	Lead, mm		1.9	1.65	1.4	1.2	1.0	0.75	0.5	0.3	0	0
Noncontrolled	Lead, mm		2.65	2.4	2.2	1.95	1.7	1.5	1.25	1.0	0.8	0.5
Controlled	Concrete, inch		5.9	5.2	4.6	4.0	3.3	2.7	2.1	1.6	1.0	0.4
Noncontrolled	Concrete, inch		8.0	7.3	6.7	6.0	5.4	4.8	4.1	3.5	2.9	2.2
			SECONDARY PROTECTIVE BARRIER THICKNESS									
Controlled	Lead, mm		0.55	0.4	0.2	0.1	0	0	0	0	0	0
Noncontrolled	Lead, mm		1.2	1.0	0.8	0.6	0.45	0.25	0.1	0	0	0
Controlled	Concrete, inch		1.9	1.4	0.8	0.2	0	0	0	0	0	0
Noncontrolled	Concrete, inch		3.8	3.2	2.6	2.1	1.5	1.0	0.4	0	0	0

*W—workload in mA· min/week, U—use factor, T—occupancy factor.

as both a primary and secondary barrier. All the factors that played a role in calculating barriers for the useful beam will have to be reconsidered in determining secondary barriers, except for U. U is really a beam direction factor and, because stray radiation goes in all directions, U is always 1.

Protection From Scatter Radiation. To determine primary barrier thickness, we make numerous estimates and allow a generous margin for error. Secondary barrier calculations are even less precise. The two most important factors, the intensity and energy of the scatter radiation, are both unknown. Therefore, before we can go any further, we must make two assumptions.

First, the energy of the scatter radiation is assumed to be equal to that of the primary radiation (provided the primary is less than 500 kVp). This assumption is reasonably accurate, especially below 100 kVp, where little energy is lost in Compton scattering, and where the secondary beam is hardened (its mean energy increased) by passing through the patient. If the assumption errs, it errs on the side of conservatism.

Second, the intensity of 90° scatter radiation, relative to the primary beam, is reduced by a factor of 1000 at a distance of 1 m for a field size of 400 cm². The 1-m distance is measured from the center of the beam on the patient's surface. When radiation can be forced to scatter more than once, for example with a maze, its intensity is reduced to inconsequential levels, well below permissible exposures, so we will not concern ourselves with multiple scatterings.

Field size is one factor that controls scatter radiation, so it is not surprising that it plays a role in determining secondary barrier requirements. The other two factors that control scattering, peak kilovoltage and patient thickness, are ignored. Field size is measured at the patient's surface. A correction factor is used for fields other than 400 cm².

$$\text{Correction factor} = \frac{F}{400}$$

F = actual field size (cm²)
400 = control field size (cm²)

The correction factor has no units, because both F and 400 are in square centimeters, and they cancel each other. For fields smaller than 400 cm², the correction factor is less than 1; for larger fields, it is greater than 1. For example, with 200 cm², the correction factor is

$$\text{Correction factor} = \frac{200}{400} = 0.5$$

The roentgen output of the x-ray tube (exposure in R/mA · min at 1 m; i.e., $\bar{E}$), workload (W), and occupancy factor (T), are the same as they were for the primary barrier calculations. Inverse square attenuation is also the same except that the distance is measured from the center of the patient rather than from the center of the x-ray tube. The use factor is dropped because it is always 1. A correction factor is added for field size, and the total exposure is divided by 1000 for right angle scattering:

$$E_s = \bar{E}WT \times \frac{1}{d^2} \times \frac{1}{1000} \times \frac{F}{400}$$

E_s = weekly exposure from scatter radiation (R/wk)
$\bar{E}$ = R/mA · min at 1 m
W = workload (mA · min/wk)
T = occupancy factor (no units)
d = distance (in meters from the center of the beam on the patient's surface)
F = actual field size (cm²)

The weekly exposure is then handled in the same manner as for primary barrier calculations. Exposures are reduced to permissible levels by one of the two previously described methods (i.e., HVLs or precalculated tables).

Protection From Leakage Radiation. Leakage radiation is radiation that passes through the lead shielding in the tube housing when the beam is turned on. By law, the **maximum permissible leakage exposure 1 m from a diagnostic x-ray tube is 0.1 R/hour** with the tube operating continuously at its maximum kVp and mA. This does not refer to the maximum mA that the tube is capable of generating, but rather the maximum mA at which the tube can be run continuously without overheating. The tube may be rated at 150 kVp and 1000 mA, but it cannot be operated continuously at this level. At 150 kVp, its max-

imum mA will probably be around 500 mA, and it will only tolerate that for a few milliseconds. The maximum mA at which the tube can be run continuously must be determined from anode heat cooling charts. Figure 21–3 shows a cooling chart for a Dynamax "69" tube. The maximum continuous mA is the maximum amount of heat per second (1400 heat units in this case), divided by the peak voltage, which may be from 100 to 150 kVp. At 150 kVp, the maximum continuous mA would be

$$1400 \div 150 = 9.3 \text{ mA}$$

The Dynamax "69" is a large tube. Smaller tubes have maximum continuous loads of 3 to 5 mA. The manufacturer must build the housing to limit exposure to 0.1 R/hour at 1 m with the tube operating at peak potential, and the highest mA that does not exceed the housing's ability to dissipate heat.

In calculating exposures from primary and scatter radiation, we could look up the roentgen output at 1 m ($\bar{E}$) for each mA of workload. Both the exposure and workload involve the primary beam. For leakage radiation, we need a comparable unit of exposure (i.e., R/mA · min at 1 m), but the "mA · min" refers to the useful beam and the "R at 1 m" to the leakage radiation. Leakage occurs whenever the x-ray beam is "on." It is completely independent of the useful beam itself, and will occur even if the collimator shutter is completely closed. As long as x rays are being generated within the tube housing, leakage radiation occurs.

Figure 21–4 shows the relationship between the workload of the primary beam and the permissible leakage level of 0.1 R/hour. In the illustration, 5 mA is given as the maximum continuous current that the tube can tolerate. If the tube runs at this level for only 1 sec, the exposure is 5 mAs, which is the unit technicians use to describe radiographic techniques. To be consistent with our previous methods, however, we will continue using the unit mA · min,

ANODE THERMAL CHARACTERISTICS

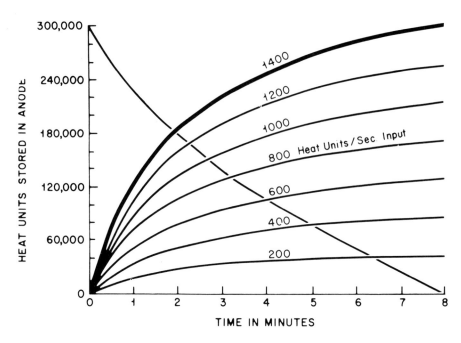

Figure 21–3 Anode thermal characteristics of a Machlett Dynamax "69" x-ray tube

which is the number of mA multiplied by the "on" time in minutes. Thus, in 1 minute of continuous operation, the output will be 5 mA · min. The leakage exposure is 0.1 R/hour at a distance of 1 m from the x-ray tube. To convert to R/min, we simply divide by 60:

$$0.1 \text{ R/hr} \div 60 \text{ min/hr} = 0.00167 \text{ R/min}$$

This is the leakage exposure that results

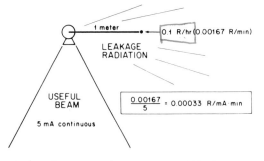

Figure 21–4 Maximum permissible leakage exposure at 1 m in R/mA · min with a maximum continuous exposure of 5 mA

from the tube being "on" for 1 minute. The workload of the primary beam for the same minute was 5 mA · min. To determine the leakage exposure at 1 m for each 1 mA · min of workload, we must divide by 5:

$$\frac{0.00167 \text{ R/min}}{5 \text{ mA} \cdot \text{min/min}} = 0.00033 \text{ R/mA} \cdot \text{min at 1 m } (\overline{E}_L)$$

Now that we have determined the exposure in R/mA · min at 1 m ($\overline{E}_L$), it is easy to calculate the exposure at some other point. We multiply the number of R/mA · min by the workload, occupancy factor, and inverse square of distance, as we did for primary and scatter exposure calculations:

$E_L = \overline{E}_L WT \times \dfrac{1}{d^2}$

E_L = weekly exposure from leakage radiation (R/wk)

$\overline{E}_L$ = leakage exposure at 1 m per mA · min of workload (R/mA · min)

W = workload (mA · min/wk)

T = occupancy factor (no units)

d = distance from x-ray tube in meters

The customary method for reducing leakage exposures to permissible levels is with HVLs of barrier. Leakage radiation is already heavily filtered by the lead in the tube housing, so the half-value method is quite accurate.

There is one last "rule of thumb" regarding radiation protection. If the difference between the barrier requirements for scatter and leakage radiation is greater than three half-value layers, use the large one and ignore the smaller one; if less than three half-value layers, add one half-value layer to the larger and ignore the smaller. For diagnostic installations, however, this rule is relatively meaningless. Leakage exposures are almost always within the permissible range without any barrier. Even more important, the walls of diagnostic rooms are almost always planned as primary barriers, and they provide ample protection from stray radiation.

Example

Figure 21–5 shows a general radiographic room with an upright Bucky mounted on the wall protecting area C. The generator, a three-phase unit, is rated at 125 kVp and 600 mA. We will calculate barrier requirements for areas A, B, and C, where A is a radiologist's office, B is the floor above a basement pathology laboratory, and C is a restroom. The distances from the points in question to the x-ray tube are given in the illustration, and note that the points are 1 ft from the wall, which is the NCRP recommendation.[4] We will assume that the x-ray tube is never directed at area A.

Because we do not know how many patients will be done in an 8-hour shift, we will accept the NCRP recommendation for a busy general radiographic room of 400 mA · min/wk for a 125-kVp installation. Then we need not concern ourselves with the generator's mA capacity, and, of course, single- and three-phase units are treated in the same way. We can look up the occupancy factors, use factors, and roentgen output at 1 m in the appropriate tables. Because the beam is never directed at area A, its use factor as a primary barrier is 0, and it will only require a secondary barrier. In actual practice, it would be better to provide a primary barrier for area A so that the room's function could be changed at a later date without the need for additional protection. We will return to

Figure 21–5 Floor plan of the general radiographic room described in the example

area A when we discuss secondary barriers. The use factor for point B, the pathology laboratory, is 1 because it is a floor, and the use factor for a floor is always 1. The table shows a use factor of 1/16 for walls, but a large number of upright chest examinations are anticipated, so we will use a use factor of 1/4 and not follow the NCRP recommendations. The occupancy factors are 1/4 for the restroom and 1 for the pathology laboratory. We will calculate primary barriers first, and in this example we will use both methods to determine barrier thickness.

Primary Barriers. *Precalculated Tables.* We will start with the table method, because it requires the least mathematics. To use the method, we must find the product of the workload (W), use factor (U), and occupancy factor (T):

$$\begin{array}{llllll}
 & W & \cdot & U & \cdot & T & = mA \cdot min/wk \\
\text{Point B:} & 400 & \cdot & 1 & \cdot & 1 & = 400 \\
\text{Point C:} & 400 & \cdot & \frac{1}{4} & \cdot & \frac{1}{4} & = 25
\end{array}$$

We can look up barrier requirements for points B and C in Table 21–12, but we have a bit of a problem, because the distances in the table are given in feet and our distances are in meters. One meter equals 39.37 in., or approximately 3.25 ft. Converting from meters to ft, we get

$$\begin{array}{l}
\text{Point B: } 3 \times 3.25 = 10 \text{ ft} \\
\text{Point C: } 4 \times 3.25 = 13 \text{ ft}
\end{array}$$

To look up the barrier thickness for point B in Table 21–12, we find 125 kVp and 400 mA · min/wk at a distance of 10 ft. Both the pathology laboratory and restroom are uncontrolled areas. The primary barrier thickness is 2.2 mm of sheet lead, or 6.7 in. of concrete, for an uncontrolled area. Because B is in a basement, we would simply make sure that the concrete floor is at least 6.7 in. thick. Point C is done similarly, but 13 ft is not shown in the table so we have to extrapolate between 10 and 14 ft. At 25 mA · min/wk, a lead thickness between 1.25 and 1.0 mm, say 1.20 mm, would be needed for an uncontrolled area. No secondary barrier would be required

for these walls, because the primary barrier would provide ample protection from stray radiation.

Half-Value Layers. To use HVLs, we must calculate the potential exposure at the points in question. The roentgen output at 1 m ($\bar{E}$) is 1.4 R/mA · min (Table 21–8):

$$\begin{array}{lllllllll}
 & E & = & \bar{E} & \cdot & W & \cdot & U & \cdot & T & \cdot & 1/d^2 \\
\text{Point B: } E & = & 1.4 & \cdot & 400 & \cdot & 1 & \cdot & 1 & \cdot & \frac{1}{3}^2 & = 62 \\
\text{Point C: } E & = & 1.4 & \cdot & 400 & \cdot & \frac{1}{4} & \cdot & \frac{1}{4} & \cdot & \frac{1}{4}^2 & = 0.154
\end{array}$$

The pathology laboratory and restroom are both uncontrolled areas with maximum permissible exposure levels of 0.01 R/wk. The exposures to both points are excessive (i.e., above permissible levels), so our next step is to determine the number of HVLs required to reduce them to permissible levels.

$$\begin{array}{lll}
\text{Point B:} & \text{Exposure} & \text{— HVLs} \\
 & 62 \text{ R/wk} & \text{— } 0 \\
 & 31 & \text{— } 1 \\
 & 15.5 & \text{— } 2 \\
 & 7.75 & \text{— } 3 \\
 & 3.88 & \text{— } 4 \\
 & 1.94 & \text{— } 5 \\
 & 0.97 & \text{— } 6 \\
 & 0.48 & \text{— } 7 \\
 & 0.24 & \text{— } 8 \\
 & 0.12 & \text{— } 9 \\
 & 0.06 & \text{— } 10 \\
 & 0.03 & \text{— } 11 \\
 & 0.015 & \text{— } 12 \\
 & 0.01 & \text{— approx. 12.6 HVLs} \\
 & 0.007 & \text{— } 13
\end{array}$$

If the number of half-value layers does not come out evenly, we can extrapolate as we did above, but it is simpler to use the whole number that reduces exposures below the permissible level (13 in this case), a practice that errs on the side of conservatism. Table 21–10 shows the HVL for 125 kVp to be 0.27 mm for lead and 0.8 in. for concrete. We multiply these values by the 12.6 HVLs required to attenuate the beam to permissible levels:

$$\begin{array}{llll}
\text{Lead:} & 0.27 & \times 12.6 & = 3.4 \text{ mm} \\
\text{Concrete:} & 0.8 & \times 12.6 & = 10 \text{ in.}
\end{array}$$

Because B is the floor, we would probably use the 10 in. of concrete. Following the same procedure for point C:

Point C: Exposure — HVLs
              0.14 R/wk — 0
              0.07   — 1
              0.35   — 2
              0.17   — 3
              0.10   — approx. 3.3 HVLs
              0.085   — 4

Lead: 0.27 × 3.3 = 0.89 mm
Concrete: 0.8   × 3.3 = 2.6 in.

The barrier thicknesses are different for the two methods (tables and HVLs), but this is not important because our purpose here is to explain principles. Also, the differences emphasize the fact that radiation protection is not a precise science.

Secondary Barriers. Wall A protects a radiologist's office and will require a secondary barrier. It is a controlled area with a maximum permissible exposure of 0.1 R/wk, and because it is a controlled area, its occupancy factor is 1. For convenience, we will calculate the exposures for both leakage and scatter radiation at a distance of 2 m as shown in Figure 21–5.

Precalculated Tables. Table 21–12 gives both primary and secondary barrier requirements. We simply multiply the workload (W), use (U), and occupancy (T) factors (WUT), and find the barrier thickness for the appropriate distance:

W   · U · T = mA · min/wk
400 · 1 · 1 = 400 mA · min/wk

Converting the distance of 2 m into feet, we get a little over 6 ft. At 125 kVp, the secondary barrier thickness for a controlled area is 0.55 mm of lead for 5 ft and 0.40 mm for 7 ft. We will need a thickness between these two, say 0.5 mm, and this would handle both the leakage and scatter radiation. In other words, we would be finished. But we will go on to make the calculations for scatter and leakage radiation separately using half-value layers.

Half-Value Layer Method for Scatter Radiation. The workload will be the same as it was for the primary barrier: 400 mA · min/wk at 125 kVp. The occupancy factor is 1 because it is a controlled area. The exposure is 1.4 R/mA · min. This exposure

is at 1 m, which we will assume is the patient's surface. This is a reasonably accurate assumption because most films are taken from a distance of 40 in. We will estimate an average field size of 14 × 14 in. (196 in.^{2}). There are approximately 6.5 cm^2/in.^{2} (2.54 × 2.54 cm), so our field will be 1270 cm^2 (6.5 cm^2/in.^{2} × 196 in.^{2}). We will also assume one right angle scattering:

$$E_s = \bar{E} \cdot W \cdot T \cdot 1/d^2 \cdot 1/1000 \cdot F/400$$
$$E_s = 1.4 \cdot 400 \cdot 1 \cdot 1/2^2 \cdot 1/1000 \cdot 1270/400$$

$$E_s = 0.45 \text{ R/wk}$$

Using the HVL method to reduce this exposure to the permissible level of 0.1 R/wk:

The HVL at 125 kVp is 0.27 mm
of lead and 0.8 inch of concrete.

Point A: Exposure — HVLs
              0.45 R/wk — 0
              0.225   — 1
              0.113   — 2
              0.10   — 2.3 HVLs
              0.056   — 3

Lead: 0.27 × 2.3 = 0.62 mm
Concrete: 0.8   × 2.3 = 1.8 in.

Half-Value Layer Method for Leakage Radiation. We will assume that 6 mA is the maximum continuous exposure the tube will tolerate without overheating. To determine the R/mA · min ($\bar{E}_L$), we divide the 0.1 R/hour permissible leakage exposure by 60 min/hour and 6 mA · min/min:

$$(0.1 \div 60) \div 6 = 0.00028 \text{ R/mA} \cdot \text{min}$$

The weekly leakage exposure at point A will be

$$E_L = \bar{E}_L \cdot W \cdot T \cdot 1/d^2$$
$$E_L = 0.00028 \cdot 400 \cdot 1 \cdot \tfrac{1}{2}^2 = 0.028 \text{ R/wk}$$

An exposure of 0.028 R/wk is less than the permissible level for a controlled area, so no barrier is required for leakage radiation. The total secondary barrier would be the 0.62 mm of lead required for scatter radiation.

SHIELDING REQUIREMENTS FOR RADIOGRAPHIC FILM

A secondary objective of radiation protection is "to prevent damage or impairment of function of radio-sensitive film or equipment."[4] We will limit our discussion to x-ray film. "An exposure of 1 milliroentgen (mR) over a portion of a film may produce undesirable shadows."[4] For protection purposes, an exposure of 0.2 mR is considered safe. This is the maximum permissible exposure that the film should receive during its entire storage life.

Protective barrier calculations for film are exactly the same as those for controlled and uncontrolled areas, with one exception. The permissible exposure for the film varies with storage life. For one week of storage, the customary time interval for protection calculations, the permissible level is 0.2 mR. For monthly storage (4 weeks), the film is only permitted a weekly exposure of 0.05 mR (0.2 mR ÷ 4 weeks). The number of HVLs of lead and concrete must be sufficient to bring exposures to the appropriate level. Barrier thicknesses can also be determined from a table similar to Table 21–12.

SUMMARY

Man has lived with, and tolerated, natural radiation since the beginning of time. Evidence is accumulating, however, that small doses of radiation can cause both mutations and neoplasms. No one knows just how much radiation is tolerable. The effective dose equivalent (H_E) attempts to relate exposure to risk. The National Council on Radiation Protection's recommendations are designed to protect both the general public and radiation worker. Many of the recommendations have been turned into laws. The most important recommendations are those involving maximum permissible doses, which are currently 5 rem/ year for a radiation worker and 0.5 rem/ year for the occasionally exposed individual. Three parameters are available to reduce radiation exposures: time, distance, and barriers. Time plays its role in three ways: in the amount of time that the machine is turned "on" at a particular current, expressed as mA · min/wk, and called the

"workload"; in the amount of time that the beam is directed at a particular area, called the "use factor"; and in the amount of time that an area is occupied, the "occupancy factor." Distance attenuates the beam by the familiar inverse square law. If time and distance fail to bring exposures to permissible levels, then the third method, a barrier, is required. Barriers are usually constructed of either sheet lead or concrete, depending on which is cheaper.

Protection must be provided against three types of radiation: the primary, or useful beam; scatter radiation; and leakage radiation. The latter two together are called "stray" radiation. If the useful beam can be directed at a wall, the wall must be a primary barrier. If the useful beam cannot be directed at a wall, it is a secondary barrier and need only protect from stray radiation. Primary barriers serve a dual function as both primary and secondary barriers.

The exposure from the primary beam can be calculated by multiplying the workload, use factor, occupancy factor, and inverse square of the distance by an R output at 1 m for each mA of workload. If this exposure, expressed in R/wk, exceeds permissible levels, then a barrier is required. Barrier thicknesses can be calculated in two ways: 1) with precalculated tables or 2) with HVLs of lead or concrete. A secondary barrier protects against stray radiation and is only required when the useful beam cannot be directed at a particular wall. Secondary barriers protect against scatter and leakage radiation. For scatter radiation, the exposure is assumed to be attenuated by a factor of 1000 (i.e., reduced to 0.001 at a distance of 1 m for each right angle scattering), and it is also assumed that its quality does not change. A correction factor is added for field size and the use factor is always 1, because scatter and leakage radiation go in all directions. Otherwise, the calculation is the same as for the primary beam. The R output at 1 m for each mA · min of workload is multiplied by the workload, occupancy factor, and inverse square of the distance, a conversion factor for field size, and 0.001 for a right angle scattering.

The exposure from leakage is based on the law that the maximum radiation level at 1 m is 0.1 R/hour, or 0.00167 R/min. This exposure must be converted to R/mA · min. The maximum operating mA for continuous exposure at maximum kVp is determined from anode heat rating charts, and it is usually about 5 mA. The conversion to R/mA · min is accomplished by dividing the 0.00167 R/min by the maximum continuous mA. This exposure at 1 m is multiplied by the occupancy factor and inverse square of distance to determine the leakage exposure at the point in question. If the barrier requirements for scatter and leakage differ by more than 3 HVLs, the larger suffices; if less than 3 HVLs, add 1 HVL to the larger.

REFERENCES

1. Buschong, S.C.: The Development of Radiation Protection in Diagnostic Radiology. Cleveland, CRC Press, 1973.
2. Dalrymple, G.V., Gaulden, M.E., Kollmorgen, G.M., and Vogel, H.G., Jr.: Medical Radiation Biology. Philadelphia, W.B. Saunders, 1973.
3. Hall, E.J.: Radiobiology for the Radiologist. Hagerstown, MD, Harper & Row, 1973.
4. Medical X-Ray and Gamma-Ray Protection for Energies up to 10 MeV—Structural Shielding Design and Evaluation. Washington, D.C., National Council on Radiation Protection and Measurements, NCRP Report No. 49, 1976.
5. Ionizing Radiation Exposure of the Population of the United States. National Council on Radiation Protection and Measurements, 7910 Woodmont Ave, Bethesda, MD 28814. NCRP Report No. 93, 1987.
6. Pizzarello, D.J., and Witcofski, R.L.: Basic Radiation Biology. 2nd Ed. Philadelphia, Lea & Febiger, 1975.
7. Schultz, R.J.: Primer of Radiation Protection. 2nd Ed. New York, GAF Corporation. X-Ray Products Division, 1969.
8. Recommendations on Limits for Exposure to Ionizing Radiation. National Council on Radiation Protection and Measurements, 7910 Woodmont Ave, Bethesda, MD 28814. NCRP Report No. 91, 1987.

22 *Digital Radiography*

The field of digital radiography has developed to its present state by the implementation of largely conventional radiographic techniques using digital electronic apparatus. No unfamiliar basic physics principles need to be introduced in describing the operation of digital radiographic systems currently in use. Most techniques (including intravenous injection for arteriography) have already been used with film-screen systems, so there is considerable common ground between digital radiography and the more familiar film-screen techniques. We will emphasize these sometimes striking similarities between digital radiography and more conventional radiography. In addition, the discussion of digital techniques offers an opportunity to demonstrate clearly some fundamental limits on radiographic imaging systems. The main topic remaining is an extension of the understanding of computer image manipulations as discussed for computed tomography (CT), without having to consider the complicated reconstruction mathematics. Finally, because there are so many promising areas for development in this field, we will take a brief look at some current research.

A DIGITAL FLUOROSCOPY SYSTEM

The most common type of digital radiography system at present is digital fluoroscopy (DF). Such a system can be used to demonstrate most digital radiography principles, so we will begin with a general system description that will be of subsequent use. At the block diagram level, the design of a DF system can be considered to be a fairly conventional fluoroscopic unit, with an added digital image processing unit.

Fluoroscopy Unit

Figure 22–1 shows a fluoroscopic unit suitable for digital applications, and obviously it is only the block diagram of a conventional unit with several minor additions. Digital applications, however, place some special demands on a fluoroscopy unit.

Mask Subtraction Application. For instance, consider intravenous injection an-

Figure 22–1 Block diagram of a fluoroscopic unit

giography, in which subtracted images are displayed on a 512 × 512 pixel matrix. We will call this technique "mask subtraction." Currently it is the most commonly used technique in digital radiography, and it is one of the methods of performing digital subtraction angiography. **Digital subtraction angiography (DSA) is the generic term for any digital radiographic method of implementing subtraction angiography.** We will discuss several other methods later.

Mask subtraction is the DSA technique that most closely resembles film-screen angiography. The patient is prepared and a catheter is placed under fluoroscopic control. The patient is then injected, either intravenously or intra-arterially, with an x-ray contrast material that contains a high atomic number element such as iodine. Individual x-ray exposures are made at a typical rate of one exposure/second or more. The exposure series begins before the contrast material is expected to arrive in the vessels of interest, and extends past the time when the contrast material is expected to have cleared the vessels. Each individual pulsed exposure forms a single image within the series. A precontrast mask and a contrast-containing image are roughly equivalent to an angiographic film pair. The subtraction of the mask image from the contrast-containing image is the basis of this mask subtraction technique. If a peripheral venous injection is used, the contrast material reaching the arteries is so diluted that only small attenuation differences exist between contrast- and non-contrast-filled arteries. The x-ray exposures needed for producing acceptable images in this situation are similar to those used for serial photospot camera images, or perhaps even higher.

A good x-ray generator and x-ray tube of conventional design are probably adequate for the mask subtraction procedure, but an excellent image intensifier is required, and the television system must be of higher quality than normally needed for routine fluoroscopy.

X-Ray Generator and X-Ray Tube. The principal function of the generator is to provide very repeatable exposures. **A small difference in the x-ray tube current or kilovoltage** supplied by the generator for two exposures in a series **will result in an improper mask subtraction** of the images of unchanged areas of the body. This improper subtraction may obscure the visualization of the actual structures of interest (such as opacified vessels), which have very small subject contrast differences on the two images. The digital image processing unit generally has some control over the generator. In the case of mask subtraction, this control can be limited to the initiation and termination of the individual exposures in a series. The generator connections required for this type of control are usually rather simple, and are similar to those needed for rapid film changers.

An x-ray tube similar in design to one that might be used in film angiography is appropriate for most DF applications. The primary beam magnification and x-ray tube loading parameters in typical digital angiographic procedures are quite similar to those encountered in film angiographic procedures, so specially designed x-ray tubes are currently unnecessary. In the specific application of the mask subtraction example, a 512- × 512-pixel image matrix was specified. This places resolution limitations on the final image that make the use of very small focal spots (such as those used in magnification radiography) unnecessary. We will discuss these resolution limitations shortly. In fact, very small focal spots are undesirable for this application because of the x-ray tube heat loading requirements.

Image Intensifier. A high quality image intensifier is needed for digital applications, but all the necessary image intensifier (II) characteristics are also desirable for some more conventional applications. **A very high contrast ratio is needed,** which mandates use of a recently designed II. In the case of our 512- × 512-pixel matrix, however, high spatial resolution is not needed for the II, so a thick input phosphor can be used for high x-ray detection efficiency. The power supply for the II must be quite stable, because small changes in accelerating potential for the electrons can produce changes in the brightness gain of the II. The power supply fluctuations are more likely to occur at radiographic tube current levels than at fluoroscopic tube current levels because of loading of the generator. The resulting change in II intensity might not be detectable in photospot or cine images, but two images from a digital series may not subtract properly.

Light Diaphragm. To this point, all components have been of a type that might be found in routine use for fluoroscopy or photospot imaging. For instance, we might have chosen a modern three-phase twelve-pulse generator, angiographic x-ray tube, and high-contrast II from those available for other uses. The selection of components that would not be part of the system were it not for our mask subtraction application begins with the light diaphragm.

The light diaphragm is used to control the amount of light from the II that reaches the TV camera tube, exactly as in the case of changing photographic f stops. In a typical procedure, the patient first undergoes some fluoroscopy with an x-ray tube current of about 2 mA at some given kVp. Subsequently, the patient undergoes a serial digital procedure in which 200 mA may be used to reduce quantum mottle. Let us choose light diaphragm sizes so that the amount of light reaching the TV camera tube for a single television frame will be approximately the same in either the fluoroscopic or the serial portion of the study. If we do not make the right choice, we will either saturate the TV camera tube with light during our high mA serial exposures, or we will use only a small portion of the TV camera tube's range for display of fluoroscopic images. In this example we

will collect a large fraction of the light from the II output phosphor for fluoroscopic images, and about 1% of that fraction for the serial images. In actuality, a combination of different sizes of light diaphragms and different electronic video gains may be employed. There is also some advantage in using a light diaphragm that is adjustable over a range for serial exposures, because this increases the flexibility of the system.

Television Image Chain. The second component of a type not normally found in fluoroscopic systems for nondigital use is **a special TV chain, one of the most critical components in the entire DF system.** The II tube absorbs a certain fraction of the incident x-ray photons and produces a quantity of light proportional to the number of incident x-ray photons. The basic function of the TV chain is to produce an electronic video signal from this light. The size of this signal should be directly proportional to the number of x-ray photons that exit the patient. Eventually this video signal will be fed to the digital image processing unit, where it will be digitized. At present, **a TV camera tube with a lead oxide vidicon target (plumbicon) is favored.** A plumbicon tube of this type has low lag and has a video output that is directly proportional to the light input.

As noted in Chapter 12, a TV camera with high lag will produce a smeared ghost that follows a rapidly moving object on the TV image. A ghost is objectionable in any procedure. The most desirable type of TV camera tube (all other factors being equal) would be one in which the image on the input phosphor is completely erased during the readout of each frame. In the case of images for digital subtraction, a tube with excessive lag can cause a situation in which the "current" frame actually has residual information that properly belongs in the past. **A TV camera tube with low lag is desirable,** especially in dynamic studies in which rapid image changes are encountered.

Perhaps the most important property

that **the TV chain must possess** is **extremely low electronic noise.** In fluoroscopy at 2 to 3 mA, there is so much quantum mottle in the image that relatively high electronic noise can be tolerated. As we shall see later, however, the combination of a much larger number of x-ray photons and working with subtracted images requires use of a different (and expensive) TV camera tube to avoid having electronic noise obscure low-contrast structures.

Television Scan Modes. Another feature that is sometimes desirable for digital fluoroscopy is a choice of television scan modes. Most television systems operate in an **interlaced mode.** In the United States, each 262.5-line field is scanned in 1/60 sec, so that the entire 525-line frame is scanned in 1/30 sec. This scan choice is adequate to avoid the perception of flicker, but it does have drawbacks for some digital applications. As normally employed, the TV tube scans continuously. When an x-ray exposure begins, first the generator and all other components must become stable, during which time the TV system continues to scan. In digital mask subtraction these stabilization frames must be discarded for several reasons. For instance, during the time the exposure is increasing, there would be no brightness in the first portion of the TV frame and considerable brightness in the last portion of the frame. This would produce objectionable flicker between the two fields of the frame and, for most of the frame, the TV camera tube would not be operating in its optimum brightness region. Another reason for discarding the early frames is the very severe demands that would be placed on all components. Each component would have to reach exactly the same operating point in the same amount of time for each exposure to ensure good subtraction. The net result of throwing away some TV frames is that the patient may be given some unnecessary x-ray exposure. There are a number of solutions to this particular problem, one of which is to change to a different x-ray exposure and TV scanning mode.

The pulsed progressive readout method involves two steps for obtaining a single TV frame image. First, TV camera scanning is halted and an exposure is made. Second, the TV camera target is operated in a **progressive scan mode,** which means that every line is read out in order, rather than in a field-interlaced fashion. Now we only need to ensure that each exposure in a series is reproducible. The exposure may be of any duration up to several seconds, and all the dose is used to form the image. Because this mode must allow time between frames for the exposures (and perhaps also for "scrubbing" any residual image off the camera target), framing rates are somewhat slower than in the interlaced mode. There is no reason why continuous progressive framing cannot be employed, but the same stabilization time penalty described for interlaced scanning will be applicable.

Another method of scanning the television target that would be unsatisfactory for real-time visual presentation is a **slow scan mode.** This method is currently being used for implementing fairly large (1024- × 1024-pixel) digital fluoroscopic matrices. Implementing a 1024 × 1024 matrix on a 1050-line television system running in interlaced mode at 30 frames per second would require an increase in the band width of the television system to four times that for a 525-line system (see Chap. 12 for an explanation of television band width). If we do not insist on 30 frames per second, each TV line can be scanned twice as long as in the 525-line system (thus doubling horizontal resolution), and twice as many lines can be scanned (doubling vertical resolution) without increasing the video band width. This limits the framing rate (7.5 frames per second) to one fourth of "real time" (30 frames per second). There are two advantages over the 30-frames-per-second approach. First, the television chain electronics and the digitizer section can have the same band width as a 525-line system, which significantly simplifies system design. Second, **at high band width, electronic noise is significantly increased,** which is avoided by slow scan. Naturally, the television camera tube must be inherently capable of higher spatial resolution than that needed for a 525-line system. Also, there are some sources of electronic noise that are worse at the higher resolution and that are not helped by the use of slow scan techniques.

Digital Image Processor

A typical digital image processor for DF is shown in Figure 22–2. This block diagram is a functional one, because different image processor units may have different physical configurations. Therefore, unlike the fluoroscopic unit, we may not be able to indicate a particular component and say that it corresponds to a particular block of our diagram. Nevertheless, all DF image processors are intended to have the same basic functions, and the same basic principles apply. Their major functions are 1) digitizing TV frames and processing them into digital images, 2) storing the digital

images for later recall, 3) displaying digital images on a TV monitor and photographing these images, and 4) manipulating digital images (e.g., averaging, subtracting, changing contrast scales).

Basic Operation. A rough description of the functions of the individual blocks in Figure 22–2 seems to be in order before discussing them individually in more detail. The central control computer is in charge of all the other components of the image processor (and, we hope, is absolutely subservient to us). Suppose we tell the computer to run a series of a certain number of exposures and to store each image of the series in digital form for later use. During the run the computer is to use the first image as a mask and is to display each subsequent image in subtracted form. We set exposure techniques on the generator and instruct the computer to begin. The computer informs the generator when to start and to stop each exposure. It sets up the digitizer (analog-to-digital converter) to convert an entire TV frame into a digital image, and starts the digitizer at the appropriate time. Meanwhile, the computer has instructed the arithmetic unit on

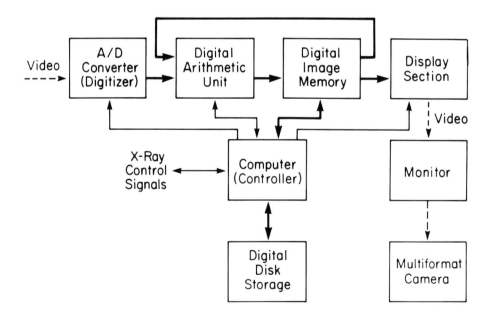

Figure 22–2 Block diagram of a digital image processor unit

what to do with the first digitized image, which is simply to place the image in appropriate form and to store it in a particular block of image memory. The computer tells the digital disc where that particular block is located in image memory, how big the image is, and when to start storing the image. Similar instructions are given to the display section.

To handle the second exposure, the control computer issues the same commands as before to all components except the arithmetic unit and display section. The arithmetic unit must handle the incoming digitized data, and stores this "raw" data in a block of image memory that the digital disk will access. Simultaneously, the arithmetic unit must access the previously stored first image (the mask), subtract the mask from the incoming second image, and store the result in a third block of image memory that the display section can access. The computer has already set the display section for contrast levels appropriate for subtracted images and has told the display section which block of image memory to show. For the third and subsequent exposures, the computer has no new tasks to perform. It only has to pay attention to coordinating the subordinate activities until the run is complete or until we abort the run from the generator.

Note that in our system the control computer only tells its subordinates what to do and coordinates their actions, a strictly managerial task. As previously indicated, the block diagram is functional rather than physical. The actual computer that is incorporated may be very primitive and without much control, so that the subordinates operate very much in a preset fashion. Conversely, the computer may be quite complex and take over most of the menial tasks from the subordinates. Both approaches have some merit. A complex general purpose computer can be very flexible and perform virtually any current or future task that may be required for digital fluoroscopy. Of course, an ingenious pro-

grammer may be required to implement the task. On the other hand, we shall see that high calculation speeds are required for even routine operations. A general purpose computer capable of such speeds can be very large and expensive. It makes sense to have less expensive specialized machine cretins that do very simply routine tasks at the required speeds, provided that the system as a whole is able to do the entire job. New applications may not be easily implemented, however, if the system is too inflexible. The present trend seems to be use of a flexible but not extremely fast general purpose computer for control and complex tasks, and use of a set of fairly flexible subordinate units for fast or more mundane work.

Analog-to-Digital Conversion. The analog-to-digital converter (ADC) converts the video images from the TV chain into digital form. Figure 22–3A is a photograph of a displayed video image of a skull. The format is a frame consisting of 525 TV lines

Figure 22–3 A TV frame of the image of a skull phantom (A) and the video signal from one line of the frame (B)

from two interlaced fields. If we consider only one of the horizontal TV lines through the center of the image from the II, the electronic video signal that defines the line for the monitor will resemble that shown in Figure 22–3*B*. The video signal has a voltage that varies during the scan from left to right along the line. The voltage is initially low, indicating a dark region on the camera input face. The voltage then rises sharply in a brighter region, drops again in a darker region, and so forth. The size of the voltage at any point along the scan should directly represent the number of x-ray photons that struck the corresponding point on the II input phosphor. The time required to scan along the line from left to right is a little over 60 μsec for standard TV in this country.

The only portion of the video frame that needs to be digitized is the portion that contains the II image. To digitize the central TV line, the digitizer notes the start of the line, waits an appropriate amount of time until the first point on the edge of the II is expected, and then measures the voltage. The measurement is simply a number that the digitizer sends along to the waiting arithmetic unit. The digitizer immediately grabs the next point along the line, measures its voltage, and passes this second number to the arithmetic unit. After all 512 points along this line have been digitized, the digitizer sits back and waits for the next line to come along. When the digitizer has performed the same operation on 512 appropriate lines of the 525 available, the entire frame has been digitized. The video image has been converted into digital form, and the digitizer can wait for the next TV frame. Digitizers are seldom given awards for high intelligence.

Matrix Size. In the above example, each television frame has the image from the II digitized into a 512- × 512-pixel matrix. It is important to note that the choice of **matrix size limits the spatial resolution** that can be achieved by the system. This is analogous to matrix size in CT. Consider the

number of line pairs that can be displayed on a 512- × 512-pixel matrix. To define a single pair of lines aligned along the vertical dimension, at least two pixels in the horizontal dimension are required, one for the bright line and one for the dark line of the pair. Thus, the 512 horizontal pixels can define (at most) 256 line pairs. This limitation can be applied to the size of the image represented by the matrix, which is roughly the II input mode size (Fig. 22–4). If the II image represents about 12.5 cm (about 5 in.) in diameter, then 125 mm into 250 line pairs gives us a limit on system resolution of 2 line pairs per mm, assuming no primary beam magnification. So, even with a small field of view, a 512- × 512-pixel matrix will be expected to be the most important limiting factor on resolution, given reasonable focal spot sizes and primary beam magnifications. **The limitation becomes more severe for larger II input sizes.** With an II operating in a 25-cm (about 10 in.) mode under the same conditions, resolution would be limited to about 1 line pair per mm at the II input face. Similarly, displaying a 50-cm diameter image of a chest would result in maximum resolution of only 0.5 line pair per mm. Naturally, if the matrix size is in-

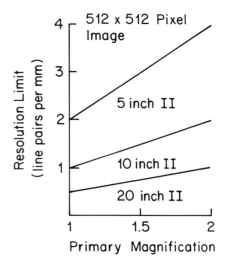

Figure 22–4 Resolution limits imposed by a 512 × 512 pixel matrix

creased to 1024 × 1024, the limitations imposed by matrix size will not be as great, and system resolution will be potentially double.

Binary Number System. We need to digress for a moment to review the binary number system. Those who speculate on such things suggest that the decimal number system is one inevitable counting method for beings with ten fingers, and that a being with eight fingers (or their equivalents) would probably have an octal number system; perhaps the argument is valid. But humans are beginning to use a binary as well as a decimal system because of computers. The validity of this statement can be checked easily by asking a bright 10-year-old.

Table 22–1 compares the binary and decimal number systems. A binary (base 2) "digit" can assume only one of two values, rather than one of ten as for a decimal (base 10) digit. So, binary counting (with the decimal counterpart in parentheses) is in the following sequence: 0 (0), 1 (1), 10 (2), 11 (3), 100 (4), 101 (5), 110 (6), 111 (7), 1000 (8), 1001 (9), 1010 (10), 1011 (11), 1100 (12), and so forth. With one **binary digit, or bit,** any whole number from 0 through 1 may be counted only two discrete values. Two bits allow the representation of 00 (0), 01 (1), 10 (pronounced one-oh, not ten; decimal 2), and 11 (pronounced one-one; decimal 3), a total of four discrete values. We note that 2^2 is 4. Three binary digits allow eight discrete values, or 2^3. We would correctly expect that with n binary bits, some 2^n discrete values could be counted. Most DF display units handle individual pixels with eight-bit accuracy for displayed brightness (we will discuss the brightness scale later). An individual pixel can therefore have any brightness value from 0 through 255 decimal, a total of 2^8 (decimal 256) possible brightness values. The bottom of Table 22–1 provides an example of how to calculate the decimal value of a binary number. The decimal representation of the number 26 can be interpreted to mean that the value of the least significant

Table 22–1. Comparison of Number Systems

	DECIMAL	BINARY
Allowed values of a single digit counting sequence	0, 1, 2, 3, 4, 5, 6, 7, 8, 9	0, 1
	0	0
	1	1
	2	10
	3	11
	4	100
	.	.
	.	.
	.	.
	255	11111111
	256	100000000
	.	.
	.	.
	.	.
	1023	1111111111

Calculation of decimal values

	10^3	10^2	10^1	10^0		2^5	2^4	2^3	2^2	2^1	2^0
$\cdots$	0	0	2	6	$\cdots$	0	1	1	0	1	0

$(0 \times 10^3) + (0 \times 10^2) +$
$(2 \times 10^1) + (6 \times 10^0)$
$= 0 + 0 + 20 + 6$
$= 26$

$(0 \times 2^5) + (1 \times 2^4) + (1 \times 2^3) +$
$(0 \times 2^2) + (1 \times 2^1) + (0 \times 2^0)$
$= (\text{decimal } 16 + 8 + 0 + 2 + 0)$
$= (\text{decimal } 26)$

digit (6) is multiplied by 10^0 (note that 10^0 = 1). The second significant digit (2) is multiplied by 10^1 (10). The third significant digit (not stated, but actually 0) is multiplied by 10^2 (100), and so forth. The actual number is the sum of the values represented by each digit (0 + 0 + 20 + 6 = 26). The decimal representation of a binary number may be calculated in the same fashion, except that the digits are multiplied by powers of 2 rather than by powers of 10. For the binary number 011010 (pronounced oh-one-one-oh-one-oh), the value of the least significant digit is 0×2^0. The value of the second digit is 1×2^1, and so forth. The result is 0 + 16 + 8 + 2 + 0 = 26.

Digital information is any information that is represented in discrete units. Analog information is any information that is represented in continuous, rather than discrete, fashion. The common meaning of the term "digital" is beginning to drift toward a usage associated only with electronics, computers, and the binary number system. We wish to use the perhaps outmoded meaning, however, to indicate the difference between analog and digital information. A video signal is an analog voltage representation of the quantity of light that strikes the input face of a TV camera tube. If this voltage analog of light intensity has a total range between 0 and 1 V, then any quantity of light from zero intensity to some maximum intensity can be represented exactly (ignoring such things as electronic noise for illustration purposes). On the other hand, if a decimal digital system with two digits is chosen to represent the amount of light, only discrete values between .00 and .99 (a total of 100 values) are possible. The error caused by using digital representation can be as great as 0.005. The 0.005 is 0.5% of the maximum value. The error as a percentage of the true value can be greater than this. For instance, a value of 0.0151 would be represented as .02, an error of more than 30% of the true value.

Digitization Accuracy. There are many different types of digitizers. The actual principles of operation of each type are rather simple, but it does not seem worthwhile describing the operation of any of them. What counts in this case is the result. A comparison of analog video voltage and digitized values is shown in Figure 22–5. The analog video indicates that a smooth variation in brightness occurs from completely dark at left to maximum brightness at right. (There would actually be some irregularities caused by noise.) The digitized values of brightness represent the output of a two-bit digitizer, so there are only two binary digits of precision. The values that the digitizer will obtain are .00 (at the left), then .01, .10, and finally .11 (at the right). Three-bit digitization would provide a stairway with smaller steps and less error, and four bits would be still better. As more bits of digitization are added, eventually the steps become so small that the changes between steps are almost completely hidden in the electronic noise from the video chain.

The statistical fluctuations in the number of x-rays that strike a small area of the II input screen can also be considered to be a source of noise, as will be discussed a little later. **Noise limits the accuracy of the image, and an appropriate digitizer will add very little to the inaccuracy.** An appropriate digitizer will have enough bits so that noise hides the steps (typically about ten bits). A very large number of bits, how-

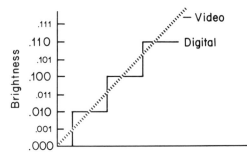

Figure 22–5 Comparison of analog video voltage and digitized values

ever, will add essentially nothing to the overall accuracy. It is easier and frequently much cheaper to build digitizers, arithmetic processors, and other system components if they only have to manipulate a small number of bits at a time. The argument extends to image memory and to digital disc storage, because useless bits are as expensive to store as significant ones.

DIGITIZED IMAGE

There are many tradeoffs that must be made in the formation of any radiographic image, and this is particularly apparent in a digital fluoroscopic image. X-ray and video chain equipment must be chosen with the digital application in mind, and all the conventional tradeoffs regarding such factors as patient dose and spatial resolution are still present. The equipment chosen and the image manipulations employed will have great influence on the diagnostic usefulness of the final image, but there is very little that is fundamentally different between a digital radiographic image and a film radiographic image. In general, the choices made in conventional film radiography and in digital radiography will have similar consequences.

Brightness Versus Log Relative Exposure Scale

We have been careful so far to maintain a linear relationship between the number of x-rays exiting the patient and the magnitude of the digital value that is measured. If the image is displayed on a monitor, as illustrated in Figure 22–6A, adding a given number of x-rays adds a constant amount of brightness to the image. At present, almost all digital fluoroscopic images are changed from this linear relationship to a logarithmic one. In the logarithmic relationship, increasing log relative exposure by a given amount will increase brightness by a constant amount (Fig. 22–6B). This type of relationship is a familiar one. Specifically, the H & D curves of film-screen systems are plotted as density versus log

relative exposure. The brightness scale under discussion is quite similar to the density scale of film-screen systems. In fact, we will use brightness as being almost synonymous with film density. (Many authors speak of a "gray scale," which is the same as our "brightness scale.") This is one of many instances in which there is a striking parallel between digital and film-screen images.

In the film H & D curves of Figure 22–7 (same as Fig. 11–15), the relationship is density versus log relative exposure. A long contrast scale is achieved in the broad latitude film B, while A has a much smaller latitude in its exposure range. Of course, the short latitude film will result in higher contrast within the exposure range in which its H & D curve is steepest. A given change in log relative exposure anywhere within this more or less straight line portion of the curve will give about the same change in density. The size of the change will be small for film B, indicating low contrast, and will be large for film A, indicating high contrast. An increase in speed would be seen over film A if an H & D curve of similar shape were drawn to the left of the H & D curve for film A.

Windowing. The analogy becomes more exact if we digress for a moment to discuss windowing. The selection of window widths and levels is familiar from the discussion of CT displays, and serves the same fundamental purpose in digital radiography. As shown in Figure 22–8, if the original digitized image were displayed following logarithmic conversion, a broad latitude of log relative exposure values could be seen (*solid line*). The windowing operation selects only a certain range of log relative exposure values to display, and uses the full brightness scale of the TV monitor to display only that selected range of log relative exposures (*dashed line*). A narrow log relative exposure range, or window, is roughly analogous to use of a high-contrast film. Moving the window to the left has the same general effect as choosing a faster film. In principle, **it is possible for**

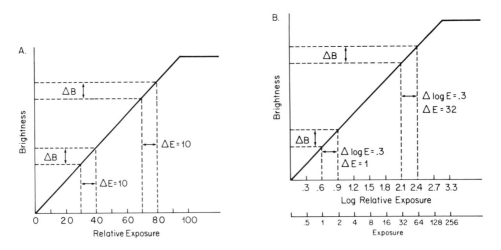

Figure 22–6 Comparison of a linear brightness scale *(A)* with a logarithmic brightness scale *(B)*

the digital system to produce almost any shape of response curve, or to **mimic the shape of an H & D curve almost exactly** if that seems desirable. The implication is that we are making a single exposure and then changing the brightness of each point in the image to make the image appear different. The fact that it is possible to make images with film-screen systems with different H & D curves causes no conceptual difficulty, so we will not allow a change in the brightness curve to cause us difficulty.

A brightness scale is analogous to the density scale for a film H & D curve. Stating that a point on a TV monitor has a certain brightness level is akin to stating that a particular point on a film has a certain density. The brightness scale is not defined as rigidly as the density scale for a particular film, of course. The brightness scale may be changed according to the DF user's pref-

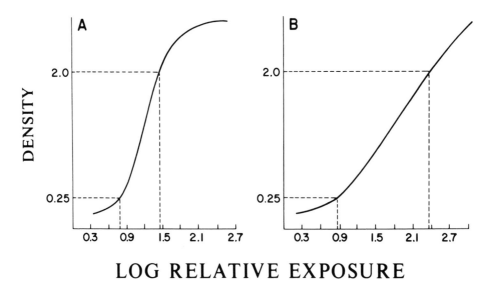

Figure 22–7 Film H & D curves

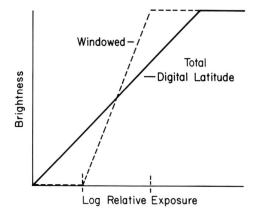

Figure 22–8 The selection of a window to display a smaller exposure latitude

erence. Conceptually, we might speak of a given structure as having a density of 2 on radiographic film. Equivalently, the same structure might have a brightness of 200, for example, on a DF image.

The importance of this analogy is that most manipulations being performed in DF have the same basic effect as those done with film. Thus, knowledge of film-screen radiographic imaging can be used directly, rather than considering a digital system as performing some new magic. Now we can return to a discussion of why the transformation to a logarithmic scale is useful.

Logarithmic Transformation. On a film radiograph a vessel of a given size will appear at about the same contrast with its background, regardless of where on the image the vessel appears. Without worrying about whether this is the most satisfactory situation, we can note that most DF images are displayed with similar characteristics. **Logarithmic transformation ensures that equal absorber thickness changes will result in approximately equal brightness changes, whether in thin or thick body parts.** The consequence of linear and logarithmic brightness relationships will be illustrated with the aid of subtracted DF images from a phantom, and an example will be offered to explain the relationships.

Figure 22–9A is a photograph of a phantom that will help to illustrate several points in the following discussion. The phantom consists of a step wedge of tissue-equivalent material, with crossing bars of bonelike material in its base. A shelf on top of the phantom makes it easy to add small structures for later subtraction. Figure 22–9B is an image of this phantom made on a DF system. Figure 22–9C is an image of only a small region of the phantom from the upper right quadrant made with the fluoro collimator jaws closed down to define only a small area. The image of this region will be used frequently, generally in conjunction with subtraction, and with photographic enlargement to show detail.

Figure 22–10 presents two subtracted digital fluoroscopic images for comparison of linear and logarithmic conversions. The subtracted image of Figure 22–10A was formed by a three-step process: (1) a mask image was obtained using logarithmic conversion; (2) a second image with some added "vessels" was obtained in an identical fashion; and (3) a subtraction of the two images was performed. This is the actual method used to implement the mask subtraction technique described previously. The subtracted image is displayed using a rather narrow window (read "high-contrast film" if you wish) to enhance contrast. There is no apparent difference in the vessel brightness (read "film density difference") between thin and thick phantom regions. (The differences in quantum mottle will be discussed later.) The image of Figure 22–10B was made in the same way, except that no logarithmic conversion was performed on the mask or second original image. The difference in vessel brightness between thick and thin body regions is obvious.

Figure 22–11 offers a numerical illustration for the difference in appearances of the images in Figure 22–10. A phantom with two different thickness parts has two vessels of equal size that can be filled with radiographic contrast material (Fig.

Fig. 22–9 A phantom for tests of a DF unit

Figure 22–10 Subtracted images using logarithmic conversion (*A*) and no logarithmic conversion (*B*)

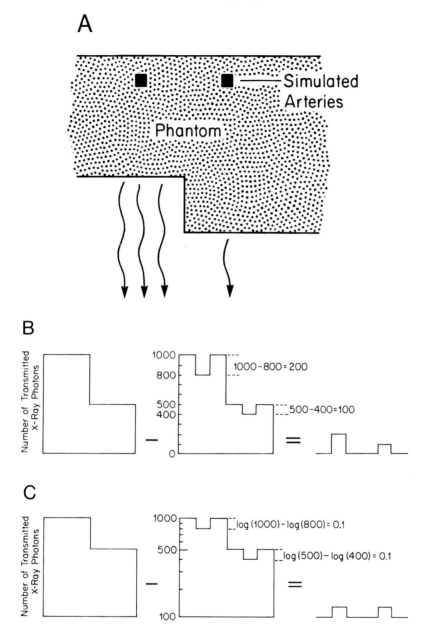

Figure 22–11   Phantom *(A)* used for numerical illustration of linear subtraction *(B)* versus logarithmic subtraction *(C)*

22–11*A).* Either vessel will absorb about the same fraction of the x-ray beam that strikes it. But, as seen in Figure 22–11*B* (a linear relationship), the difference in the absolute number of photons transmitted by the contrast-filled vessels is greater for the thin than for the thick part. The result of the linear relationship, after subtraction, is that the vessel within the thin part appears to have been denser than the vessel in the thick part. The logarithmic relationship of Figure 22–11*C* makes equal fractional changes in the number of x-ray photons result in equal brightness changes. The same percentage change, therefore, whether for a large number of photons (the thin phantom region) or for a small number of photons (the thick region), will provide the same apparent vessel density after subtraction.

Subsequently, we will see that some other sources of image degradation may make some modification of the strictly logarithmic shape advisable, but the assumption of a logarithmic conversion will be adequate for our present purpose.

There are many ways in which the individual pixel brightness values can be converted from a linear exposure relationship to a logarithmic exposure relationship. The exact method, provided that the end result is obtained in a reliable manner, does not really matter. There is one interesting method that illustrates a common type of computer data manipulation. Before the advent of the hand calculator, we used tabulated values instead of calculating trigonometric and logarithmic functions. Of course, there is a way to calculate the value of a logarithm from scratch, but none of us could remember many details beyond the fact that it was not too much fun. A logarithmic table for looking up two decimal digits of precision would only need 100 entries ($10^2 = 100$). A typical DF system might digitize to ten bits (binary digits) of precision, and thus would need a table with only a little over 1000 entries ($2^{10} = 1024$). The advantages are the same for the machine as for a human: simplicity and speed. Computers take advantage of tables quite a bit in the "calculation" of values from data with limited precision. All that is necessary is for the arithmetic processor to look up the logarithmic value of pixel brightness furnished by the digitizer, and to store that value in its image memory. If we do not like a logarithmic transformation, we can put anything we want into the table and the machine will never know the difference. Note that when it is time to convert from digital pixel values back into analog video levels, an appropriate table can tell

what analog level to assign to what digital value. Thus, it is easy to change window levels and widths, or to make other changes in the shape of the display response curve (nominally brightness versus log exposure) without altering the values stored in memory.

Image Noise

Our ability to measure any quantity in the real world is ultimately limited by noise. The statement sounds something like, "If nothing else kills you, a meteor will." Unfortunately, noise is an important problem throughout imaging. This is especially true in the case of radiographic imaging, in which x-ray photon statistics are always a problem. The addition of electronic image chain noise further complicates matters for digital radiography. The quantum noise in digital subtraction angiographic images is particularly prominent, as is true for images from CT and nuclear medicine.

Most important sources of noise in radiographic imaging are random in nature. By comparison, an image basically consists of a distribution of densities or brightness variations arranged in some set spatial pattern. Random noise, as the name implies, does not have a set spatial pattern. Mathematically, random noise and all that it produces can be described statistically. An expanded discussion of some statistics of random noise seems to be in order here. (The authors reluctantly concede that a love of statistics is not necessarily prima facie evidence of mental instability.) Our emphasis is practical, and the discussion is mandated by recent developments in medical imaging. We will present an example of DF images degraded by different amounts of noise, followed by several examples explaining different aspects of noise degradation effects.

The major sources of random noise in a digital fluoroscopic image are electronic noise from the television chain and quantum noise from statistical fluctuations in x-ray photon density. The digital portion of the system should not further degrade the image by the addition of still more noise. A well-designed digital system can meet this responsibility, so there is nothing inherent in digital radiography that necessarily leads to more noisy images.

Quantum Mottle. Quantum mottle, caused by the statistical fluctuations in the number of photons that exit the patient, is ultimately a limiting factor for all x-ray imaging. If quantum mottle is regarded as fluctuations in the brightness or density of the image, the effects of the mottle become a bit easier to describe. The concept is illustrated in Figure 22–12. Figure 22–12A, B, and C are the mask-subtracted images of simulated blood vessels superimposed on the region of the phantom shown in Figure 22–9C. Each image is heavily dominated by quantum mottle, and electronic noise is negligible. Subtracted images shown in Figure 22–12A, B, and C are displayed using the same window width and level. The image in Figure 22–12A was made with each individual unsubtracted frame taken at fluoroscopic dose levels (about 0.1 mAs at 80 kVp). The image in Figure 22–12B represents about four times

that dose, and the image in Figure 22–12C has 16 times the dose of Figure 22–12A. Note how smaller detail becomes visible on the subtracted images as dose is increased. Figure 22–12D is the same as Figure 22–12C, except that the window has been narrowed to increase contrast and to show more clearly that even the smallest vessel is now visible. **The visual prominence of noise increases as the display window is narrowed.**

Standard Deviation. One x-ray exposure is not identical to a second x-ray exposure, even though the same x-ray tube, generator, kVp, mA, and time are used. Also, the number of photons incident on different areas of the patient is not identical for a single exposure, simply because the production of x-rays is a random statistical process. The concept of standard deviation (SD) was introduced in Chapter 14. The standard deviation (SD) for x-ray photon statistics can be calculated by

$$SD = \sqrt{N}$$

where N is the number of photons involved. For instance, suppose that an aver-

Figure 22–12 The effect of quantum mottle on mask-subtracted images. Images have relative exposures of 1 (A), 4 (B), and 16 (C). The image in D is the same as in C, but is windowed to enhance contrast

age of 10,000 photons per mm² exit a phantom and are incident on the face of an II during the time of one TV frame. (An actual pulsed DF image might contain 100,000 photons/mm² or more. We are using 10,000 photons/mm² to simplify arithmetic.) The standard deviation in 10,000 photons is SD = $\sqrt{10,000}$ = 100. The calculation is simple, but the practical meaning of standard deviation requires more explanation.

The statistics of random processes allows us to calculate the probability of occurrence of certain situations. Table 22–2 presents some probabilities based on standard deviations. The first line of Table 22–2 indicates that, about two out of three times, a particular value will be within 1 SD of the average value. For the case in point, a particular 1-mm² area on the face of the II will be expected to have between 9,900 and 10,100 photons incident on it about two out of every three TV frames, if there is no change in the phantom or x-ray beam parameters. Another valid interpretation is that, for a phantom of uniform thickness, about two out of every three randomly chosen 1-mm² areas of the II will have between 9900 and 10,100 incident photons.

Suppose that a nodule with a 1-mm² cross-sectional area absorbs about 1% of the photons that strike it (Fig. 22–13A). This is the same as saying that the average subject contrast between this nodule and its surroundings is 1%. The addition of the nodule to the phantom will result in the absorption of 100 of the 10,000 photons that would otherwise strike the II face, on the average (Fig. 22–13B). Our chances of examining one TV frame and detecting

that the nodule has been added are very poor. According to Table 22–2 (column 3), statistical fluctuation causes 1/3 of all the 1-mm² areas of the TV screen to have more than 10,100 or less than 9900 incident photons. About 1/6 of the areas that are the same size as the added nodule will actually be darker than the area beneath the nodule (column 4). We must also keep in mind that, for a given TV frame, the added object may produce more or less actual subject contrast with its surroundings. The average fraction of the photons absorbed is equal to the average subject contrast (1%), because 100/10000 = 0.01, or 1%. In fact, the number of photons beneath the object (average of 10,000 − 100 = 9900) will be between 9800 and 10,000 photons only about 2/3 of the time. The situation improves rapidly with increasing x-ray absorption.

Subject Contrast. Higher subject contrast lessens the importance of noise. A 1-mm² nodule that absorbs 2% of the photons incident on it (2% average subject contrast) will exhibit an average of two standard deviations difference (200 photons, or 2% of 10,000) with its surroundings (Fig. 22–13C). About 19 out of 20 1-mm² areas will be within two standard deviations of the average of 10,000 photons. Only one area in 40 will be less than 9800 photons (i.e., 2 SD below the average, line 2 of Table 22–2). There are so many 1-mm² areas on the II face that the addition of a 1-mm² nodule with 2% subject contrast still cannot be reliably detected, using our 10,000 photons per mm² example.

A nodule that has an average subject contrast of 4% has a very good statistical chance of being detected reliably in this

Table 22–2. Some Probabilities Based on Standard Deviations

NUMBER OF STANDARD DEVIATIONS	AVERAGE FRACTION OF READINGS		
	WITHIN	OUTSIDE	BELOW
1	2/3	1/3	1/6
2	19/20	1/20	1/40
3	997/1,000	3/1,000	3/2,000
4	99,994/100,000	6/100,000	3/100,000

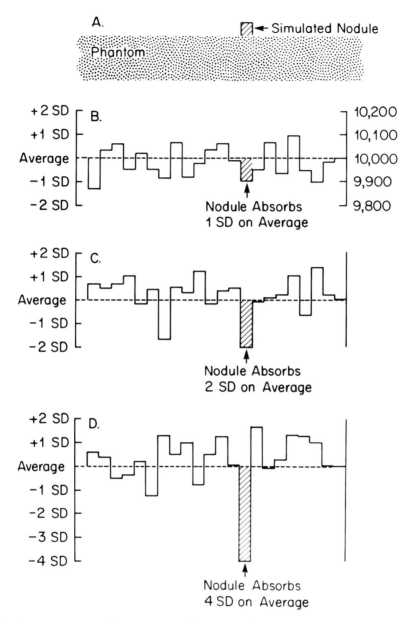

Figure 22–13 Increasing subject contrast with a constant noise level

situation (Fig. 22–13D). A 4% contrast level represents 400 photons, or 4 SD. Only three 1-mm² areas of 100,000 such areas will have less than 9600 photons. Therefore, the chance that statistical fluctuations will mimic a 4% contrast 1-mm² nodule is only three per 100,000 in our example using 10,000 photons per mm².

Increasing Exposure. Increasing ex-posure reduces quantum mottle. Figure 22–14 illustrates quantum mottle at different exposure levels. Figure 22–14A corresponds to the situation in Figure 22–13B. Suppose that exposure (in milliampere seconds) is increased fourfold. In the example just discussed, with 1% subject contrast for a nodule of 1-mm² area, quadrupling the exposure increases the number of photons

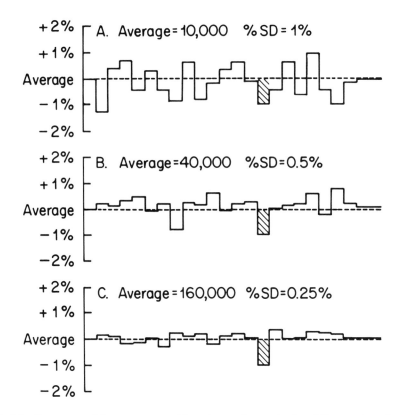

Figure 22–14   Constant subject contrast with a decreasing noise level (increasing dose)

per square millimeter from 10,000 (where the SD was 100) to 40,000/mm². Figure 22–14*B* shows this increased number of photons. The standard deviation of 40,000 photons is SD = $\sqrt{40,000}$ = 200. Another way to calculate this is to note that the new SD = $\sqrt{4 \times 10,000}$ = $\sqrt{4} \times \sqrt{10,000}$ = $\sqrt{4} \times 100$ = 2 × 100. The obvious extension of this is to increase mAs by 16 times (Fig. 22–14*C*). Thus, the SD = $\sqrt{16} \times \sqrt{10,000}$ = 4 × 100 = 400.

There appears to be a problem here. We know that increased dose means less quantum mottle, yet the number of photons in one standard deviation is larger for larger doses. The solution to the quandary is to consider the average number of photons removed by the nodule. Because 1% of 40,000 photons is 400 photons, a 1% contrast level represents 400 photons when there are 40,000 photons in the region of interest. The standard deviation of 40,000 is only 200, which means that the number of standard deviations represented by the 1% contrast level is 400/200 = 2 (Fig. 22–11*B*). Increasing the mAs fourfold increases the number of photons by four (from 10,000/mm² to 40,000/mm²), which increases the number of photons absorbed by four times (from 100 to 400) but only increases the standard deviation by $\sqrt{4}$ = 2 times. Statistical fluctuations (quantum mottle) now represent a smaller percentage of the total number of photons (200/40,000, or 0.5%), and are therefore less likely to be confused with the nodule (1% average subject contrast). For simplicity, we will regard this as being equivalent to reducing quantum mottle to half of its previous level. Figure 22–14*C* represents 16 times the dose of Figure 22–14*A*. The quantum mottle is reduced to one fourth (i.e., $1/\sqrt{16}$) of the original value. **Increas-**

ing the dose M times reduces quantum mottle by $\sqrt{M}$ times.

Noise and Observer Performance. In practice the relationship of image statistics to the performance of an observer is qualitative rather than quantitative. Improving statistics in a particular imaging situation does improve visibility to the point where other imaging limitations such as resolution become more important. It may be possible to state that increasing dose will improve the visibility of small low-contrast objects in DSA images of a particular body region. It would not be valid to declare that mammograms are "better" than chest radiographs because the former has more photons. Direct comparisons are valid only when such parameters as background structures, size of image features, and contrasts are reasonably similar. For instance, we can legitimately compare the effects of increasing contrast with the effects of increasing dose in DSA images. Reducing noise (quantum mottle, in this case) by half (by increasing dose by four times) has the same effect on detection probabilities as doubling subject contrast. In fact, a subtracted image of the high-dose example using a narrow window would be virtually indistinguishable from a subtracted image of the high subject contrast example using a broader window.

Noise and Subtracted Images. At first glance the quantification of the effects of noise on subtracted images seems to be a more difficult concept. One simple consideration, however, allows us to describe noise in subtracted images in a very straightforward way. The key is to consider the total number of photons within the region of interest for both the mask and the contrast-containing frame. Again, using 10,000 photons per mm^2 within a single frame for an example, a subtracted image requires at least two frames, one for the mask and one for the contrast-containing image. The final subtracted image is formed by using about 20,000 photons per

mm^2 in the regions that contain no contrast material, and SD $= \sqrt{20,000} = \sqrt{2} \times 100$. Only one of the original images contains contrast material. If the contrast-containing object absorbs 1% of the incident x-ray photons (in compliance with our first example), an average of 100 photons will represent the subject contrast in the final image. The statistical fluctuations are higher ($\sqrt{2} \times 100 = 141$) than for a single frame, yet the contrast-containing structure is represented by the same number of photons as in a single frame. **The noise in subtracted images is worse than in either the mask or in the contrast-containing image.**

Noise and Object Size. The importance of quantum mottle tends to be much greater for small objects than for large ones. In the example of a 1-mm^2 lesion, which absorbs 1% of the 10,000 incident photons, we noted that there is about one chance in six that any randomly chosen 1-mm^2 area of the image could be mistaken for the lesion itself. The situation with a 4-mm^2 lesion is much better. **Quantum mottle is much less significant for detecting large structures than for detecting small ones because the larger structures have both higher inherent subject contrasts and cover larger areas.** The diameter is doubled, so the area is four times that of the 1-mm^2 lesion and attenuation is twice as great. The x-ray attenuation of the 4-mm^2 lesion is 2%, and there are about 40,000 photons within the area; thus, an average of 800 photons is absorbed. The SD of 40,000 is only 200, so the lesion should produce an average difference with its surroundings of about four standard deviations (800/200 $=$ 4). The probability of occurrence of statistical fluctuations with four standard deviations is much less than for one standard deviation, as previously noted. Table 22–2 indicates that only about three lesion-sized areas out of 100,000 will be expected to have statistical fluctuations that could cause an incorrect identification of quantum mottle as being the 4-mm² lesion in this case. In a clinical situation observer performance would be improved, but not nearly as much as these simple statistics would suggest.

Independent Noise Sources. Every source of image noise contributes to image degradation to some extent. For the most common types of random noise, the total degradation can be calculated by using the percentage standard deviations of the individual noise sources. For our purposes, the percentage standard deviation (% SD) can be defined as the percentage fluctuation in the brightness (or density) of an image. For instance, the percentage standard deviation caused by x-ray photon statistics with 10,000 photons is 1% (100 is 1% of 10,000). In the case of DF, the major noise sources are random electronic noise from the TV system (% SD_{TV}) and quantum statistical fluctuations in the number of detected x-rays (% SD_Q). An equation for calculating the composite percentage standard deviation (% SD_C) for this situation is

$$\%SD_C = \sqrt{(\%SD_{TV})^2 + (\% SD_Q)^2}$$

The result is that the % SD (the magnitude of image fluctuations) is greater than would be seen as a result of either of the two noise sources operating alone. This is consistent with our overall convention of considering noise as fluctuations in the final image.

A poor TV system for DF use might have random noise at a midbrightness level with a % SD_{TV} of 1%. This is the percentage fluctuation in the image that would be produced by electronic noise alone. If the quantum noise at some x-ray exposure level has a % SD_Q of around 0.4%, then % $SD_C = \sqrt{(1)^2 + (0.4)^2} = 1.077\%$. The composite image noise in this case is only a little worse than that of the TV chain alone. One common method of reducing the noise in DF images is to increase the exposure per frame. That clearly will do no significant good here, because even re-

ducing the quantum noise to a small fraction of the 0.4% level will produce little improvement in image quality.

A better TV chain might have random noise at a midbrightness level with a % SD_{TV} of around 0.2%. Under the same exposure conditions, % $SD_C = \sqrt{(0.2)^2 + (0.4)^2} = 0.45\%$. The image is dominated by quantum noise, and the system is good enough to make efficient use of patient dose. Note that for very low exposures per frame such as are typically seen in routine fluoroscopy (about 0.1 mAs per frame), the quantum noise will be much worse than for pulsed DF exposures (perhaps 10 mAs per frame), and even the "poor" TV system might be perfectly adequate.

Frame Integration. Another common method of reducing the noise in DF images is to average or to add together several frames, sometimes called frame integration. Frame integration reduces the effect of all types of random noise. The composite % SD_C is reduced by $\left(\dfrac{1}{\sqrt{M}}\right)$ where M is the number of frames averaged together. The specific equation is not of much interest to us. Whether M frames are averaged together or the dose per frame is increased by M, the final image represents the same number of x-ray photons. The difference is that **increasing the dose per frame reduces only the x-ray quantum noise effects, but integrating frames reduces both electronic and quantum noise effects.** Exposure levels and TV chain quality determine whether this distinction is important. On the practical side, averaging also has the advantage of reducing the importance of the x-ray exposure used during the stabilization time (if any). Of course, frame integration has the disadvantage of longer exposure times.

X-Ray Scatter

X-ray scatter produces the same fundamental types of degradation in digital radiographic applications as in any other radiographic applications. Some potentially valuable techniques in digital radiography, however, impose severe demands on an imaging system. Therefore, effects that were not especially significant in past applications now become more limiting. **Scatter has three major effects that degrade images:**

1. Scatter reduces radiographic contrast.
2. Scatter causes small structures with equal attenuation to appear to have different contrasts with their surroundings, depending on whether the structures are in thin or thick body regions, even after logarithmic conversion.
3. Scatter raises the patient dose required to obtain a given x-ray photon statistical confidence level.

The action of scattered x-ray photons in reducing subject contrast has been discussed in Chapters 8 and 14, so we will concentrate on the second and third effects.

Figure 22–15 illustrates the effect of scatter on contrast in different thickness body regions for subtracted images. The region of the phantom in Figure 22–15A has tight collimation to define a very small x-ray field and thereby to reduce scatter. Figure 22–15B was made with a wider collimator opening and was then photographically cropped to show the same region. The unsubtracted image in Figure 22–15C is darkest in regions of greatest thickness, as has been our custom to this point. The simulated vessels produce less contrast in thick body part areas than vessels in the thin region. The effect occurs because scatter tends to appear as the addition of a uniform x-ray background all across the image. The explanation of the effect requires an examination of the logarithmic conversion that was performed during the collection of these images.

Scatter was not discussed in the section on logarithmic conversion. We implicitly assumed that a structure that attenuated

Figure 22–15   Effect of scatter on contrast. *(A),* Low scatter. *(B),* High scatter. *(C),* Unsubtracted image is shown for comparison some fixed fraction of the number of incident photons would remove that fixed fraction of the number of photons from the final image. Unfortunately, that assumption is not valid. Figure 22–16 shows the situation when a uniform background of scattered x-ray photons is added to Figure 22–11B. Recall that the transformation of Figure 22–11B to a logarithmic scale produced Figure 22–11C, in which each opacified vessel caused a change of 0.1 with respect to local background. The familiar effect of the addition of scatter is that contrast is reduced. This can be seen by using a calculator, and noting that in the thick body region of Figure 22–16, log 2000 − log 1800 = 0.046 instead of 0.1 Another effect of scatter is that the vessels in thin and thick regions no longer produce the same contrast change. Note that log 1500 − log 1400 = 0.03, which is less than the change produced by the vessel in the thin region (0.046). In other words, when equal amounts of scatter are added to all parts of an image, the removal of a small number of photons from the thick area will not produce as large a percentage difference as the

removal of a larger number of photons from the thinner area.

The most obvious potential solution to force thin and thick body parts to display true attenuation is to subtract out the scatter. Unfortunately, the amount of scatter depends on such x-ray beam parameters as kVp and field size. Scatter also depends on the composition, thickness, and location of the structure being imaged. Finally, scatter is not really uniform across the entire image. It is not feasible, therefore, to correct an image completely for scatter by simply subtracting the same fixed fraction of photons from every image. In practice, an attempt to correct for scatter partially is often employed with DSA images. A modification to the "logarithmic table" (or an equivalent method) is commonly employed.

Scatter also makes quantum noise worse, which leads to the discussion of the third major effect. Our well-worn example of 10,000 photons per mm² (primary) will serve one last time. If 30,000 photons per mm² of scatter are added (not unreasonable), the quantum noise in the image is caused by 40,000 photons per mm² (i.e., primary plus scatter), but the useful image is still formed by using only 10,000 photons per mm² (primary only). Small low-contrast objects still attenuate the same number of primary x-ray photons. The vessel that attenuates 1% still removes about 100 photons. The standard deviation with scatter is 200, and without scatter it is only 100. Thus, quantum noise is worse by a factor of two in this case with scatter present. Even if it were feasible simply to subtract scatter after it was detected, the discussion of subtracted images suggests that the worsening of quantum noise by scatter would still persist.

Other solutions are feasible. Increasing dose by four times will reduce quantum noise by $\sqrt{4}$, or twice. This means that 160,000 photons per mm² (scatter plus primary) will give the same statistical confi-

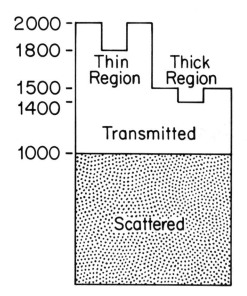

Figure 22–16 Effect of a constant scatter background on thin and thick body regions

dence level in the final image as for 10,000 photons per mm² without scatter. Increasing dose is not only bad for the patient, but the II-TV chain would have to handle 16 times as many x rays. The TV chain would also need better noise characteristics to handle the smaller percentage contrast differences without degradation of the image.

Note the implication that less dose is required for images with an x-ray grid as opposed to images without a grid for the same low-contrast detectability. This option is not easily implemented with film-screen radiography because enough x-rays must be absorbed to expose the film to usable densities.

The best solution to all problems caused by scatter is to eliminate all scatter completely, if possible. X-ray grids and primary beam magnification help to some extent. Another particularly effective method of eliminating scatter will be discussed in a later section.

Veiling Glare

There are other effects that also contribute to a reduction in image contrast. For instance, image intensifiers reduce image contrast because of light scatter and other phenomena within the II (see Chap. 13). "Veiling glare" is a term used in optics to describe the light that is scattered and reflected within a lens system. For convenience, consider image veiling glare to consist of all those processes except x-ray scatter that produce a similar result in a DF system. The II contributes most of this veiling glare, and the remainder is contributed by the optical coupling to the TV chain and even the TV chain itself. Veiling glare becomes worse at larger field sizes. The effects of veiling glare on the image are similar in some respects to those of x-ray scatter. The addition of a background brightness to the image provides the same problem of thickness-dependent contrast levels following simple logarithmic conversion. The correction of an image for veiling glare is similarly difficult, and of course

image contrast is somewhat reduced. Veiling glare, however, does not significantly affect x-ray photon statistics. Thus, images with and without veiling glare will need about the same patient dose for equivalent confidence levels, based on x-ray photon statistics alone.

DIGITAL SUBTRACTION TECHNIQUES

We have defined digital subtraction angiography (DSA) as the generic term for any digital radiographic method of implementing subtraction angiography. Many techniques may be applied to DSA: we will discuss four. These are (1) mask subtraction (previously described), (2) dual energy subtraction, (3) time interval differencing, and (4) temporal filtering. Each technique is mentioned under several names in the current literature, so our choice of terminology is somewhat arbitrary. Mask subtraction is by far the most common at present, but each of the other three techniques is beginning to see clinical use. The field of digital radiography is advancing rapidly, and any or all of these specific techniques may be supplanted before they are widely used.

Mask Subtraction

The general method by which mask subtraction is implemented was described at the beginning of this chapter. We have since noted a number of limits on radiographic imaging systems in general, and a few that apply specifically to digital radiographic systems.

The image spatial resolution at present tends to be limited by the digital matrix sizes used. The ability to resolve low subject contrast objects is limited by the number of x-ray photons used (quantum mottle) and by the electronic noise of the video chain. Quantum mottle may be reduced by increasing the x-ray tube mA, thereby increasing the number of x-ray photons in each frame. Frame averaging is often employed to reduce the effects of video chain noise (as well as quantum noise) in forming a single image in the series. Scattered x rays and image veiling glare also reduce contrast and cause other problems. Patient motion between the time the mask is taken and the time the contrast-containing image is taken is a severe problem that does not have any optimal solution at present. The discussion of partial solutions to this motion artifact problem will be deferred for now.

Dual Energy Subtraction

Another technique for performing DSA is dual energy subtraction, a method that does not require the acquisition of images before and after the arrival of contrast material. In dual energy subtraction, two images are taken within a very short period, during which time there is no change in the patient. These two images are obtained by making exposures with different x-ray energy spectra as would be obtained, for instance, from a high-kVp exposure and a low-kVp exposure.

Film-Screen Method. We will first offer an idealized example of dual energy subtraction using a film-screen system. This example will illustrate the basic principle of how to eliminate soft tissue, leaving only bone. Figure 22–17A shows the exposures transmitted through different thicknesses of soft tissue at high kVp, and the resulting densities recorded on a high-contrast film-screen system. The x-ray attenuation is low at high kVp, and the difference in log relative exposure values between the thinnest body part and the thickest body part is 0.5 (log relative exposures of $1.7 - 1.2 = 0.5$). The high-contrast film records soft tissue over a density range of 1.5 (densities of $2.5 - 1.0 = 1.5$). Figure 22–17B shows the exposures transmitted through the same soft tissue thicknesses at low kVp (and higher mAs). Low kVp inherently provides higher subject contrast than high kVp, so a low-contrast film was chosen to record the low-kVp image. The low kVp and mAs would have to be adjusted experimentally

to give the desired density range for a particular patient, so our example is not very practical. In principle, though, this could be done. The difference in log relative exposures between thin and thick body parts is 0.8 for the low kVp but, as a result of the choice of a low-contrast film for low kVp (and our judicious tinkering with x-ray technique factors), the thinnest soft tissue part is displayed at the same density (2.5) as on the high-contrast film used in the high-kVp image. The thickest part is also displayed at the same density (1.0) on both images.

Recall that successively adding equal thicknesses of tissue will cause equal changes in density within the straight line portion of the H & D curve. This means that an intermediate soft tissue thickness will also give the same film density (1.75) on either the high- or low-kVp image. The net result is that the high-kVp image (recorded on high-contrast film) may be subtracted from the low-kVp image (recorded on low-contrast film), and soft tissue structures will cancel. What about bone?

It is no surprise that the differential attenuation between bone and soft tissue at low kVp is much greater than their differential attenuation at high kVp, a point made in Chapter 5. Perhaps the best practical example is high-kVp versus low-kVp chest films. The bone contrast in the high-kVp films is reduced much more than is the soft tissue contrast. For review, bone has the higher atomic number, and thus has a lot more attenuation because of the photoelectric effect. Because the photoelectric attenuation drops off very rapidly as kVp is increased, bone attenuation changes much more than soft tissue attenuation. Figure 22–18 has the same soft tissue thicknesses as the previous figure, but a small bone has been added to the object. In the regions that do not contain bone, soft tissues still cancel, but bone attenuation has changed more than has soft tissue attenuation. Regions that contain bone will not cancel completely. Thus, the final

Figure 22–17 Film in *A* was selected to have soft tissue contrasts at high kVp equivalent to contrasts of film in *B* at low kVp

image consists of only bone plus the inevitable noise. If soft tissue film contrasts are made equivalent between low- and high-kVp images, bone contrasts will not be equivalent.

Digital Method. The dual energy subtraction operation can be implemented in practice using digital image processing.

The basic principle is the same, so consider the example just presented using film-screen subtraction. Figure 22–19*A* corresponds closely to Figure 22–18*A*. The same three thicknesses of soft tissue and the same added bone, kVp, and so forth are illustrated. The digital brightness scale has been modified so that the windowed digital

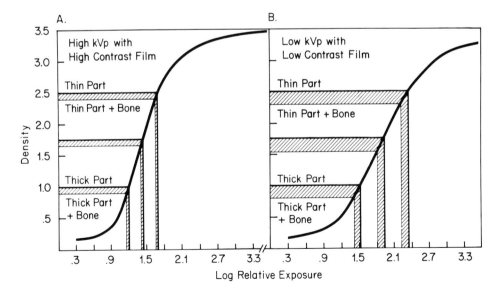

Figure 22–18 Dual energy subtraction principle. Bone contrasts change more with kVp than do soft tissue contrasts

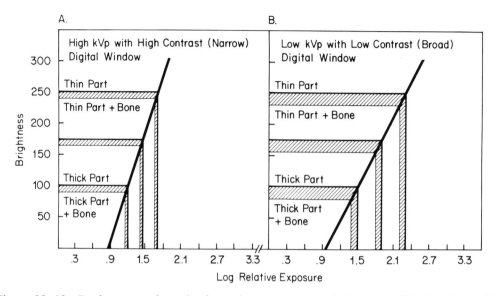

Figure 22–19 Dual energy subtraction by setting appropriate windows on a digital radiographic system

line and straight line portion of the film H & D curve would superimpose. Similarly, the low-kVp digital window depicted in Figure 22–19B and the film H & D curve in Figure 22–18B are essentially identical. The brightness levels of thick (50), thin (250), and intermediate (175) soft tissue regions that contain no bone are the same either on the narrow window (high display contrast), high-kVp image, or on the broad window (low display contrast), low-kVp image. Soft tissues will cancel except for noise. As before, the final image will consist of bone only. The small bone reduces brightness by 20 whether in thick (100 − 80 = 20), thin, or intermediate regions of the low-kVp image. But the same bone only reduces the brightness by 10 in the high-kVp image.

Implementing dual energy subtraction by film-screen systems is very difficult. The advantage of the digital approach is flexibility. The beam energies and x-ray doses can be chosen with comparatively little concern for whether a good subtraction will result. The "windows" are chosen after the images are acquired (conceptually equivalent to choosing film types before expo-

sure), and can be readily modified for the patient's requirements. A set of windows appropriate for the subtraction of bone rather than soft tissue can obviously be used if desirable for a particular problem. A single high-kVp and low-kVp image pair can yield chest images of either bone only, soft tissue only, or both. It should be noted that our use of display windows is for explanation, and that the technique is implemented by hardware performing functionally equivalent operations internally.

Problems of Dual Energy Subtraction. There are inevitably some disadvantages attached to this approach to imaging. All the problems associated with radiographic imaging in general and with DSA in particular are still present, except perhaps for anatomic motion. There are also some special problems unique to the use of dual energy subtraction.

First, the high-kVp image still has some bone within it. When the soft tissue densities are eliminated by subtracting windowed high- and low-kVp images, some of the bone density is also reduced. This implies that to obtain the same contrast differences as with a mask subtraction technique, more display contrast enhancement would be necessary with the dual energy scheme. As always, enhancing display contrast also increases the visibility of noise. More patient dose is required to suppress the visibility of this quantum mottle for dual energy subtraction.

Second, a more complex x-ray machine is indicated. An x-ray generator capable of switching kVp and mAs rapidly is needed to overcome problems with anatomic motion. Also, bone contrast in the subtracted image is greatest with two x-ray beams of greatly different energy spectra. The energy spectra can be varied even more by several methods. For instance, very different peak voltages can be employed, and extra filtration can be added to the higher kVp beam. The additional filtration adds some load to the x-ray tube that would not otherwise be necessary. Some mechanism for rapidly changing filters between exposures is also necessary.

Third, we actually made an invalid assumption in our example. A polychromatic x-ray beam is in fact hardened as it traverses the body. Beam hardening is the term used to describe the preferential removal of the lower energy x rays as the beam traverses a thick body structure (see Chap. 5). The main cause of beam hardening is the photoelectric effect, which drops off rapidly at higher photon energies. The net effect is that the effective energy of the beam increases as it passes through thick body parts. Note that the photoelectric effect is greater in higher atomic number materials, so higher atomic number materials have a greater beam hardening effect. Also, higher kVp x-ray beams will have different beam hardening as compared to lower kVp beams. Beam hardening does not cause much of a problem in the simple mask subtraction technique, because only one x-ray beam energy is employed. The amount of beam hardening caused by bone and soft tissue is the same for each image, and small quantities of contrast material have only a small ad-

ditional beam hardening effect. Unchanging structures still cancel without leaving residual images. The situation with dual energy subtraction is more complex because of the two beam energies employed. If each beam exhibited exactly the same amount of beam hardening in each region of the body, proper subtraction of bone and soft tissue would not be significantly affected. The broad range of thicknesses of soft tissue and bone, however, affect the two beams differently. A final image that should contain soft tissue structures only may in fact have significant amounts of residual bony structures that were improperly subtracted.

Finally, three different beam spectra are required to handle three substances with greatly differing atomic numbers. This might be termed "three-energy subtraction." The reason that three images at different beam energies are necessary can be understood by some simple algebra. Each pixel in a single image has information about unknown thicknesses of soft tissue, bone, and contrast material. Each of the three energies gives up independent (i.e., different) information about the thickness within that pixel. So, we have three unknown thicknesses and three equations that can be used to solve for the unknowns. For most angiography work using energy subtraction techniques alone, three exposures would be necessary to yield a subtracted image of iodine only. The iodine contrast would be even lower than for a dual energy subtraction, and the third image would contribute still more quantum noise. The display window would need to be narrowed even more than for the dual energy subtraction technique. The increased quantum mottle in the contrast-enhanced final images would become more prominent. Three exposures per image implies an increase in dose over the two exposures per image used for dual energy subtraction.

Other Dual Energy Subtraction Methods

K-Edge Subtraction. A technique called "K-edge subtraction," using film-screen systems, received considerable research interest several years ago. Interest waned partly because of the difficulty of using film as the recording medium. The technique was named because of the K-shell absorption edge seen on a photoelectric attenuation curve. Figure 22–20 summarizes a method of using K-edge absorption x-ray filters to improve dual energy subtraction for contrast materials such as iodine. One of the two images should have the highest possible iodine x-ray contrast, and the other image should have little or no iodine x-ray contrast.

Iodine attenuates diagnostic x-rays almost entirely by the photoelectric effect. One method for achieving high iodine subject contrast is removal of all x-rays from the beam except those that lie just above the K-shell binding energy of iodine (about 33 keV). An x-ray filter made of the rare earth named cerium can do this quite well. Figure 22–20A shows the x-ray tube brems-

strahlung spectrum to be filtered. As can be seen from Figure 22–20B, the K-edge photoelectric absorption of cerium begins at about 40 keV (binding energy of cerium's K-shell electrons). A thick filter of cerium inserted into the beam will remove most of the x rays above 40 keV by the K-shell photoelectric effect. Many x rays in the range of 30 to 40 keV will get through the filter. The x-ray spectrum through this filter will have its highest intensity just above the K-shell binding energy of iodine (Fig. 22–20C). This spectrum is nearly ideal for providing the highest possible x-ray subject contrast for iodine. This is the advantage of K-edge filtration, whether or not the technique is to be used with dual energy subtraction.

The image to be subtracted (roughly equivalent to a mask) should have little or no iodine subject contrast. The appropriate x-ray spectrum should contain few x rays that could be absorbed by iodine (Fig. 22–20D). If a thick iodine filter is placed in the beam, then almost all the x rays that could be absorbed by iodine have been absorbed before reaching the iodine within the patient. The resulting image will have very low iodine subject contrast.

The K-edge subtraction to form the final image is still a type of dual energy subtraction, and is accomplished by a method similar to that previously described. The problems with dual energy subtraction images, including incomplete bone-soft tissue cancellation with only two beam spectra, are still present, but the very high and very low subject contrast iodine images make most of those problems somewhat less important. The exception is that the technique is most effective with thick filters that remove most of the original beam intensity, and the high mAs required as a result makes x-ray tube load problems much worse. There are other problems, including those regarding patient dose and choice of materials for the most efficient filters, which we will not discuss.

Hybrid Subtraction. Another promising use for dual energy subtraction techniques

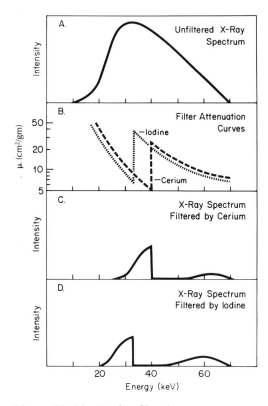

Figure 22–20   K-edge filtration

is hybrid subtraction. A simple mask subtraction technique is combined with dual energy subtraction (thus "hybrid"). The technique is designed for the situation in which anatomic motion is expected to be a problem. The data are collected much as in simple mask subtraction, with images being collected at about 1-sec intervals over the course of the passage of contrast material through the vessels. The difference is that where each single image of the series is collected for mask subtraction, a high-kVp/low-kVp image pair is collected for hybrid subtraction. If there is no patient motion, the low-kVp image series can be used as if a simple mask subtraction had actually occurred.

Very little patient motion can be tolerated in simple mask subtraction between the time the mask is taken and the time the contrast material arrives in the vessels of interest. The soft tissues (large structures without sharp edges) cancel properly if patient motion is not too great, but bone edges cause severe artifact problems. Consider the subtracted images to consist of only two atomic number materials, iodine and bone. The hybrid subtraction technique produces two sets of subtracted images, one from the low-kVp and the other from the high-kVp series that were collected simultaneously. The same bone and iodine structures are present on both sets. Dual energy subtraction can now be used to eliminate bone, leaving only iodine. The final image will have lower contrast and more noise than if the dual energy operation had proved unnecessary, but the critical diagnostic information may be saved.

Dual energy and three-energy subtraction techniques have so much promise that they may be successful in spite of their obvious problems. First, the elimination of either bone or soft tissue by dual energy subtraction may be worthwhile, especially in chest radiography. Second, hybrid subtraction may be helpful in imaging situations in which normal anatomic motion is expected, as well as in the case of the uncooperative patient. Third, it may be possible in some instances to obtain the same diagnostic information in three exposures with a three-energy technique that would require about 20 exposures in temporal mask subtraction. Finally, there is the promise of obtaining subtraction images of contrast material for such procedures as laminography and cholecystography where the time span between pre-contrast and post-contrast images is long.

Time Interval Differencing

Time interval differencing (TID) is another digital subtraction technique, and it has seen some application in cardiology. The technique is closely related to simple mask subtraction. In simple mask subtraction an early image is chosen as the mask, and this single mask is subtracted from each succeeding image of the series to form the series of subtracted images. In the TID technique, a new mask is chosen for each subtraction.

For simplicity, assume that images are collected and stored at the rate of 30 images per second for several seconds. Choose image 1 as the first mask, and subtract the mask from image 7 (0.2 sec later in time) to form the first subtracted image. Next, choose image 2 as the second mask, and subtract from image 8 (again, 0.2-sec time interval) to form the second subtracted image. The third subtracted image is a subtraction of image 3 from image 9, and so on. **Each subtracted image is the difference between images separated by some fixed interval of time.** The successive subtracted images are frequently displayed in a rapid sequence that is repeated to show dynamic function.

Each individual image of the series might have rather poor statistics that can be improved by frame integration at the expense of increased blurring caused by anatomic motion. For four-frame integration, images 1, 2, 3, and 4 are added together to form the first mask. Frames 7, 8, 9, and 10 are added together, and the first mask is subtracted from the result to form the first subtracted image. The second subtracted image uses frames 2, 3, 4, and 5 as the mask, subtracted from the sum of frames 8, 9, 10, and 11. This particular TID technique involves adding a number of images to form a mask that represents information about one time period, and subtracting the mask from the sum of another group of images that represents information about another time period. In principle this is very similar to another digital subtraction technique called temporal filtering.

Temporal Filtering

Time interval differencing can actually be considered to be a temporal filtering technique. The word "temporal" means of or limited by time, and clearly applies. We will not attempt a mathematical description of filtering either here or later in the examples of spatial filters. The description of the TID filtering operation is sufficient to explain the principle for present purposes. A set of final data (images) was formed from a set of original data (also images) by applying a consistent set of rules. Each successive final image was formed in exactly the same fashion, except for a shift along the time axis of the data. This operation of adding and subtracting part of a set of data together according to a set of rules to get one answer, and then shifting and repeating to get the next answer, is a filtering operation.

Time interval differencing is not usually regarded as a filtering technique, but of course it is actually a valid example. Temporal filtering is very general, and there are temporal filters that can be used to perform DSA (sometimes the awesome term "temporal filter" is even used). A simple example will show the general operation.

The passage of contrast material through an artery following intravenous injection will result in a contrast dilution curve with the general shape shown in Figure 22–21. Suppose that we wish to use our knowledge regarding the curve to perform DSA. The first step is to inject a bolus of contrast material intravenously. A second step might be to operate the x-ray tube in a continuous fashion at 10 to 20 mA, during which time individual frames are collected and stored at 30 frames per second. Now for the final step. One obvious approach is to choose either an early or a late frame with no contrast material present as a mask, and to subtract later frames from the mask as was done for simple mask subtraction. Unfortunately, the low mA leads to very high quantum noise in single frames. Another almost equally obvious approach is to add together several of the early frames and several of the late frames to form the mask. An equal number of frames that contain contrast can be added together to form a contrast-containing image. DSA is now accomplished by subtraction of the low-noise mask from the low-noise contrast-containing image.

In other words, individual images (single TV frames) are added together or subtracted from each other to form a composite image. The exact time of arrival of the contrast material is sometimes difficult to predict in reality, so the manual selection of the most appropriate frames to use for the individual steps could be quite time-consuming. Perhaps it would be better to allow the computer to do the selection using some consistent set of rules, and then to generate a large number of individual composite DSA images so that the best may be chosen. We now have a filter for doing DSA. Again, this filter generates one final image by adding and subtracting some of the original images together, and then shifting and repeating to form the next image. Obviously a temporal filter of almost any shape can be selected. The one used in this example was chosen for simplicity of didactic explanation, and is not the optimal shape for the application.

One advantage of the temporal filtering approach is that less severe demands are placed on the video image chain than for simple mask subtraction, because the x-ray tube can be operated at much lower tube current values. Typically, mask subtraction requires around ten times the tube current needed by temporal filtering for comparable contrast detectability. An obvious disadvantage is that a large number of indi-

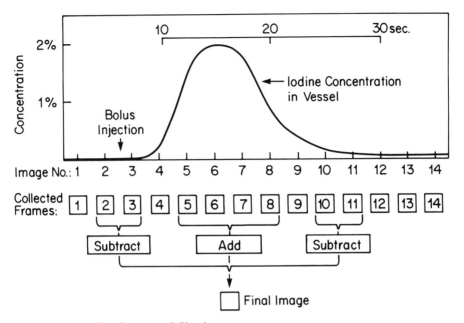

Figure 22–21   Principle of temporal filtering

vidual frames must be handled for temporal filtering.

Comparisons of patient dose and the sensitivity of the system to artifacts caused by patient motion are difficult to make at the present stage of development. Both patient dose and anatomic motion sensitivity are highly dependent on the way in which the techniques are implemented.

DIGITAL IMAGE PROCESSING

The field of image processing has received much attention since about the mid-1970s. Much of the impetus for this attention has come from the space program. The startling images from satellites are typically manipulated by digital image processing techniques prior to being photographed for presentation to the public. Clearly, it is possible to manipulate medical images by computer in a manner analogous to the way in which these satellite images are manipulated. Nuclear medicine images in particular have had increasingly sophisticated digital processing techniques applied to them for years. At this point, digital x-ray image processing must be regarded as being in its infancy. No attempt

will be made here to survey the rapidly growing field of digital x-ray image processing, but some discussion of present techniques and areas receiving attention is appropriate. Our examples will be linked to simple illustrations of a few general types of manipulations, rather than to specific complex (and changeable) processing operations now in use.

There are many ways to classify types of image manipulations (image processing operations). Engineers tend to classify on the basis of the type of mathematical operation that is implemented. We will classify them on the basis of the fundamental purpose of the manipulation.

First, there are manipulations that are intended to correct a deficiency in the imaging system or to place the information in a form more suitable for later processing. This might be termed "preprocessing," and it is usually performed during or immediately after data collection. Second, preprocessed images may be further manipulated by such methods as subtraction to form viewable images of the type desired for a particular application. Enough examples of these manipulations have been given in the discussion of DSA methods to illustrate this point. Third, there are manipulations employed to enhance the visibility of certain types of structures or certain features of images. Finally, certain manipulations are not intended to result in an improved visible image at all, but rather are aimed at allowing the computer to extract information such as projected crop yields in Canada, volcanic activity on Jupiter's moons, or the probability that a patient has cardiac insufficiency. A single type of mathematical operation may find application in all four of these types of image manipulations. Similarly, a single application may require all four general types of image processing.

For instance, several processing steps are applied in the mask subtraction technique of DSA. The individual images are first preprocessed by a logarithmic or similar conversion. Next, individual images are subtracted from each other to remove structures that are not of interest. A narrow display window is then selected to increase displayed vessel contrast. The first of these manipulations falls most conveniently into the preprocessing category. Subtraction provides a viewable image suitable for the application (DSA), our second category. The increase of displayed contrast by windowing is an example of image enhancement. Numerous researchers are working on methods for extracting numerical information regarding blood flow from DSA images, which would fall into our fourth general category. Obviously, categorization of image processing operations by intended purpose of the operation is somewhat arbitrary, because an argumentative person could successfully place a given manipulation into some category other than the one which we have chosen.

Image Correction and Preprocessing

In general, preprocessing of images is done to increase the value or accuracy of the data for later processing steps. The utility of a preprocessing step is very dependent on the later use to be made of the images. For instance, one of the most useful features of logarithmic conversion is that equal-sized vessels appear equally dense after the later subtraction.

An operation that would be immediately useful is the correction of images for x-ray scatter and image system veiling glare. Such corrections are needed to increase the utility of numerical densitometry techniques (to be mentioned shortly). In another area, the II-TV system introduces geometric distortion in the image. This geometric distortion causes few problems in simple image viewing, but makes exact evaluation of spatial relationships somewhat difficult. Generally, the specific operations employed for preprocessing are not intended to compensate for all problems in the original data exactly. The common approach is to use approximate methods to attack only those problems most important to the application. Something similar to logarithmic conversion is very important for DSA, and scatter and veiling glare corrections would be helpful, but geometric corrections would be superfluous for most DSA applications.

Image Enhancement

For our purposes, image enhancement operations are performed at the viewer's option after the basic image of a particular type has been formed. This might be termed "postprocessing of images." There are so many image enhancement methods available that books on the subject survey only a small fraction of the available techniques, and are obsolete before they are published. Three postprocessing operations that are common in digital radiography are mask reregistration, noise smoothing, and edge enhancement. A common feature of these three operations (and enhancement operations in general) is that "enhancement" is actually the suppression of information that the viewer deems to be unnecessary for a particular problem.

Mask Reregistration. Mask reregistration is sometimes useful when there is patient motion between the time the mask is taken and the time that contrast material arrives in the vessel of interest. The problem is illustrated in Figure 22–22, in which portions of the two digital images are shown. Each pixel is represented by a number (brightness level) in a digital matrix. Bony structures within the patient that should subtract on the two images are not recorded in the same position on the mask frame as the same structure on the contrast-containing frame. The subtracted image of Figure 22–22A shows the misregistered bony edges that produce motion artifacts whose magnitudes are greater than the magnitudes of the contrast-containing vessels of interest. The same problem occurs in film-screen subtraction angiography, in which the mask and contrast-containing image are aligned by eye until the "best" subtraction is obtained. This may be considered to be a form of manual reregistration, and is successful when patient motion is moderate. A similar approach will work for DSA. When the reregistered mask is subtracted from the contrast-containing image, Figure 22–22B does not contain the motion artifact. The aim is to throw away the information represented by the motion artifact.

The reregistration of the mask may be accomplished either manually (viewer-controlled) or automatically (computer-controlled). Manual reregistration is similar to alignment of the films. The viewer rotates the mask and translates it vertically or horizontally while viewing the subtracted image until a satisfactory subtraction is obtained. Automatic reregistration depends on computer calculations, and may be done in several ways. One method is first to calculate the sum of the "absolute values" of all pixels in a subtracted image. The absolute value of a negative number (-5, for instance) is just the number without the negative sign (5), and is the same as the absolute value of the same positive number. The sum of the absolute values of -5 and $+5$ is 10.

Now an observation can be made. The contrast material is present on a subtracted image whether the mask is properly registered or not. In the case in which the image is properly registered, the only image features present are contrast and noise. Misregistration adds such factors as bony edges to the subtracted images, and the sum mentioned above should be higher

Figure 22–22 Mask reregistration. *(A)* Poor registration. *(B)* Good registration of mask and contrast-containing image

than for a properly registered mask. The computer can therefore try numerous positions for reregistration, calculate the sum of absolute pixel values for each, and pick the reregistration position for which the sum is a minimum. Under good conditions, this minimum sum position will produce acceptable subtracted images.

There are numerous situations in which mask reregistration will be of limited value. The patient is three-dimensional, and mask reregistration operations are effective only for motions confined to a plane. Upper structures project onto different lower structures when the patient rolls onto one side as compared to being flat on his back. Reregistration cannot exactly compensate for this type of motion. The motion of structures within the patient (especially bowel gas and larynx) also changes the relative positions of prominent structures, and again reregistration cannot compensate exactly. In the case of automatic reregistration, there are numerous situations in which the minimum sum position of the mask (or some other calculation criterion) is not the position that even the most forgiving viewer would judge to be optimum for subtraction.

Noise Smoothing. Noise smoothing is an attempt to decrease the visual prominence of noise so that low-contrast objects of moderate to large size may be better appreciated. All methods of smoothing x-ray quantum noise sacrifice some resolution in the process of smoothing the image. One method is illustrated in Figure 22–23. The technique operates by reducing the statistical fluctuations in each pixel by averaging the pixel with its closest neighbors. The first pixel in the smoothed image is formed by averaging the nine nearest neighbors in the upper left corner of the original image (rows 1, 2, and 3). The second pixel in the smoothed image is formed by shifting one column to the right in the original image and averaging, and the process continues until the entire first row has been formed. The second and subsequent rows are formed similarly. One shifts down a row in the original image and averages the nine

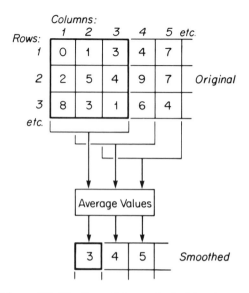

Figure 22–23 Smoothing noise by blurring an image

adjacent pixels (rows 2, 3, and 4 of the original) to form the first pixel in the second row. The final image is a blurred version of the original. The visual prominence of noise has been suppressed through the process of averaging noise within small areas, but the disadvantage is that resolution is decreased.

The operation just described is a filtration operation. A final image was generated by applying a consistent mathematical operation to the original image to form the first pixel, and then shifting and repeating to form subsequent pixels. The operation of the filter suppressed small structures (high spatial frequencies) and had little effect on large structures (low spatial frequencies). This type of operation is sometimes called "low-pass spatial filtering," indicating that low spatial frequencies are passed and high spatial frequencies are filtered out. For general information, the specific mathematical operation described in the preceding paragraph is a convolution. We note in passing that the literature contains references to "spatial domain" filtering (of which the above is an example) and "frequency domain" or "Fourier" filtering as mathematical approaches. The specific mathematical approach is largely a matter of computational convenience, because a given filter can generally be implemented either by Fourier methods or by spatial domain methods. With that, we put the mathematics of filters to rest.

Edge Enhancement. Edge enhancement is intended to increase the visibility of small structures with moderate to high contrast. The basic goal is to discard most of the information about the large structures and keep the information that relates to small structures. The appearance of a xeroradiograph is very familiar to most radiologists. The principal features of the xeroradiograph that distinguish it from film radiographs and DF images are that the xeroradiograph has a very broad latitude but still shows edges at high contrast. Problems with the xeroradiograph are that the necessary patient exposure becomes significantly higher as the kVp is increased. Also, once xeroradiography is chosen, it becomes difficult to display these images as the more conventional film radiographs. For these and other reasons, xeroradiography is not widely used for general radiographic applications.

If a conventional radiograph could be processed into an image that resembled a xeroradiograph in appearance, then it might be possible to have the advantages of both methods readily available. The combination of the blurred (low-pass filtered) image just described and the original image contain everything necessary to implement edge enhancement and mimic a xeroradiograph. The low-pass filter contains only the information about large structures and has low noise, while the original image contains additional information about the edges plus noise. The subtraction of the low-pass filtered image from the original yields an image in which edges and small structures remain. Edge enhancement is accomplished by suppressing information regarding large structures. Unfortunately, noise is also prominent in this edge-enhanced image. The final image has effectively been high-pass filtered, and the operation is sometimes referred to as a blurred mask subtraction. Many other specific mathematical operations could be used to perform exactly the same overall operation.

Information Extraction

A most promising area in digital radiography is the extraction of numerical or graphic information from images. The extraction of such information from nuclear medicine images is now routine in some applications. Many nuclear medicine blood flow measurements and similar dynamic techniques can be implemented using DF images. The development of useful methods for extracting information from DF images is still in its infancy at present.

It might be useful to have a technique that could accurately measure both the quantity of contrast material contained within some organ and the way in which the quantity of contrast changes with time. A DSA series of images contains the needed information. A somewhat trivial technique (not workable as described here) begins when a viewer circles the region of interest on one of the images. The brightness level in any given pixel in the subtracted image is directly proportional to the quantity of contrast material in the patient volume imaged onto the pixel for the idealized case (ignore scatter, veiling glare, geometric image distortion, and magnification). The total quantity of contrast within the region of interest could be calculated by simply adding together the contributions from all the individual pixels. Successive images of the same region of interest could be processed in the same way to produce the information needed for a graph of time versus total contrast material. Unfortunately, all the factors that were ignored are important to the accuracy of the results. The person charged with the resolution of these technical problems may have an easy task as compared to the person who is responsible for evaluating the technique for efficacy.

FUTURE EQUIPMENT DEVELOPMENTS

Alternate Image Receptor Systems

At present, digital radiography is almost synonymous with digital fluoroscopy in clinical use. A large fraction of DF systems are installed on C-arm units, and almost all are limited to use in one room or in two closely adjacent rooms. The average DF unit utilizes a 9-in. II and is capable of generating digital images on a 512- × 512-pixel matrix. Most manufacturers now offer 1024 × 1024 matrices as options, and 12- to 14-in. IIs are available for C-arm use. Both the large matrices and the large IIs are expensive. In addition to limitations on field of view and matrix-imposed resolution, we have discussed sources of image degradation inherent in conventional x-ray IIs and in TV video cameras and chains.

There are many alternatives to the conventional II-TV-based imaging chain. These have been investigated for many years, but digital x-ray imaging lends new urgency to the search for new imaging systems. Image receptor systems for three areas of application are receiving most of the research attention. The first is slit radiography using linear detector systems. The second is two-dimensional detectors for replacement of film-screen cassettes. The third area now uses automatic film changers. We are short on crystal balls, so each example offered has been chosen to illustrate a diversity of approaches rather than to predict an ultimate winner of the technologic sweepstakes for that area.

One-Dimensional Image Receptors.

Most radiographic imaging utilizes two-dimensional image receptor systems. An entire volume of the patient is projected onto the two-dimensional receptor (typically a film-screen cassette or II) during a single exposure to form the final image. In a technique called "slit radiography," the x-ray beam is collimated into a fan-shaped beam so that a thin line is defined on the final image. Postpatient collimation is used to define further the line of the final image that is being formed, and to reject scatter that would strike other regions of the image receptor. A long x-ray exposure is used, during which the beam-defining collimator slit and the scatter rejection postpatient slit are swept in synchrony from the head to the foot of the patient.

The single most important reason for the development of slit radiography is the very high scatter-rejection characteristics of the technique. Figure 22–24 compares scatter rejection for a slit radiography system and a two-dimensional film-screen imaging system with a grid. The only radiation reaching the image receptor during the exposure for slit radiography is that portion of the primary radiation that does not undergo any interactions within the patient, and radiation that is scattered over very small angles. Radiation scattered over wide enough angles to miss the postpatient slit and almost all multiple scattered radiation are absorbed before reaching the image receptor. The gridded system also rejects singly scattered photons, although perhaps somewhat less efficiently than for slit radiography. Also, multiple scattered photons may reach the image receptor. The importance of scatter for radiographic imaging in general, and digital radiography in particular, has been discussed in detail. Scatter rejection increases contrast, increases dose efficiency by reducing x-ray quantum requirements, and provides a final image that reflects true attenuation in thin or thick regions more accurately.

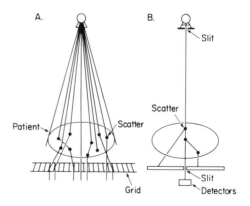

Figure 22–24 Comparison of scatter rejection for a grid (*A*) and for slit radiography (*B*)

Detector systems commonly in use for x-ray CT may be considered to be one-dimensional. Experiments with slit radiographic techniques were done with some of the earliest CT scanners. Many modern CT scanners have some type of scout image capability (such as the GE Scoutview), which is in fact slit radiography. GE calls the technique "scanned projection radiography." The biggest problem is that, because of the size of individual detector elements, spatial resolution is poor for general radiographic work. A typical scanning slit imaging system with a single-line image receptor currently being applied to chest radiography digitizes the line into 1024 separate pixels. There is controversy over whether 1024 elements in one dimension is adequate for chest radiography, and image matrix sizes of greater than 1024×1024 may be necessary.

The slit radiography approach that depends on a single-line image receptor does have some significant drawbacks. Each individual line of the image requires that enough x-rays be detected to define that line. It is true that fewer x rays (and less patient exposure) are required to arrive at the same contrast detectability in the absence of scatter, and it is also true that the detector system might be more efficient in stopping x rays. The slit radiography system, however, still requires that a certain minimum number of x rays be delivered to each line of the system. For a 1024-line image, this essentially amounts to making 1024 separate exposures. Each exposure will be considerably less than required for a single film-screen radiograph, but the sum of all individual exposures will still be quite large.

The net result is that the x-ray tube must deliver about 100 times the radiation for the single-line slit radiography system as would be required for a film-screen exposure with similar photon statistical contrast detectability characteristics. These exposure requirements can be met in a dedicated chest imaging system. The problem becomes more acute when higher exposures are needed, as in abdominal imaging. Also, much more time is required to obtain an image. Inaccuracy in collimating the beam and in moving the beam-defining slit increases patient dose. Some of the most valuable types of dynamic digital subtraction angiographic procedures, therefore, are clearly impossible. The extension to a larger image matrix would make the x-ray tube load and exposure time drawbacks even more significant.

There are some extensions to the technique that might help to solve some of these problems. For instance, the slit might be made larger, and several lines of detectors might be used to increase the number of lines defined per exposure. Unfortunately, this tends to increase the complexity and consequently the cost of the system. Slit radiography was originally developed on a film-screen system, which is a two-dimensional image receptor. There may be little net advantage for digital radiography in using a receptor system that is inherently one-dimensional versus using one that is inherently two-dimensional.

Fixed Two-Dimensional Image Receptors. For fixed systems there are alternatives to IIs and TV cameras. An old idea for replacement of conventional x-ray IIs was to use optical coupling of the light image formed on an x-ray screen, followed by light amplification. Each absorbed x ray produces so much light than an efficient lens system can guarantee that each x ray will be detected in the light amplifier. It is easy to amplify the light enough so that the presence of the x ray is detected in the final image. Compared to a small x-ray II, the solution is both bulky and expensive. For larger field sizes, however, the approach does have some merit. The input x-ray screen can be flat if that is desirable. Good optical systems with low veiling glare characteristics can be designed.

Alternatives to conventional TV cameras are also under development. One of the most promising, which has a light-sensitive region about the size of the input phosphor on a conventional TV camera tube, is similar in appearance to a large semiconductor electronic chip. A two-dimensional array of light detectors is embedded in this light-sensitive area. Each element of the array defines a single pixel of the image, and is essentially independent of all other pixels. The advantages, in addition to size, are that the system is more light-sensitive than most types of conventional TV tubes, and has much lower electronic noise.

Film-Screen Cassette Replacement. The benefits of having an image receptor that can be carried to remote locations and used with virtually any existing radiographic x-ray machine are obvious. An image receptor similar to a film-screen cassette in portability, resolution, and x-ray detection efficiency will eventually be developed for use in digital radiography. There are many possibilities. For instance, xeroradiographic plates initially accumulate an image in the form of a charge distribution that has been altered by the absorption of x rays. Several methods have been proposed and tried for scanning this charge distribution to convert the charge image into an electronic video image directly. Cassettes similar to xeroradiographic cassettes could be used at any convenient location and then brought to a central facility for "processing" and storage as digital images.

Archiving and Display of Large Image Matrices

At present, almost all DF display matrices are 512 × 512 pixels. Archiving is usually accomplished by recording the video display of the DF images onto film.

The development of a digital radiography apparatus that uses larger image matrices will require better display systems than those presently in use. Some expensive display systems are available with resolution of 2048 × 2048 pixels or better, but currently these are expensive and not very reliable. Presumably a radiology department that handles all images in digital format will require a large number of such display consoles, each with a moderate amount of image postprocessing and enhancement capability. Each console will probably need some rapid method of transferring images from a central area for display of recently acquired radiographs, and a somewhat slower method for transferring images from archival storage.

The digital archive storage problem appears to be intractable with currently available technology. Given 2048 × 2048 images, each image would require the storage of about 4,000,000 pieces of data. Digital discs capable of storing 250 such images are becoming more economical (larger and more expensive discs are also available), but storage of even 1 week's radiographs for a sizable radiology department would be prohibitively expensive. Other digital disc technology (such as the much publicized optical or laser discs) is under development. Archiving large numbers of images in digital form presents a formidable challenge.

Fortunately, medical imaging is not the only area with the need for better digital displays and storage retrieval methods. Applications as diverse as robotics, earth resources satellites, and computer games are adding impetus to development of the necessary technology. There no longer seems to be a question about whether an all-digital radiology department will be possible. The question now is how long it will be before such a department actually comes into being.

SUMMARY

The most common type of digital radiography system is digital fluoroscopy (DF). A DF system requires an image intensifier (II) with a high contrast ratio and a TV chain with low lag and low electronic noise. The TV system may be operated in an interlaced, progressive, or slow scan mode.

The digital image processor performs four basic functions: forming the image, storing the image, displaying the image, and manipulating the image.

An analog-to-digital converter converts the analog video image into digital form. The computer handles numbers in binary form. Digital information is any information represented by discrete units. Analog information is any information represented in continuous, rather than discrete, fashion.

Manipulating the window width of the digitized image changes image contrast in a manner analogous to changing film gamma in routine radiography. Changing the digital window level is analogous to changing film-screen speed. Logarithmic transformation of the digitized image ensures that equal absorber thickness changes will result in approximately equal brightness changes, whether in thin or thick body regions. Film-screen radiographs inherently contain an analogous transformation.

The major sources of noise in a digital fluoroscopic system are electronic noise and quantum noise. Higher subject contrast, increased patient exposure, large object size, and frame averaging all reduce the prominence of noise.

X-ray scatter rejection increases contrast and dose efficiency by reducing x-ray quantum requirements, and provides a final image that reflects true attenuation in thin or thick body regions more accurately. Veiling glare reduces contrast.

We have described four techniques for digital subtraction angiography:

1. Mask subtraction (most common)
2. Dual energy subtraction
3. Time interval differencing
4. Temporal filtering

Digital image processing is intended to accomplish one or more of four basic functions:

1. Image correction and preprocessing
2. Formation of viewable images appropriate to the application
3. Image enhancement
4. Image information extraction

Exciting new types of hardware are being developed. Many technical problems must be overcome before all medical images are routinely acquired and manipulated by digital computers.

REFERENCES

1. Brody, W.R., and Macovski, A.: Dual-energy digital radiography. Diagnost. Imag., *18*: 1981.
2. Foley, W.D., Lawson, T.L., Scanlon, G.T., Heeschen, R.C., and Bianca, F.: Digital radiography using a computed tomography instrument. Radiology, *133*:83, 1979.
3. Frost, M.M., Fischer, H.P., Nudelman, S., and Rohrig, H.: Digital video acquisition system for extraction of subvisual information in diagnostic medical imaging. SPIE *127*:208, 1977.
4. Kruger, R.A., Mistretta, C.A., Crummy, A.B., Sackett, J.F., Riederer, S.J., Houk, T.L., Goodsit, M.M., Shaw, C.G., and Flemming, D.: Digital K-edge subtraction radiology. Radiology, *125*:243, 1977.
5. Mistretta, C.A., and Crummy, A.B.: Digital fluoroscopy. *In* The Physical Basis of Medical Imaging. Edited by G.M. Coulam, J.J. Erickson, F.D. Rollo, and A.E. James. New York, Appleton-Century-Crofts, 1981, p. 107.
6. Mistretta, C.A., Crummy, A.B., Strother, C.M., and Sackett, J.F.: Digital Subtraction Arteriography: An Application of Computerized Fluoroscopy. Chicago, Year Book Medical Publishers, 1982.
7. Ovitt, T.: Noninvasive contrast angiography. Proceedings of a Conference on Noninvasive Cardiovascular Measurements. Palo Alto, CA, Stanford University Press, 1978.

CHAPTER

23 *Nuclear Magnetic Resonance*

Nuclear magnetic resonance (NMR) is a powerful technique for the investigation of chemical and physical properties at the molecular level. Since its inception in the mid-1940s, it has been used extensively as an analytical tool for biologic studies as well as for physical and chemical investigations. The first imaging technique is attributable to Lauterbur.[2] In 1972, at Stony Brook, New York, he was able to generate the first two-dimensional NMR image of proton density and spin lattice relaxation time. Lauterbur coined the term "zeugmatography" (from the Greek *zeugma*, meaning that which joins together) for his technique. Joined together are a radio frequency magnetic field and spatially defining magnetic field gradients that produce the NMR image. (If you try to pronounce the word, or even spell it, it is easy to see why "NMR imaging" is used more extensively.) We will use the term Nuclear Magnetic Resonance (NMR) to indicate the physics of nuclear magnetic resonance phenomena (there is also an electron spin resonance that has not yet appeared in medicine). In the next chapter, we will use the term Magnetic Resonance Imaging (MRI) to indicate the way that NMR is used to produce a medically useful image. MRI will be introduced in this chapter and expanded in the next chapter. We do not feel strongly about these terms, but note that most physics texts discuss NMR while medical texts discuss MRI. The physics is the same; it's difficult and beautiful.

Perspective

We are going to look in detail at the physics (without the mathematics) of NMR. Note that the physics of NMR is completely different from anything that has been introduced and used in the radiological sciences. This very fact is going to make NMR more difficult to understand than was, for example, CT. For CT scanning we already understood the principles of x rays, detectors, and attenuation; all we needed to learn were image reconstruction, computer capabilities, and how to read the cross-sectional images. For NMR we need to start with the very basic concepts of the nucleus and proceed from there.

So the road is clear, if somewhat rocky. We must describe nuclear structure and nuclear angular momentum, and then discuss gyroscopic behavior (beautifully illustrated by the toy top). The combination of angular momentum and gyroscopic effects will lead us to the resonance (R) part of NMR. Resonance here refers merely to the change in energy states of the nuclei caused by absorption of a specific radio frequency (RF) radiation (but not of RF radiation at any other frequency). The resonance concept is one that we have already seen in characteristic x-ray production. Finally, we will find that resonance can occur in an external magnetic field, which of course is the magnetic (M) part of NMR.

We are going to try to convince you in the next few pages that a proton in a magnetic field will **precess** about the magnetic field because it has **spin angular momentum** and a **magnetic dipole moment.** There are three terms in the last sentence that we have not introduced before in the field of radiology. Before we discuss them in relation to the hydrogen nucleus, or the proton if you prefer, we would like to explain these three terms by using the earth as an example.

We are all familiar with the day-night rotation of the earth, or at least we ought to be. We are aware that the earth rotates about an axis which we call the north-south axis (the two ends being the north pole and south pole). In discussing rotation, it is necessary to discuss that rotation relative to some axis. The day-night rotation of the earth is analogous to the "spin rotation" of the nucleus (proton). The earth also has a magnetic field, with the north pole of that magnetic field fairly close to the spin axis of the earth. We call the north pole of the earth the magnetic north pole. Because the earth has two magnetic poles (north and south) it is a magnetic dipole. The earth is a spinning magnetic dipole. As the earth spins on its axis it also precesses. Precession is change in the direction of the axis of rotation. The earth's precession will cause the axis of the earth's rotation to move so that Polaris will no longer be the North Star. In 12,000 years, the North Star will be Vega.

The proton precesses a bit faster than the earth, but it is still the **precession of the proton that allows magnetic resonance imaging.** And for this reason, it is necessary that we investigate these strange things that we call "spin angular momentum" and "magnetic dipole moment." With the earth we do not see resonance because we cannot make the earth flip on its axis. So our analogy falls down on the resonance part. For continued well being of the human race, we do not want to see resonance of the earth.

We will present a brief discussion of nuclear physics, quantum mechanics, some electromagnetic theory, and even a bit of classical mechanics. (Normally six graduate physics courses cover this material.) One of the biggest problems we will find as we go along is to represent three-dimensional entities with two-dimensional drawings; some of the drawings are more successful than others, but we have tried our best.

ANGULAR MOMENTUM

The description of NMR must be made in terms of the **angular momentum of the nucleus,** so let us introduce the concept of angular momentum now. Angular momentum is one of the sacred cows of physics because, like energy, it is a constant of motion. **Angular momentum describes the rotational motion of a body.** Unlike energy, **angular momentum has direction (it is a vector) as well as magnitude.**

The angular momentum of a body may be changed by applying a torque on the body. Torque is a force that tends to rotate the body, rather than moving it in a straight line. Sometimes the change in angular momentum increases or decreases the rotational motion of the body. Sometimes the change in angular momentum merely changes the direction of the axis about which the body is moving. Later we will see these statements illustrated by the spinning top.

There are two types of rotational motion, **orbital** and **spinning.** As you might guess, there is an angular momentum associated with each of these motions. The earth and sun are good examples. The earth is orbiting the sun in a stable (unchanging) orbit and completes an orbit in 1 year. The angular momentum caused by orbiting, the **orbital angular momentum,** depends on the earth's mass and velocity and on the radius of the orbit. In addition, the earth is rotating (spinning) about its own axis. This rotation, or spin, produces the day-night period; there is one complete rotation about its axis in 1 day. We wish to emphasize the difference between rotational angular velocity and angular momentum.

Angular velocity is simply a measure of the rate of rotation. Rotational angular momentum is the angular velocity times the moment of inertia. The moment of inertia is just a description of the mass and how the mass is distributed over the body (a disc and a wheel, though they have the same mass, will have a different moment of inertia). In nuclear physics we call the day-night rotation "**spin**," which has a **spin angular momentum** associated with it. The spin motion is an intrinsic property of the earth and does not depend on its interaction with the sun. If the sun were to disappear, the earth's orbital motion would cease; it would move off in a straight line but would continue to rotate on its axis. Of course, that would matter little to us since we would all be frozen very quickly.

Electron Angular Momentum

We will briefly discuss electron angular momentum even though electrons are not involved in NMR. The electrons in atoms have both orbital and spin rotation. The electron's orbital angular momentum depends on its relative motion to the nucleus (i.e., which shell it is in), but the electron's **spin angular momentum is an intrinsic property** that it has by existing. The total electron angular momentum is some combination of the spin and orbital angular momenta. The value of the spin angular momentum of every electron in the cosmos is the same. The detectable spin angular momentum of an electron equals the spin quantum number multiplied by a constant. The spin quantum number (usually more simply called "electron spin") is given the symbol s, and s always equals $\frac{1}{2}$. The constant is given the symbol $\hbar$ and equals h/2π (h = Planck's constant = 6.6×10^{-34} joule · seconds). The symbol $\hbar$ is pronounced "h-cross."

In Chapter 1, the value of h was given as 4.13×10^{-18} keV · sec. Both keV and joules are energy units, so that the difference in the value of h is just a matter of the size of the energy unit we are using. In

Chapter 1, h was introduced in its relation to the energy of a photon. In this chapter, h is introduced as the fundamental unit of angular momentum. It is the same constant in both of these applications. (Isn't it astounding that the same constant can be used to express both the energy of a photon and the angular momentum of a particle?)

Two interacting electrons always exist in the lowest possible energy state unless they are disturbed from the outside world. **The lowest energy state for the interaction is when the spin angular momenta are in antiparallel directions.** The direction of the spin is along the axis of rotation. Imagine a ball with a sharpened pencil through it (Fig. 23–1A). Now rotate the ball about the pencil so that the fingers of your right hand curl in the same direction the ball is rotating and your thumb points to the sharp end of the pencil. In this simple model, the pencil represents the spin angular momentum of the electron (represented by the ball. Physicists really don't like to think of electrons as spherical particles, but for this text the picture is acceptable). The point of the pencil is aimed in the direction of the spin angular momentum of the electron. With two balls representing two electrons (Fig. 23–1B), the lowest energy state exists when the pencils are parallel but pointing in opposite directions (i.e., the spin angular momenta are in antiparallel directions). This configuration of the lowest energy state between electrons is usually called **spin-pairing,** a term we will use frequently in this chapter. In the helium atom, there are two K-electrons. These two electrons are spinning in opposite directions, called by physicists **"spin-up"** and **"spin-down."** We suspect that if there were two earths in the earth's orbit, the sun would rise in the west and set in the east on the other earth. This certainly represents the concept of spin-up and spin-down. In atomic structure, electrons will nearly always pair up with one spin-up and one spin-down. **The**

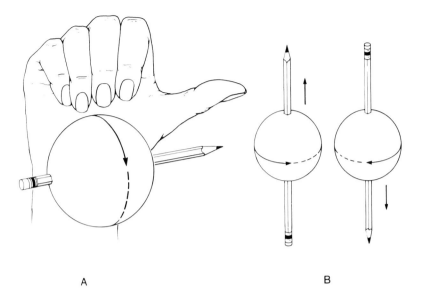

Figure 23–1 Spin angular momentum direction (A) and spin pairing (B)

net spin angular momentum for a spin-up and spin-down pair is zero.

There are a few exceptions in which the lowest energy state of a group of electrons is not produced by spin pairing. Nonspin pairing results in ferromagnetic materials, of which iron is the best-known example. The very strong magnetic properties of iron are caused by nonpairing electrons.

Nuclear Angular Momentum

The nucleus is composed of neutrons and protons. Recall from Chapter 2 that protons have one unit of positive charge (equal to the unit of negative charge on the electron) while the neutron has none. Their mass is about the same, about 1836 times larger than the electron's mass. The collection of protons and neutrons, called collectively nucleons, is confined to a very small volume called the nucleus.

It should be obvious that the nucleus is not held together by an electrostatic force (i.e., Coulomb force, which is the force between charged particles), because the like charges of the protons would be expected to repel each other. There is a nuclear force, much larger in magnitude but shorter in range than the Coulomb force,

that holds the nucleus together. (The origin of the nuclear force will not be discussed here.) The concept of the protons and neutrons maintaining their identity while in the nucleus is acceptable although not entirely correct. This concept most readily allows discussion of nuclear magnetism, and is the picture that we will use. Therefore, we have the nucleus with protons and neutrons being contained in a small volume by large nuclear forces.

One further step is required. The nucleons (both protons and neutrons) do, in some fashion, orbit about the center of the nucleus and have **orbital angular momentum.** The orbital motion of the nucleons is actually caused by the spinning motion of the entire nucleus rather than by independent orbital motion of the individual particles within the nucleus. An analogy is Mount Everest orbiting about the earth's axis of rotation. **In addition, both protons and neutrons have the same spin and therefore the same spin angular momentum as does the electron.**

Furthermore, there are energy levels for the nucleons very similar to the electronic levels (shells) in atomic structure. By now it comes as no surprise that the protons will fill these energy states by pairing them-selves with spin-up and spin-down, or that the neutrons do the same. A proton will not pair with a neutron. This pairing of protons or neutrons produces cancellation of their spin angular momentum. The nu-cleus, however, does have angular momen-tum. **The angular momentum of the nu-cleus is determined by the spin of the unpaired neutrons and protons and by the orbital angular momentum of the neu-trons and protons.** Something very inter-esting happens here. The combination of all these functions produces a very simple number for the value of the nuclear spin, designated by the letter I. The maximum detectable nuclear angular momentum is $I\hbar$. The letter I is called the nuclear spin (analogous to s, the electron spin).

Maximum detectable nuclear angular momentum = $I\hbar$

I = nuclear spin

$\hbar$ = h/2π (h is Planck's constant)

The nuclear spin, I, is always either zero, multiples of $\frac{1}{2}$, or whole numbers. (Note that this is a bit more complicated than with electrons, for which s is always $\frac{1}{2}$.) **Thus there are only three kinds of nuclei as far as the spin is concerned:**

1. If the mass number A (protons plus neutrons) is odd, the nuclear spin, I, is a multiple of $\frac{1}{2}$ ($\frac{1}{2}$, $\frac{3}{2}$, $\frac{5}{2}$, $\frac{7}{2}$)
2. If the mass number A and the atomic number Z (protons) are both even, I is 0
3. If the mass number A is even but the atomic number Z is odd, I is a whole number (1, 2, 3, 4, or 5)

There are no other possibilities. Al-though the concepts concerning the nu-clear angular momentum are difficult, the nuclear spin I that gives the value of the nuclear angular momentum is rather an uncomplicated number.

Why do we include angular momentum? Angular momentum is a physical quantity that describes the rotational motion of a body (i.e., a spinning nucleus has angular momentum). Why is angular momentum of the nucleus important to NMR? Without angular momentum, a nucleus would not precess when placed in a magnetic field. Without precession there would be no res-onance, and the R part of NMR would not exist. We hope this introduction to angular momentum will help you develop a better understanding of nuclear resonance.

Up to this point we have discussed the fact that the charged nucleus is spinning and has angular momentum. Now we must investigate the magnetic effects caused by this spin. We will introduce the subject by using illustrations involving electrons flow-ing in a wire.

MAGNETISM AND THE MAGNETIC DIPOLE MOMENT

Magnetic Field Due To Electron Flow

To see how magnetism occurs in the nu-cleus, and also in the orbiting electrons, we need to retreat from the world of tiny par-ticles to the more conventional world. Con-sider electrons flowing through a wire. The electron flow will produce a magnetic field (H) surrounding the wire. The direction of the magnetic field can be determined by a left-hand rule (Fig. 23–2A). With the thumb of the left hand pointing in the di-rection of electron flow, the fingers will curl in the direction of the magnetic field. (Note that most physics tests define current in terms of positive charge motion. For such a definition, all the left-hand rules become right-hand rules.) When the wire is formed into a circle, the same electron flow will produce a magnetic field upward inside the circle and a field downward outside the cir-cle (Fig. 23–2B). The magnetic field about the loop of wire looks very much like the field surrounding the short bar magnet of Figure 23–3A. Note that Figure 23–3B is the same as Figure 23–2B.

Of more immediate interest is what hap-pens if both the bar magnet and the wire loop with electrons flowing through it are placed in another (or external) uniform

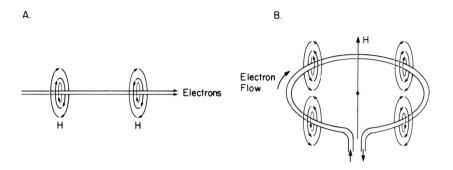

Figure 23–2   Magnetic field (H) caused by electron flow

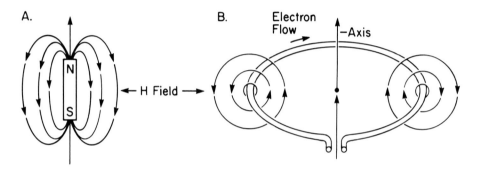

Figure 23–3   Magnetic field (H) comparison between bar magnet (*A*) and loop of electron flow (*B*)

magnetic field. In Figure 23–4*A*, the bar magnet will have equal but opposite forces on the ends (actually, nearly the ends where the magnetic poles are located), and therefore will have no net force (a net force would cause the bar to move up or down). Each pole has a torque, however, that will cause a rotation about the center of the bar.

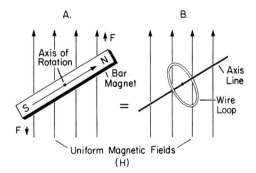

Figure 23–4   Effect of external field on bar magnet (*A*) and wire loop (*B*)

The rotation will be such that the arrow from the S pole to the N pole will align with the arrows representing the magnetic field. We say that the magnet aligns itself along the field. As the magnet moves to align along the field, the torque decreases to zero when the bar is parallel to the field. We have just described a magnetic compass.

The loop with electrons flowing in it will also have a net torque and will rotate to align the loop itself perpendicular to the field. The axis line is defined as a line that is perpendicular to the plane of the loop and that passes through the center of the loop (Fig. 23–4*B*). This axis is analogous to the axle of the wheel. When the loop is aligned perpendicular to the magnetic field, the axis line is along the field, just like the bar magnet in Figure 23–4*A*. The loop alignment in a field is the principle on which voltmeters and ammeters operate.

Magnetic Dipole Moment

The **magnetic dipole moment (MDM)** is a property of a magnet or of a loop of wire with electrons flowing through it. **The reason for introducing the MDM is that the nuclei we use in NMR also have a magnetic dipole moment.** If we understand the effects of the MDM for these large bar magnets, we can more easily understand the effects for the smaller, invisible nuclei.

Perhaps the best way to describe the MDM is to say that **it is that property or characteristic of a magnet (or wire loop) that indicates how quickly the magnet will align itself along a magnetic field.** For a bar magnet, the stronger the magnet, the more quickly it will align with the field. In addition, the length of the magnet is significant: long magnets will align faster than short ones, all else being equal. For the loop of wire, the larger the electron flow, the more quickly the loop will align itself. In addition, larger area loops will align faster than smaller loops for a given electron flow.

If we were clever, we would define the MDM so that the direction or orientation of the MDM would give us the orientation of the object possessing the MDM. It seems obvious that the MDM for a bar magnet would give the orientation of the bar magnet if the MDM were along the length of the magnet. For the loop, however, we cannot draw a single line along the entire loop, but we can draw a line through the center of the loop. If that line were perpendicular to the loop, that line would give the orientation of the loop. In Figure 23–4A the MDM for the bar is a line going through the S and N poles and pointing out the N end. For the loop the axis line becomes the line of the MDM. The MDM, however, can be along the axis in one of two directions. The proper direction is obtained by another left-hand rule: curl the fingers of your left hand in the directions of electron flow, and your thumb will give the direction of the MDM. Test yourself on Figure 23–3A.

Magnetic Dipole Moments for Rotating Charges.

Please note that a single electron orbiting about the nucleus constitutes an electron flowing in a circle (loop); it has a MDM. If the electron orbit is the smallest possible orbit (K shell), the MDM is called a **Bohr magneton.** For an electron in a higher shell (e.g., L, M), the MDM is the orbit number (L = 2, M = 3, etc.) multiplied by the Bohr magneton.

In addition to its orbital rotation, the electron has intrinsic spin. This spin rotation also represents a rotating charge. **The electron has a MDM of one Bohr magneton associated with the spin (this is in addition to the Bohr magneton associated with orbital motion).** We will give the value of the Bohr magneton (μ_B) in two systems of units:

$$\mu_B = 9.27 \times 10^{-24} \text{ J/tesla (SI units)}$$
$$\mu_B = 9.27 \times 10^{-21} \text{ erg/gauss (cgs units)}$$

We include cgs units because NMR magnets are sometimes described in terms of gauss rather than tesla. Remember that a joule or an erg is a unit of energy, and tesla and gauss are units of magnetic field strength (really units of magnetic induction; see "Addendum" for a discussion of H and B at the end of this chapter.) One tesla = 10^4 gauss, and 1 J = 10^7 erg. Refer to Chapter 1 for a brief description of SI units.

If spinning electrons represent a rotating charge, a nucleus must also be a rotating charge. The differences between a proton and electron are the sign of their charge and their mass. In deriving the Bohr magneton, the electron mass shows up in the equation (not shown here). If we merely replace that electron mass by the proton mass, we have the nuclear magneton. The nuclear magneton is designated by the symbol μ_N.

Let us consider the meaning of this term "magneton." **A magneton is a unit used to express the value of the magnetic dipole moment.** There are two units (these units are related in a manner analogous to inches and feet):

1. The Bohr magneton is used to express the MDM of electrons.
2. The nuclear magneton is used to express the MDM of nuclei.

The MDM of nuclei are not calculated, but instead are measured for each individual nucleus. These values are then expressed as a certain number of nuclear magnetons. Similarly, the MDM of the proton or neutron is measured in the laboratory and found to be different from the nuclear magneton. Even more strange, the MDM of the nuclei cannot be calculated by adding up the MDM of all the protons and neutrons in the nucleus. What all this teaches us is that nuclei, protons, and neutrons are not the simple structures we once thought them to be. To be complete, we will list the values of the nuclear magneton (μ_N), the MDM for the proton (μ_p), and the MDM for the neutron (μ_n):

$$\mu_N = 5.05 \times 10^{-27} \text{ J/tesla}$$
$$\mu_p = 2.7928\mu_N$$
$$\mu_n = -1.9128\mu_N$$

where μ_N is the nuclear magneton, μ_p is the proton MDM, and μ_n is the neutron MDM.

For spinning particles, the MDM is always along the spin axis. (We described the spin axis as the pencil passing through the center of a ball, Figure 23–1.) A positive value indicates that the MDM and the angular momentum (remember the ball, pencil, and right-hand rule) are in the same direction. A negative value indicates that the MDM points in the opposite direction from the angular momentum.

Magnetic Dipole Moments of Nuclei. The MDM of nuclei depend on the number and arrangement of the protons and neutrons. We have already seen, though, that the protons and neutrons produce spin-up-spin-down pairs in the nucleus. The nuclear MDM is not just a simple addition of the MDM of the nucleons. In fact, the MDM of nuclei have been measured. We

can note that if the nucleus has no spin (I = 0; i.e., it has no angular momentum), it will have no MDM. **Nuclei with no MDM will not be detectable by NMR.** Therefore, all nuclei whose mass number A (protons plus neutrons) and atomic number Z (protons) are both even cannot be used in NMR studies. Table 23–1 presents a number of elements that are of interest in medical NMR.

Alignment of Nuclear MDM in a Magnetic Field

We have tried to show you and to explain why some nuclei have spin angular momentum and a magnetic dipole moment. **The term MDM can be translated,** if you are so inclined, **to "tiny magnet."** MDM might be considered as that property of a nucleus that causes it to behave like a tiny magnet (if the tiny magnet is spinning around its north pole-south pole axis, it will possess spin angular momentum). When placed in a magnetic field, the tiny magnets will try to align along the field. Unfortunately, things in the tiny world don't always behave as we anticipate. In the present example, **the tiny magnet is allowed only a limited amount of alignment in the field.** Here we have a quantum rule very similar to the electronic condition in atomic structure that electrons can only be in certain energy shells.

We must digress a moment and mention quantum physics. Quantum physics dictates certain rules that govern the behavior of objects the size of electrons and nuclei. Large objects, such as our examples of balls, bar magnets, and wire loops, are not limited by these quantum rules, which is why the analogy between magnets and spinning nuclei is not always precise. For example, magnets are able to align themselves exactly with a magnetic field, but spinning nuclei are limited in their alignment (Fig. 23–5). The possible alignments (orientations) are shown for nuclei with positive MDM and I = ½ (Fig. 23–5A) and I = 1 (Fig. 23–5B). (We really don't think

Table 23–1.   Table of Nuclear Properties

ISOTOPE	MDM × NUCLEAR MAGNETON	SPIN, I	GYROMAGNETIC RATIO (× 10⁷ Hz/T)	LARMOR FREQUENCY FOR H = 1 T MHz/T
n	− 1.91	$\frac{1}{2}$	− 18.3	29.16
¹H(p)	2.79	$\frac{1}{2}$	26.8	42.58
²H	0.85	1	4.1	6.53
¹³C	0.70	$\frac{1}{2}$	6.7	10.70
¹⁴N	0.40	1	1.9	3.08
¹⁹F	2.63	$\frac{1}{2}$	25.3	40.05
²³Na	2.21	$\frac{3}{2}$	7.1	11.26
²⁷Al	3.64	$\frac{5}{2}$	7.0	11.09
³¹P	1.13	$\frac{1}{2}$	10.8	17.24

Example: MDM of ¹H = 2.79 × 5.05 × 10⁻²⁷ joules/tesla
Gyromagnetic Ratio of ¹H = 26.8 × 10⁷ Hz/T

that medical NMR will be applicable to nuclei with higher values of I, with the possible exception of Na.) Refer to Table 23–1 for some nuclei that might have medical applications.

The nucleus with I = ½ can spin in either of the two orientations shown in Figure 23–5A, but no others. The nucleus cannot come into exact alignment with the magnetic field. The bar magnet and wire loop would sooner or later come into exact alignment, because they are too large to be dominated by the quantum rules. Figure 23–5B shows that there are three orientations for the I = 1 nuclei.

Suppose we have a large number of nuclei of spin I = ½. With no applied magnetic field H, the nuclei (and MDM) would be in random orientation in all directions. By applying a magnetic field, all the MDM would move into the two orientations, with some in one and some in the other (Fig. 23–5A). As might be expected, the two orientations have two different energy values. The up orientation has the lower energy, and the down orientation a slightly higher one. The number of nuclei that move into the lower energy state (up orientation) is only a little greater than those that move into the higher energy state (down orientation). The ratio of the numbers is determined by the difference in energy between the two states, the magnetic field, and the temperature. For instance, in a population of 2,000,000 nuclei, 1,000,000 + 1 might go to the lower energy state, while 1,000,000 − 1 might go to the higher state. This isn't very much difference. For a sample with about 10²³ nuclei, the difference in the population of the two states would be about 10¹⁷ nuclei. The NMR signal is produced only by the 10¹⁷ excess nuclei. **Therefore, of all the nuclei, very few participate in the NMR signal.**

When the little magnets reach the orientation allowed by the quantum rule, the magnetic field is still trying to move them into exact alignment. This means that there is still some torque on each of the little magnets. In the next section, we will see that this remaining torque is responsible for the MDMs precessing about the magnetic field.

Why do we include a discussion of magnetic dipole moment? First, it gets us thinking of certain nuclei as tiny (nuclear-sized)

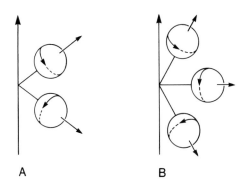

Figure 23–5   Nuclear alignment in a magnetic field

magnets. Second, we can see how these tiny magnets align themselves in an external magnetic field. Now that we understand this, we have the M part of NMR.

Angular Momentum and Precession

We have just described a nucleus with spin angular momentum and a MDM in a magnetic field. The nucleus still has some torque on it. In this section we need to describe the effect of this torque on the motion of the nucleus. We feel, and most other experts agree, that the best way to visualize the motion of the nucleus is to describe the motion of a spinning top in a gravitational field. Once again we are trying to use a large object to illustrate a quantum-sized object. Fortunately, in this example, we will not find a discrepancy in the analogy because of the size of the two objects. One of the most interesting motions in the world is the motion of a tilted spinning top. (We should really be talking about spinning jacks because one of us (JED) could never wrap a string around a top, throw it down, and get it to spin. His always just bounced off the floor. But he could really spin those jacks with his thumb and finger.) A top that is spinning at some tilted angle (we normally define tilted as being at some angle to up and down that we automatically define as the direction of gravity) will continue to spin with its axis at the tilted angle, but the axis of rotation will move in a circular path about the direction of gravity. The motion of the axis about the direction of gravity is called **precession.**

The precessional path of the center of the top is shown in Figure 23–6A as the circle at the apex of the top. Of course, this point (apex) is just exactly where the spin axis (L) emerges from the spinning top. (In physics texts the letter L is used to represent angular momentum, so we use it here.) Remember, the spin angular momentum is also along the spin axis and, in this case, will point up from the top (along L). We know that a toy top will slow down and that the precessional circle will get larger until

the side of the top touches the floor. (That's when it goes rolling across the floor.) The slowing down is a result of frictional forces at the point of rotation (and even frictional forces between the top and air molecules). Two assumptions have been made that are rather subtle: 1) there is sufficient frictional force to hold the tip of the top in place; and 2) the top is symmetric about the spin axis. If the first were not true, we would see something other than a top spinning on a fixed tip. More than likely, the tip would be moving in a circle on the floor. If the second assumption were not true, there would at least be wobble in the precessional motion and, very likely, no spinning about a single axis. We would really hate to try to spin a top with chewing gum on its side.

We are tempted to explain why a spinning top precesses but a nonspinning top falls off its tip. As a matter of fact we tried, but got bogged down in such matters as perpendicular vectors called torque, weight, angular momentum, and the change in angular momentum. Therefore, we are going to assume that you believe that a spinning top will precess when in a gravitational field, and that a nonspinning top will fall over onto its side.

Larmor Frequency

When we wrote this section we used H instead of B to indicate the magnetic field. Please feel free to substitute B for H if you wish. Most other MRI texts use B, while many physics texts use H.

All we need for precessional motion is a **symmetric body with spin angular momentum and some torque that is perpendicular to the angular momentum.** We have just that situation with a spinning nucleus in a magnetic field (Fig. 23–6B). Furthermore, there is no frictional force, so the nucleus will not slow down and fall sideways. The frequency of precession, called the **Larmor frequency,** is of fundamental importance in NMR. You will recall from Chapter 1 that the Greek letter ν (nu) was used as the symbol for frequency. Sim-

A.

B.

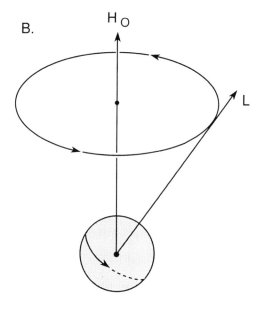

Figure 23–6   Precession

ilarly, ν_L is the symbol for the Larmor frequency (sometimes the letter f is used for frequency). The Larmor frequency depends on the magnetic field and the gyromagnetic ratio, γ (gamma). This relationship is expressed by

$$\nu_L = \gamma H/2\pi$$
ν_L = Larmor frequency
γ = gyromagnetic ratio
H = magnetic field

(We sometimes see the Larmor frequency written as $\omega = \gamma B$. Here omega, ω, is really the angular velocity, and $\omega = 2\pi\nu$.) We assume that this nucleus is in the presence of other nuclei so that we can use the magnetic induction, B, rather than the magnetic field, H. If the nucleus were in the region by itself, we would properly use the magnetic field (H), since there would be no induction. And, as we say in the addendum at the end of this chapter, in the body B and H are so nearly the same that the terms can be used as synonyms (even though such use is not correct in terms of the physics of the situation).

The gyromagnetic ratio (also called the magnetogyric ratio) is the ratio of the

MDM to the nuclear spin angular momentum I$\hbar$. Therefore,

$$\gamma = \frac{\mu}{I\hbar}$$
γ = gyromagnetic ratio
μ = MDM
I = nuclear spin
$\hbar$ = h/2π, h is Planck's constant
h = 6.6 $\times$ 10^{-34} joules $\cdot$ sec

The values of γ are included in Table 23–1. The gyromagnetic ratio is a unique value for each type of nucleus. For example, the γ values of the hydrogen isotopes (^{1}H, ^{2}H, ^{3}H) are all different from each other, and also different from the γ values of helium isotopes.

Now we have gotten where we promised we were going. The mysterious spin angular momentum and magnetic dipole moment have formed a ratio called the gyromagnetic ratio. The gyromagnetic ratio and magnetic induction (from our imaging magnet) produce the Larmor frequency of precession. Hydrogen nuclei (protons) precessing at their Larmor frequency form the basis of clinical magnetic resonance imaging (proton imaging).

The defining equation for the Larmor

frequency shows that **each type of nucleus will precess at a unique frequency in a given magnetic field.** Two different nuclei will precess at two different frequencies in a given field. Therefore, **the Larmor precession is a process that, for a given field, can distinguish between nuclear types.** We also need to note that a given type of nucleus will precess at different frequencies when in different magnetic fields.

For example, a hydrogen nucleus (proton) has a gyromagnetic ratio of 26.8×10^7 1/tesla-sec (Hz/tesla). In a magnetic field of strength 0.2 tesla, the proton will precess at a frequency of about 8.5 MHz (8,500,000 cycles/sec). Calculate this yourself using the equation $\nu_L = \gamma H/2\pi$, being careful to keep track of units and powers of 10. Similar calculations show that the Larmor frequency for the proton in a 1-tesla field is about 42.58 MHz, as listed in Table 23–1. We can find the resonance (Larmor) frequency of any of the nuclei listed in Table 23–1 in any magnetic field strength simply by multiplying the field strength (in tesla) by the listed value of the Larmor frequency in a 1-tesla field (last column of Table 23–1). Remember the conversion from gauss to tesla: 1 tesla = 10^4 gauss. Tesla and gauss are units of magnetic induction, but we are are going to use the term "magnetic field."

Of course, the magnetic field need not vary much over a group of identical nuclei for those nuclei to precess at detectably different frequencies. **This concept of identical nuclei in slightly different magnetic fields is the concept on which a great deal of NMR work is based.** The chemical shifts, measured so extensively in chemistry laboratories, are just instances of identical nuclei finding themselves in slightly different fields because of local environmental perturbations on the applied magnetic field. Of more interest in NMR imaging is the purposely varied field to help establish different Larmor frequencies for a given nuclear type (usually hydrogen)

across the object to be imaged. We will return to this imaging method later.

Figure 23–6B shows a nucleus (I = ½) spinning in the spin-up orientation. Note that in the spin-down orientation (not shown), the nucleus, as far as the magnetic field is concerned, has reversed its direction of spin. (Note the direction of the arrows in Figure 23–5A and B.) The torque on both spin-up and spin-down nuclei, however, is the same. Therefore, both spin-up and spin-down nuclei precess in the same direction.

Energy States for Nuclear Spin Systems

We feel compelled to return to a discussion of the energy states associated with the spinning nucleus in a magnetic field. We have already mentioned that there are two energy states for an I = ½ nucleus that finds itself in a magnetic field. Remember that the spin-up orientation has the lower energy.

When this chapter was originally written, we included a calculation for the energy of a bar magnet when placed in a magnetic field. That calculation is not really difficult, but we feel it would be sufficient for our purpose to give the results. When a bar magnet is aligned with a field, as in Figure 23–4A, its energy (potential energy) is just $E = -\mu H$ (μ = MDM), while in the reversed orientation its energy is $E = \mu H$. The difference in energy between these two orientations is $2\mu H$. This is also true for the loop.

The energy of a nucleus may also be written in exactly the same way. Figure 23–7A shows the two energy states for the I = ½ nucleus. Remember that spin angular momentum has direction as well as magnitude. We use the direction of spin to indicate whether a nucleus is in the spin-up or spin-down state. In this example, I = ½ indicates spin-up and I = −½ indicates spin-down. Note that the spin-up (I = ½) state is lower in energy than the spin-down (I = −½) state. The energy (E) of these states ($E_1 = \mu H$ and $E_2 = -\mu H$) may be

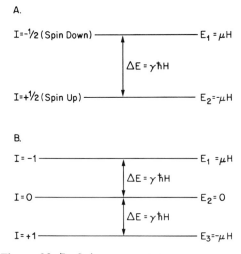

Figure 23–7 Spin energy states

expressed in terms of the gyromagnetic ratio (γ). Because the equation defining the gyromagnetic ratio contains the terms I and μ (MDM), such an expression can be obtained with a little simple algebra (i.e., $E_1 = \mu H = \gamma I \hbar H$). With this substitution, the difference in the spin-up and spin-down energy states, as illustrated in Figure 23–7A, may be expressed as $\Delta E = \gamma hH$. $E_1 - E_2 = \gamma I_1 \hbar H - \gamma I_2 \hbar H$. For E_1, $I_1 = +\frac{1}{2}$; for E_2, $I_2 = -\frac{1}{2}$. Substituting these values for I, we obtain $E_1 - E_2 = \frac{1}{2}\gamma\hbar H - (-\frac{1}{2})\gamma\hbar H = \gamma\hbar H$.

Now let us use this expression to describe how Larmor frequency relates to the frequency of the transition radiation between these two spin states. Transition radiation refers to the energy absorbed by the nucleus when it flips from the lower energy state to the higher energy state. This is analogous to the photoelectric effect when electrons absorb energy and go from a lower energy level to a higher energy level (e.g., from the K shell to the L shell).

There is a reason for all this. If the nucleus flips from the lower energy state to the higher, it must absorb an amount of energy equal to the energy difference. We have certainly seen this concept before. Remember that the production of characteristic x rays looks like this. Consequently, if

a nucleus flips from the lower to the higher energy state, it must absorb this amount of energy from somewhere. When it returns to the lower energy state, it must give up this amount of energy. (We will see later that the emission of a photon is not the principal means of energy transfer when the nucleus returns from the higher to the lower energy state.) For x rays the emission was electromagnetic radiation that we called a photon. For nuclear transitions the energy is transformed to the lattice (the material structure surrounding the nucleus). This type of transition is called a radiationless transition, and usually heats the surrounding material (lattice).

In Chapter 1, we showed that the energy of a photon was given by $E = h\nu$ (Planck's constant multiplied by frequency). Because we have the energy difference between the two nuclear spin states ($E = \gamma\hbar H$), we can find the frequency of the photon absorbed to produce a spin state transition. That is, the energy ($h\nu$) of the photon producing the spin state transition must be exactly equal to the difference in energy ($\gamma\hbar H$) between the two spin states. Let us write this statement in the form of an equation, and then solve the equation for the frequency (ν) of the photon producing the transition:

$$E = h\nu = \gamma\hbar H$$
$$\nu = \gamma H/2\pi$$

E = energy of photon absorbed
ν = frequency of the photon
γ = gyromagnetic ratio
H = magnetic field
h = Planck's constant ($\hbar = h/2\pi$)

This equation for the frequency of the photon producing the transition should look familiar. It is exactly the same as the Larmor frequency of precession of nuclei about a magnetic field. **The Larmor frequency of precession is exactly equal to the frequency of radiation absorbed in a transition from one spin state to another.** In the literature, statements about the radiation of transition are referred to as radiation at the Larmor frequency. Now we know why that is acceptable.

As an example, the Larmor frequency of a hydrogen nucleus (proton) in a 1-tesla (10^4-gauss) magnetic field is about 42 MHz (42,000,000 Hz). Let us compare this to more familiar electromagnetic radiation: the frequency of 300-nm (3000 A) visible light is about 10^9 MHz, and a 124-keV x-ray photon has about 10^{13} MHz. Inspection of the electromagnetic radiation frequency spectrum reveals that 42 MHz falls within the radio frequency range. All NMR studies are performed in the radio frequency range (about 1 KHz to 100 MHz).

For interest, the energy states of an I = 1 nucleus are shown in Figure 23–7B. But be careful; there are three, one of which is zero. Only the two transitions shown are possible. The transition from the upper state (I = −1) to the lower state (I = 1) is impossible; it is one of those "forbidden" transitions from quantum physics. Note that the allowed transitions give an energy difference just like the I = ½ nucleus. Thus, we are back to Larmor frequency for the absorbed radiation.

The basis of NMR is to induce transitions between these energy states by the absorption and transfer of energy. Whatever description is used to picture NMR, here or elsewhere, the whole concept basically deals with the transitions between these spin states. NMR is nothing more than the flooding of a sample with radiation at the Larmor frequency, and then measuring the Larmor frequency signal coming from the sample.

Earlier we said that for a sample with some 10^{23} nuclei, only about 10^{17} nuclei would be involved in the NMR process (these are the excess nuclei). Only 10^{17} nuclei! We cannot even image 10^7, let alone 10^{17}, nuclei. It is impossible to visualize what these nuclei are doing. Normally, then, we replace all these individual nuclei having individual MDMs by a single vector termed the **"magnetization,"** and give it the symbol M. We will discuss magnetization in the next section.

NMR PARAMETERS

Magnetization Vector

Recall that, in a normal-sized sample, there is an extremely large number of nuclei and, in a magnetic field, only a little more than half are in the spin-up state precessing at the Larmor frequency. A little less than half are in the spin-down state, also precessing at the Larmor frequency. Remember that each nucleus has a MDM and an angular momentum that are parallel, and that each nucleus looks like a tiny magnet. If we add up the MDM of all these tiny magnets, the resulting sum is the magnetization, M, of the sample. Because the nuclei have a spin angular momentum parallel to the MDM, there will also be a net angular momentum parallel to M.

In Figure 23–8A, we attempt to show several of the large number of nuclei (these are identical nuclei), some spin-up, some spin-down. Each MDM can be considered

Figure 23–8 Effects of nuclear spins in an external field, H to have one part along the field and one part perpendicular to the field. (Because the MDM is a vector, it has components parallel and perpendicular to the field.) This is illustrated in Figure 23–8B, in which μ_1 is the component of the MDM perpendicular to the magnetic field, H, and μ_2 is the component of the MDM parallel to the magnetic field. There are similar components of the spin angular momentum. All the MDM components along the field for the spin-up nuclei add together and give a net result that is pointing up. The sum of components along the field for the spin-down nuclei also add together, but give a net result that is pointing down. When these two results are added together, there is a net result that points in the direction of the field because there are more nuclei in the spin-up than in the spin-down state. Effectively, then, **the excess nuclei in the lower energy state give a net MDM component along the field.**

Figure 23–8C attempts to show the top view of Figure 23–8A. What we see are the components (the μ_1 components of Fig. 23–8B) of the MDMs that are perpendicular to the field. Even with this small sample of nuclei, the tendency for these components to add up to zero (or to average to zero) may be seen. **For all nuclei, the perpendicular components of the MDM for both spin-up and spin-down add up to zero.**

We can replace all the nuclei in the sample by the single vector that is the sum of the components of the MDM for the excess nuclei. This vector is called the magnetization, M, for the sample. **The magnetization behaves like a magnet that has a spin angular momentum.** That is, the magnetization can precess about a magnetic field if the magnetization and the magnetic field are not parallel.

Precession requires spin angular momentum and a torque perpendicular to the angular momentum. Because the magnetization, M, as shown in Figure 23–8B, is exactly parallel to the magnetic field, H, no

torque will be acting on M. This means that M cannot precess about H (a difficult concept, because the individual nuclei that make up M continue to precess). Without precession we are unable to detect any spin angular momentum of the magnetization vector, even though such spin angular momentum is present. If M were to be displaced from H, M would precess about H because there would now be a torque on M. In the next sections we will see 1) how to displace M from H and 2) how to observe and measure the resulting precessional motion of M.

RF Magnetic Field (Radio Frequency)

We would like to displace M from its direction along H and watch M as it tries to go back to its alignment along H. In the next few paragraphs we will discuss the method by which M can be displaced. It is not as easy as it sounds to make M move away from H because, as soon as M is displaced, it starts precessing about whatever magnetic field is present. If, by some means, M were displaced a bit from the H direction, M would precess about the H field with the Larmor frequency (Fig. 23–9A).

One way to displace M would be to apply a second magnetic field, H_1, but this second field H_1 would have to have a particular characteristic. Suppose H_1 were a constant (static) field. All we would see is the little dipole magnets realigning themselves and beginning to precess about the net magnetic field, which would become the vector sum of H and H_1. Of course, H_1 could be turned on and off quickly, in which case we would get a small displacement of M and it would then precess about H and gradually realign itself along H (Fig. 23–9A).

Or, we could have H_1 rotating about H at the Larmor frequency. In this case H_1 would follow M in the precessional motion about H. At this point most authors introduce a rotating coordinate system to discuss the motion of M and H_1. We can il-

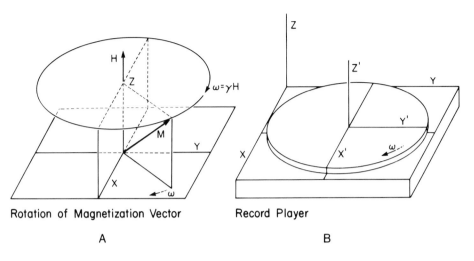

Figure 23-9 Rotating coordinate system compared to a record player

lustrate a rotating coordinate system by using mathematics, a merry-go-round, or a record player. We feel a record player would be best to use (because we can't draw horses).

Suppose we draw two perpendicular lines on a record and set the record on the turntable. Now our coordinate system would be the two perpendicular lines (x^1 and y^1) on the record, and the vertical line through the spindle (z^1) of the turntable (Fig. 23-9B). When the record player is turned on, x^1 and y^1 will rotate with the turntable at the angular velocity ω (instead of the familiar rate of 33⅓ rpm, we are talking about a few million revolutions per second). Note that z^1 is not rotating. Compare that to the fixed coordinate system (x, y, z) of Figure 23-9B. Of course, z and z^1 do not change relative to each other, but x^1 and y^1 move relative to x and y. If we were to place z^1 along the H field and rotate the player at the Larmor frequency, we would have a system that would rotate with the same frequency as M, if M were slightly displaced from H so that it could precess. **Therefore, M would not seem to be moving in the $x^1y^1z^1$ system while it precessed about H.**

The situation with the merry-go-round analogy would be the same. A person standing on the ground (a fixed coordinate system such as xyz in Figure 23-9B) would see the little horses moving around and around. When he stepped onto the merry-go-round (a rotating coordinate system such as $x^1y^1x^1$ in Fig. 23-9B), the little horses wouldn't seem to be moving (of course, the rest of the world would be whizzing by).

In NMR studies, H is normally much larger than H_1, so the precession of M about H is much faster than M about H_1. Remember that the Larmor frequency will be greater in a larger magnetic field for identical nuclei: $\nu_L = \gamma H/2\pi$. Figure 23-10A attempts to show the spiral path that the tip of M will follow when both H and the rotating H_1 are present. This drawing represents the path seen from a fixed coordinate system, which represents the laboratory and the observer. The number of spiral loops is determined by the sizes of H and H_1.

The reason for choosing this particular rotating coordinate system (rotating at the Larmor frequency) is that the effective magnetic field appears to be zero (H appears to disappear) prior to applying the H_1 field. When we apply the H_1 field, it is the only magnetic field that the magnetization vector sees. This is why the mag-

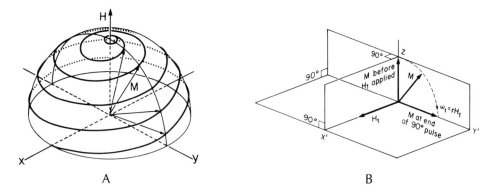

Figure 23–10 Beehive path of the magnetization vector, M, during a 90° pulse *(A)* and path of M during a 90° pulse as seen from a rotating coordinate system *(B)*

netization vector, M, will leave its original direction (along H) and precess about the applied H_1 field. In any other rotating coordinate system (with H_1 rotating with it), part of the original field H would still be affecting M. At most, what we would see would be a perturbation of the magnetization precession about the H field. More than likely, M would continue to be along H and we would see nothing new because of the H_1 field.

We had better reconsider the last paragraph. We said that if we rotate around a magnetic field, H, at the Larmor frequency of a precessing nucleus, the magnetic field will disappear as far as the precessing nucleus is concerned. That sounds like magic and, indeed, physicists use the term "fictitious forces" when discussing rotating coordinates (and you thought we weren't going to get into science fiction).

Consider the analogy of a boy whirling a ball on a string. If you are standing near the boy, you will see the ball going around and around, faster if the boy applies more force on the string (this force is normally called tension) and slower with less tension. The tension in the string is analogous to the magnetic field, H. Now suppose you can make yourself very small and that you jump onto the ball (and have enough frictional, not fictitious, force so that you will stick to the ball). An amazing thing happens; from your new vantage point (your

coordinate system) the ball is no longer moving. Because it was the force that the boy applied to the string that caused the ball to move in a circle as you looked at it from the ground, your new assumption must be that the boy is no longer applying any force to the string. Of course, your friends on the ground still see the ball whirling around (and you now see them whirling around while you stand still). By whirling around at the same speed as the ball, therefore, you no longer detect a force that makes the ball whirl. You really detect no net force, but because the boy is still applying tension by the string, some new force must have arisen to counteract that tension. That new force is the fictitious force, and appears only because you are on a rotating coordinate system. We may use the term "fictitious," but you can certainly feel these forces. Jump on a merry-go-round and right away you are trying to slide away from the center; if you don't hold on you will indeed fall off.

We do the same sort of thing by standing on the earth. The earth is moving rapidly, but we have the sensation of standing still. This allows us to extend the analogy a bit further. Standing on the moving and rotating earth, we do not detect the force causing the motion. If another force comes along (such as a strong wind), however, we respond to the new force. Similarly, in our coordinate system rotating at the Larmor frequency, the nuclear magnets no longer detect the H field, so they are able to respond to the new H_1 field as if it were the only one present. Note that if the speed of rotation is not at the exact Larmor frequency of the nucleus in question, some of the H field will still be detected by its interaction with the magnetization vector, M.

You might think of this detectable part of H in terms of chasing the whirling ball in a tiny airplane. If your speed is exactly the same as that of the ball (i.e., if your airplane is moving in a circle with the ball), the ball will appear stationary relative to you. If your circular speed is a little slower or faster than the ball, however, the ball will appear to move ahead or behind you. This motion of the ball would be your detection of a portion of the original tension (force) applied to the string. Now back to the magnetization vector.

Because M cannot detect H in a coordinate system rotating at the Larmor frequency, M is free to interact with H_1 as if H_1 were the only magnetic field present. If H_1 is also rotating at the Larmor frequency, H_1 will appear to be a constant (unchanging) magnetic field. If H_1 is applied so that it is perpendicular to H, then Figure 23–10B represents the precession motion of M about H_1. This precession motion is much easier to see than is the spiral motion of M as seen in the fixed laboratory system. We must remember, though, that the coordinate system $x^1y^1z^1$ and the entire Figure 23–10B is rotating about z^1 at the Larmor frequency $\nu_L = \gamma H/2\pi$. All that said and done, it is still within the fixed coordinate system that we actually observe the motion of M. Indeed, we will see M move in the "beehive" motion shown in Figure 23–10A.

The spiral path concept of M moving from being parallel to H to being perpendicular to H is hard to visualize, so we would like to give an analogy before continuing. Consider a jeep perched on top of a steep mountain. Obviously, you cannot drive the jeep straight down the side of the mountain. Rather, the jeep must circle down and around and around the mountain in a gradual descent. Similarly, M leaves H and moves along a spiral path until it reaches the plane perpendicular to H and parallel to H_1 (for 90° motion, at least). A little later we will allow M to return parallel to H; it will move "up the mountain" in a spiral path, but the path will be a different spiral from that used on the downhill trip (see Fig. 23–11A).

When M finally reaches the xy plane, we have an interesting condition. There is no magnetization component along the z axis, which means that the spin-up-spin-down states are equally populated. The entire M vector is a result of the little magnets (nuclear magnetic dipole moments) grouping together as they precess about H. In Figure 23–8C, this would be seen as an excess number of nuclei on one side of the circle. We might call this grouping together as being "in phase." Note that the transverse component of M (that component perpendicular to H) is produced by the in-phase grouping of the dipoles. The parallel component of M (that component parallel to H) is produced by the population ratio of the two spin states. (We will return to a more complete discussion of in phase later.)

We need to determine how to produce H_1 so that it will rotate at the Larmor frequency about H and be perpendicular to H. Fortunately, a sinusoidally varying magnetic field that is perpendicular to H will look exactly like a constant field in the rotating coordinate system, and this is what we want. We can then produce the H_1 field by a conductor with electrons flowing through it if we design the conductor configuration in such a way that H_1 is perpendicular to H. (We will present more on this structure later; see "Radio Frequency Coils.") Remember that H_1 must rotate at the Larmor frequency, which is in the radio frequency range. Therefore, the electron flow in the RF coil must vary at the Larmor frequency (thus the term RF [radio frequency] magnetic field).

If this discussion of the precession of M about H_1 is sufficient, we can define two more terms before describing NMR parameters. If H_1 is on long enough to rotate M by 90°, we have what is called a **90° pulse.** If H_1 stays on twice as long, so that the precession of M carries M all the way to the $-z$ axis, we have rotated M by 180°. The RF pulse necessary to produce the 180° rotation is called a **180° pulse.**

Free Induction Decay

We are now ready to discuss NMR parameters, which are those quantities that are measurable with the NMR technique. It is important here to state that the NMR signal cannot be described in terms of photon emission alone, as we do with x-rays. Rather, we must move M away from the H direction and observe M moving back along H. We are going to describe the parameters first and then discuss some possible reasons for observing what we do.

Recall that we can rotate M away from H by applying an RF field at the Larmor frequency. If M precesses about the varying RF field by 90°, we have applied a 90° pulse (see Fig. 23–10B). Suppose we apply a 90° pulse; the RF field is on until M is entirely in the plane perpendicular to H, and then H_1 is turned off. Thus, we see that a 90° pulse is simply the length of time that H_1 is turned on (the time will be different for different values of H_1). When H_1 is turned off, M will continue precessing about H. At the same time, the dipole magnets (spinning nuclei) will start returning to the equilibrium distribution (i.e., the distribution that existed before H_1 was turned on). In other literature you may encounter the term **thermal equilibrium;** this is exactly the same thing that we have called equilibrium distribution.

So, we have M precessing about H and moving back toward the direction of H. Figure 23–11A shows the path along which M returns to H. The coil shown in Figure 23–11B is an RF coil (more than likely the one used to produce the field H_1). Remem-

ber that M can be considered to be a magnet. When the end of the M magnet sweeps past the windings of the RF coil, a current (electron flow) is induced in the coil. For all jeep drivers, you may visualize Figure 23–11A as though you were in a helicopter hovering exactly over the top of a mountain while watching the jeep make its spiral climb back up the mountain. In Figure 23–11B, M at 1 is not inducing a current; at 2 the induced current has a maximum value; it is zero at 3; and at 4 the induced current is again a maximum but in the opposite direction from that at 2. It is the opposite direction because M is sweeping the loops in opposite directions at 2 and 4. Remember that M is getting closer to H between 1 and 4 (the jeep is getting closer to the top of the mountain, so it will appear to be closer to the center top of the mountain), so the current at 4 has a smaller maximum than at 2. For each trip of M around H we have the same shape of induced current, with the maximum values getting smaller. This decreasing induction continues until M is along the H direction.

The total signal induced in the coil is shown in Figure 23–12A. What we see is an alternating voltage (produced by the induced current) that has the Larmor frequency. It also decays to zero (at least, to background noise) exponentially. (X-ray beams decay exponentially. At least, a monochromatic beam would be attenuated exponentially by some attenuating material.) This signal produced by the free return of M to the H direction is called the **free induction decay (FID).**

When we discuss MRI in the next chapter, we will use M_{xy} to indicate the magnetization vector in the xy imaging plane. In the current discussion it is more correct to use the term M_y to indicate the 90° rotated M vector in a rotating coordinate system.

The return of M to the H direction is accomplished by two different mechanisms. Note that as M returns to the H direction, the component of M along y^1

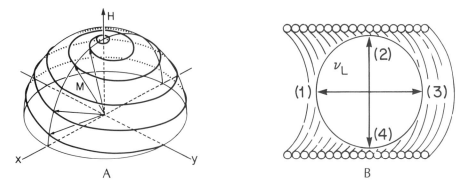

Figure 23–11 *A.* Beehive path of M during free induction decay. *B.* Generation of the FID signal

(called M_y in Figure 23–12*B)* decreases to zero. The M_z component (the component of M along H), however, increases from zero during the FID. **We will need to discuss these two components as separate topics. They produce two other parameters of NMR, namely T_1 and T_2, the relaxation times.**

Spin-Spin Relaxation Time (T_2). Having mentioned the FID, it would be appropriate here to introduce the concept of spin-spin relaxation time, T_2, **because T_2 is closely related to the FID.** Before explaining what T_2 represents, we need to discuss what happens after a 90° pulse to get M pointing back along H.

Refer back to Figure 23–8*C*, which showed that the little magnets (the nuclear MDM) were precessing about H so that their components perpendicular to the H field added up to zero. Obviously, this is not the case after a 90° pulse. We can visualize the little magnets as being placed in phase by the 90° pulse.

Figure 23–12*B* and *C* attempt to show how the nuclei are in phase at the end of a 90° pulse when M_y is greatest. As M_y decreases with time, the nuclei are resuming the random distribution that existed before the 90° pulse (H_1) was applied. The drawing represents an extreme case in which all the nuclei group together in phase, which is hardly to be expected in actuality. (The next paragraph will explain why the nuclei (dipoles) return to a random distribution

after the 90° pulse.) Going in phase may be compared to closing one of those old-fashioned folding fans that high-society matrons used to carry to the opera, and going out of phase is analogous to opening the fan. In fact, some authors use the term "fanning out" instead of going out of phase.

When the 90° pulse is ended, the little dipole magnets start precessing about H, each with a Larmor frequency. The Larmor frequency for each little magnet is not necessarily the same because of local magnetic fields that are produced by the environment (the material structure surrounding the dipole) and by poor H-field uniformity. Remember, the Larmor frequency will vary if the magnetic field varies. The in-phase dipole magnets start to separate, because some precess faster than others (we will later call these fast and slow dipoles). When the M vector is back along H, we again have a random distribution of the dipoles about H. The return to random distribution from the in-phase distribution is an exponential function of time. T_2 is the time constant for this exponential function when only the interaction between the dipoles is considered. The exponential function is presented in Figure 23–12*A* as the dashed line connecting to the tops of the peaks. We would like to draw that function again in Figure 23–13.

Note that T_2^* is introduced in Figure

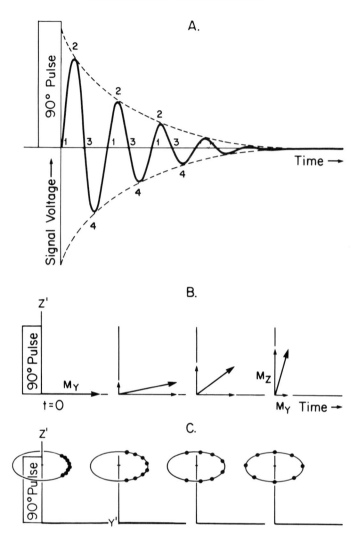

Figure 23–12 *A*. FID signal. *B*. Components of magnetization along y' and z' axes following a 90° pulse. *C*. M_y decreases with increasing dephasing

Figure 23–13 Graphic representation of the decay constant T_2^*

23–13 as a constant in the exponential portion of the equation

$$M_y = M_Y e^{-t/T_2^*}$$

M_y = component of M along the y axis

M_Y = component of M along y at the end of the 90° pulse

t = time following the 90° pulse

T_2^* = decay constant for randomization of the in-phase dipoles

We do exactly the same thing in x-ray attenuation where we introduced the attenuation coefficient, and we do the same thing in radioactive decay by introducing the disintegration constant. With these two constants we then proceeded to find the half-value layer and the half-life. We would like to do something slightly different here. Consider the exponential expression from Figure 23–13, e^{-t/T_2^*} If time (t) is made equal to T_2^*, then $t/T_2^* = 1$ and the exponential becomes e^{-1} (remember that $e^{-1} = 1/e$). Therefore, at $t = T_2^*$, the value of the magnetization in the y^1 direction has decreased to $1/e$ of its maximum value at $t = 0$. (In this paragraph, e is the base of the natural log; it is not the electronic charge. $1/e$ has the value of 0.37.) In Figure 23–13, **T_2^* is the time required to reduce the value of magnetization along the y^1 axis (the transverse magnetization) to $1/e$ of its value following the 90° pulse.**

Therefore, T_2^* is the decay constant for randomization of the in-phase dipoles. T_2^* relates to randomization analogous to the way in which an isotope's half-life relates to the decay of the radioactive sample. It takes several T_2^* periods for the in-phase dipoles to approach randomization. The dispersion of the dipoles is determined by the local Larmor frequency, which is determined by the local magnetic field. The local magnetic field depends on, first of all, the applied field, H. The variations in the local field, however, depend on the fluctuating fields produced by neighboring charged particles and on permanent inhomogeneity in the applied field, H. The permanent inhomogeneity in the H field simply means that it is impossible to make a perfect magnet. If the applied field, H, were perfectly uniform (no inhomogeneity), the T_2^* would be exactly equal to the spin-spin relaxation time, T_2. Because this is never the case, we will see later (see "Spin-Echo Technique") that T_2 is measured experimentally by procedures designed to eliminate the effects of the field inhomogeneity. T_2^* is very much shorter than T_2. The T_2 relaxation time of most tissues ranges from about 50 to 350 ms, while T_2^* is only a few ms. Thus, T_2^* is a

response to inhomogeneity in the magnetic field, and T_2 is a characteristic of the material under investigation. In general, T_2 of abnormal tissue is longer than T_2 of normal tissue.

During the dephasing of the dipoles, energy may be transferred from one dipole to another, but no energy is transferred to the surrounding material. The transfer of energy to the surrounding environment brings about the return of the nuclear dipole to the lower energy spin state. There is another time constant for the return of the dipoles to the lower energy spin state.

Spin-Lattice Relaxation Time (T_1). Recall that at equilibrium in a magnetic field, the spin-up (lower energy) population of nuclei contain about 1 in 1,000,000 more nuclei than are contained in the spin-down (higher energy) population. The excess nuclei in the spin-up state are responsible for producing the component of the magnetization vector, M, that is parallel to the magnetic field, H.

At the end of a 90° pulse, the two spin states of the nuclei are equally populated, and there is no component of the magnetization vector (M_z) in the H direction. This means that some (half) of the excess nuclei in the lower energy state have absorbed energy and have flipped to the higher energy state. At the end of the 90° pulse, those nuclei (or their relatives) transfer energy to the structure (called the lattice) that surrounds them, and return to the lower energy state. As they return to the lower state, the component of M along H is reestablished as the equilibrium distribution of the nuclei is reestablished. Here again, we find that the number of excess nuclei remaining in the higher energy state as time passes is an exponential function of time. (Remember that the number of x-ray photons remaining in a beam is an exponential function of absorber thickness.) Therefore, the number of nuclei that have returned to the lower state is obtained by subtracting those remaining in the higher energy state from the total number of excess nuclei that were

in the higher state at the end of the 90°
pulse. (This is exactly analogous to the
number of x-ray photons removed from
the x-ray beam.)

As always, we have a constant for this
exponential function (like the attenuation
coefficient for x rays) that we call $\mathbf{T_1}$, the
spin-lattice relaxation time. T_1 is the time
for 63% of the nuclei to return to the lower
energy state following a 90° pulse. The
equation for the return to equilibrium following a 90° pulse is

$$M_z = M_z (1 - e^{-t/T_1})$$

M_z = component of M along H at time t
M_z = component of M along H at equilibrium
t = time following a 90° pulse
T_1 = spin-lattice relaxation time

When t is equal to T_1, we have $e^{-t/T_1} = e^{-1}$
= 0.37.

One more interpretation of T_1 might be
in order. $\mathbf{T_1}$ is a rate constant. The rate
(the number of nuclei per unit of time) at
which the nuclei are flipping from the
higher to lower energy state depends on
the number of nuclei available for the transition and on some constant, T_1, that is a
function of the environment in which the
nuclei find themselves. Thus, the number
of nuclei per unit of time that undergo a
transition approaches zero because fewer
nuclei are available to make the transition.
(This again is completely analogous to
x-ray attenuation or radioactive decay.)

Figure 23–14 shows the return to equilibrium population following a 90° pulse in

terms of the component of M along H, M_z.
Note that we are close to the equilibrium
population after a time of 4 to 5 T_1 has
passed.

Things have been going too well in the
discussion of T_1 and T_2. So it's time for a
small problem. The return of the nuclei to
equilibrium distribution does not give an
NMR signal (Remember that T_2^* could be
measured by the FID signal produced by
the transverse M_y.) This means that T_1 cannot be measured directly by NMR techniques. But, more importantly, it means
that at the end of the FID signal, there may
still be some excess nuclei in the higher
energy state. In general, the nuclei will dephase (remember the T_2 discussion) before
all the nuclei return to the equilibrium distribution following a 90° pulse, or time $\mathbf{T_1}$
will be longer than time $\mathbf{T_2}$. Sometimes T_1
and T_2 are nearly the same, as in liquids,
and sometimes T_1 is much longer than T_2.
For example, in a 1-tesla field, cerebral spi-
nal fluid has a T_1 of 3000 ms and T_2 of
2000 ms, whereas muscle has a T_1 of 750
ms and a T_2 of 55 ms.

There are several ways to measure T_1.
Probably the simplest is to use an RF pulse
sequence of a 90° pulse followed by a short
latent period, followed by another 90°
pulse (Fig. 23–15A). Pulse sequences are
used extensively in NMR, with each designed to provide some particular bit of
information. The sequence given above
may be written as $90° - \tau - 90°$. (A sequence
is normally notated by some shorthand notation such as this.) In the $90° - \tau - 90°$ sequence, the first 90° pulse rotates the M
vector. During the time, τ, relaxation occurs as some of the nuclei flip from the
higher to the lower energy state. Another
90° pulse is used to produce an FID that is
made by fewer nuclei (because we are not
at thermal equilibrium at the start of this
pulse). The ratio of the FID amplitudes
immediately after the two 90° pulses is a
measure of how many nuclei flipped from
the higher to lower state during the time,
τ, between the pulses. This procedure is
repeated for various values of τ, and T_1

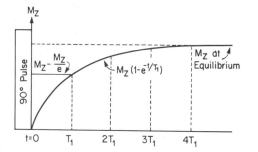

Figure 23–14 Graphic representation of the
time constant T_1

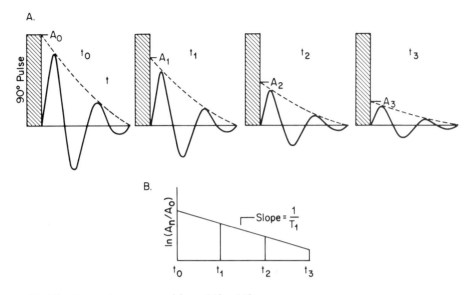

Figure 23–15 T_1 can be measured by a $90°$-τ-$90°$ sequence

can then be calculated from the data (Fig. 23–15*B*). Many people may prefer using a $180°$ pulse sequence: $180° - \tau - 90°$.

Spin Density. The density of the spinning nuclei is proportional to the amplitude of the FID. Density here means the number of identical nuclei per unit volume that are found in an identical environment or, if you prefer, the number of nuclei per unit volume that have the same Larmor frequency. We would expect the magnetization to increase with an increased number of nuclei simply because there would be more dipoles to help form the magnetization. As the magnetization vector sweeps past the RF coil to produce the FID, we have already seen that the induced signal size depends on the size of the transverse component of the magnetization. Therefore, we would expect larger values of magnetization to produce larger FID amplitudes.

Because the number of nuclei at the Larmor frequency determines the size of the FID signal, we need only measure the FID amplitude to obtain the spin density. We must ensure that no other effect is changing the amplitude of the FID. For example, the nuclei must be in the equilibrium dis-

tribution before applying the $90°$ pulse to evoke the FID. Usually, for NMR measurements, we use more than one pulse to help improve the signal-to-noise ratio (S:N). That means that a repetitive pulse sequence is normally used to form the final NMR signal.

MECHANISMS FOR RELAXATION

We have said that photon emission alone cannot explain the spin-lattice relaxation time, T_1. (This is different from the production of characteristic x rays, which we described entirely as photon emission.) Consequently, we must discuss what methods can be used by the nuclei to get rid of energy so that they can flip from the higher to the lower energy state.

For a proton in a 1-tesla magnetic field, the energy separation between the two spin states is only 1.759×10^{-7} eV. We generally think in terms of kiloelectron volts when dealing with x rays which means that the energy state separation for proton spins is some 10^{-10} smaller than the energy separation of the inner atomic electrons. (You can try this calculation if you use 1 tesla = 1 kg/C $\cdot$ sec, 1 MHz/tesla = 1 C/kg, 1 eV = 1.6×10^{-19} J, and h = 6.6×10^{-34} J $\cdot$

sec). Look up the gyromagnetic ratio of a proton in Table 23–1, and remember the formula $\Delta E = \gamma \hbar H$.

When there are two quantum energy states (either spin states or electron energy shells), there is competition between photon emission and radiationless transfer of energy to the environment (sometimes called the lattice). For the nuclear spin flips, most transitions occur by radiationless transfer of energy to the lattice.

There are several ways, depending on the lattice structure in which the nuclei find themselves, by which the nuclei may transfer their energy to the lattice. The main requirement is that the nuclei be in the presence of locally fluctuating magnetic fields produced by the environment. Therefore, any means by which varying magnetic fields can be produced can be a means to transfer energy. The larger the field, the more quickly the energy can be transferred.

In no way do we intend to leave the impression that the T_1 interactions are simple and easy to catalog. Much of the work in NMR is in the area of trying to understand the interactions that produce the T_1 time. **We should note that the time T_1 is an indication of the environment in which the dipole is located.** This is useful in NMR imaging. In tissues, T_1 can be as short as about 200 ms for fat, or as long as 3,000 ms for cerebrospinal fluid and free water. In the brain, gray matter and white matter differ in water content by only about 10%, but their T_1 times differ by a factor of almost 1.5 (in a 1-T field, the T_1 of white matter is about 390 ms and gray matter about 520 ms). In general, the T_1 of abnormal tissue is longer than the T_1 of normal tissues.

Spin-Echo Technique

We have seen that the dephasing (T_2^*) of the nuclear dipoles following a 90° pulse is determined by two quantities, 1) the spin-spin relaxation time and 2) the H-field inhomogeneity. We should keep in mind that

the H-field inhomogeneity is built into the magnet and is undesirable but unfortunately quite permanent. Furthermore, the field inhomogeneity varies from point to point within the H field. **The spin-echo technique was developed to remove the effect of the H-field inhomogeneity.**

The spin-echo process starts with a 90° pulse along the x^1 axis (Fig. 23–16A) so that M will precess about x^1 to the y^1 axis. Remember that x^1 and y^1 are rotating at the Larmor frequency. Of course, at the end of the pulse, dephasing starts among the spin dipoles. Some dipoles will be in a field larger than the H field because of local fields adding to the H field. They will precess faster than the M vector, which is precessing at the Larmor frequency. Some will be slower than M because they are in a smaller field than H. Remember, the frequency of precession is related to the strength of H:

$$\nu = \frac{\gamma H}{2\pi}$$

We can refer to these dipoles as fast and slow dipoles. In Figure 23–16B, the $x^1 y^1$ coordinate is rotating at the Larmor frequency and, therefore, M appears not to be rotating. Those slow dipoles will then appear to be rotating in the $-y^1$ direction (i.e., they appear to be falling behind M) while the fast dipoles appear to be rotating in the $+y^1$ direction (they appear to be pulling away from M). That is, the fast and slow dipoles are rotating in opposite directions relative to M.

So, we have the 90° pulse. After a time, τ, a 180° pulse is applied along the x^1 axis. (Remember again that $x^1 y^1$ are rotating at the Larmor frequency. Our electronics must keep track of how far the x^1 axis has rotated during the time, τ, so the 180° pulse can be applied along the x^1 axis.) The 180° pulse simply inverts the magnetization components. For the spin-echo technique, the component along H (M_z) is of no consequence. The spin grouping, however, is inverted about the x^1 axis for the transverse

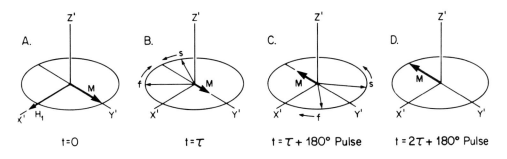

Figure 23–16 Spin-echo sequence

components by precession about the x^1 axis.

It is noteworthy that, after the 180° pulse, the fast dipoles are behind M and the slow ones are ahead of M (Fig. 23–16C). After a time, τ (the same as before), the fast dipoles will catch up with M at the same time that M catches up with the slow dipoles. Everything will again be in phase, and the magnetization, M, along the y^1 axis will be maximal (Fig. 23–16D).

The effect is similar to that of a group of runners starting a mile run. Because they run at different speeds, the runners spread out as they get farther from the starting line. If, at an arbitrary time, τ, they are suddenly told that they are going the wrong way, they will turn around and head back for the starting line. The fast runners will be farther from the starting line than the slow runners. Because the runners who are the farthest away are the fastest, all will arrive back at the starting line together at a time equal to 2τ (assuming that everyone runs back at a constant speed). This analogy would be more accurate if we kept the runners going in the same direction all the time. By magic, at time t we would interchange the fast and slow runners. Then, at time 2τ, the fast runners would exactly catch up with their slower companions. Of course, the dipoles (as would the runners) immediately start dephasing again as the fast dipoles pass the slow ones. As the dipoles come together (we get a reverse FID) and separate (another FID), we get a pulse that looks like 2 FIDs back to back (Fig.

23–17). **This back-to-back FID is the spin-echo.** Because we have used a 180° pulse, we effectively remove the H-field inhomogeneity from the dephasing.

The dephasing caused by spin-spin relaxation, however, would continue. The amplitude of the echo is smaller than the initial FID. The decrease in amplitude is an exponential function of T_2, the spin-spin relaxation time. T_2 can be measured by repeating the 180° pulse every 2τ and by measuring the time constant of the decrease of the amplitude of the echoes. This type of pulse sequence has the name Carr-Purcell echo sequence, and it (or some modification) is usually used to measure T_2.

Fourier Transforms

We have previously mentioned Fourier transforms (FT) in connection with the modulation transfer function and computed tomography reconstruction methods. The application of the FT to magnetic resonance is very straightforward, perhaps somewhat easier to understand than our previous examples. The signal received from NMR (the FID, for instance) is in the

Figure 23–17 Spin-echo signal

form of amplitude versus time. The FT of a signal of this type is in the form of signal strength versus frequency.

For instance, consider a simple sine wave, which has a time for one complete cycle period of T (Fig. 23–18A). This sine wave has only one frequency (f), so the FT of the sine wave is only a single line in the plot with a height that is proportional to the total strength of the sine wave (Fig. 23–18B). (Of course, in any practical situation, we cannot obtain a true single-frequency sine wave because additional frequencies result from starting and stopping the wave form.) It is interesting to note that both curves of Figure 23–18 contain the same information and that, given one, we can get the other by means of the FT. Note that two sine waves with different frequencies would add together to give a complicated-looking signal in the "time domain" (before the FT of the signal), but would simply be two lines in the "frequency domain" (after the FT of the signal) whose heights would represent the relative strengths of the sine waves.

The sine curve looks something like an FID, except that the FID decays to zero. Thus, we might expect the FT of the FID to be something like the FT for the sine curve. If the FID is composed of dephasing nuclei in similar environments, the Larmor frequency of the FID is essentially a single-frequency decaying sine curve. We might expect the local environmental magnetic fields to cause the dipoles to precess at slightly different frequencies. Furthermore, we might expect that those slightly different frequencies would show up in the FT of the FID.

Figure 23–19 gives an FID and its FT. There are some points to note about the FT curve. First, it is a Lorentzian shape. (We make this observation only because you may have read this elsewhere.) The term "Lorentzian" is used to provide information (to mathematicians) about the symmetry of the line about the Larmor frequency. The second point is that the line width at half its maximum value (called the FWHM, the full width at half-maximum) is $2/T_2^*$. This result is verifiable by mathematics but is a terrible task involving integral calculus. Remember that $2/T_2^*$ has the unit of 1/time, which is the same unit that the frequency has.

Suppose we have a sample with two groups of nonidentical nuclei. If their gyromagnetic ratios were different, there would be two Larmor frequencies. (Remember, $\nu_L = \gamma H/2\pi$, where ν_L = Larmor frequency, γ = gyromagnetic ratio, and H = applied magnetic field.) In such a case, the FID would be the sum of the two exponentially decaying sine waves, one at each of the Larmor frequencies. If, by chance, **we had two groups of identical nuclei in different magnetic fields, we would also see the composite FID of the two Larmor frequencies.** We will depict the two Larmor frequencies (Fig. 23–20A), the

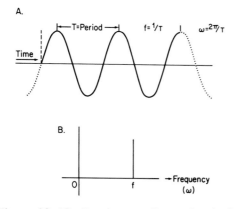

Figure 23–18 Fourier transform of a single-frequency sine wave

Figure 23–19 Fourier transform of a single FID

composite FID (Fig. 23–20*B)*, and the FT of the FID in Figure 23–20. Note that Figure 23–20*B* shows a time function and, by use of the FT, this has been converted in Figure 23–20*C* to a frequency function.

We can see from these examples that the **FT of the FID can reduce a rather complicated signal to relatively simple frequency lines that indicate the spin density at each frequency.** This is an important concept for NMR imaging. In some NMR imaging, we purposely vary the field across the subject so that the resonance Larmor frequency will be different for points across the subject. Figure 23–21 diagrams the effects of varying the field for three samples of identical nuclei. The single received signal (composite FID), when the FT is taken, shows us that there are three groups of nuclei. Furthermore, we are told that the three groups have equal spin density (i.e., the same number of nuclei per unit volume in all three samples).

Now, if we relate the Larmor frequency back to the magnetic field, we know that group 1 is where H_1 exists, and so forth. If we happen to make the change in the magnetic field a linear change, then we know the value of the field everywhere along the sample. This allows us to transform the information given in terms of frequency to sample location in spatial coordinates, and that is exactly what we need to do for spatially imaging a sample. If we could do all these simple steps, we could image, at least, a one-dimensional spatially varying sample.

INSTRUMENTATION

Magnets

It would seem from the foregoing discussion that there are several pieces of apparatus that are essential for the production, detection, and display of an NMR signal. These include a magnet to produce the H field, some equipment to produce the varying H_1 field, a device to detect the

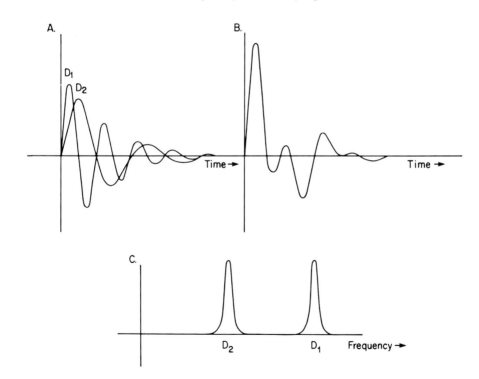

Figure 23–20 Fourier transform of a composite FID

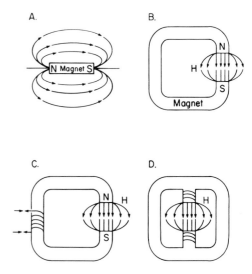

Figure 23–21   Fourier transform of three groups of identical nuclei in different magnetic fields

FID of M, and the electronics to assimilate and display the NMR signal.

In NMR, producing and holding H constant is one of the most difficult jobs. Generally, the H-field value should be as large as possible because the signal-to-noise ratio (S:N) of the output information depends on H. The higher the value of H, the larger the S:N ratio. We must be aware that NMR requires an RF magnetic field that must penetrate tissue to image a body in cross section. A higher H value requires an increase in the RF frequency, which does not penetrate the body as well as low-frequency RF. A higher H-field value may present problems with skin penetration by the RF field. In addition, H must be uniform (i.e., have the same strength and direction) over the entire volume of sample under investigation. Of course, when we make statements like the last two, we have to amend them immediately. We will probably find that stronger fields can improve the S:N ratio just so much, and then we see no further improvement with larger and more costly magnets. There will always be a tradeoff between field strength, unifor-

mity, and magnet cost. We have always been in that position, however, when considering new imaging equipment.

Bar Magnets and Electromagnets. When discussing magnets we feel that it would be instructive to start with an iron bar magnet and to work forward and upward from there. In Figure 23–22A, the lines labeled

Figure 23–22   Configuration of magnets

"H" represent the magnetic field. The lines are usually called the "magnetic lines of force," and indicate the direction of the magnetic field at each point along the line. If we are careful, but not too rigid, the lines may also indicate the field strength: the closer the lines are together, the larger the field strength. (More formally, the field strength at a point is the number of lines passing through a unit area centered at this point.) With this notation, a uniform field would be represented by straight lines evenly spaced. Obviously, if our drawing is any good at all, there is no uniform field area around the bar magnet.

Note the space called the "gap" of the C magnet in Figure 23–22B. There the lines are fairly straight and evenly spaced in the middle region. Toward the outer regions of the gap the lines become curved, which would indicate that the field is no longer uniform. The gap region of the C magnet could be used as the H field for NMR studies, but the sample to be investigated should be entirely within the uniform field area. Of course, bar magnets could be bent into a horseshoe shape to give a uniform field in the gap. Permanent magnets can be used for NMR imaging if they are big enough. Permanent magnets with field strengths of about .05 to 0.3 T (500 to 3000 gauss) have been designed for use in NMR imaging.

Figure 23–22C and D indicate the fields produced by two configurations of electromagnets. The field strength depends on the current; larger currents produce larger fields. Physics and chemistry laboratories worldwide use magnets based on the "yoke"-type construction for NMR studies (Fig. 23–22D). The magnets vary in size and construction, but all have one common property: the space between the pole faces is small, being at most a few inches wide. The restricted space between the pole faces restricts the size of the sample that may be investigated. (People will certainly not fit within the pole gap of commercially available electromagnets that have iron cores.)

Resistive Coil Air Core Magnets. Magnetic fields can be produced by current-carrying conductors. (This concept was discussed earlier in this chapter.) Suppose we have a coil of wire with current (electron flow) passing through it. In Figure 23–23A we have current (I) passing through a coil of wire (more than one loop), which produces the magnetic field (H) indicated. In Figure 23–23B the coil of wire is pulled out to form a solenoid (resembles a wire spring). The field inside the solenoid is fairly uniform, while outside the solenoid the field looks like the field around a bar magnet.

Further investigation would reveal that the field uniformity could be improved by a pair of Helmholtz coils, although the field strength might be somewhat lower than for a comparable solenoid. Figure 23–24A represents a pair of Helmholtz coils. A Helmholtz pair of coils consists of two parallel coils in which the current is flowing in the same direction.

The coil arrangement in Figure 23–24B consists of two sets of Helmholtz coils that can be used to produce sufficiently uniform fields with ample room for NMR imaging. A person could be placed in this field by sliding him in the direction of H through the opening in the coils. With the four coil arrangement (two sets of Helmholtz coils), field uniformities of one part per thousand over about a 50-cm diameter can be achieved. Field strength, H, is somewhere in the half-tesla region. **This type of magnet is called a resistive coil air core magnet.** The resistive coil part of the name implies that current must be supplied during the entire time that the magnet is activated. Therefore, electrical power is consumed during the entire time that the magnet is producing the magnetic field.

Superconducting Magnets. An alternative to the resistive coil magnet is the superconducting magnet. **"Supercons,"** as they are called, **take advantage of the zero resistance that certain materials have at very low temperatures.** At zero resistance

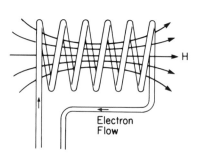

Figure 23–23 Magnetic field in a solenoid

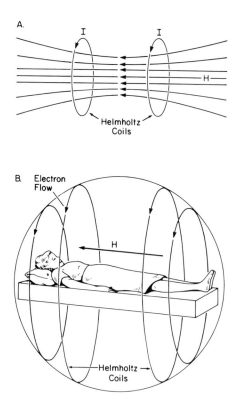

Figure 23–24 Magnetic field of a Helmholtz pair (*A*) and a resistive coil air core magnet (*B*)

a current, once started, will continue to flow without further power input. That means that supercons are initially connected to a power supply, brought up to the design field strength, and then disconnected from the electrical power source. The current continues and the magnetic field remains constant. There is just one little problem! **The entire magnetic system must be maintained at about 4° K,** which makes the North Pole look like Palm Springs. This low temperature can be maintained if the magnetic coils are submerged in liquid helium.

The supercon contains a solenoid of superconducting material, perhaps NbTi, in the form of filaments embedded in a copper matrix. The solenoid is surrounded by liquid helium; around the liquid helium is a vacuum (a very poor heat conductor). The helium must be in a container (stainless steel) surrounded by another container. A vacuum is hopefully maintained between these two containers. A double-walled container designed to hold low-temperature material is called a Dewar. Next to the vacuum region is a layer of liquid nitrogen, then another vacuum, perhaps some insulation, and an outside polished container.

Note that the entire structure outlined above is designed to keep heat energy from being transferred from the room temperature around the magnet to the liquid helium inside the magnet. Such structures are not perfect, and some heat will get to the liquid helium. The heat energy will convert some liquid helium to helium gas (liquefied gases have very low boiling points). If all the liquid helium is "boiled away," the temperature of the superconducting material will start to increase. If the temperature increases above that temperature at which superconductivity starts, the magnet will lose its field. **It is most important to keep liquid helium in the magnet.** Therefore, about once a week, the magnet must be filled with liquid helium (and nitrogen, too).

We are not good enough artists to draw the inside of a supercon, but we can present some photographs. Figure 23–25 shows a 5-in. bore supercon. The bore is the diameter of the center area into which the sample to be investigated is inserted (with all the RF coils necessary to make the meas-

urements). The bore of the 5-in. magnet is vertical, and the samples must be inserted from the top or bottom. The small cylinders on top are tubes with which to fill the magnet with liquid nitrogen and helium and to monitor the temperatures and liquid levels inside the magnet. The field strength, H, is 5 tesla at the center of the bore (along the center line halfway from top to bottom), and the field homogeneity is one part in 10^7 over a 2-cm^3 volume. Obviously, this magnet is used for laboratory investigations and not for imaging.

Some cautionary measures are in order. If the temperature of any segment of the solenoid goes above the temperature for superconduction, that segment will then have some resistance. Power loss in this resistance ($P = I^2R$) would be converted to heat, and the adjoining segments would be raised to nonsuperconducting status. This would continue until the entire solenoid would no longer be superconducting and the net result would be loss of current and liquid helium. "Quench" is the term used to describe this disaster. There is a reason, therefore, for putting superconducting filaments in a copper matrix: the copper hopefully keeps the filaments from melting down during a quench. In addition, a disturbance in the fringing fields (the magnetic field outside the magnet that we cannot remove) can induce a quench of the magnet. Therefore, no large steel object should be moved around close to the magnet. Don't put these magnets close to elevators or parking lots. Although these two would probably not produce a quench, they would disturb the field and produce unreliable results. **Don't use steel rolling carts in the area. Don't use steel tools near the bore of the magnet.** They might well be sucked up into the bore. (This would be extremely dangerous, obviously, if there happened to be a patient in the magnet at the time.) Also, don't allow people with pacemakers to wander freely about the area. The fringing fields could affect the pulse timing of the pacemaker. Finally,

Figure 23–25 A 5-in. bore superconducting magnet

there is one other warning. **When a magnet undergoes a rapid quench, there is a tremendous amount of helium gas released in a very short time,** and this gas could make breathing difficult for patients. In an imaging system room, a large exhaust system must be available to remove the gas quickly.

Most commercial NMR imaging magnets are permanent or superconducting magnets. Let us briefly consider the advantages or disadvantages of these two magnets.

Permanent magnets are available with field strengths of about 0.05 to 0.3 tesla. Because they do not require cooling, these magnets are relatively inexpensive to operate. The magnets are stable and have good field strength homogeneity. Low acquisition and operating costs are probably the major advantage of permanent magnets. The main disadvantage is weight. A large iron core magnet is very heavy (up to 200,000 lbs). Another disadvantage is that these magnets must be kept at a very constant temperature to maintain stability of the magnetic field.

Superconducting magnets are available with field strengths of about 0.3 to 2.0 tesla. High field strength with excellent stability and homogeneity are the main advantage of supercons. The major disadvantage of superconducting magnets is the high cost of the liquid nitrogen and helium. The high field strength limits the area in which a magnet can be located. Site preparation costs can be high.

Radio Frequency Coils. Now that the magnetic field, H, can be established, the next thing to do is to produce the varying H_1 field. Remember, H_1 must be perpendicular to H and must vary sinusoidally with the Larmor frequency. For H fields obtainable and gyromagnetic values that nuclei possess, the Larmor frequency will be somewhere in the radio frequency range (1–100 MHz). **The device that produces H_1 is called a radio frequency coil.**

There are several types of RF coils that may be used. Figure 23–26 shows repre-

Figure 23–26   Configuration of RF coils

sentative coil configurations of two commonly used types.

The saddle-shaped coil illustrated in Figure 23–26A is really a Helmholtz pair as shown in Figure 23–24A. The difference is that the saddle-shaped coil has been curved to fit in the round bore of the magnet and has been made rectangular rather than round. The saddle-shaped coil will yield an H_1 field that is perpendicular to H_0 of a superconductive magnet. The geometry is such that the patient, lying on a bed, is placed with H_0 along the length of the body.

On the other hand, the solenoidal coil illustrated in Figure 23–26B is a nice companion for the permanent magnet. Notice that the main field of the permanent magnet is from face of magnet to face of magnet. The solenoidal coil, when placed as indicated in Figure 23–26B, provides the proper direction for H_1. The patient is placed in the magnet with the main field (H_0) transverse to the body.

At this point, we should note that the RF coils so far have been used to produce the magnetic field, H_1. There is one other requirement: The NMR signal must be detected. The device should be one that detects low energy signals at the Larmor frequency, which sounds like an RF coil, doesn't it? Indeed it is. Because we use a pulsed H_1 field, the H_1 RF coil may be used to detect the NMR signal during the time when it is not producing the H_1 field. It is only during this time that we can detect the NMR signal, however, so we can use one RF coil to produce the H_1 field and to detect the NMR signal. There may be times when we prefer to use two RF coils, one to produce H_1 and the other to detect the signal (this is the usual situation when surface coils are used). If we do this, the two RF coils are normally placed in the magnetic field perpendicular to each other (and, of course, with H_1 still perpendicular to H).

Electronics

The job that the electronic devices must perform is to apply an RF voltage in pulsed sequence across the RF coil, detect the NMR signal (the free induction decay or spin-echo for the pulse sequence), and record or display the information in the desired form. With imaging, the electronics must also control the gradient coils (to be described later) and construct the image from the data.

Suppose we have a sample (for NMR analysis, not for imaging) within an RF coil, and both the sample and coil are within a magnetic field, H. If we knew the Larmor frequency, we could apply a single frequency to the RF coil to invoke the NMR signal, at least from those nuclei with a Larmor frequency equal to the one applied. There is the problem of local magnetic environment at each nucleus, which requires a slightly different Larmor frequency. To observe these slightly different Larmor frequencies, we must apply a range of frequencies to the RF coil (or, as in many physics experiments, slightly vary the magnetic field). Thus, we need a device to generate a sweep of RF frequencies about the Lar-

mor frequency that we would have if there were no environmental effects. "Sweep" is really not the right word. If we apply a square wave pulse (such as that shown in Figure 23–12A for the FID), the pulse contains all the frequencies needed to excite the nuclei of interest. We need a pulse generator that can vary the RF frequency to obtain the Larmor frequency, fix the pulse width, and develop the pulse sequence. The pulse generator may not produce sufficient power, so we normally use an RF amplifier to feed the RF coil. The combined pulse generator and amplifier is sometimes called the "transmitter."

At the end of a pulse, we would like the RF coil to detect the NMR signal. Remember that the detection is accomplished by the decaying M vector inducing a current (voltage) at the Larmor frequency in the RF coil. We want the NMR signal to go into an RF amplifier that will not distort the signal. The NMR signal is considerably smaller than the input RF pulse. After the amplifier, there are several ways to proceed. Because we have described the Fourier transform method of producing the NMR spectrum, we will use that. If so, we need to digitize the signal and then use FT. The FT of the signal is what we would like to see displayed as the NMR information. Therefore, after the FT, we either display the signal or store it for later use. Figure 23–27 presents a basic block diagram of the NMR system.

But matters are hardly ever this simple. We must be able to keep track of or choose the phase of the RF pulse and the NMR signal. Furthermore, we use repetitive pulsing to improve the S:N ratio. A computer is not absolutely necessary, but most systems have one. Figure 23–28 shows the console for the 5-in. bore magnet, which has lots of knobs on it. This is representative of the control console for an NMR system that can measure the NMR signal for an entire small sample. (Things are not going to get any simpler, though, when we start imaging.)

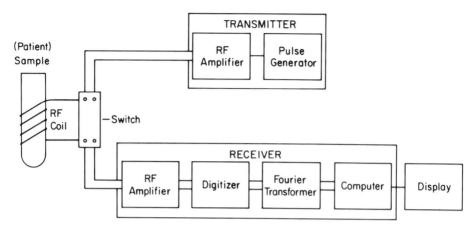

Figure 23–27 Schematic drawing of a nonimaging NMR system

NMR Spectrum

Figure 23–29 is a phosphorus (^{31}P) NMR spectrum of muscle in the human forearm. Dr. Ray L. Nunnally, of our Radiology Department, was kind enough to supply this spectrum with the following words:

A high-resolution phosphorus-31 NMR spectrum from the flexor carpi radialis and pal-maris longus muscles of the human forearm. The peaks resolved are inorganic phosphate (P_i), phosphocreatine (PCr), and the α, β, and γ phosphorus atoms of adenosine triphosphate (ATP). PCr and ATP constitute the reserve and direct chemical species (respectively) which yield energy to support cellular functions. This spectrum required two minutes of signal averaging using the standard pulse Fourier transform method. It was ob-

Figure 23–28 Console for a 5-in. bore supercon

Frequency (Hz)

Figure 23–29 NMR spectrum for ³¹P. (Courtesy of Dr. Ray L. Nunnally, University of Texas Health Science Center at Dallas, Radiology Department)

tained on an Oxford Instruments 30-cm horizontal bore superconducting magnet operating at a field of 1.9 tesla.

ADDENDUM

In the material on NMR, we have used the symbol H to represent the applied magnetic field. Other discussions on NMR will sometimes use B to represent the magnetic field, which may be called the magnetic induction. These two symbols are used universally for H = magnetic field and B = magnetic induction. We feel the need for a few words on these two quantities.

A device such as a supercon does indeed produce a magnetic field, H. If we put some material in the magnetic field, however, the internal organization of the material may be changed so that the magnetic effects in the material are increased. That is, the magnetic field inside the material is larger than the magnetic field outside the material. We have induced an additional magnetic field (or we have, at least, increased the magnetic field) in the material. Therefore, we call the field inside the material the magnetic induction, B.

It is not hard to imagine that the magnetic induction in soft iron is greater than the magnetic induction in copper. In fact, we use soft iron in transformers simply to increase the magnetic field produced by the primary winding. The magnetic field,

H, and the magnetic induction, B, are related very simply by B = μH, where μ is the magnetic permeability. It might be better to consider μ as the magnetic conductivity (because we have already discussed conductors). In a vacuum, which contains no material, μ = 1 and B = H. In iron, μ can be as high as 1000. In air, μ = 1.0000004. Consequently, we can discuss the magnetic field in the bore of a supercon, rather than the magnetic induction, with 0.00004% correctness. We doubt if we should worry too much about this error.

SUMMARY

Nuclear magnetic resonance (NMR) is a new modality for obtaining dynamic studies of certain physiologic functions and for imaging proton density (and perhaps that of other nuclei) in the body. As the name suggests, NMR is the resonance transition between nuclear spin states of certain nuclei in an external magnetic field. As a prominent radiologist, R.H. Epstein, once said, "NMR is like sex: the first time you hear about it, you just can't believe it."

Only certain nuclei, those with a net spin angular momentum, can be observed by NMR techniques. The maximum observable spin angular momentum is given by $I\hbar$, where I is the "nuclear spin" and has a simple value for each elemental nucleus. Nuclei with I = 0 cannot be used in NMR studies. For most NMR studies, nuclei with I = ½, including the proton, are investigated.

The spin angular momentum is important because it represents a spinning charge. A spinning charge will always produce a magnetic dipole moment (MDM, given the symbol μ), which makes the spinning charged nucleus behave like a tiny bar magnet. The MDM is a measure of the strength or size of the tiny magnet. The MDM is related to the spin angular momentum by

$$\mu = \gamma I\hbar \ (\gamma = \mu/I\hbar)$$

where γ is the gyromagnetic ratio. (The

gyro part is $I\hbar$; the magnetic part is μ. Because μ is on top in the definition of γ, the ratio is sometimes called the magnetogyric ratio.) The gyromagnetic ratio has a unique value for each nuclear type.

If the tiny nuclear magnet is placed in a magnetic field, H, the tiny magnet will try to align itself along the magnetic field. Quantum physics rules prohibit exact alignment and, as a matter of fact, will allow only certain specified alignment orientations. There is a specific energy with each of these orientations. The nucleus may make a transition from one energy state to another by gaining or losing energy in an amount exactly equal to the energy difference between the two states. Whether there are two energy states $(I = \frac{1}{2})$, three energy states $(I = 1)$, or more, the difference in energy that the nucleus must gain or lose is always $\Delta E = 2\mu H$. (Or, if you prefer, $\Delta E = \gamma\hbar H$.) NMR is nothing more than the induced transitions between spin states.

The inexact alignment in an H field of the tiny nuclear magnets causes the tiny magnets to precess about the magnetic field. The frequency of precession is called the Larmor frequency, and is given by

$$\nu_L = \gamma H/2\pi$$

(If we consider $\Delta E = h\nu$, which represents a photon, the frequency of the photon is exactly equal to ν_L. This means that a nucleus, in order to go from a lower energy spin state to a higher energy spin state, must absorb energy equal to that of a photon with frequency ν_L.)

In a sample of observable size, there are a very large number of nuclei. For a nuclear type for which $I = \frac{1}{2}$, some nuclei are in the lower spin state and some in the higher state. At room temperature and in normal (available) magnetic fields, the number in each state is nearly the same, with about one nucleus per million more in the lower energy state. It is these "excess" nuclei that give an NMR signal.

We represent all these excess nuclei by a single quantity called the magnetization, M. It is easier to describe NMR signals in terms of M rather than of the excess individual nuclei (about 10^7 per mole). In a magnetic field, M will normally be exactly along H. It is the function of NMR to make M move away from H, and then to observe its return to alignment along H. (Remember, the nuclei are still changing spin states.)

The M vector is made to precess about a second field, H_1, that is effectively rotating about H (and perpendicular to H) at the Larmor frequency. The second field, H_1, is generated by applying an alternating voltage (alternating at the Larmor frequency) to an RF coil surrounding the sample. While H_1 is on, M will precess about H_1 at a frequency of $\gamma H_1/2\pi$. If H_1 is on long enough for M to rotate through 90°, we have applied a 90° pulse; if M rotates through 180°, we have a 180° pulse. When H_1 is turned off, M precesses about H and returns to its orientation along H. This motion of M, described as a beehive motion, induces a signal in the RF coil (again at the Larmor frequency). This induced signal is the NMR signal.

Following a 90° pulse, the signal induced in the RF coil is called the free induction decay (FID). M is free to return along H; it induces a signal in the RF coil that goes from a maximum value to zero (below noise, at least). The reduction in the signal is an exponential decay characterized by a decay time, T_2^*. T_2^* is determined by magnetic field inhomogeneities and by the dephasing of the nuclear spins.

The return of M along H following a 90° pulse is made up of two parts. The component of M along H grows from zero to some value while the component of M perpendicular to H (the transverse component) decays from some value to zero. Both are exponential functions characterized by two time constants called the "relaxation times." T_1 is the time constant for the component along H, and is called the "spin-lattice relaxation time." T_2 is the time constant for the transverse component, and is called the "spin-spin relaxation time."

T_1 is determined by how quickly the nuclei can transfer energy to their surroundings (lattice) and return to the lower energy state. T_2 is determined by how quickly the nuclei can interact (transfer energy among themselves) to produce random distribution of the precessing nuclei about the H field. These are two NMR parameters that are of interest in describing the environment in which the nuclei are found. Nuclear spin densities are indicated by the amplitude of the FID.

The Larmor frequency is determined by the local magnetic field, and may vary from one environment to another for otherwise identical nuclei. NMR spectra are merely representations of identical nuclei that are found in slightly different magnetic fields because of local environmental effects.

For NMR imaging, the local magnetic fields are purposely varied in some pre-scribed fashion so that identical nuclei in different spatial locations will have different Larmor frequencies, thus producing FIDs with different Larmor frequencies. Imaging requires a measurement of the spin densities (amplitude of the FID with a particular Larmor frequency) and a method of relating the Larmor frequency to a spatial position.

The instrumentation for NMR requires a large magnet to produce the H field, radio frequency electronics to produce the RF pulse and to record the resulting NMR signal and, of course, sufficient electronics and computer power to store, manipulate, and display the NMR information.

REFERENCES

1. Fukushima, E., Roeder, S.B.W.: Experimental Pulse NMR—A Nuts and Bolts Approach. Addison-Wesley Publishing Co., Reading, Mass., 1981.
2. Latebur, P.C.: Image formation by induced local interactions: Example employing nuclear magnetic resonance. Nature, 242:190, 1973.
3. Slichter, C.P.: Principles of Magnetic Resonance. 2nd ed. Springer-Verlag, Berlin, 1978.

24 *Magnetic Resonance Imaging*

In this chapter we will work our way through the acquisition of an image using nuclear magnetic resonance, concentrating on the spin-echo technique. This procedure is called "magnetic resonance imaging (MRI)." We assume the student has read and studied the preceding chapter and is familiar with the basic physical concepts of nuclear magnetic resonance (NMR).

We have used the term "NMR" to indicate magnetic resonance measurements from all the material in a sample. In MRI we would like to collect resonance information from only a small volume within the sample, and be able to change which small volume is being observed. **To accomplish this task we must set resonance conditions in the small volume, and non-resonance conditions in the rest of the sample.** If we can set these conditions, any resonance signal detected by the receiving RF coil will originate in the small volume in which the resonance condition has been established.

The resonance conditions can be set in a small volume. In reality, we observe Larmor frequencies from many small volumes all at once with only one echo pulse (more details later). This is accomplished by varying (very slightly) the magnetic field strength throughout the sample. We set slightly different conditions in each of many small volumes throughout the patient. The frequencies contained in the RF pulse will then determine which of the small volumes will produce a Larmor frequency signal. The variation of the mag-

netic field is accomplished very nicely by three sets of electromagnetic coils called "gradient coils." **The gradient coils must be able to produce small spatial variations in the magnetic field in the direction of the magnetic field produced by the main magnet.** The magnet fields produced by the gradient coils are not perfectly aligned with the main field. Those components of the gradient field not aligned along the main field may fortunately be ignored since they are so small relative to the main field. In the rest of our discussion, we will consider that the gradient coils produce perfectly aligned magnetic fields, and indicate those fields by arrows in the direction of the main field (some may be in the reverse direction). You may not understand the relevance of this paragraph until you have studied the section on gradient coils that follows. **Don't despair.** Now that this little dab of physics is out of the way, let's get on with forming an image.

A sequential approach to forming an image will be used. First, we will use RF pulses to form a signal using the FID as the detected signal (recognizing that imaging is never done this way). Second, we will use gradient coils and variations in RF pulse frequency to divide the patient's anatomy into cross sectional slices, and divide the slices into voxels. Next, we will add the spin-echo pulse sequences to the image and discuss TE and TR. In a fourth section we will discuss how pulse sequences are used to produce T_1- and T_2-weighted images. Some authors designate the relaxation times by T1 and T2, but they are exactly the same as our T_1 and T_2. The fifth section will examine noise in the image, and the many factors that influence noise. **Noise is important because it limits contrast resolution, and contrast resolution is the principal advantage of MRI.** Finally, several other topics will be explored briefly. MRI has developed so rapidly in the last few years that one chapter in a general text cannot deal with all aspects.

BASIC MAGNETIC RESONANCE IMAGING

Basic MRI requires three steps:

1. Place the patient in a uniform magnetic field
2. Displace the equilibrium magnetization vector with an RF pulse
3. Observe the signal as the magnetization vector returns to equilibrium

Our illustration assumes a 1-tesla imaging magnet. When a patient is placed in a 1-tesla (1T) magnet, the hydrogen nuclei in her body will align themselves in the magnetic field (we will use symbol H for the magnetic field). This alignment produces a net magnetization vector (M_0) in the direction of the magnetic field. M_0 is called the "equilibrium magnetization." Figure 24–1 illustrates H, z, and M_0. By convention, the direction along the magnetic field is called the "z coordinate." Magnetization along z may be designated as M_z. Net magnetization, M_z, exists, but may

sometimes be zero. M_z does not process. M_z cannot be detected.

A note about M_0 and M_z. When the patient is placed inside the imaging magnet, the magnetization vector along the z axis appears and is called M_0. M_0 is the equilibrium magnetization vector. As soon as we begin to manipulate the magnetization vector, the value of the vector in the z axis begins to change. M_z is the strength of the magnetization vector along the z axis at any time. Any time the magnetization vector is displaced from the z axis it is no longer M_z (there may still be an M_z component). The displaced magnetization vector will be called M. M_z can never be greater than M_0, and is almost always less than M_0. Recognize that M_0 is a special condition of M_z. To jump a bit ahead, what is M_{xy}? When the magnetization vector (M) is displaced from the z axis, the component of the magnetization vector (M) that is in the xy plane is designated by the term M_{xy}.

Notice that step two mentions the magnetization vector M. The previous chapter led us into a detailed discussion of magnetic dipole moments, nuclear spins and spin energy states. These parameters are replaced with the magnetization vector M. In this chapter you will not encounter any discussion of MDM, spins, etc.—only the resulting magnetization vector. We hope our readers understand that the magnetization vector we so casually rotate about the main magnetic field is not simply a magic arrow that appears from nowhere. The magnetization vector is the result of some beautiful physics. Enough said, we return to the magnetization vector as a simple arrow that we will flip around with RF pulses and gradient fields.

The second step in MRI requires that we displace M so that it does not line up with H. In our discussion we will deal exclusively with imaging of hydrogen nuclei (protons). The magnetization vector, M, can be displaced by applying a second magnetic field which we call H_1. H_1 must be rotating at the Larmor frequency of hydrogen nuclei

H=1 TESLA

Figure 24–1 A patient in a 1-tesla magnetic field that is aligned along the Z axis. M_0 = longitudinal magnetization at equilibrium

in a 1-T magnetic field, which is 42.58 MHz. (Our choice of a 1-T magnet is arbitrary; it makes a nice even number). Where do we find a magnetic field that is varying 42,580,000 times per second? We turn on a radio transmitter and tune it to transmit at a frequency of 42.58 MHz (your FM radio works at a frequency of 88 to 108 MHz), hence the term "radio frequency (RF) pulse." **RF radiation is a form of electromagnetic radiation (EM).** In the first chapter of this book we remind you that EM radiation is made up of an electric field and magnetic field that mutually support each other. The magnetic field of RF radiation is exactly what we need. One chooses an RF pulse of proper frequency, strength, and duration to cause the M vector to rotate 90° relative to the z direction (a 90° pulse).

A note about which direction is which. By convention we use the letters x, y, and z to indicate directions in three dimensions. Refer to Figure 24–2. The z direction goes through the patient from foot to head (horizontal). The x direction goes across the patient from side to side (transverse). The y direction cuts through the patient from back to front (vertical). It is difficult to draw and visualize three dimensional lines on a sheet of paper. That is why we will often include a view of our patient in which we are looking directly at the top of her head.

At the end of a 90° RF pulse the magnetization vector will be oriented in the xy plane (this is 90° to the z axis). **We will call the component of the M vector in the xy plane M_{xy}.** At the end of a 90° pulse, the magnetization vector (M) is entirely in the xy plane, so that $M = M_{xy}$ and $M_z = 0$. Figure 24–3 shows a 9-voxel slice after a 90° pulse. Notice that all M_{xy} vectors have the same orientation (they are in phase), and the same frequency of precession.

Now step two is complete. A magnetic field, H_1, rotating at the necessary Larmor frequency, has rotated M away from z and into the xy plane. It is now time to shut off the H_1 magnetic field.

Step three is the signal-producing step, and begins when H_1 is turned off. The displaced M vector (M_{xy}) now sees only the magnetic field of our MR magnet (H), which is one T in our example. M_{xy} precesses around H at its Larmor frequency. Also, M returns to its equilibrium position along Z as M_{xy} diminishes toward zero and M_z increases from zero. How long does this processing and return to equilibrium take? The magnetization vector in the xy plane (M_{xy}) disappears very fast, gone in a few milliseconds. The recovery of M_z to equi-

Figure 24–2 Illustration of the x, y, and z planes from the longitudinal (A) and axial (B) perspectives

90° RF PULSE ON
Z (slice) GRADIENT ON

→ = M_{XY} MAGNETIZATION VECTOR

∿ = FREQUENCY OF PRECESSION
OF M_{XY} (Larmor frequency)

Figure 24–3 Slice selection with the Z gradient. All voxels have M_{xy} in phase and same frequency

librium magnetization takes much longer (up to about 15 sec for water) and varies with different tissues.

So here we are. The H_1 RF pulse is turned off. M_{xy} exists. M_{xy} can be detected. M_{xy} is precessing around the main magnetic field H at the Larmor frequency. **Only M_{xy} can be detected; the regrowth of M_z cannot be detected.** As M_{xy} precesses it constitutes a rotating magnetic field. This rotating magnetic field is detected by the same RF coil that was used to produce the H_1 field. After the 90° RF pulse, the RF coil is switched from the transmit to the receive mode. **The rotating M_{xy} magnetization vector induces a signal in the RF coil while the coil is in the receive mode.** The signal will be a radio frequency signal at the Larmor frequency. The signal decreases in intensity with time as M_{xy} decays. This signal is called the "free induction decay (FID)." Two facts about the FID are important. The FID is a very weak signal

compared to the 90° RF pulse. The FID decays very fast. Even though the RF coils can be switched from the transmit to the receive mode rapidly, much of the FID is lost before it can be detected. Because of these two problems (weak strength and rapid decay of the FID), special pulse sequences are used in MRI. We will discuss the spin echo sequence in some detail.

It is obvious that recording the FID from a large anatomic area of the patient does not produce an image. Our next chore is to divide the patient into voxels, and record the information from each voxel and display it as a pixel. This is roughly analogous to the way CT generates a cross section image. In CT one uses multiple detectors and a moving x-ray tube with a collimated beam to create voxels. In MRI nothing moves, so a different approach is required. We now consider gradient coils and varying the frequency of the RF pulses as the means of dividing the patient into slices, the slices into voxels, and displaying voxels as pixels. How the gradient coils and RF pulses produce voxel selection is the subject of the next few sections.

MAGNETIC FIELD GRADIENT COILS

Producing an image from the NMR signals (i.e., MRI) requires that a specific slice within the patient's body be examined, and that voxels be designated within the slice. The following discussion refers to transaxial imaging. Three functions select the slice and voxels:

1. A magnetic field gradient along the z axis is the slice selection gradient.
2. The Y-gradient produces phase encoding within the slice.
3. The X-gradient produces frequency encoding within the slice.

Slice Selection

Preparation for slice selection is done with a pair of magnetic field gradient coils. The coils produce a gradient along the z axis of the patient.

Typical gradient coil magnetic field strengths are 0.2 to 1.0 gauss per cm (.00002 to .0001 tesla per cm). Consider a 30-cm imaging volume, a 1-tesla magnet, and a gradient field of 1.0 gauss per cm. Magnetic field strength will vary from .9985 T toward the patient's feet, to 1.0015 toward the head, and will be 1.0000 T in the center of the imaging volume. Figure 24–4 shows the configuration of a pair of Z-gradient coils with a patient ready to be placed inside the coils. Remember that these coils are inside the bore of the magnet. The arrows on the coils indicate current flow. Use the right hand rule to convince yourself that the magnetic field induced by the left coil opposes (and thus weakens) the main H field, while the field induced by the right coil will reinforce the H field. These statements are valid only for the volume between the two coils, and inside the cylinder defined by their circumferences. Imaging is strictly limited to that portion of a patient's anatomy that is located within this sensitive volume between the coils. Figure 24–5 shows the Z-gradient coils surrounding a patient in a uniform 1-tesla magnetic field. When current flows in the coils, the Z-gradient exists. Our example of a 30-cm field with a gradient of 1.0 gauss per cm results in a .9985-T field strength in the plane of the left (caudad) coil, and a 1.0015-T field in the plane of the right (cephalad) coil.

The obvious question is now ready for an answer. How do we use the Z-gradient to pick a slice in the patient? Remember that the Larmor frequency is the product of the gyromagnetic ratio and magnet field strength:

$$\nu_L = \gamma H$$
ν_L = Larmor frequency (MHz)
γ = gyromagnetic ratio (MHz/T)
H = magnetic field (T)

We are only considering protons (hydrogen nuclei) for this imaging discussion. The gyromagnetic ratio of the proton is 42,800,000 cycles per second in a 1-T field (42.58 MHz/T). In a 1-tesla field, the Larmor frequency of the proton is:

$$(42,580,000) \times (1) = 42,580,000 \text{ Hz}$$

Now consider what the Z-gradient has done. It has put protons in slightly different magnetic fields, depending on the location of the proton in the patient. All protons in the plane of the left coil will be in the same (slightly reduced) magnetic field. Look at Figure 24–5. Protons in the 0.9985-T field will have a different Larmor frequency than those in the 1.0015-T field:

$$(42,580,000) \times (.9985) = 42,516,130 \text{ Hz}$$
$$(42,580,000) \times (1.0015) = 42,643,870 \text{ Hz}$$

Finally we are getting somewhere because protons (hydrogen nuclei) in different areas of the patient's body are behaving in

Z GRADIENT COILS
(Slice Selection)

Figure 24–4 Z-gradient coils

H=1 TESLA   1 cm CROSS
             SECTION SLICE

Z GRADIENT
COILS

.9985 TESLA ← → 1.0015 TESLA
      Z GRADIENT

SLICE

Hz Hz

Figure 24–5 Z-gradient coils change the magnetic field along the z axis. This gradient is used for slice selection

different ways. We can take advantage of this difference.

Remember that a proton precessing at a certain Larmor frequency will respond to an RF pulse only if the RF pulse frequency is exactly the same as the Larmor frequency.

The mechanism for slice selection is now clear. Apply a Z-gradient so protons in one slice precess at a unique Larmor frequency, different from all other protons in the imaging field. Tip the resulting magnetization (M) vector with a 90° RF pulse that matches the unique Larmor frequency. In Figure 24–5, the gradient is 1.0 gauss (.0001 T) per cm. Assume a 1-cm thick slice. Calculate the Larmor frequency along each side of the slice if the magnetic field varies from 1.0010 T to 1.0011 T across the slice:

$$(42{,}580{,}000) \times (1.0011) = 42{,}626{,}838 \text{ Hz}$$
$$(42{,}580{,}000) \times (1.0010) = 42{,}622{,}580 \text{ Hz}$$

In our example, a 1-cm slice is represented by a Larmor frequency difference of 4258 Hz (or 4.258 kHz). To select the slice in question, the RF transmitter is tuned to

transmit frequencies from a low of about 42.6226 mHz to a high of about 42.6268 mHz. A 90° pulse transmitted at this frequency range will cause the m vector to rotate 90° in only the 1-cm slice in question. In a 1-tesla magnet with a gradient of 1.0 gauss per cm, an RF pulse width of 4.258 kHz will select a 1-cm wide slice, whereas a 2.129-kHz pulse width will select a 0.5-cm wide slice. **Thus, the frequency of the RF pulse selects the location of slice, and the band width of the RF pulse selects the thickness of the slice.**

We hope it is now quite clear how the H field, the Z-gradient field, and the RF pulse work in harmony to select the level and thickness of a cross-sectional slice of the patient's anatomy. The Z-gradient is tiny compared to the field strength of the main magnet (0.1 to 1 gauss per cm. versus 10,000 gauss in our example). This is the reason that MRI magnets must have such perfect fields. Very small variations in field strength of the large magnet would obscure the small additions or subtractions caused by the weak gradient field. As we will explore in a few pages, gradient coils must be switched on and off rapidly during an MRI sequence. Coils are resistive electromagnets. The clicking sound heard during MRI is produced by the switching of gradient coils.

Another note about RF pulses is in order. We speak of pulse band width as if it were controlled to within 1 Hz of the desired frequency. In fact, the RF pulse is not so precise. Some frequencies above and below the desired frequency span will be contained in the pulse. These undesired frequencies will cause tissues outside the intended slice volume to respond to the RF signal. The undesired signal resulting from this "slice crosstalk" will degrade the image. For this reason, it is common practice to always leave a gap between slices in MRI (recall that CT scans frequently use contiguous slices or even allow slice overlap). As a general rule, a gap of about 30% is often used for 5 mm or thicker slices, and a gap of about 50% for slices less than 5 mm thick.

Let us review where we are in the formation of an image using the spin echo technique. The patient is in a uniform H field. Use of a Z-gradient electromagnetic coil and an RF 90° pulse of appropriate frequency range has tipped the magnetization vector 90° in a specific slice. Figure 24–3 is a diagram of a slice after slice selection. The slice is divided into 9 voxels (a 3 × 3 matrix). Notice that in each voxel the M_{xy} magnetization is pointed in the same direction (M_{xy} is in phase in all voxels), and the frequency of precession of M_{xy} is exactly the same in each voxel. It is now time to examine how we can change the phase and frequency of precession to give each voxel a unique signal. Keep in mind that a clinical image may be a slice that contains 256 × 256, or 65,536 voxels.

What is phase? We feel that a brief explanation of phase will allow a better concept of what phase encoding means.

First, look at Figure 24–6. The solid lines represent an M_{xy} vector that is rotating (clockwise) in a circle in the x-y plane. If the size of M_{xy} remains constant during this rotation, the tip of the vector will subscribe a circle. We can represent the position of the tip in time as a sine wave function. Note in Figure 24–6 we have to choose where the tip is at time equal zero (we have chosen point A to represent time equal zero). The figure indicates the position during one complete circle (rotation is in the direction of A to B to C). Notice that the solid M_{xy} vector is pointed toward 0° at time equal 0, and the sine wave generated by this vector begins at the intersection of the x and y axes on the graph. (Had we chosen D as the starting point, a cosine function would be generated and would be just as valid. If you don't know the difference between sine waves and cosine waves don't worry about it.)

The concept of phase is used to describe the relative position, or direction, of two vectors. So let us put in another M_{xy} vector as a dashed line in Figure 24–6. At time 0, the angle between the solid M_{xy} vector and the dashed M_{xy} is 45°. The phase difference between solid M_{xy} and dashed M_{xy} is 45° (one may also say that the phase angle between these two vectors is 45°). The dashed M_{xy} vector (rotating in a clockwise direction) generates the dashed sine wave in Figure 24–6. Since the two vectors are rotating at exactly the same frequency and have exactly the same magnitude, the generated sine wave curves differ only in phase (and the phase difference is the same at any point along the curves). **So, phase does nothing more than define the relative position of the vectors at a given time.** This is exactly the situation that exists at the end of a phase encoding pulse, as illustrated in Figure 24–7. Assume that each M_{xy} vector in Figure 24–6 rotates inside an RF coil in which each vector induces an alternating electric current. The electronics that detect these currents are able to detect and keep

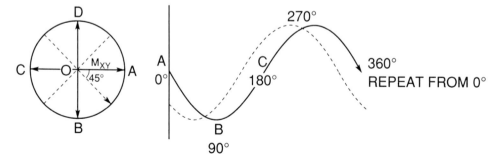

Figure 24–6 Sine curves A and A′ are 45° out of phase

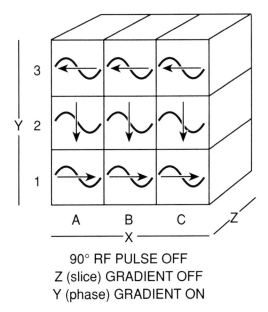

90° RF PULSE OFF
Z (slice) GRADIENT OFF
Y (phase) GRADIENT ON

Figure 24–7 Phase encoding with the Y gradient. All voxels have the same frequency. Each row (1,2,3) has a unique phase

track of the phase angle difference between the two signals. This phase angle difference is the reason for phase encoding. **Phase encoding is the first step in dividing a slice into voxels for purposes of image reconstruction.**

Phase Encoding

The unusual shape of the Y- (and X-) gradient coils is dictated by two considerations. First, one must maintain cylindrical symmetry so we can place a patient inside the coils. Second, this design allows us to have a field in the z direction that changes values along y (the Y-gradient). The configuration as shown in Figure 24–8 is called

a "Goley coil." The effective gradient is confined to the gap between the two pairs of coils.

A glance at Figure 24–7 will allow a preview of what phase encoding in the y-axis will accomplish. Direct your attention to rows 1, 2, and 3. Notice that the phase (direction) of the M_{xy} vector has changed in rows 2 and 3. Each row has a unique phase, and each voxel in one row has the same phase. We no longer have identical voxels.

Within the strict limits of our example, the Y-gradient is the phase-encoding gradient. The purpose of phase encoding is to set different phases throughout the slice. Figure 24–7 suggests that MRI divides a slice into individual voxels just like CT. Such a picture allows one to develop a mental picture of image formation, but the picture is really not correct. In MRI the computer stores phase and frequency information as it is accumulated, then reconstructs the image by mathematical manipulation of the data. It is a complex process that does not lend itself to simple illustration. In the next section, a gradient in the x direction will complete the division.

A y-axis magnetic field gradient is applied in a fashion similar to the z-axis gradient. Two pairs of Y-gradient coils (4 coils total) are positioned as shown in Figure 24–9 (the Z-gradient required only one pair of coils). You may right hand rule the arrows in Figure 24–8 to verify the gradient shown in Figure 24–9. Alignment of the coils changes the magnetic field strength from the back to the front of the patient. When the Y-gradient coils are on, the protons near the front of the patient

Figure 24–8 Y-gradient coils

Figure 24–9 Y-gradient coils change the magnetic field through the patient from back to front. This gradient is usually used for phase encoding

will precess faster (because they are in a higher magnetic field) than those protons near the back of the patient. The Y-gradient is turned on at the end of the 90° RF pulse, and is left on for a short time (about 3 to 5 ms).

The purpose of the Y-gradient is to change the phase of the magnetization vectors in each row of the slice being imaged. Look at Figure 24–9. When the Y-gradient is on, protons near the front of the patient are in a stronger magnetic field than those near the back of the patient. In Figure 24–7, row 1 is assumed to be about in the middle of the patient (where there is little or no gradient), and row 3 near the front of the patient where the gradient is positive and at a maximum. Since row 3 is in the strongest magnetic field, all its protons will precess faster than will the protons in row 2 or row 1. We show the effect by showing the M_{xy} in row 2 is 90° ahead of row 1, and the M_{xy} vector in row 3 is 180° ahead of row 1. Now the Y-gradient is suddenly turned off. Immediately, all protons in rows 1, 2, and 3 begin to precess at the same rate (determined by the main magnetic field H). But, each M_{xy} vector "remembers" and maintains the phase at

which it was precessing at the end of the Y-gradient pulse. This row-by-row phase difference has divided the previously uniform slice into horizontal rows. **At the end of a Y-gradient pulse, all M_{xy} vectors are precessing at the same rate, but not all M_{xy} vectors are in the same phase.**

Frequency Encoding

The Z-gradient allowed slice selection. The Y-gradient allowed each slice to be phase encoded.

Now an X-gradient is going to allow each slice to be divided by frequency encoding.

The X-gradient coils look like the Y-gradient coils, rotated 90° (Figure 24–10). The purpose of the X-gradient is easy to understand. At the end of the Y-gradient all M_{xy} vectors return to precessing at the Larmor frequency associated with the main magnetic field, H. The purpose of the X-gradient is to change, very slightly, the magnetic field in the imaging volume to create a gradient along the x axis (Figure 24–11). In our illustration, the main magnetic field is reduced on the patient's right side and increased on the left side. The X-gradient will cause the protons in different vertical columns (columns A, B, and C in

Figure 24–10 Frequency encoding with the X gradient. Each voxel now has a unique M_{xy}. Each row (1,2,3) has a unique phase, each column (A,B,C) has a unique frequency

Figure 24–12) to experience slightly different magnetic fields. Protons in different magnetic fields will precess at different frequencies. This is shown in Figure 24–12, with the magnetization vectors in column A precessing slower than those in column B.

The X-gradient is the frequency-encoding gradient. In our example, frequency encoding provides a way to divide the slice into vertical columns. The Y-gradient uses phase encoding to divide the slice into horizontal rows.

We can now select a slice, and phase and frequency encode the slice. The next task is to combine the gradients (X, Y, and Z) with RF pulses in order to obtain resonance information that can be used to form the image. **The way in which the RF coil and gradient fields are turned on and off is called a "pulse sequence."** We will next describe the pulse sequence for the spin echo technique.

THE SPIN ECHO IMAGING SEQUENCE

It is now time to assemble the RF pulses and magnetic field gradients into a temporal package that will allow acquisition of an image. The spin echo pulse sequence with 2D-FT transformation is most commonly used in clinical imaging. Abbreviations to be used in this section include:

RF = radio frequency pulse
G_z = z axis magnetic gradient (slice selection)
G_y = y axis magnetic gradient (phase encoding)
G_x = x axis magnetic gradient (frequency encoding)

Figure 24–11 X-gradient coils

90° RF PULSE OFF
Z (slice) GRADIENT OFF
Y (phase) GRADIENT OFF
X (frequency) GRADIENT ON

Figure 24–12 X-gradient coils change the magnetic field through the patient from side to side. This gradient is usually used for frequency encoding and is the readout gradient

Look at Figure 24–13. This is a line diagram of the timing of the components of the spin echo sequence. For convenience, the sequence is divided into 5 segments for purposes of ease of discussion.

The pulse sequence begins during segment 1 (Figure 24–13). Notice that the slice selection Z-gradient (G_z) is applied slightly before the 90° RF pulse tips the magnetization vector into the xy plane. Remember, **G_z and the 90° degree RF pulse working as a team control the level and thickness of the axial slice of tissue** from which the image will be formed. At the end of the 90° pulse, slice selection is complete and G_z is removed. Remember that the RF must be at the resonance (Larmor) frequency of the selected slice in order to tip the magnetization vector. Therefore, the RF pulse will tip M only in one slice.

When G_z is removed, the 90° tipped magnetization vector in each voxel will begin to precess at the Larmor frequency dictated by the main magnetic field, H. However,

the phase encoding gradient (G_y) is immediately applied (segment 2, Figure 24–13) to allow phase encoding along the y-axis. The peculiar way G_y is drawn in Figure 24–13 serves to remind us that the magnitude of G_y is changed many times during an entire image acquisition (we show only 2 G_y values). One complete spin echo image, using a 2D-FT 256 × 256 matrix, will require 256 separate spin echo sequences. (The reason for 256 will be discussed later.) Each sequence requires a different value of G_y. The gradient pulses G_z and G_y are on for a short time; a time of about 5 ms for each would be a very rough typical estimate.

During segment 1 of the spin echo pulse an RF pulse and G_z allow slice selection. During segment 2, G_y produces phase encoding. When G_y is turned off, protons once again begin precessing about H at the Larmor frequency. Dephasing of protons begins as a result of T_2^*, and an FID is produced. But we choose not to detect the FID. Instead, preparation for an echo is made by applying a 180° pulse (the 180° pulse occurs in segment 3, Fig. 24–13).

For the spin echo sequence, the NMR signal that is acquired to make an image is the **"echo"** which occurs after the 180° pulse. A couple of considerations make the echo attractive as the detected signal. First, the echo occurs a considerable time after the RF pulse, which gives time for appropriate electronic switching. Second, the time of echo formation (TE) is determined by the time between the 90° and the 180° pulse, which allows producing images that contain T_1 and T_2 information (much more on this topic will follow).

Return to Figure 24–13. Note that the 180° RF pulse is applied during segment 3 of the pulse sequence. The slice selection gradient (G_z) is on during the 180° RF pulse. The echo is detected during segment 4 of the pulse sequence. During echo detection, the frequency encoding gradient, G_x, is turned on. Since G_x on during de-

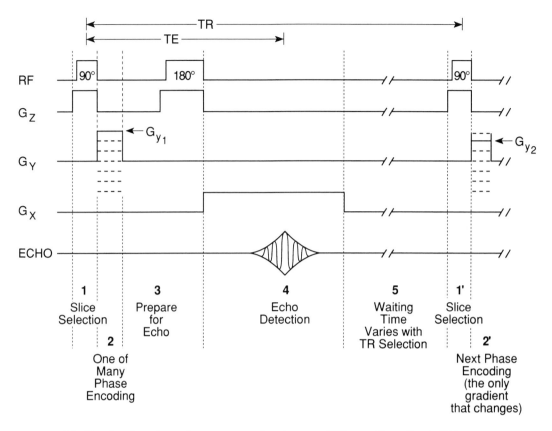

Figure 24–13 A spin echo pulse sequence showing two different Y gradients (G_y)

tection, or "reading," of the echo; **G_x is often called the "readout gradient."**

Segment 5 of Figure 24–13 is the long interval following the readout of the echo, before another 90% pulse starts the sequence all over again. Figure 24–13 shows segment 5 to be a time of inactivity. In real life, this is a time of frantic activity which we will explore under the heading of multiple slice acquisition. Times 1' and 2' start another pulse sequence with a different G_y. Many, up to 256, pulse sequences provide data for a single image.

TE and TR

TE and TR are such important parts of the spin echo sequence that we give them their own special heading. The significance of these two terms is, fortunately, easy to understand.

The time interval between each 90° pulse in an imaging sequence is called the "TR interval." TR is shorthand for time of repetition. TR is measured from one 90° pulse to the following 90° pulse. In most clinical spin echo pulse sequences, the TR interval varies between roughly 500 ms (0.5 sec) and 2000 to 3000 ms (2 to 3 sec). Actually, anything over 2000 ms is a very long TR. The TR interval has an important influence on tissue contrast, and we will examine this later in the chapter. The TR interval also determines the time required to acquire an image. Let's look at TE, then return to image acquisition time.

TE is shorthand for time to echo. **The TE time is the time from the middle of the 90° RF pulse to the peak of the detected echo** (see Fig. 24–13). The time from the middle of the 90° RF pulse to the middle of the 180° rephasing RF pulse is exactly TE/2. This means that it takes as long for the protons to rephase as the time they were allowed to dephase. Therefore, TE is selectable by selecting the time between the 90° pulse and the 180° pulse. Typical TE times vary from 30 ms to about 150 ms in most clinical imaging. Thus, TE intervals are much shorter than TR intervals. The TE time is, like TR, an important determinant of contrast in the MR image.

How long does it take to acquire one complete MR image? The answer depends on how the image is acquired. Remember that a single echo acquisition does not provide enough information to reconstruct an image. Consider an image displayed using a 256 × 256 matrix (displayed as 65,536 pixels). The mathematics of the image formation process require that a 256 × 256 matrix be produced by 256 different signal acquisitions. The word **different** is vital. Not only must one complete image be formed from 256 signal acquisitions, it must be formed from 256 different signal acquisitions. Now we return to the function of the phase encoding gradient, G_y. Recall that G_y is varied each time a new signal (i.e., a new spin echo sequence) is generated. This means that one complete image is formed from 256 different spin echo acquisitions, each spin echo acquisition differing from the others in the magnitude of the G_y magnetic field gradient. The spin echo sequence shown in Figure 24–13 would be repeated 256 times to allow formation of one cross sectional image. To calculate the time needed to acquire 256 signal acquisitions, one must obviously multiply the time for one signal acquisition by 256. How long does it take to acquire one signal? The answer is that it requires one TR interval. An example may help.

How long does it take to acquire a spin echo image using a 256 × 256 matrix and a TR of (a) 500 ms and (b) 2000 ms?

(a) 256 × 0.5 sec = 128 sec = 2 min 8 sec
(b) 256 × 2.0 sec = 512 sec = 8 min 32 sec

Now the influence of TR on imaging time becomes easy to understand. A long TR means a long time to acquire an image. In clinical practice, two (sometimes four or more) signals are averaged to provide the final image. Averaging provides a better signal-to-noise-ratio, a topic for more discussion later in this chapter. Averaging two signals will double imaging time. An image using a TR of 2000 ms and two signal averaging will require about 17 min to acquire using a 256 × 256 matrix. To summarize acquisition time:

$$\text{Time} = G_y \text{ steps} \times \text{TR} \times \text{Averages}$$

Image Reconstruction

The entire process of MRI is obviously the formation of an image. The imaging technique that we have discussed is a two-dimensional Fourier transform (2D-FT) spin echo technique. This technique includes phase encoding, frequency encoding, and the spin echo pulse sequence. The big trick is to perform a Fourier transform in the frequency direction and then a Fourier transform in the phase direction (these are the two dimensions of the 2D-FT). These transforms are performed within the system computer. Since computers work on a binary system, we normally expect the computer to give us information in a pixel format that is based on powers of two (2^n). For example, the computer may digitize the continuously varying frequency in the echo signal into 256 discrete frequency values ($256 = 2^8$). To obtain equal resolution throughout the image, it is necessary to have 256 different phase divisions as well as the 256 frequency divisions. These phase divisions are accomplished by varying the G_y gradient 256 times per image. From these two transforms the computer can form the final image, and assign display values to selected pixel sizes. We realize that this is a superficial description of the computer's task, but we do not apologize for not going into it in more detail.

There are other display formats than 256 × 256, but all are based on powers of 2. The most common is a 128 × 128 format

$(128 = 2^7)$. There is a hybrid matrix of 128 × 256 that is sometimes used because it requires only 128 phase-encoded echoes (fewer echoes saves time). These power-of-2 numbers are also used to determine the display matrix of CT images, even though CT and MR images are collected in entirely different fashions (the computer is the same in both).

By convention, a strong MR signal is displayed as white on the CRT or film, whereas a weak MR signal is displayed as dark gray or black. Pixel brightness is a term used to indicate the strength of the MR signal assigned to each pixel. Pixel brightness can be manipulated by the operator in the choice of TR and TE values.

MULTISLICE IMAGING

As we have already mentioned, the time required for acquisition of an image may be quite long. For example, the time to acquire an image using a 256 × 256 matrix, a TR of 2.0 sec and two signal averages is:

256 × 2.0 sec × 2 signals = 1024 sec
= 17 min 4 sec

One might shorten acquisition time by acquiring only one signal, but this increases noise (more about noise shortly). One may also shorten scan time by using a shorter TR, but this would change contrast and might result in a less desirable image. A smaller matrix (128 × 128) will also shorten scan time, but decreases resolution by using larger voxels.

Assume we are struck with a 17-min scan time. A typical MRI head scan will contain at least 10 slices, often more. Obtaining 10 slices one at a time would require 170 min, or about 3 hours of scan time.

There is a way to acquire all the slices at one time, called "multislice imaging." This technique takes advantage of the long waiting time required by the TR interval. If the TR interval is 2000 ms, and the TE is 90 ms, there is about 1900 ms of free time between the end of the echo and the next 90° pulse. It is this long wait, imposed by the long TR, that allows multislice imaging.

Since the Z-gradient is turned on during both the 90° RF and 180° RF pulse, only the one slice (where Larmor resonance exists) is excited by these two RF pulses. All other regions in the imaging volume remain undisturbed by these two RF pulses. After the echo is detected (in our example with TE of 90 ms, the echo develops after 90 ms), one may obtain an image from another slice while waiting for the TR time to pass. Turn the Z-gradient back on and apply a 90° RF and 180° RF pulse with an appropriate Larmor frequency for the new slice. Of course, the appropriate phase encoding and frequency encoding gradients must be applied for each slice. In fact, it is possible to image many slices in consecutive fashion during the long TR interval. This is why we mention period 5 of Figure 24–13 as a time of frantic activity. Figure 24–14 is a simplified drawing showing the RF pulses and echoes for three slices using the multislice spin echo technique. The illustration does not show the application of the gradients.

The number of slices that can be obtained with the multislice technique depends on both TR and TE. A new slice cannot be excited until the echo from the previous slice has been completely detected. Use of a long TE or a short TR will mean less time for multiple slices. The precise number of slices that can be acquired in one sequence varies with different instruments. Three examples used in our department will illustrate the principles.

TR (ms)	TE (ms)	Multiple Slices
500	40	7
2000	90	16
2000	120	14

Multislice techniques are a trick that can be used to acquire multiple consecutive image slices during the time required for a single slice. Total imaging time is shortened tremendously with the technique.

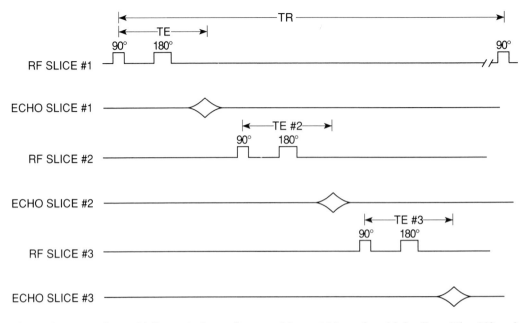

Figure 24–14 The multislice technique allows rapid acquisition of multiple slices. The 90° and 180° RF pulses have appropriate Larmor frequency for each slice

Unfortunately, the excitation process causes some spillover that involves protons in adjacent slices. "Slice crosstalk" was discussed earlier in this chapter. Often, a gap is left between slices to eliminate the overlap area. The image is degraded when the spillover areas are included in the imaging volume of a slice. As a general rule, a gap of about 30% is used between slices for 5 mm or thicker slices, and a gap of about 50% for slices less than 5 mm thick. For 10-mm thick slices, a gap of about 3 mm of nonimaged tissue between slices is commonly allowed.

MULTIECHO IMAGING

It is often useful to have a series of images made with different spin echo (TE) times. For example, one of the most common head imaging techniques used in our department calls for a TR of 2000 ms with TE of 30, 60, and 90 ms, and two image averaging. Acquisition time for this image (TR = 2000 ms, two image averaging) requires 17 min. If a new image were acquired for each of the three TE times,

imaging times would be prohibitively prolonged.

A technique called "multiecho imaging" allows one to obtain two or three images with different TE times during the same time interval required for one image (the TR is the same for all images).

Figure 24–15 is a simplified diagram of a multiecho acquisition using a TR of 2000 ms, and TE of 30, 60, and 90 ms. Exactly 15 ms after the 90° RF pulse a 180° RF pulse is given, providing an echo at 30 ms (TE = 30 ms). Then exactly 15 ms after the first echo, another 180° pulse is given and a second echo is produced at 60 ms. Similarly, a third echo is produced at 90 ms by an appropriately timed third 180° RF pulse. All the 30 ms pulses (256 pulses with a 256 × 256 matrix) are collected to make one image, the 60 ms pulses a second image, and the 90 ms pulses to make a third image. All three images can be obtained in the same imaging sequence.

Notice in Figure 24–15 that the amplitude (i.e., signal strength) of the echo decreases with lengthening TE time. This is

Figure 24–15 The multiecho technique allows acquisition of more than one TE echo from one slice during one TR time period

the effect of continued T_2 dephasing. Because the early echo yields the strongest signal, the early echo will have the best signal-to-noise ratio. Images obtained from echoes with longer TE intervals will contain more noise, but will show greater image contrast. Contrast and noise are such important aspects of the MR image that we will devote the next two sections of this chapter to these topics.

Use of the multiecho technique does not preclude the simultaneous use of the multislice technique of image acquisitions. In fact, most imaging pulse sequences routinely use both techniques. The most common imaging pulse sequence used in MRI is multislice, multiecho spin echo imaging.

CONTRAST

All NMR signals are a measure of the value of M_{xy} (the transverse magnetization) at the time of detection. Anything that will influence the size of the M_{xy} magnetization vector will influence the NMR image. It seems rather obvious that the value of M_{xy} will depend on the number of protons that contribute to the total detected magnetization vector. Some protons respond to the RF signals, but their return to equilibrium is so fast that we do not notice the NMR signal in clinical imaging sequences. For ex-

ample, bone cortex shows no signal, but bone cortex contains protons. These cortical protons do respond to the NMR conditions, but have very short T_1 and T_2 times and are back in the equilibrium state before our imaging system is ready to respond to the signal. With clinical NMR pulse sequences, one is generally imaging protons that are present in biologic liquid states. **The concentration of detectable hydrogen nuclei in a biologic tissue is usually termed the spin density of the tissue.** The strength of M_{xy} is also determined by its decay characteristics (this is characterized by T_2), and how long after its formation it is detected (this is determined by TE). One other thing we need to notice is that the initial magnitude of M_{xy} is determined by the number of excess protons that are in the low energy (spin-up) state. This number is different from the equilibrium condition if we have disturbed the spin densities (i.e., following a 90° pulse before M_z has returned to its equilibrium condition). This is the reason that T_1 and TR play a role in the image formation.

In an MR image the intensity of the signal obtained from a tissue is related to:

PROTON DENSITY

T_1 TIME

T_2 TIME

The single most important advantage of MRI is excellent contrast resolution. Differences in proton density, T_1, and T_2 between tissues are significantly greater than differences in electron density and x-ray linear attenuation coefficients between the same tissues. This discussion will be limited to the spin echo technique. We must examine how differences in T_1 and T_2 relaxation times of tissues combine with the TR and TE times of the pulse sequence to create a pixel with a large signal (white) or a small signal (black). Examples will be mostly limited to differences between brain tissue and cerebrospinal fluid (CSF).

Spin echo images are not purely spin density or T_1 or T_2 images. All images have contributions from all three of these parameters, but images may have a predominance of T_1 or T_2 information. It is customary to refer to these as T_1-weighted and T_2-weighted images. It is a complicated problem, but let's give it a try.

Proton Density

When a patient is placed in an imaging magnet, hydrogen nuclei (protons) align in the magnetic field to produce the equilibrium magnetization vector M_0. For any tissue, the magnitude of M_0 will depend on the number of protons per unit volume that the tissue contains. This proton concentration is called the "proton density" of the tissue.

A related term is spin density. **Spin density is a measure of the relative concentration of protons that contribute to the detected MR signal.** In clinical imaging, spin density is the important characteristic. Figure 24–16 is a diagram showing a rough approximation of the spin density of CSF, brain white matter, and gray matter. All spin densities are compared to water.

Spin density is the basis of the NMR image (without protons there is no signal). Since T_1 and T_2 also determine the magnitude of M_{xy}, one cannot predict the image brightness of a tissue by knowing its relative proton density. The pulse sequence also

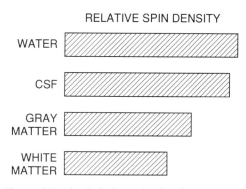

Figure 24–16 Relative spin density

has a great deal to do with the detected signal. With the pulse sequence used in the spin echo technique, the TR time is of such a length that most spin densities do not have a chance to return to equilibrium. This means that M_z is going to be somewhat less than M_0. As a matter of fact, after about 4 spin echo pulse sequences, a new equilibrium value for the longitudinal magnetization of each tissue is established (that is, M_z is less than M_0). The new equilibrium is determined mainly by the TR of the pulse sequence and the T_1 of the tissue.

> Spin density determines M_0
> Spin density, TR, and T_1 determine M_z
> M_z determines the magnitude of M_{xy}

Figure 24–17 is a spin density weighted image (TR 3000 ms, TE 40 ms) of the brain. Notice that the gray matter has a brighter signal than white matter. This reflects the fact that gray matter has a proton density about 20% higher than white matter. All spin echo images contain a proton density contribution. As this section progresses we will try to explain why a TR of 3000 ms and TE of 40 ms produces a spin density weighted image.

T_1 and T_2 Weighted Images

Spin echo pulse sequences can provide images that reflect mainly the T_1 values of tissues, or images based mostly on T_2 values. The images are usually very different.

What is T_1? Recall from Chapter 23 that T_1 is a reflection of the time required for

Figure 24–17 A proton density weighted image showing gray matter (20% higher spin density) to have a stronger signal than white matter

the longitudinal component of magnetization to regrow following a 90° RF pulse. At equilibrium, the M vector will be at a maximum value (M_0). After a 90° RF pulse, the M_z vector becomes zero (and M_{xy} is at a maximum). When the 90° RF pulse stops, the M_z vector begins to return. If M_z regrows to its original value, M_z will equal M_0. T_1 is the time required for the regrowing M_z vector to regain 63% of its original value. The number 63% results from the regrowth being exponential. For example, in tissue with a T_1 of 1000 ms, M_z will obtain 63% of the value of M_0 in 1 sec. A T_1 of 500 ms will regrow to 63% of M_0 in ½ sec, and a T_1 of 2000 requires 2 sec to regain 63%. Table 24–1 lists the percent regrowth of M_z after a time interval of 0.5, 1, 1.5, 2, 3, 4 and 5 T_1 periods. This concept of regrowth of M_z with time is very important.

A few examples will emphasize the concept.

Assume a tissue has a T_1 value of 500 ms. After a 90° pulse, what fraction of M_z will have regrown after (a) ½ sec, (b) 1 sec, (c) 2 sec?

(a) ½ sec = 1 T_1 = 63% regrowth
(b) 1 sec = 2 T_1 = 86% regrowth
(c) 2 sec = 4 T_1 = 98% regrowth

Table 24–1. Regrowth of Longitudinal Magnetization, M_z, Relative to T_1 Periods (after a 90° pulse)

NO. OF T_1 INTERVALS	REGROWTH OF M_z
0.5	39%
1.0	63%
1.5	78%
2.0	86%
3.0	95%
4.0	98%
5.0	99%

Now it is time to relate T_1 and the TR time of a spin echo pulse sequence. A 90° RF pulse starts the spin echo sequence. At the end of the 90° pulse M_z is zero. During the period TR (i.e., the time until the next 90° pulse), the M_z vector regrows toward equilibrium. When the next 90° RF pulse is applied the magnitude of M_{xy} will be directly related to the magnitude of M_z at the time the pulse was applied. A higher strength M_{xy} means a stronger echo signal.

Let's go to an example to explore what effect T_1 and TR have on the signal strength from two tissues. Brain tissue has a T_1 of about 500 ms, and CSF has a T_1 of about 3000 ms (in an 0.5 T magnet). Using a TR of 2000 ms, what will be the relative magnitude of M_z for brain and CSF at the end of a TR time of 2000 ms? In 2000 ms, brain tissue will recover for about four T_1 periods, or about 98% of its M_z maximum. On the other hand, CSF will have had time to recover for only ⅔ of one T_1 time, which amounts to about 49% of its maximum M_z value. Since both brain tissue and CSF have about the same spin density levels, a spin echo pulse sequence using a TR of 2000 ms will allow brain tissue to show about twice the signal strength as does CSF (if only T_1 is considered). Fat has a T_1 of about 200 ms, so fat will regain M_z strength at a very fast rate after a 90° pulse. Table 24–2 lists fat (T_1 = 200 ms), brain (T_1 = 500 ms), and CSF (T_1 = 3000 ms) and compares the regrowth of M_z for TR times of 500 to 10,000 ms.

Consider Table 24–2. Notice at a short TR (500 ms) there is a large difference in the M_z regrowth of the three different tissues. At a TR of 1000 ms, fat and brain are close to the same, and at a TR of 2000 fat

and brain are the same. CSF, with its very long T_1, is quite slow to regrow. M_z does not reach 96% until 10,000 ms, which is 3⅓ T_1 times. Some basic facts emerge as one studies Table 24–2:

1. With a short TR, tissue T_1 differences are reflected in different signal strengths.
2. With a long TR, tissue T_1 differences have little influence on relative signal strengths.
3. Tissues with a short T_1 recover signal strength rapidly after a 90° RF pulse.
4. Tissues with a long T_1 recover signal strength slowly after a 90° RF pulse.

A spin echo sequence that allows tissue T_1 values to influence the strength of the echo signal is called a T_1-weighted sequence. **A spin echo sequence with a short TR will produce a T_1-weighted image.** A sequence using a a short TR (such as 500 ms) will be T_1-weighted. Tissues with a short T_1 time (such as fat and brain) will produce bright signals in short TR sequences. Figure 24–18 is a sagittal view of the head obtained with a TR of 500 ms. Notice that the subcutaneous fat (T_1 of 200 ms) has a very bright signal. Brain (T_1 of 500 ms) has a moderately bright signal. CSF (T_1 of 3000 ms) is black because it produces almost no signal.

Ail this stuff about T_1 and TR is fine. Unfortunately there are still T_2 and TE to consider. These two parameters can produce change in the image as dramatic as the T1-TR parameters. Understanding MR images is difficult because the T_1-TR pair causes one influence, and the T_2-TE pair another influence on the final image. We will move on to T_2 in a minute.

Table 24–2. Regrowth of M_z as a Function of Tissue T_1 Time and Pulse Sequence TR Time

	T_1 VALUE (ms)	REGROWTH OF M_z TR (ms)					
		500	1000	2000	3000	5000	10,000
Fat	200	92%	99%	99%	99%	99%	99%
Brain	200	63%	86%	98%	99%	99%	99%
CSF	3000	22%	28%	49%	63%	81%	99%

Figure 24–18 A T_1-weighted image reflects the T_1 values of fat (200 ms), brain (500 ms), and CSF (3000 ms)

Table 24–3 lists some T_1 values contained in the literature. The values are listed for both 0.5-tesla and 1.0-tesla magnet strengths. We fudged a bit in giving fat a T_1 value of 200, and brain a T_1 of 500. Notice that T_1 may be longer in a stronger magnetic field. The T_1 value of fat is minimally influenced by magnetic field strength.

T_1 Weighted Images. A T_1-weighted image allows tissue T_1 values to play the

Table 24–3. Tissue T_1 Characteristics

	T_1 (ms)	
TISSUE	0.5 TESLA	1.0 TESLA
Fat	220	220
Brain	600	860
CSF	3000	3000

major role in determining whether the tissue develops a bright or dark image. Tissues with longer T_1 values (relative to TR) will produce darker images than those tissues with a shorter T_1. Remember that both TR and TE times must be selected to make an image. We will deal with the selection of TE later in the chapter. Brightness in the image is related to a strong echo signal. If T_1 is to determine the brightness with which the tissue is displayed, then T_1 must influence the signal strength. We would like to examine how T_1 can influence the size of M_{xy}, the producer of the signal.

T_2-Weighted Images. A T_2-weighted image allows tissue T_2 values to play the major role in determining whether the tissue develops a bright or dark image. Tissues with long T_2 values will produce brighter images than those with shorter T_2 values (note the difference between this and T_1 weighting). If T_2 is to determine the brightness with which a tissue is displayed, then T_2 must influence the strength of the signal. We will now examine how T_2 can influence the size of M_{xy}, the producer of the signal (you read this same thing at the beginning of the T_1 weighting section).

After a 90° RF pulse, the magnetization vector M is tipped 90° into the xy plane. The FID generated by M_{xy} is ignored, and the echo generated after the 180° refocusing pulse is detected. The TE (time to echo) is the time from the 90° RF pulse to the peak of the detected echo (review Fig. 24–13). TE is selected by determining when to apply the 180° rephasing pulse. Typical TE times are between 30 and 120 ms. We have said all this before, but a little repetition never hurts.

What happens to M_{xy} when the 90° RF pulse is turned off? M_{xy} precesses about H at the Larmor frequency with decreasing strength because of T_2 dephasing. How fast does M_{xy} decrease? M_{xy} decays in an exponential fashion with a time constant T_2 (the spin-spin relaxation time). Use of the spin echo sequence allows us to deal with T_2 rather than T_2^*. How long is T_2? T_2 is different for different tissues. T_2 is generally not dependent on magnetic field strength. For a given material, T_2 will vary from magnet to magnet. Published values of tissue T_2 times will show considerable variation. Table 24–4 lists some typical T_2 values for fat, brain, and CSF. (Notice that we do not separate brain into white and gray matter for simplicity.) In biologic tissues, T_2 is always shorter than T_1. At the end of one T_2 time period there will be 37% of the initial M_{xy} remaining (this is also described as a 63% loss of M_{xy}). Decrease of M_{xy} to 37% of its maximum value will require 60 ms for fat, 70 ms for brain, and 2000 ms for CSF (see Table 24–4). M_{xy} of brain tissue will decrease to 37% of maximum in 70 ms, to 14% (.37 × .37) of max-

Table 24–4. Tissue T_2 Characteristics

TISSUE	T_2 (ms)
Fat	60
Brain	70
CSF	2000

imum in 140 ms, and 5% of maximum in 210 ms. Table 24–5 lists the value of M_{xy} for increasing numbers of T_2 time periods.

Now it's time to relate T_2 spin-spin relaxation time (decay of M_{xy}) to the spin echo pulse sequence TE time. After the 90° RF pulse, M_{xy} is at its maximum value (the maximum value of M_{xy} depends on the value of M_z at the time the 90° pulse is applied). When the 90° pulse is turned off, M_{xy} immediately begins to decay. **The rate of decay of M_{xy} depends on the T_2 time of the tissue being imaged.** At some time (TE) after the 90° pulse, an echo signal is detected. The signal strength of the echo depends on the magnitude of M_{xy} at the time the signal is detected. During the TE time (from 90° pulse to echo), M_{xy} has decreased. **The percent decrease in M_{xy} depends on:**

T_2 time of the tissue
TE time of the spin-echo sequence

The value of M_{xy} will be about the same for most tissues immediately after the 90° RF pulse. The value of M_{xy} will begin to differ among tissues as M_{xy} decays with time. Some tissues lose M_{xy} rapidly (those with a short T_2), while others lose M_{xy} slowly (these with a long T_2). Thus, T_2 influences

Table 24–5. Decrease of M_{xy} Signal Intensity Relative to T_2 Periods (this is strictly an exponential decay)

NO. OF T_2 PERIODS	RELATIVE M_{xy} SIGNAL INTENSITY
0	100%
0.25	78%
0.50	61%
0.75	47%
1	37%
2	14%
3	5%
4	2%

the relative value of M_{xy} among tissues. Long TE intervals give more time for T_2 relaxation to reduce M_{xy}. Remember, we are using a spin echo pulse sequence.

A short TE minimizes T_2 differences because there is little time for M_{xy} to decay, no matter how short or long the T_2 of the tissue.

A long TE maximizes T_2 differences because there is time for M_{xy} to decay. The rate of decay of M_{xy} will be rapid for short T_2 tissues (fat), intermediate for intermediate T_2 tissues (brain), and slow for long T_2 tissues (CSF).

A spin echo sequence using a long TE will be a T_2-weighted sequence. In general, a short TE means 30 or 40 ms, whereas a long TE means 90 to 120 ms.

Figure 24–19 is a T_2-weighted image of the brain (TE = 120 ms). Notice that CSF gives a very bright (white) signal, while the brain signal is dark (weak). This reflects the rapid loss of M_{xy} in brain tissue (a T_2 of 70 ms will retain only 18% of M_{xy} at 120 ms) compared to the slow loss of M_{xy} in CSF (a T_2 of 2000 ms will retain 94% of M_{xy} at 120 ms). While T_2 has profoundly influenced the image of brain and CSF in Figure 24–19, there is also some influence from T_1 and spin density in the image. Let us remind you that MR images are produced by a combination of spin density, T_1, and T_2. Further, T_1-weighted images or T_2-weighted images are just that: weighted in favor of T_1 or T_2 but not formed exclusively by T_1 or T_2 information.

Figure 24–19 A T_2-weighted image of the brain (TE = 120 ms) shows a strong CSF signal and a weak brain signal

Recapitulation. A spin echo MR imaging sequence may produce images that are:

Spin-density weighted
T_1 weighted
T_2 weighted

Figure 24–20 illustrates a set of curves that show the regrowth of M_z of CSF (T_1 = 3000 ms) and brain (T_1 = 600 ms) after a 90° RF pulse. Notice that the 100% line is higher for CSF than for brain, reflecting the higher spin density of CSF. Spin density always influences an MR image.

Figure 24–20 illustrates how the TR interval of the pulse sequence and the T_1 recovery time of tissue combine to produce an image which may magnify or obscure T_1 differences (i.e., whether or not the image is T_1-weighted). First, consider a 500 ms TR. At 500 ms, M_z of CSF has had little time to recover (M_z is 15% of maximum), while M_z of brain has recovered a lot (M_z is 56% of maximum). If a 90° RF pulse is applied at 500 ms, the M_{xy} of brain will be strong, while the M_{xy} of CSF will be only about ⅓ as strong. The echo produced using a 500 ms TR will show a lot of signal difference between brain and CSF because of T_1 differences; the signal is T_1-weighted. **A short TR produces T_1-weighted images.** Figure 24–18 is a T_1-weighted image (TR = 500 ms). Notice the fairly bright (white) signal from brain, and the very weak (black) signal from CSF. Fat, with a very

short T_1 of 220 ms, has recovered 90% of its M_z in 500 ms and produces the brightest signal in Figure 24–18.

Figure 24–21 illustrates a set of curves that show the decay of M_{xy} after a 90° RF pulse for CSF (T_2 = 2000 ms) and brain (T_2 = 70 ms). Drawing the curves in Figure 24–21 presents a problem because we must choose a maximum value of M_{xy} from which to start each decay curve. Figure 24–20 indicates that the value of M_z (and therefore, M_{xy} after a 90° pulse) for CSF and brain depends on the TR interval being used in the spin echo pulse sequence. We will use the relative values of M_{xy} as derived from the 2000 ms TR point on the curve of Figure 24–20 (a typical T_2-weighted image uses a TR of 2000 ms). At a 2000-ms TR, the M_{xy} of brain will be roughly ⅓ stronger than that of CSF. Therefore, in Figure 24–21, the value of M_{xy} of brain is greater than the value of M_{xy} of CSF at time zero.

Study Figure 24–21 carefully. Notice that at a TE interval of 20, 30, or 40 ms the M_{xy} strength of brain and CSF is about the same. But the strength of M_{xy} of brain tissue is losing ground fast. By a TE of 60 ms, brain produces a much weaker signal than CSF, and the difference becomes even greater with longer TE intervals. At a TE of 120 ms, the CSF signal retains over 90% of its original value, while the brain M_{xy} value is only 18% of its original value. The

Figure 24–20 Recovery of M_z for brain and CSF as a function of time TR of the pulse echo sequence and T_1 recovery time of brain and CSF

Figure 24–21 Decay of M_{xy} for brain and CSF as a function of the time TE of a pulse echo sequence and the time T_2 of brain and CSF long TE interval results in a marked difference in signal between brain and CSF because of T_2 difference between brain and CSF. **A long TE produces a T_2-weighted image.** Figure 24–19 is T_2-weighted (TR 3000 ms, TE 120 ms). Notice the bright signal from CSF.

To summarize:

1. A short TR enhances T_1 differences
2. A long TR minimizes T_1 differences
3. A short TE minimizes T_2 differences
4. A long TE enhances T_2 differences

And the same thing in another format:

		TR	
		SHORT	LONG
TE	SHORT	T_1-WEIGHTED	SPIN DENSITY
	LONG	NOT USED	T_2-WEIGHTED

And the same thing again:

SPIN DENSITY: LONG TR   SHORT TE
T_1-WEIGHTED: SHORT TR   SHORT TE
T_2-WEIGHTED: LONG TR   LONG TE

And once again:

> A spin-density-weighted image uses a long TR to minimize T_1 tissue differences, and a short TE to minimize T_2 tissue differences.
> A T_1-weighted image uses a short TE to minimize T_2 tissue differences.
> A T_2-weighted image uses a long TR to minimize T_1 tissue differences.

As a general rule, the T_2 time of abnormal tissues is longer than that of normal tissues. Images with T_2 weighting are most commonly used when looking for tumors. T_1-weighted images are more commonly used to display anatomy.

MULTIPLANAR IMAGING

MRI can image in axial, sagittal, coronal and oblique planes. Multiplanar imaging with MRI requires collection of data unique to the plane being imaged. This is unlike CT, which uses data from a transaxial image to reconstruct sagittal or coronal images. Our discussion of axial imaging continuously referred to the z axis as

the slice selection gradient. If the slice selection gradient is along the x axis, a sagittal image will result. Obviously, using the x-axis gradient coils for slice selection requires that the y- and z-axis gradients be used for phase and frequency encoding. This emphasizes the fact that the gradient coils do nothing more than produce a gradient magnetic field. How these gradient fields are used in imaging is determined by the pulse sequencing. Slice selection with the Y-gradient produces coronal images. Slice orientation is under control of the operator.

INVERSION RECOVERY PULSE SEQUENCE

Interest in the inversion recovery pulse sequence is growing. We will present a few basic observations about the inversion recovery pulse sequence, but will not attempt a comprehensive review of this interesting imaging technique. Inversion recovery images are produced by repetitions of a 180° RF pulse followed by a spin echo (signal generating) sequence. Gradient fields are required for imaging, just like with spin echo, but we will not discuss this technical detail.

The Inverting RF Pulse

The inversion recovery sequence begins with a 180° RF pulse that inverts the magnetization vector, M_z, from the $+z$ axis to the $-z$ axis. A 180° RF pulse does not change the magnitude of M_z, it just turns M_z upside down so that $+M_z$ becomes $-M_z$. The slice selection gradient must be on during the 180° RF pulse, so that M_z is inverted in only the slice to be imaged.

When the 180° RF pulse is turned off, $-M_z$ begins to recover back toward $+M_z$. The rate at which $-M_z$ returns toward $+M_z$ depends on tissue T_1 relaxation time. Look at Figure 24–22, which shows $-M_z$ recovering toward $+M_z$. After one T_1 time, $-M_z$ has recovered to $+26\%$ M_z; after 2 T_1 periods, $+73\%$ M_z (etc.). The recovery curve of Figure 24–22 gets quite interest-

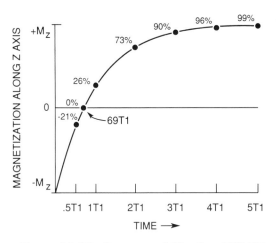

Figure 24–22   Recovery of M_z after 180° RF pulse

ing at a time equal to 0.69 T_1 and less. **Notice that at time equals 0.69 T_1, the magnitude of M_z is zero.** This is a fascinating aspect of the inversion recovery pulse sequence that we will explore in more detail (this is the same value M_z has after a 90° pulse). At times less than 0.69 T_1, the value of M_z is negative, representing a radical departure from M_z values encountered in the spin echo pulse sequence.

Where are we now? A 180° RF pulse has turned M_z upside down. Turning off the 180° RF pulse allows $-M_z$ to begin to recover toward $+M_z$. The absolute value of M_z will at first decrease ($-M_z$ approaches 0), then begin to increase (M_z increases from 0 toward $+M_z$). This **biphasic** change in the value of M_z contributes to the fascination and complexity of the inversion recovery sequence. It is not possible to detect M_z. What do we do? We begin what amounts to a spin echo pulse sequence following the 180° RF pulse, detecting an echo whose magnitude is directly proportional to the value of M_z.

Forming the Signal

Since M_z is not detectable, the magnetization vector must be tipped away from the z axis, in order to produce an M_{xy} vector that can induce a signal in the receiving RF coil. We have said this enough times that M_{xy} no longer comes as a surprise.

Signal generation after the inverting 180° RF pulse is nothing more than a spin echo sequence. The strength of M_{xy} for a particular tissue will be proportional to M_z of the tissue at the time the spin echo sequence starts.

Look at Figure 24–23. At a time TI (for time of inversion) after the 180° pulse, a 90° pulse rotates the magnetization vector into the xy plane (which starts the spin echo sequence). The magnitude of M_{xy} for a particular tissue is determined by how much M_z has recovered during the TI time period. M_{xy} is detected as an echo following a rephasing 180° pulse, exactly as we have discussed in the spin echo sequence. The time TE is the time from the 90° RF pulse to the time of echo detection, again exactly as in a spin echo sequence.

How long will TR, TI, and TE be in an inversion recovery sequence? Times are quite variable. In general, TR times are in the 1000- to 1500-ms range. TE times are generally quite short, on the order of a few tens of milliseconds (perhaps 20 ms to 50 ms is a reasonable range). The TI time can vary from as short as 100 ms to as long as about 700 ms. It is possible to apply the 90° pulse before M_z of a tissue has recovered to a positive value. In fact, this is exactly what is done with short TI imaging. This now causes no problem, but was a source of complication in older instruments and may cause confusion when one reads the literature. Return to the rotating coordinate system a moment. If the 90° RF pulse is applied along the x axis, M_{xy} will appear along the $+y$ axis if M_z is positive, and along the $-y$ if M_z is negative. Thus, the M_{xy} resulting from a negative value of M_z will be 180° out of phase compared to M_{xy} resulting from a positive value of M_z. A technique called "quadrature detection" allows the computer to distinguish between a positive M_z and a negative M_z.

In the past, inversion recovery sequences got a lot of bad press because a long TI

Figure 24–23 Inversion recovery pulse sequence

precluded multislice acquisition. For example, with a TR of 1500 ms and a TI of 700 ms, only two simultaneous slices could be imaged. Such a limit greatly prolongs total imaging time if multiple slices are required for a complete examination. A short TI time (100 ms) will allow multislice imaging, as we will describe in the next section.

Short TI Inversion Recovery

The short TI inversion recovery pulse sequence is usually called a **STIR** sequence (for short TI IR sequence). The nature of this text does not allow us to discuss many sequences in detail. We feel the STIR sequence illustrates some interesting physics, and the sequence shows the promise of becoming very useful in clinical MRI.

What is a STIR sequence? A STIR sequence is an inversion recovery sequence that uses a short value of TI (around 100 ms). A typical STIR sequence in our department (0.35-T magnet) is 1500/30/100 (TR = 1500 ms, TE = 30 ms, TI = 100 ms). This shorthand way of expressing inversion recovery sequences is common, but the order of the numbers may vary. We chose to write in the order of TR/TE/TI.

The STIR sequence allows an interesting manipulation of tissue images. It is possible to choose a TI time that causes the value of M_{xy} of a particular tissue to be zero at the time of the 90° RF pulse. Look at Figure 24–24 and note that the M_z regrowth curve of fat passes through zero at 138 ms (assuming fat has a T_1 of 200 ms). The M_{xy}

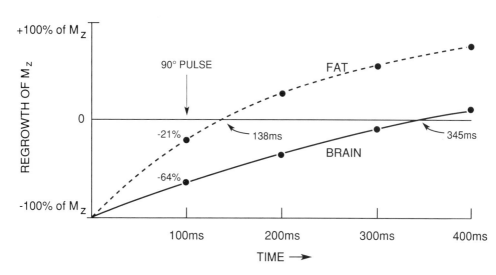

Figure 24–24 Regrowth of M_z for fat (T_1 = 200 ms) and brain (T_1 = 500 ms) after an inverting 180° pulse

value of a tissue will be zero at a TI time that equals a value of $0.69 T_1$ for the tissue ($0.69 \times 200 = 138$). **STIR sequences can be used to eliminate the signal of selected tissues.** A TI of 100 ms or a little greater will suppress (or partially suppress) the signal of fat. Eliminating the strong signal from fat may allow better visualization of pathology. Specific examples include the orbit, where fat signals can hide optic nerve pathology, and vertebral body bone marrow, where fat in the marrow may hide or mimic signals due to osteomyelitis.

Use of STIR to reduce fat signals will cause all tissues with a T_1 longer than fat to have a negative value of M_z at the time of the 90° RF pulse. This is all right because contemporary MR machines can keep track of negative and positive M_z values.

There is another advantage of the STIR sequence (compared to IR sequences with a longer TI interval). **A short TI interval allows multislice imaging comparable to spin echo sequences.**

To summarize, the STIR pulse sequence may be useful because:

1. Selective suppression of a tissue signal is possible
2. Multislice acquisition is possible

SIGNAL-TO-NOISE RATIO

A magnetic resonance image is a composite of the RF signal induced from each voxel in the imaging volume. Voxels with a strong RF signal are displayed as white pixels. Body tissues also produce random RF fluctuations that influence the RF signal. **This random variation in signal intensity is called noise.** Noise in MRI is just like noise of radiographs: **noise limits the visibility of low contrast structures.** Good images require a high intensity signal and low intensity noise, i.e., a good signal-to-noise ratio. A number of factors influence the signal to noise (S/N) ratio.

Voxel Size

The size of a voxel depends on the size of the imaging matrix. Large voxels pro-

duce large signals for each pixel in the image. A 128×128 matrix produces voxels that are four times as large as those in a 256×256 matrix. Similarly, thick tissue slices produce voxels larger than thin tissue slices because of increased voxel length. Large voxels produce better S/N ratios, but large voxels limit spatial resolution. Voxel size also influences the time required to acquire an image. A 128×128 matrix requires only half the time (half as many phase encoding gradients) as a 256×256 matrix.

To summarize:

VOXEL SIZE	
SMALL	LARGE
Worse S/N	Better S/N
Better resolution	Less resolution
Longer time	Shorter time

Number of Averages

Noise is a random event. Sometimes noise variation will increase the signal from a voxel; sometimes noise will decrease the signal. If a voxel is averaged for several imaging sequences, the effect of noise will be reduced. The effect of signal averaging can be calculated. Let A represent the number of images averaged. Signal strength will increase as a linear function of A, but noise will increase as a linear function of the square root of A. Therefore, $S/N = A/\sqrt{A} = \sqrt{A}$ (do you remember that $\frac{x}{\sqrt{x}} = \sqrt{x}$?). Thus, S/N improves only as the square root of the number of averages. Averaging 2 images improves S/N by $\sqrt{2}$ or 1.4, whereas averaging 4 images improves S/N by $\sqrt{4}$, or 2.

As always, one pays a price for improving S/N by image averaging. The price is time. A spin echo sequence using a 256×256 matrix and a TR of 1000 ms requires 4¼ min for one signal, 8½ min for two signal averaging, and 17 min for four signal averaging.

To summarize:

AVERAGING

MORE	LESS
Better S/N	Worse S/N
More time	Less time

Time of Repetition (TR)

Signal strength from a tissue is proportional to the magnitude of the longitudinal magnetization (M_z) at the time the 90° pulse is applied during a spin echo sequence. A long TR interval allows for more regrowth of M_z. Of course, the tissue T_1 value influences how fast M_z will regrow. S/N ratios are improved when a long TR is used. Changing TR also changes contrast in the image, influences the number of simultaneous slice acquisitions possible, and influences image acquisition time. TR influences a lot of things.

To summarize:

TR

SHORT	LONG
Worse S/N	Better S/N
More T_1 weighted	Less T_1 weighted
Less time	More time
Fewer slices	More slices

Time to Echo (TE)

The TE time is used to influence the amount of T_2 information contained in the image. A long TE produces a T_2-weighted image. During the TE interval the strength of the M_{xy} (signal-producing) magnetization vector is decreasing because of T_2 dephasing. An image with a short TE will have a stronger signal than an image with a long TE. A short TE produces an image with a better S/N ratio than an image produced with a long TE. Images that are T_2-weighted (long TE) will be noisy because of decreased signal strength. Look at Figure 24–25, *A* and *B*. Both images were made using a TR of 3000 ms. Figure 24–25*A* was obtained with a TE of 40 ms (a spin density image), and displays little noise; it is a nice "smooth" image. Figure 25–25*B* was obtained with a TE of 120 ms (a T_2-weighted image). Notice the mottled appearance of the T_2-weighted image, a reflection of increased brightness fluctuation in each pixel caused by statistical variations in signal strength (noise). Students of this text are permitted to exchange knowing smiles and nudge each other with elbows when their less sophisticated colleagues refer to "grainy" images rather than noisy images. TE does not influence image acquisition time, but may limit the number of multislice acquisitions permitted.

To summarize:

TR

SHORT	LONG
Better S/N	Worse S/N
Less T_2-weighted	More T_2-weighted

Surface Coils

A surface coil is a special type of RF coil. Such a coil usually consists of multiple turns of wire enclosed in a plastic material. The coils come in a variety of sizes and shapes and are designed to be placed directly on the patient's body. A surface coil is used as a receiver only. The RF coil of the imaging magnetic is the transmitting coil.

The main advantage of a surface coil is improved spatial resolution. Surface coil images a comparatively small volume of tissue. Thus, for same size matrix reconstruction, pixel size for a surface coil is less than that for whole body imaging.

Surface coils also improve the S/N ratio of the image. The amount of random RF noise generated by body tissues is related to the volume of tissue contained within the sensitive field of the RF coil. Larger whole body coils detect more noise and have a lower S/N ratio.

The disadvantages of surface coils are a limited field of view and difficult positioning. To maximize the signal received from the small volume being imaged, the coils must be carefully oriented with respect to the x and y planes. Slight malpositioning can result in significant loss of signal strength.

Figure 24–25 Influence of TE on noise. Both images have a TR of 3000 ms. Image (A) TE = 40 ms, image (B) TE = 120 ms

To summarize:

SURFACE COILS RELATIVE TO WHOLE BODY COILS
Better S/N
Better spatial resolution
Limited field
Harder to use

FAST IMAGING TECHNIQUES

Considerable effort is being directed toward developing MRI techniques that allow imaging times of a few seconds rather than a few minutes. Most of these techniques use a reduced flip angle and a short TR. Only a few basic principles will be presented. Numerous variations of this theme exist. Some of the catchy acronyms used to describe the various sequences are:

FLASH (fast low angle shot)
FFE (fast field echoes)
GRASS (gradient-recalled acquisition in the steady state)
FAST (Fourier acquired steady-state technique)
FISP (fast imaging with steady precession)

And a few simply use the term "partial flip angle MR imaging." Unfortunately, no consistency of nomenclature for this type of echo sequence has yet been developed. It has been proposed that the term "gradient echo" is both explanatory and unambiguous.

Reduced Flip Angle

A routine spin-echo imaging sequence begins with a 90° RF pulse. After this pulse, the M_z (longitudinal) magnetization is zero. Magnetization along the z axis (M_z) recovers to a varying degree during the TR period (depending on the length of TR and tissue T_1 time). The relatively long TR time causes imaging times to be long.

Figure 24–25. *Continued*

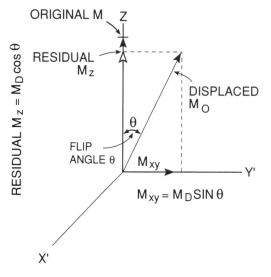

Figure 24–26 A reduced flip angle allows a reasonably large M_{xy} while retaining a large M_z

Reduced flip angle techniques displace M by less than 90°, with angles as small as 5° being used. The concept of a reduced flip angle is illustrated in Figure 24–26. If longitudinal magnetization is large, the M_{xy} component of the slightly displaced vector (M_D) will be reasonably large, allowing a reasonable FID or echo signal. Equally important, a very large longitudinal component of the magnetization vector persists (unlike a 90° pulse, in which the longitudinal component becomes zero). The M_{xy} component of the displaced magnetization vector (M_D) is proportional to the sine of the flip angle, while the remaining longitudinal component is proportional to the cosine of the flip angle. Assume a flip angle of 15°. M_{xy} will correspond to 26% (sine 15° = .26) of M_D, whereas 97% (cosine 15° = .97) of M_D will remain along the z axis. This is the key to reduced flip angle imaging. **Longitudinal magnetization remains large at all times,** which allows the signal-producing M_{xy} vector to be reasonably large with small angles of displacement. One is not obliged to wait for M_z to recover, so short TR intervals (as short as 10 to 20 ms) can be used.

Gradient Sequences

A spin echo pulse sequence uses a 180° refocusing RF pulse to "turn the system around" and form an echo. Small flip angle sequences cannot use a 180° RF pulse because such a pulse would serve to invert the M_z vector as it does in an inversion recovery sequence. Another type of approach to turning around the M_{xy} vector to form an echo is used. After the small flip angle RF pulse, a negative magnetic gradient is applied in the readout gradient axis. The negative readout gradient is applied for a few milliseconds, during which time there is dephasing of spins. The negative readout gradient is followed by a positive readout gradient which causes rephasing of spins and generates an echo. A simplified diagram of a gradient reversal sequence is shown in Figure 24–27. Since TR times can be made very short, imaging times can be correspondingly short. For example, a 256 × 256 matrix image (requiring 256 acquisitions, each with a different phase gradient), using a TR of 20 ms, could be obtained in $(.02)$ $(256) = 5.12$ sec.

Potential of Fast Imaging

Let us turn from being scientists to being mystics. The potential for fast imaging techniques is exciting. Images acquired with these techniques reflect complex relationships involving T_1, T_2, T_2^*, TE, TR, and flip angle.

FLASH images are reported to exhibit T_1 contrast superior to that obtained with spin echo images. At this time, T_2 contrast has not been as good as with the spin echo sequence. One technique reported to achieve good T_1 contrast in a 1-T magnet

uses a TR of 40 ms, TE of 8 ms, and a 50° flip angle.

Fast imaging techniques are being used to acquire the large numbers of image slices required for computer reconstruction of 3D images. Fast acquisition times allow multiple thin slices to be obtained in about the same amount of time required for one spin echo image. Since images are collected rapidly, artifacts due to patient motion are minimized. Obviously, 3D reconstruction will be impossible if the patient moves while the composite slices are being obtained. Once the computer has the information from a set of contiguous thin slices taken in one plane, additional manipulation of the data can reconstruct images oriented in any other plane or in 3D.

The potential for fast imaging techniques to become a routine clinical imaging tool is real. It is possible to obtain real time images of moving structures, such as the heart or aorta, and replay the images as a cine display.

SAFETY CONSIDERATIONS

We will consider two aspects of MRI safety:

Human exposure to magnetic and RF fields
Hazards associated with strong magnetic fields

Human Exposure Considerations

Potential health hazards of MRI lie in the area of the

Static magnetic field
Gradient magnetic field
RF electromagnetic fields

Available data indicate that these fields, as used in clinical MRI, are free of deleterious bioeffects.

Magnetic Fields. In 1982 the Food and Drug Administration (FDA) established guidelines setting maximum permissible limits for the static and variable magnetic components, and the RF electromagnetic fields, of MRI. The guidelines are regarded by the FDA as "interim and somewhat arbitrary in nature."

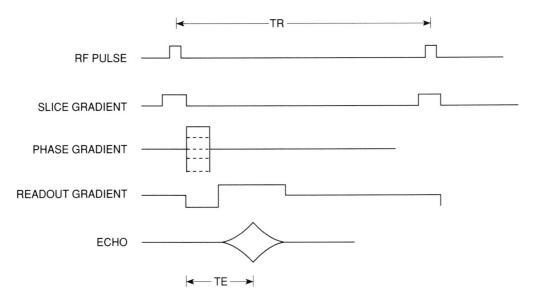

Figure 24–27   Example of a fast image sequence using readout gradient reversal to generate the echo

The suggested limits for magnetic fields are:

> Static Magnetic Field:
> 2.0 tesla
> Rate of Varying Magnetic Fields:
> 3.0 tesla/sec

What does a varying field of 3 tesla/sec really mean? Consider a gradient field that uses a 1-gauss-per-cm gradient applied over a 50-cm field of view (this is a large gradient). At the edge of the field of view, the gradient magnetic field will vary from 0 to +25 gauss or from 0 to −25 gauss each time a gradient is applied. The cm of tissue at the extreme edge of the field will observe a rapid magnetic field change of 25 gauss. How rapid is the change? Gradient fields have a "rise time" that varies with the equipment used. An approximate rise time is in the order of 1 ms. This means a change of 25 gauss in 1 ms at the outer edge of the imaging area. With careful unit conversions, one finds that 1 gauss per ms is equivalent to 0.1 tesla per sec. So, 25 G/ms is the equivalent of 2.5 T/sec, which puts us in the ballpark of the guideline limit. Remember that we have used an extreme case and estimations in this example.

Below these suggested guidelines no documented permanent adverse biologic effects have been observed. The only biologic effect associated with exposure to a static magnetic field is augmentation of the T-wave amplitude observed on an electrocardiogram. The T-wave amplitude is directly proportional to the strength of the static magnetic field. Augmentation of the T-wave is not believed to present any significant health problem.

Time varying magnetic fields (gradient pulses) induce currents in the patient. The currents can produce mild cutaneous sensations, involuntary muscle contractions and cardiac arrhythmias. Subjective visual effects, light flashes known as magnetophosphenes, may result from stimulation of the retina.

Radio Frequency Fields. The measure of dose of RF energy is the specific absorption rate (SAR). The units of SAR are watts per kilogram (W/kg). SAR is a measure of power absorbed per unit mass. SAR is to MRI what the gray (old "rad") is to ionizing radiation (i.e., a unit of absorbed dose).

The measure of exposure to RF is expressed in units of power (watt) per meter². **Exposure is measured in W/m².** W/m² is to MRI what coulombs/kg (C/kg) is to ionizing radiation (old term "roentgen," which is not an SI unit).

To summarize:

	IONIZING RADIATION	MRI
EXPOSURE	C/kg (roentgen)	W/m²
ABSORBED DOSE	gray (Gy) (rad)	W/kg

The main effect of RF exposure is an increase in body temperature.

Federal guidelines set limits on RF exposure to the whole body, and local exposure averaged over any one gram of tissue.

SAR LIMITS
Whole Body:
0.4 W/kg
Absorbed by any 1 g of tissue:
2.0 W/kg/g

What does 2.0 W/kg/g mean? An absorbed dose of 2.0 W/kg/g means any 1 g in the body may absorb .002 W. This is an acceptable absorption for the 1 g. Other areas in the body must experience sufficiently lower doses so that the average whole body absorption does not exceed 0.4 W/kg.

Exposure to an SAR up to 0.4 W/kg should produce no temperature increase. However, additional evaluations are needed for heat sensitive organs such as the testes and eyes.

MRI During Pregnancy. In general, MRI is not believed to be hazardous to the fetus. However, a variety of mechanisms have the potential to produce harmful interactions between electromagnetic fields and a fetus. Additional work is needed to study such interactions.

The Food and Drug Administration requires labeling of MRI systems to indicate that "the safety of MRI when used to image fetuses and the infant has not been established." It is considered inadvisable to use MRI routinely in pregnant women until more information regarding potential haz-

ards becomes available. MRI during pregnancy may be indicated if ultrasound cannot provide the needed information or if the clinician feels it is necessary to avoid exposure to ionizing radiation.

Magnetic Field Hazards

A superconducting magnet is on full strength at all times. Safety considerations exist at any time any person or any object is near the magnet.

Fringe fields exist around magnets. The 0.5-mT field extends about 8.5 m (about 28 ft) from an 0.5-T magnet, and to about 11 m (about 36 ft) from a 1.0-T magnet. These fringe fields are modified with shielding, so the fringe fields around an individual magnet will depend on magnetic strength and shielding.

One of the greatest potential hazards around a magnet is the missile effect. Objects with iron (ferromagnetic) in them can be pulled into or toward a magnet and injure persons within or near the magnet. Small objects (hammers, screwdrivers, wrenches) and large objects (vacuum cleaners, oxygen tanks, tool chests, and crash carts) are equally hazardous.

Hazards also exist for patients who have medical devices implanted in their bodies. Patients who should be excluded from a magnet include those with:

1. Cardiac pacemakers
2. Cerebral aneurysm clips
3. Shrapnel or other metallic foreign bodies
4. Implanted electrodes, such as neurostimulators and bone growth stimulators
5. Internal drug infusion pumps

Some neurosurgical clips are magnetic and some are not. It is a good general rule to exclude all patients with neurosurgical clips from the magnet, then make exceptions if the clip is absolutely known to be nonmagnetic. Surgical clips in sites outside the head are not considered to pose a significant threat, especially since such clips are usually nonmagnetic.

At times, radiographs may be required if a patient has a questionable history of a metallic foreign body. Some feel that sheet metal workers should be excluded from MRI because of the danger of movement of small metal particles near the orbit (one such case is reported).

Most middle ear prostheses are nonmagnetic, but exceptions may exist. Be cautious.

Most metallic bioimplants pose no significant risk to the patient. Implants located in an imaged area may produce significant artifacts, an example being hip prostheses that can preclude MRI of the pelvis.

Any time a question exists, testing or consultation should be obtained before a patient with an implant of unknown composition is placed in a magnet.

Much of the equipment used for cardiopulmonary resuscitation cannot be used near a magnet. Management of medical emergencies that occur while a patient is in the MR scanner will be difficult, and will often require that the patient be removed from the magnet room before resuscitation begins. Recently, devices for cardiac and respiratory monitoring during MRI have become available. These devices can operate during MRI and produce no image artifacts.

Objects that may be damaged by a 0.5-mT field includes watches, credit cards, tape recorders, calculators, and cameras. Magnetic materials may exist in jewelry, limb braces and support shoes, various hairpieces, and dentures.

Safety considerations related to the magnetic field include:

Projectile effects
Effects on surgically implanted devices
Magnetic foreign bodies
Life support devices

Contraindications to placing a patient in the magnetic field include:

Cardiac pacemakers
Intracranial clips and implants
Metallic foreign bodies
Implanted electrodes

Caution should be exercised with:

Middle ear prostheses
Metallic bioimplants

Careful screening of anyone (workers, patients, visitors) having access to the magnet is required.

The safety of MRI during pregnancy has not been established.

SUMMARY

Basic MRI requires:

1. A uniform magnetic field
2. Displacement of M by an RF pulse at the proper Larmor frequency
3. Observe the signal generated by M_{xy}

Most MR imaging uses the pulse echo sequence and 2D-FT image transformation. Magnetic field gradients allow images to be formed by producing gradients leading to:

1. Slice selection
2. Phase encoding
3. Frequency encoding

Variables in the pulse echo sequence that influence image contrast are:

1. TR (time of repetition)
2. TE (time of echo)

Image acquisition time is related to:

1. The TR time
2. Matrix size
3. Number of averages

Image contrast is related to:

1. Proton (spin) density
2. Tissue T_1 time
3. Tissue T_2 time

A spin echo spin density-weighted image is produced using a short TR and a short TE. A spin echo T_1-weighted image is produced using a long TR and a short TE.

A spin echo T_2-weighted image is produced by using a long TR and a long TE.

Most MR imaging is produced using multislice, multiecho spin echo techniques.

Inversion recovery techniques are more T_1-sensitive and may require more imaging time.

Image quality in MRI is noise limited. Noise is decreased by:

1. Large voxel size
2. Large number of averages
3. Long TR
4. Short TE
5. Surface coils

Fast imaging techniques used reduced flip angle and gradient echo techniques.

Safety considerations include:

1. Human exposure to static and varying magnetic fields
2. Human exposure to RF fields
3. Magnetic field hazards

BIBLIOGRAPHY

1. Balter, S.: An introduction to the physics of magnetic resonance imaging. RadioGraphics, 7:731, 1987.
2. Bushong, S.C.: Magnetic Resonance Imaging Physical and Biological Principles. C.V. Mosby Co., St. Louis, 1988.
3. Fullerton, G.D.: Magnetic resonance imaging signal concepts. RadioGraphics, 7:579, 1987.
4. Haase A., Frahm, J., Matthaei, D., et al.: FLASH imaging. Rapid NMR imaging using low flip-angle pulses. J. of Magnetic Resonance, 67:258, 1986.
5. Merritt, C.R.B.: Magnetic resonance imaging—a clinical perspective: image quality, safety and risk mangement. RadioGraphics, 7:1001, 1987.
6. Pavlicek, W.: MR instrumentation and image formation. RadioGraphics, 7:809, 1987.
7. Runge, V.M., Wood, M.L., Kaufman, D.M., et al.: FLASH: Clinical three-dimensional magnetic resonance imaging. RadioGraphics, 8:947, 1988.
8. Shellock, F.G., Crues, J.V.: Safety considerations in magnetic resonance imaging. MRI Decisions, 2:25, 1988.

INDEX

Page numbers in *italic* refer to illustrations, numbers followed by the letter "t" refer to tabular matter.